# Pathology of
# Pseudoneoplastic
# Lesions

# Pathology of Pseudoneoplastic Lesions

Editors

**Mark R. Wick**
*Professor of Pathology*
*Washington University School of Medicine*
*St. Louis, Missouri*

**Peter A. Humphrey**
*Associate Professor of Pathology*
*Washington University School of Medicine*
*St. Louis, Missouri*

**Jon H. Ritter**
*Assistant Professor of Pathology*
*Washington University School of Medicine*
*St. Louis, Missouri*

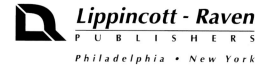

**Lippincott - Raven**
P U B L I S H E R S
*Philadelphia • New York*

Acquisitions Editor: Vickie Thaw
Developmental Editor: Melissa James
Manufacturing Manager: Dennis Teston
Production Manager: Lawrence Bernstein
Production Editor: Loretta Cummings
Cover Designer: Edward Schultheis
Indexer: Robert Elwood
Compositor: Maryland Composition
Printer: Toppan Printing

Printed and bound in Singapore.

9  8  7  6  5  4  3  2  1

**Library of Congress Cataloging-in-Publication Data**

Pathology of pseudoneoplastic lesions / edited by Mark R. Wick, Peter
    A. Humphrey, Jon H. Ritter.
        p.   cm.
    Includes bibliograpical references and index.
    ISBN 0-7817-0302-6
    1. Tumors—Diagnosis.   2. Pathology, Surgical.   I. Wick, Mark R.,
1952–    .  II. Humphrey, Peter A.   III. Ritter, Jon H.
    [DNLM:   1. Disease.   2. Diagnosis, Differential.   3. Neoplasms-
diagnosis. QZ   140   P294   1997]
RC269.P386   1997
616.07—dc20
for Library of Congress                                              96-43036
                                                                          CIP

# Contents

# Contributing Authors

**Philip B. Clement, M.D.**   *Professor, Department of Pathology, Vancouver Hospital and Health Sciences Centre and the University of British Columbia, 855 West 12th Street, Vancouver, British Columbia, Canada V5Z 1M9*

**John R. Craig, M.D., Ph.D.**   *Associate Professor, Department of Pathology, St. Luke Medical Center, 2632 East Washington Boulevard, Pasadena, California 91109-7021*

**John N. Eble, M.D.**   *Professor of Pathology and Experimental Oncology, Department of Pathology and Laboratory Medicine, Indiana University School of Medicine, 1481 Indianapolis, Indiana 46202-2884*

**Samir K. El-Mofty, D.M.D., Ph.D.**   *Associate Professor of Pathology and Otolaryngology, Lauren V. Ackerman Laboratory of Surgical Pathology, Washington University Medical Center, One Barnes Hospital Plaza, St. Louis, Missouri 63110*

**Patrick L. Fitzgibbons, M.D.**   *Department of Pathology, St. Jude Medical Center, 101 E. Valencia Mesa Drive, Fullerton, California 92635*

**Glauco Frizzera, M.D.**   *Professor and Director of Hemopathology, New York University Medical Center, 550 First Avenue, New York, New York 10016*

**Peter A. Humphrey, M.D.**   *Associate Professor, Lauren V. Ackerman Laboratory of Surgical Pathology, Department of Pathology, Barnes-Jewish Hospital at Washington University Medical Center, One Barnes Hospital Plaza, St. Louis, Missouri 63110*

**Giorgio Inghirami, M.D.**   *Director of Molecular Pathology and Professor, Department of Pathology, New York University Medical Center, 550 First Avenue, New York, New York 10016*

**George M. Kleinman, M.D.**   *Department of Pathology, Bridgeport Hospital, 267 Grant Street, Bridgeport, Connecticut 06610*

**J. Carlos Manivel M.D.**   *Professor and Director of Surgical Pathology, Box 76, University of Minnesota Health Center, 420 Delaware Street, S. E., Minneapolis, Minnesota 55455*

**Eugene Mark, M.D.**   *Professor, Department of Pathology, Massachusetts General Hospital, Fruit Street, Boston, Massachusetts 02114*

**Osamu Matsubara, M.D.**   *Professor, Department of Pathology, National Defense College, 3-2 Namiki, Tokorozawa, Saitama, 359 Japan*

**Michael B. McDermott, M.B., M.R.C., Path.**   *Fellow, Division of Surgical Pathology, Washington University Medical Center-Barnes Hospital, One Barnes Hospital Plaza, St. Louis, Missouri 63110*

**Douglas C. Miller, M.D., Ph.D.**   *Associate Professor of Neuropathology, New York University Medical Center, 550 First Avenue, New York, New York 10016*

**Jon H. Ritter, M.D.**   *Assistant Professor, Department of Pathology, Washington University School of Medicine, 660 South Euclid Avenue, St. Louis, Missouri 63110*

**Stefano Rosati, M.D.**  *Fellow of Hematopathology, Department of Pathology, New York University Medical Center, 550 First Avenue, New York, New York 10016*

**Jeffrey E. Saffitz, M.D.**  *Professor, Department of Pathology, Washington University School of Medicine, One Barnes Hospital Plaza, St. Louis, Missouri 63110*

**Paul E. Swanson, M.D.**  *Associate Professor, Department of Pathology, Washington University Medical Center/Barnes Hospital, One Barnes Hospital Plaza, St. Louis, Missouri 63110*

**Henry D. Tazelaar, M.D.**  *Professor of Pathology, Division of Anatomic Pathology, Mayo Medical School, 200 First Street, S.W., Rochester, Minnesota 55905*

**Mark R. Wick, M.D.**  *Professor, Department of Pathology, Washington University School of Medicine, 660 South Euclid Avenue, St. Louis, Missouri 63110*

**Robert H. Young, M.D., F.R.C., Path.**  *Associate Professor, Department of Pathology, Massachusetts General Hospital, Harvard Medical School, Fruit Street, Boston, Massachusetts 02114*

# Preface

The idea that an entire book should be devoted to the surgical pathology of pseudoneoplastic lesions was crystallized in a series of discussions with Dr. Stephen S. Sternberg of Memorial Sloan-Kettering Cancer Center (New York, New York, USA) in 1992. In these conversations, it became evident that pertinent facts on such pathologic entities were widely scattered in monographs and individual articles in periodical literature, and that they were not readily accessible to the practicing surgical pathologist. It was agreed that there was a need to assemble reviews which focused on the morphologic attributes and differential diagnosis of pseudoneoplastic proliferations in one reference source. Moreover, we have been impressed with the frequency with which pseudoneoplasms are considered interpretatively in the evaluation of tumefactive lesions in virtually every organ site. This fact is, understandably, a reflection of the dominance which neoplastic diseases have in the daily caseload of any surgical pathologist, regardless of their particular practice setting. It also indicates the potential that virtually all physicians share for the diagnostic confusion of true neoplasms with their biologically-innocuous simulants, a trap that has enormous consequences for the patients in question.

In that context, one realizes that the "pseudotumors" which surgeons and radiologists may encounter are not necessarily those that challenge pathologists, because of the differing means by which such lesions are detected by these respective specialists. After much deliberation, it was decided to limit the scope of this volume to mainly those pseudoneoplastic disorders that concern *surgical pathologists*. The task at hand simply would have been overwhelming if all mimics of neoplasms were considered in all potential clinical settings, and, just as importantly, many of those entities would not be germane to the problem-solving thought processes of morphologists. Even with this important restriction the differential diagnostic lists of pseudoneoplastic lesions that can be generated for any given anatomic site are impressive. Furthermore, we elected to forego much discussion of the *cyto*pathology of such disorders, a topic that is genuinely worthy of a full text in its own right.

This book has been organized by organ systems, with each chapter authored by individuals recognized as authorities in their respective fields. Such an approach was most *apropos* to the usual cerebral machinations of surgical pathologists, although one should also realize that "pseudotumors" can be categorized in a mechanistic fashion as well. The fact that a common etiological agent may elicit a sterotypical tissue response in differing anatomic locations inevitably leads to a certain degree of overlap in discussions of pseudoneoplastic lesions of those sites. Nevertheless, each chapter author has been encouraged to maintain a sense of categorical completeness in that context, while at the same time considering any possible topography-related nuances that a particular disease might have. Indeed, we believe that a particularly fascinating aspect of "pseudotumors" is represented by their partially-shared and partially-distinctive manifestations among dissimilar tissues and organs.

Hopefully, readers of this text will find the pathologic features of pseudoneoplastic diseases to be as absorbing as we did, in the preparation of the monograph. We have also intended that the book be used as a practical resource in the daily evaluation of surgical specimens by pathologists. To the extent that we might have succeeded in this goal, we are sincerely grateful to our collaborators and colleagues for their contributions and suggestions.

*Mark R. Wick, M.D.*
*Peter A. Humphrey, M.D., Ph.D.*
*Jon H. Ritter, M.D.*
*Lauren V. Ackerman Laboratory of Surgical Pathology*
*Washington University Medical Center*
*St. Louis, Missouri, U.S.A.*
*March 1995*

# Pathology of
# Pseudoneoplastic
# Lesions

*Pathology of Pseudoneoplastic Lesions,*
edited by M. R. Wick, P. A. Humphrey, and J. H. Ritter.
Lippincott-Raven Publishers, Philadelphia © 1997.

# CHAPTER 1

# Pseudoneoplastic Lesions: An Overview

Mark R. Wick and Jon H. Ritter

The term *pseudotumor* is, admittedly, an inaccurate designation. It is typically employed to connote the presence of a mass lesion (which, by definition, is a "tumor") that on clinical or pathologic grounds, or both, is thought to represent a neoplasm. Thus, the name "pseudoneoplasm" would be more à propos under such circumstances. Nonetheless, it is virtually certain that "pseudotumor" will remain in the active medical lexicon for the foreseeable future because of the difficulty that is generally encountered in challenging an established clinicopathologic rubric.

Perhaps apocryphally, ophthalmology has been cited as the first specialty area in which the related body of literature embraced the term "pseudotumor" as a useful description (1). In 1930, Birch-Hirschfeld used this designation in a discussion of orbital soft tissue lesions that were capable of producing proptosis (2). Thereafter, it was garnished with the descriptors "inflammatory," "lymphoid," "granulomatous," "xanthomatous," and "fibrous," in an attempt to subdivide the disorder in question into pathologically recognizable categories (3). To a large extent, this usage persists to the present time; however, the term "pseudotumor" has been extrapolated greatly to many histologically dissimilar lesions in a wide variety of anatomic locations and has been synonymized by such alternatives as "postinflammatory tumor" (4,5), "histiocytoma" (6), "plasma cell granuloma" (7–9), "mast cell granuloma" (10), "xanthoma" (11–14), "xanthogranuloma" (15), "plasma cell/histiocytoma complex"

(16), and, in some reports (17), "sclerosing hemangioma" as well.

This brief introductory chapter considers definitions for the term "pseudotumor" that are morphologically broader than those mentioned in the preceding paragraph and yet more restrictive than others in existing clinical applications. Because this book is directed principally to the needs of histopathologists, such definitions will generally be based on the microscopic characteristics of the lesions in question rather than on their macroscopic attributes.

## PHILOSOPHICAL AND PRACTICAL ISSUES PERTAINING TO PSEUDOTUMORS

To a certain extent, the day-to-day "images" of patients that are seen by clinical practitioners, radiologists, and pathologists are potentially quite different from one another. For example, the surgeon may believe that he or she is palpating a tangible and definable mass lesion in the breast, yet the radiologist sees little or nothing on mammography. Likewise, a pathologist asked to interpret a fine needle aspiration biopsy of the putative lesion may find no cytologic abnormalities. Under these conditions, the second and third physicians involved in the case may question the claims of the first; however, short of physically examining the patient themselves, they can never really determine whether a "tumor" (mass) is actually present or not with absolute certainty. In this scenario, the palpable lesion is indubitably a "pseudotumor" (pseudoneoplasm) in the mind of the surgeon, whereas the other consultants may conclude that it is instead an imagined condition.

M. R. Wick and J. H. Ritter: Department of Pathology, Washington University Medical Center, St. Louis, Missouri 63110.

Nonetheless, members of the latter two specialty groups are—whether they realize it or not—subject to the same tricks of nature in their own practice areas. Radiologically, it is well known that hemorrhages in hemophiliac patients may simulate neoplasms in areas where little clinical abnormality can be palpated or seen (18,19); pathologic specimens from these "hemophiliac pseudotumors" show only degenerating components of a hematoma and may therefore be difficult for the microscopist to reconcile with clinical concern over a neoplasm. Similar comments apply to roentgenographic images of "tumefactive biliary sludge" (20), "tumefactive cutaneous pneumocystosis" (21), "mucosal rosettes" of the duodenal ampulla (22), musculoskeletal anatomic variations (23), and "rounded atelectasis" of the lung (24–27). From the pathologist's vantage point, there are also similar interpretative "sinkholes" wherein histologic findings suggest the presence of a neoplasm in the face of little or no clinical or radiologic abnormality. These include unexpected adnexal nevi in skin biopsies done for other reasons (28–30), incidental cutaneous reactions to the application of Monsel's solution (a styptic preparation) (31), serendipitous inclusion of the organ of Chievitz (which may resemble a focus of carcinoma) in biopsies of the oral mucosa (32,33), and observation of the infection-related hemophagocytic syndrome (a disorder that simulates certain forms of malignant lymphoproliferation) in bone marrow or lymph node biopsies from patients with other diseases (34,35).

These discrepancies are in all likelihood destined to be a constant part of medical practice under the existing conditions in which they take place. Only by close (usually face-to-face) collegial interaction—as in the setting of a clinicopathologic conference, for example—can all accrued information on such cases be synthesized to yield a clear and correct assessment of the disease processes or anatomic-physiologic variations in question (36). Short of that investment of time and effort, disagreements between the physicians involved in any given case must serve as important clues to the existence of an unusual or unexpected condition. If they are heeded, these checks often provide the benefit of avoiding misinterpretation and mistreatment.

Lest we become too complacent that errors of this type will always be caught, it is crucial to emphasize that a large number of entities may simulate neoplasms on all levels—clinical, radiologic, and pathologic—and therefore they represent major opportunities for prognostic or therapeutic disaster. These are the clinicopathologic entities to which this book is attuned, primarily so that surgical pathologists will oppose, rather than foster, clinical and radiologic misconceptions in any given circumstance. Accordingly, a concerted attempt has been made to concentrate the discussion on histopathologic images of benign, potentially tumefactive, but nonneoplastic disorders that may be mistaken for true neoplasms by pathologists as well as practitioners in other specialties. In addition, however, other pathologic entities are included that histomorphologists alone may uniquely misinterpret as neoplasms.

In undertaking such a task, certain assumptions and determinations must be made. For example, we have arbitrarily decided that our consideration of "inflammatory pseudotumors" will—for purposes of consideration here—include entities known as "inflammatory myofibroblastic tumors," even though some authors feel that at least some of the latter lesions are, in fact, neoplastic in nature (38). Similar comments apply to the inclusion of angiomyolipoma of the kidney, which is variously and contentiously regarded as neoplastic or maldevelopmental (39–42). Conversely and just as arbitrarily, there will be no discussion of melanocytic nevi herein because most of these proliferations are, in our opinion, neoplasms rather than errors of morphogenesis (43). Finally, it should be recognized that not all entities currently thought to represent pseudoneoplastic proliferations will be proven to be definitely nonneoplastic. For example, not all pseudolymphomas represent pseudotumors; undoubtedly some cases, particularly those primarily considered pseudolymphomas in the gastrointestinal mucosa, represent lymphomas of mucosa-associated lymphoid tissue (MALTomas). This became apparent with the emergence of new technologies, namely, immunohistochemistry and gene rearrangement analyses. Our consideration of entities designated pseudotumors in this book is based on our interpretation and synthesis of the current literature. With the accumulation of new knowledge, we realize that classification of such pathologic entities as pseudotumors or true neoplasms may require revision of the concepts presented in this book.

## TOPOGRAPHIC DISTRIBUTION AND NATURE OF PSEUDOTUMORS

Given the above-cited considerations, it should come as no surprise that virtually all topographic sites in the human body may play host to lesions or malformations that simulate neoplasms. Perhaps because they are more susceptible to etiologic events that predispose to the development of pseudotumors, certain of these locations are dominant with regard to the relative frequency of their involvement by such proliferations. Such examples include the lung, the urinary tract, and the gut. It is also interesting that partially overlapping and partially distinctive groups of pseudoneoplastic lesions affect different anatomic sites (Table 1). This phenomenon may again reflect the relative influences of dissimilar pathogenetic factors, but other variables that are currently undefined must almost certainly have an influence as well. The following sections consider specific lesions in a general fashion, as related to their putative etiologic categories (Table 2).

### Idiopathic Pseudotumors

With selected exceptions, the prototypic "inflammatory pseudotumor" (IP) is of unknown causation. This lesion is perhaps the most common in the pulmonary parenchyma of

**TABLE 1.** *Listing of exemplary "pseudotumors" by organ system*

*Skin*
  Inflammatory pseudotumor
  Adnexal nevi
  Lymphoid hyperplasias
  Reactions to Monsel's solution
  Acroangiodermatitis
  Proliferating scars
  Intravascular papillary endothelial hyperplasia (Masson's lesion)
  "Spindle cell hemangioendothelioma"
  Pseudoepitheliomatous epithelial hyperplasia
  "Rudimentary meningocele"
  Mycobacterial pseudotumors
  Bacillary angiomatosis
*Soft Tissue (Including Muscle)*
  Neuromuscular choristoma
  Fibrolipomatous hamartoma
  Nodular fasciitis
  Proliferative myositis
  Myositis ossificans
  "Tumefactive fibroinflammatory lesions" (e.g., idiopathic retroperitoneal fibrosis)
  Florid (tumefactive) lymphocytic myositis
  Inflammatory pseudotumor
  "Atypical decubital fibroplasia"
  Tumoral amyloidosis (amyloidoma)
  Selected examples of intraabdominal "cystic mesothelioma"
  Paraffiruma
*Bones and Joints*
  "Fibroosseous pseudotumor" of digits
  Synovial chondrometaplasia/chondrocalcinosis
  Fibrous dysplasia and "fibroosseous lesions"
  Metaphyseal fibrous defect
  Paget's disease of bone
  Aneurysmal bone cyst
  Giant cell reparative granuloma
  Cherubism
  Avulsion fractures of ischial tuberosities
  "Brown tumor" of hyperparathyroidism (osteitis fibrosa cystica)
*Breast*
  Radial scar
  Choristoma (Hamartoma)
  Inflammatory pseudotumor
*Nervous System*
  Inflammatory pseudotumor
  Gliosis
  Active phase plaque of multiple sclerosis
  Progressive multifocal leukoencephalopathy
  Paraventricular glial nodule of tuberous sclerosis
  Malakoplakia
  Posttraumatic "neuroma"
*Endocrine System*
  Inflammatory pseudotumor of thyroid
  Hashimoto's thyroiditis
  Nodular thyroid hyperplasia
  Nodular parathyroid hyperplasia
  Nodular adrenal hyperplasia
  Chronic tumefactive pancreatitis
*Lymphoreticular System*
  Selected lymphoid hyperplasias
  Florid unilinear hyperplasia in bone marrow recovery
  Infection-related hemophagocytic syndrome
  Epstein–Barr virus–related atypical lymphoid hyperplasias
  Mycobacterial pseudotumor
  Malakoplakia
  Inflammatory pseudotumor, not otherwise specified

*Upper Airway*
  Bacillary angiomatosis
  Pseudoepitheliomatous epithelial hyperplasia
  Oral organ of Chievitz
  Necrotizing sialometaplasia
  Radiation effects on mucosal epithelia
  Benign lymphoepithelial lesion of salivary gland
  Traumatized antral/choanal polyps
  Glial heterotopias
  Benign fibroosseous lesions
  Inflammatory pseudotumor
*Mediastinum*
  Sclerosing mediastinitis
  Inflammatory pseudotumor of thymus
  Thymic dysplasia
*Lower Airway*
  Pseudoepitheliomatous epithelial hyperplasia
  Fibrohyaline plaque of pleura
  Florid mesothelial hyperplasia
  Localized tumefactive organizing pneumonia
  Lymphocytic interstitial pneumonia
  Pulmonary "pseudolymphoma"
  Pulmonary chondroid/lipomatous/muscular hamartomas
  Inflammatory pseudotumor
  Malakoplakia
*Alimentary Tract*
  Pseudoepitheliomatous epithelial hyperplasia
  Enteritis/colitis cystica profunda
  "Adenomyoma" of duodenum
  Tumefactive chronic pancreatitis
  Virally induced "pseudotumors" of small and large bowel
  Mycobacterial pseudotumors
  Bacillary angiomatosis
  Florid lymphoid hyperplasia
  Hepatic bile duct hamartoma
  Hepatic focal nodular hyperplasia
  Inflammatory "cloacogenic" polyp
  Xanthogranulomatous cholecystitis
  Malakoplakia
  Inflammatory pseudotumors
*Genitourinary Tract (Male and Female)*
  Pseudoepitheliomatous epithelial hyperplasia
  Postoperative spindle cell nodule
  Inflammatory ("fibrous") pseudotumor of kidney, bladder, and testis
  Drug effect (e.g., cytoxan cystitis mimicking CIS)
  Urethral (prostatic utricular) polyp
  Caruncle of urethra
  Renal angiomyolipoma
  Malakoplakia of kidney/bladder/testis/prostate/uterus/ovary
  Paratesticular mycobacterial pseudotumor
  Xanthogranulomatous nephritis/cystitis/orchitis/endometritis/oophoritis
  Adenomatous and basal cell prostatic hyperplasia
  Cribriform intraductal prostatic hyperplasia
  Nodular stromal prostatic hyperplasia
  Prostatic sclerosing adenosis
  Radiation effect on prostatic stroma and epithelium
  Granulomatous prostatitis
  Vaginal adenosis
  Uterine cervical mesonephric remnants
  Uterine cervical microglandular adenosis
  Arias–Stella reaction of endometrium
  Ovarian stromal hyperplasia/hyperthecosis
  Nephrogenic metaplasia of bladder and urethra
  Mesothelial cysts of the female pelvis
  Endometriosis
*Cardiovascular System*
  Cardiac inflammatory pseudotumor

**TABLE 2.** *Listing of exemplary "pseudotumors" by etiologic category*

| Idiopathic | Developmental |
|---|---|

Idiopathic
  Selected "inflammatory (fibrous) pseudotumors" of all locations
  Selected lymphoid hyperplasias
  Lymphoma-like Hashimoto's thyroiditis
  Radial scar of breast
  Selected "cystic mesotheliomas" of the abdomen
  Urethral (prostatic utricular) polyp
  Selected angiomyolipomas of kidney
  Tumefactive Paget's disease of bone
  Benign fibroosseous lesions of the head and neck
  Cutaneous "spindle cell hemangioendothelioma"
  Metaphyseal fibrous defect of bone
  Aneurysmal bone cyst
  "Tumefactive fibroinflammatory lesions" of bone and soft tissue
  Tumefactive plaques of multiple sclerosis
Reparative/Posttraumatic
  Selected "inflammatory (fibrous) pseudotumors" of all locations
  Pseudoepitheliomatous epithelial hyperplasia of all locations
  Acroangiodermatitis
  Nodular fasciitis
  Proliferative myositis
  Tumefactive lymphocytic myositis
  Myositis ossificans
  Exuberant osseous fracture calluses
  Posttraumatic "neuroma"
  Proliferating cutaneous scars
  Intravascular papillary endothelial hyperplasia (Masson's lesion)
  Giant cell reparative granuloma of bone
  Synovial chondrometaplasia/chondrocalcinosis
  Avulsion fractures of ischial tuberosities
  Necrotizing sialometaplasia
  Traumatized antral/choanal polyps of head and neck
  Pleural fibrohyaline plaques
  Radiation reactions
  Gliosis
  Nephrogenic metaplasia of urinary tract
  Xanthogranulomatous inflammation
  Urethral caruncle
  Inflammatory cloacogenic polyp
  Enteritis/colitis cystica profunda
  Tumefactive chronic pancreatitis

Developmental
  Adnexal nevi of skin
  Choristomas of all locations
  Hamartomas of all locations
  Vaginal adenosis (selected cases)
  Uterine cervical mesonephric remnants
  Selected angiomyolipomas of kidney
  Glial heterotopias of head and neck
  Rudimentary meningocele of skin
  Oral organ of Chievitz
  Fibrous dysplasia of bone
  Thymic dysplasias
  "Adenomyoma" ("Brunner's gland hamartoma") of duodenum
  Paraventricular glial nodules of tuberous sclerosis
Functional
  Nodular hyperplasias of endocrine organs
  Florid bone marrow hyperplasia in marrow recovery
  Focal nodular hyperplasia of liver
  Prostatic hyperplasias
  Arias–Stella reaction of endometrium
  "Brown tumor" of hyperparathyroidism (osteitis fibrosa cystica)
  Ovarian stromal hyperplasia/hyperthecosis
  Uterine cervical microglandular hyperplasia
Iatrogenic
  Cutaneous reactions to Monsel's solution
  Drug effects (e.g., cytoxan cystitis simulating CIS)
  Postoperative spindle cell nodules of genitourinary tract
  Vaginal adenosis (selected cases)
Infectious
  Mycobacterial pseudotumors
  Viral (EBV/CMV)–associated pseudotumor
  Malakoplakia of all locations
  Bacillary angiomatosis
  Infection-related hemophagocytic syndrome
  Progressive multifocal leukoencephalopathy
  Lymphocytic interstitial pneumonia (selected cases related to EBV infection)
  Lymphoid hyperplasia (selected examples in selected organ systems)

EBV, Epstein–Barr virus; CMV, cytomegalovirus.

children and young adults (37) (Figs. 1 and 2), but it can be seen in patients of virtually any age and in a multitude of organ sites (44–90). Some authors have, in the authors' opinion, complicated the literature on this entity by including as "IPs" some pathologic entities that are almost certainly neoplastic, namely, variants of fibrous histiocytoma (16,91). If one restricts attention to proliferations other than those, a clearer picture of such lesions begins to emerge. For example, one of the two resulting subgroups of IP in the lung probably represents unresolved and organizing pneumonia—infectious or otherwise (38) (Fig. 3)—whereas the other type is truly idiopathic and may be associated with systemic signs and symptoms that suggest production of a cytokine by the proliferating cells (37). Affected patients may develop fever, weight loss, neutrophilia, and hypochromic-microcytic anemia in that scenario (92). This same constellation of findings can be associated with non-pulmonary IP as well (90). However, what the stimulus for such lesions is and why a proportion of them appear to regress spontaneously are unanswered questions at present.

Similarly, there are several other IP variants that represent etiologically heterogeneous entities, with at least one variation of each of them being idiopathic in nature. Examples include lymphoid hyperplasias of the lung, gut, skin, various

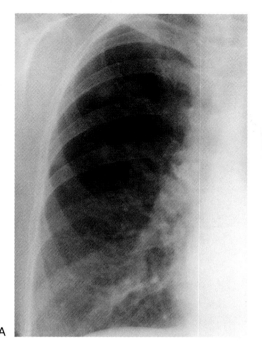
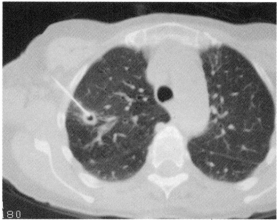

A

B

**FIG. 1. A:** Chest radiograph showing an ill-defined parenchymal density in the right lower lobe in a 50-year-old woman. **B:** Corresponding computed tomogram of the chest demonstrating a nodular lesion (into which a biopsy needle has been placed). Although fine needle aspiration biopsy was not definitive, the lesion ultimately proved to be an inflammatory pseudoneoplastic proliferation rather than a carcinoma, which had been suspected clinically.

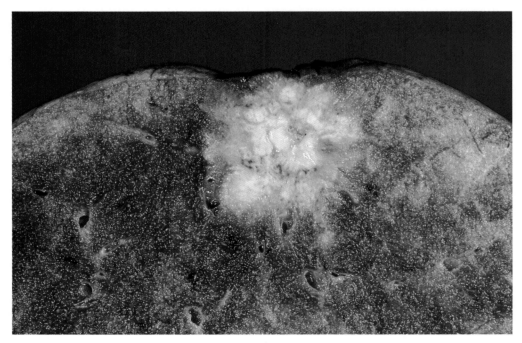

**FIG. 2.** Gross photograph of a segmentectomy specimen of lung, taken from the same patient shown in Fig. 1. The subpleural mass shown here looks remarkably like a peripheral pulmonary carcinoma, but it instead represented an "inflammatory pseudotumor."

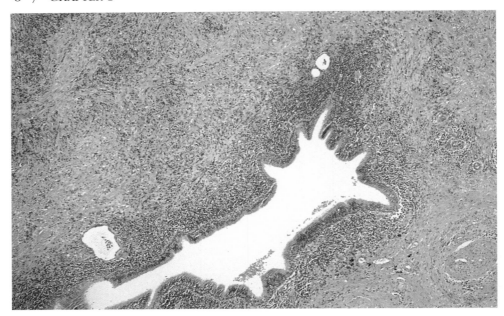

**FIG. 3.** The microscopic appearance of the lesion shown in Figs. 1 and 2 was that of an organizing and fibrotic pneumonic process, which, in this photograph, is centered on a small bronchus. Despite assiduous sampling, no neoplastic disease was observed.

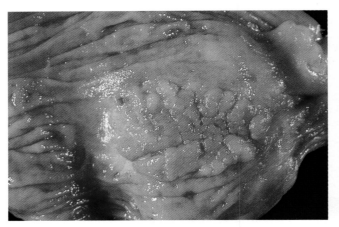

A

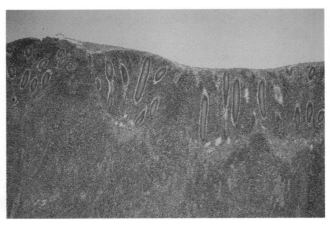

B

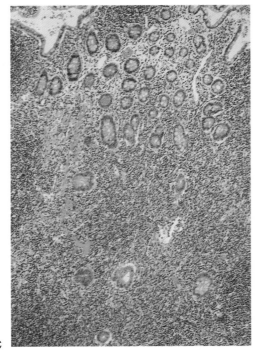

C

**FIG. 4. A:** Gross photograph of a cecal lesion seen in a bowel resection specimen taken because of abdominal trauma. There is a multinodular mucosal irregularity that was felt by the surgeon and that raised the suspicion of possible neoplasia. **B, C:** Microscopy of the specimen demonstrated entrapment and displacement of colonic glands by a dense infiltrate of lymphoid cells. These were shown to be polytypic by frozen section immunohistology, confirming the benign "pseudolymphomatous" nature of the lesion.

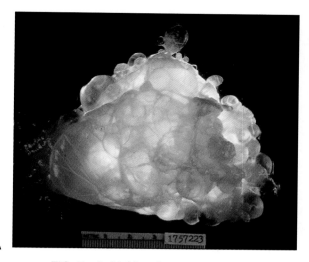 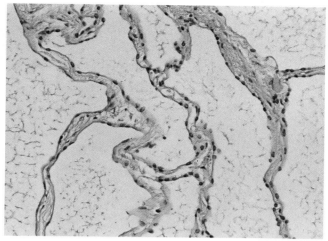

**FIG. 5. A:** Multiloculated cystic mass from the abdomen of an adult woman, with the macroscopic appearance of a "multicystic mesothelioma." **B:** Microscopic analysis shows a compartmentalized lesion that is subdivided by attenuated fibrous septa that are lined by flattened, bland mesothelial cells. (Case courtesy of Dr. Sharon Weiss, Department of Pathology, University of Michigan School of Medicine, Ann Arbor, Michigan.)

mucosae, soft tissue, and lymphoreticular system (93–109) (Fig. 4); fibroosseous lesions of craniofacial and small tubular bones (110–113); and angiomyolipomas of the kidney (40–42,114). In these three groups of disorders, definable pathogenetic factors include viral infection or autoimmune diseases (98,100,101,109); fibrous dysplasia or familial "cherubism" (112,115,116); and the tuberous sclerosis complex (39,40), respectively. However, other morphologically identical IPs in each category can be linked to no such explanatory factors and must therefore be classified as idiopathic.

Still other conditions are "quasi-neoplastic," in that they feature causally unknown (and, to some extent, autonomous) cellular proliferations in various locations with no identifiable "trigger" or stimulus. The pathologic entities known as radial scar of the breast (117–119); "cystic mesothelioma" of the abdomen (120–122) (Fig. 5); urethral (prostatic utricular) polyp (123); "tumefactive fibroinflammatory lesions" of soft tissue (124,125), metaphyseal fibrous defects of bone (126,127); and aneurysmal bone cysts (128,129) (Fig. 6) fall into this category. They differ from true neoplasms because they are self-limited or even spontaneously regressing in

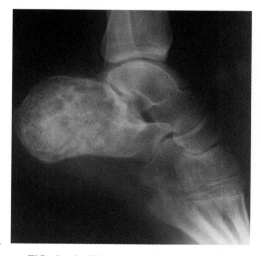 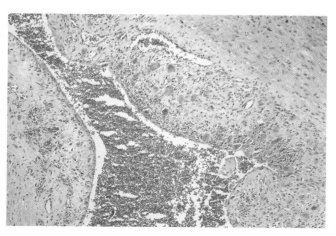

**FIG. 6. A:** This expansile lesion of the calcaneus has an internally multiloculated appearance on plain film radiography. It was associated with pain on weight bearing and was clinically suspected to represent a neoplasm. **B:** Curettage and thorough sampling of the mass showed numerous fibrous septa comprised by bland spindle cells and collagenous stroma, with numerous interposed blood lakes and roughly linear arrays of osteoclast-like giant cells in the septations. This constellation of observations is typical of an idiopathic aneurysmal bone cyst.

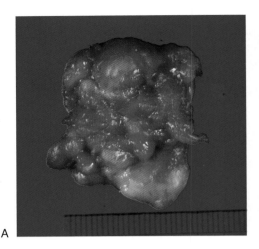
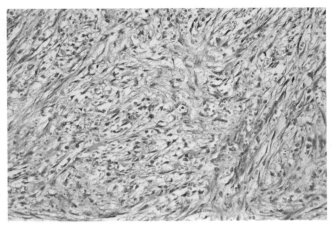

**FIG. 7. A:** Gross photograph of an excised nodule from the superficial soft tissue of the forearm in a 23-year-old man. The mass had grown rapidly over the preceding two weeks. **B:** Histologically, the lesion demonstrates a proliferation of bland spindle cells with numerous mitotic figures, prominent small stromal blood vessels, extravasation of erythrocytes into the interstitial space, and a myxedematous background. These findings are characteristic of nodular fasciitis.

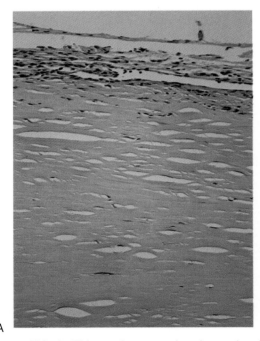
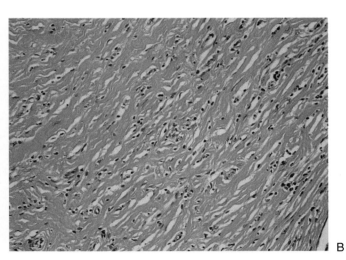

**FIG. 8.** This section was taken from a localized tumefactive nodular lesion of the right visceral pleura, which projected into the pleural space on plain film radiography. It was excised because of concern over the diagnosis of a solitary pleural fibrous tumor but instead shows the "basket-weave" pattern of a typical pleural plaque **(A)** as related to prior asbestos exposure. **(B)** Some foci in the lesion were slightly more cellular and may have caused temporary concern over an interpretation of desmoplastic malignant mesothelioma. However, both the bland nature of the proliferating cells and the macroscopically circumscribed nature of the lesion are inconsistent with the latter diagnosis.

character. However, inciting causes and molecular mechanisms governing the evolution of such processes represent uncharted conceptual territory.

Some pseudotumors included in this section do have a known cause, i.e., identification of an underlying disease process, but the etiology of the latter condition may be idiopathic. Paget's disease of bone [which may cause osteolytic, mixed, or osteoblastic lesions that simulate neoplasms (129–131)], tumor-like cerebral plaques of active multiple sclerosis (132), and lymphoma-like Hashimoto's thyroiditis (133,134) are representative examples of such disorders.

### Reparative/Posttraumatic Pseudotumors

There is little question that exaggerated host responses to injury, which may be either physical or inflammatory in nature, constitute the most common sources of pseudoneoplastic proliferations. In some instances, the injury may have been rather trivial (subclinical), and the resulting reparative process could therefore be regarded as idiosyncratic and "inappropriate." This situation would appear to apply to cases of nodular fasciitis (135–137) (Fig. 7), proliferative myositis (137,138), giant cell reparative granuloma of bone

(129,131,139,140), fibrohyaline plaques of the pleura (141–145) (Fig. 8), and xanthogranulomatous inflammation of various sites (146–148).

On the other hand, more pseudotumors are incited by tangible and documented episodes of injury, but again with an overzealous and individualistic reparative response. In this vein, pseudoepitheliomatous hyperplasias of the skin and mucosae (149–151) (Fig. 9), acroangiodermatitis (152,153), myositis ossificans (154,155) (Fig. 10), posttraumatic "neuroma" (156), "atypical decubital fibroplasia" (157), tumefactive synovial chondrometaplasia (158,159), avulsion fractures of the ischial tuberosities (131,160), exuberant osseous calluses (161), necrotizing sialometaplasia (162,163), traumatic changes in choanal sinonasal polyps (164,165), gliosis (166), nephrogenic urothelial metaplasia (167), urethral caruncles (168), inflammatory polyps of the anorectal region (169), colitis cystica profunda (170), florid but reactive mesothelial proliferations (171) (Fig. 11), tumor-like chronic pancreatitis (172), and radiotherapy-induced tissue reactions (173) all follow discrete or repetitive episodes of injury. However, why some individuals develop these exaggerated manifestations of repair and other (indeed, most) patients do not do so is an unsettled question at present.

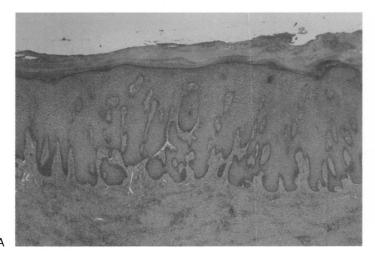

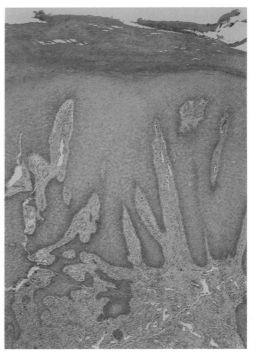

A                                                                                    B

**FIG. 9. A:** This biopsy was taken from the skin surrounding a draining sinus tract in a patient with chronic osteomyelitis. The specimen exhibits slightly irregular downward growth of the epidermal rete ridges, which show a tendency to confluence. There is moderate underlying perivascular inflammation. **B:** Although closer inspection shows irregularity in the shapes and sizes of the rete, they "respect" their interfaces with the subjacent dermis and are not associated with a desmoplastic response or localized stromal eosinophilia. These attributes are those of pseudoepitheliomatous hyperplasia rather than squamous carcinoma.

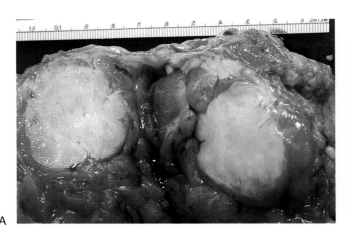
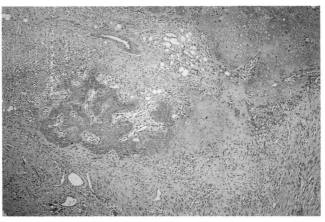

A

B

**FIG. 10. A:** Localized, "fleshy" intramuscular mass in the vastus lateralis in a 21-year-old man. It had grown substantially over a 4-week span of time and was therefore excised with a tentative clinical diagnosis of sarcoma. However, further questioning revealed that the patient had been hit in this area with a hockey puck 6 weeks previously, and microscopy of the lesion **(B)** shows the typical chondroosseous "zonation" pattern of myositis ossificans.

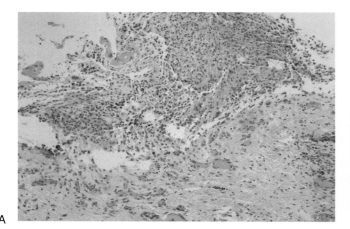
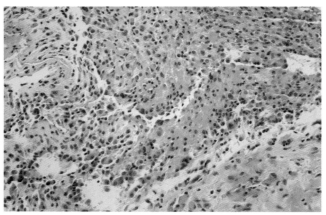

A

B

**FIG. 11. A:** Histologic examination of an inguinal herniorrhaphy specimen—taken from a hernia known to have been partially incarcerated—shows the proliferation of mesothelial cells around fibrovascular cores, with a papillary configuration. Consideration was given to the possibility of an underlying mesothelioma, but thorough sampling and closer inspection failed to show infiltration of the mesothelial cells into the subjacent stroma, significant nuclear atypia, or spontaneous necrosis **(B)**. Thus, the final diagnosis was that of secondary florid mesothelial hyperplasia.

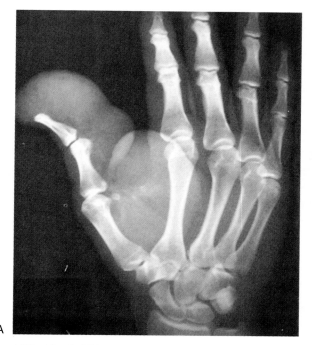

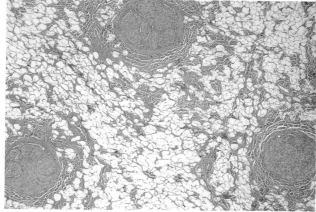

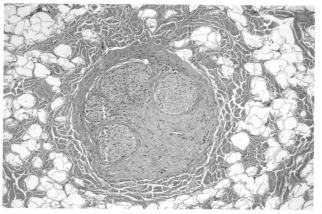

**FIG. 12. A:** This young man had had worsening localized macrodactyly of the right thumb for several years. Exploration of an associated mass in the soft tissue of the forearm showed a proliferation of bland fibrofatty tissue that was centered in the median nerve **(B)**. The neural fascicles are structurally normal **(C)**, but they are splayed apart by this fibrolipomatous neural hamartoma. (Fig. 12A reproduced from Silverman TA, Enzinger FM. Fibrolipomatous hamartoma of nerve: a clinicopathologic analysis of 26 cases. *Am J Surg Pathol* 1985;9:7–14.)

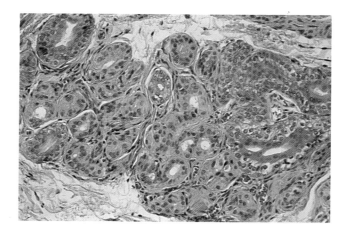

**FIG. 13.** This localized proliferation of apocrine glands was observed incidentally in a blepharoplasty specimen taken from an elderly woman. It was felt initially to represent an apocrine hidradenoma, but the identity of each of the constituent tubules with normal apocrine gland coils marks the lesion as a nonneoplastic apocrine nevus.

## Developmental Pseudotumors

From a pathologic standpoint, the most straightforward group of pseudotumors is that which relates to developmental quirks of individual organisms or, just as commonly, an ignorance on the part of the observer regarding details of organogenesis and embryology (at least, the authors certainly have had to plead guilty to the latter charge on several occasions!). One can place all choristomas (174), hamartomas (175,176), and cutaneous adnexal nevi (28–30) in the first of these two explanatory categories (Figs. 12 and 13). Such lesions are felt to lack the potential for truly autonomous growth and are instead generally classified as flaws of morphogenesis. Nonetheless, variations in their histologic characteristics may well cause confusion with neoplastic proliferations in selected cases.

Microanatomic remnants or heterotopias relating to embryologic changes in structure constitute another large group of developmental lesions. Here, some examples of vaginal adenosis (177–180), cervical mesonephric remnants (181)

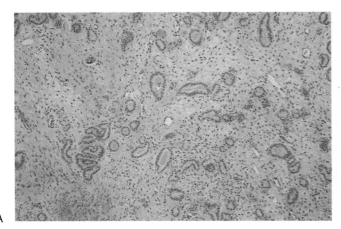

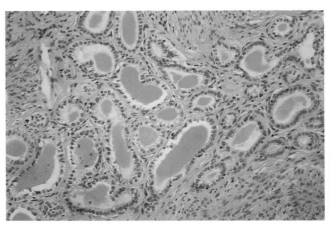

A

B

**FIG. 14. A:** A cervical conization was performed in a 35-year-old woman who had surface mucosal squamous carcinoma in situ. In the deeper matrical tissues, however, there was a disorganized proliferation of tubular ducts and gland-like structures that engendered worries over a diagnosis of adenocarcinoma. Closer inspection **(B)**, however, demonstrated a regimented basal orientation of bland nuclei within such structures, along with slightly lucent cytoplasm and dense luminal secretions. This group of findings is diagnostic of mesonephric remnants in the cervical stroma.

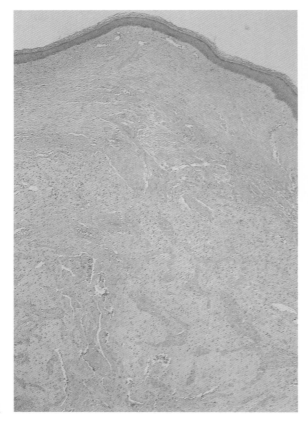

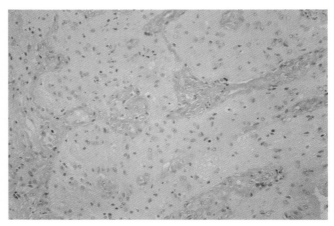

B

A

**FIG. 15.** A 15-year-old boy was found to have a slowly enlarging nodule in the skin over the bridge of the nose, which was excised. It showed a fascicular proliferation of bland, ovoid cells that were dispersed in a fibrillary matrix **(A)**. Higher power examination **(B)** demonstrated occasional, dispersed larger cells with the characteristics of neurons, identifying this lesion as a glial heterotopia (so-called nasal glioma).

(Fig. 14), "adenomyoma" ("Brunner's gland hamartoma") of the duodenum (182), "rudimentary meningocele" of the skin (183,184), and instances of glial heterotopia (185,186) of the head and neck (Fig. 15) are representative. The oral organ of Chievitz, conversely, is a normal structure rather than an embryologic vestige (32,33); however, it is so uncommonly seen in mucosal biopsies that many histopathologists fail to recognize it as a normal structure and instead may confuse this inclusion with a metastatic malignant neoplasm.

Malformations that are related to heritable Mendelian syndromes also may resemble neoplasms. As referenced above, cases of angiomyolipoma of the kidney in Bourneville's disease are appropriately included in that context (40), as are tumefactive lesions of osseous fibrous dysplasia (131,139, 187) and the paraventricular glial nodules of tuberous sclerosis (39). Although it does not produce a mass lesion, thymic dysplasia (188) may be mistaken for "microscopic thymoma" (189) in children with selected congenital immunodeficiencies.

## "Functional" Pseudotumors

Some pseudoneoplastic proliferations prove to be a manifestation of a functional pathophysiologic state, often—but not always—relating to endocrine under- or overactivity. It is well known by all pathologists that "dominant" follicular nodules often arise in the setting of diffuse parenchymal hyperplasia of the thyroid or parathyroid glands (134) and that these may simulate an adenoma or even a carcinoma microscopically. Similar comments apply to localized unilateral nodular hyperplasias of the adrenal (190), an increasing number of which are being seen as surgical pathology specimens because of the widespread use and high sensitivity of computed tomographic (CT) scans of the abdomen. Other pseudotumors are consequences of normal aging or of physiologic processes such as pregnancy, but they have an endocrine basis nonetheless. In the latter subset of proliferations, prostatic hyperplasias (191–193), focal nodular hyperplasia of the liver (194,195) (Fig. 16), ovarian stromal

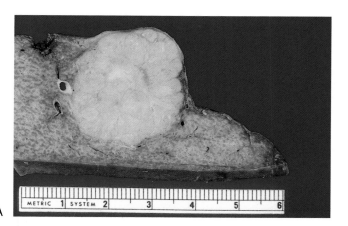

A

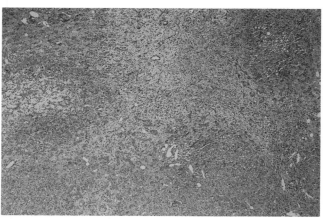

B

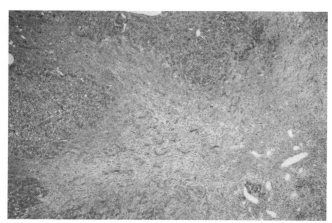

C

**FIG. 16.** This 4-cm intrahepatic mass was detected on computed tomography of the abdomen in a 36-year-old woman who had intermittent abdominal pain. The resected specimen **(A)** shows a discrete nodular lesion with a notable central fibrous zone. Histologic examination of the lesion **(B)** confirms the latter impression and demonstrates that the proliferating hepatocytes are cytologically unremarkable. Trichrome staining **(C)** confirmed the "pseudo-cirrhotic" configuration of the mass. This concatenation of observations is diagnostic of focal nodular hepatic hyperplasia.

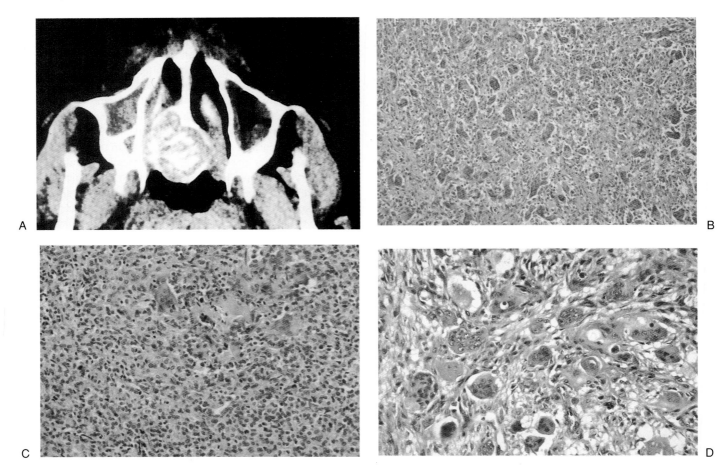

**FIG. 17.** A 46-year-old man presented with symptoms of bilateral nasal obstruction and was found to have a mass in the posterior nasal fossae on direct rhinoscopy. Computed tomography **(A)** of the head corroborated the clinical findings, and curettage of the lesion **(B–D)** revealed a cytologically bland fibroblastic proliferation that was punctuated by osteoclast-like giant cells. This mass was felt to represent a so-called giant cell reparative granuloma or a true giant cell tumor of bone until it was found that the patient had a calcium level of 11.5 mg/dl and an elevation in serum parathormone. Thus, the final diagnosis was that of parathyroid osteopathy ("brown tumor of hyperparathyroidism").

hyperthecosis (196,197), the Arias–Stella reaction of the endometrium (198,199), osteitis fibrosa cystica (osseous "brown tumor" of hyperparathyroidism) (200,201) (Fig. 17), and uterine cervical microglandular hyperplasia (202) all may develop in reaction to alterations of the systemic hormonal milieu. In predefined clinical circumstances, each of these processes has the potential to be mistaken as a neoplasm by both clinicians and pathologists.

### Iatrogenic Pseudotumors

Several surgical procedures and other therapies are capable of producing tissue reactions that may mimic neoplasms. Most of these proliferations are reparative in nature and might have been rightly included in the corresponding section cited previously. However, because of their clear iatrogenic nature, they deserve special recognition as complications of medical intervention. In the past decade, it has been recognized that instrumentation or surgery of the genitourinary tract may result in an idiosyncratic, microscopically worrisome, tumefactive proliferation of spindle cells that is known simply as "postoperative spindle cell nodule" (203,204) (Fig. 18). Over the same time, but with decreasing frequency because of changes in therapeutic practice, tissue reactions to the application of an iron salt–based cutaneous styptic (Monsel's solution) have been documented as poten-

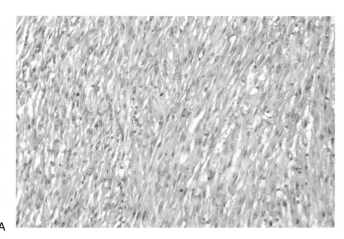
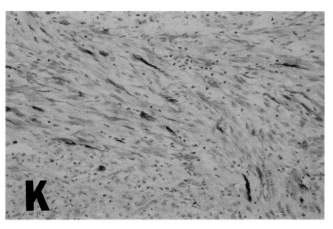

A

B

**FIG. 18.** A 66-year-old man had had removal of a grade 2/4 noninvasive papillary transitional cell carcinoma via cystoscopy. Two months later, he returned with symptoms suggesting urinary obstruction, and was found to have a 1-cm mass in the mucosa of the trigone. This was resected with the cystoscope, showing a disorganized proliferation of spindle cells with only a modest number of inflammatory cells **(A)**. Despite immunoreactivity for keratin (K) in the lesional cells, the correct diagnosis is not one of sarcomatoid carcinoma—as initially feared—but rather that of a reactive postinstrumentation spindle cell nodule **(B)**.

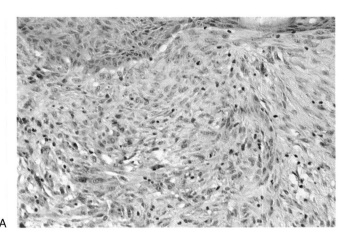
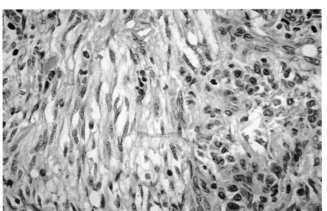

A

B

**FIG. 19. (A–C)** A 41-year-old man had had removal of a skin tumor by shave biopsy 6 weeks previously. Because the area of the latter procedure remained irregular and became slightly raised, it was excised, yielding the sample shown in **(A)**. The original lesion had been seen at another institution and was not available for review. Because of the proliferation of spindle cells seen in the excision specimen, with multifocal entrapment of erythrocytes between them **(B)**, a diagnosis of possible Kaposi's sarcoma was initially entertained. However, clumped iron pigment was subsequently found in the center of the lesion **(C)**, and it was learned that the patient had originally had a basal cell carcinoma with application of Monsel's solution (a styptic) to the base of the shave biopsy. Hence, the final diagnosis is that of a fibrovascular proliferative reaction to Monsel's solution.

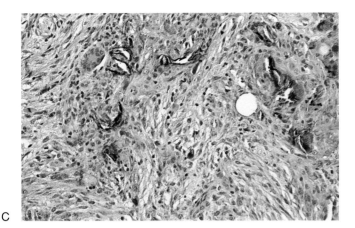

C

FIG. 19. *Continued*

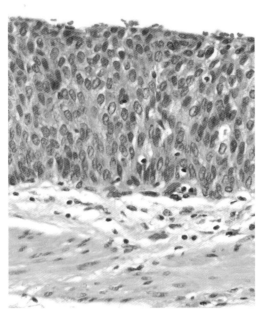

FIG. 20. A 55-year-old man presented with hematuria and was found to have irregular, hemorrhagic bladder mucosa by cystoscopy. A biopsy of the bladder (shown here) disclosed notable epithelial atypia, causing concern over a diagnosis of urothelial dysplasia or carcinoma in situ. However, it was then learned that the patient had recently been given cyclophosphamide in treatment of recalcitrant psoriasis. After the latter medication was terminated, subsequent biopsies of the bladder demonstrated no histologic abnormalities. Thus, this case exemplifies the potential for cyclophosphamide to cause pseudoneoplastic (reversible) epithelial alterations in the bladder mucosa.

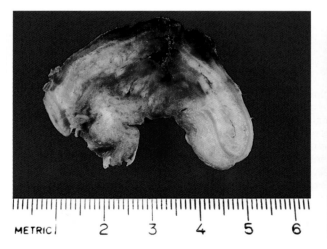

A

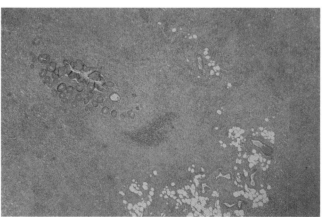

B

FIG. 21. **A:** A 47-year-old man who was infected with Human Immunodeficiency Virus developed the clinical picture of acute appendicitis. Inspection of the excised appendix by the surgeon raised concern over a possible neoplasm because of the irregular firmness and thickening that were observed in the wall of this structure. This impression was further fueled by histologic observations **(B, C)**, showing a fibroxanthoma-like mural proliferation that effaced the muscularis and extended into the periappendiceal soft tissue. Nevertheless, positive immunostains **(D)** for an "early" antigen of cytomegalovirus **(C)** indicated that the process was a virally induced "pseudotumor."

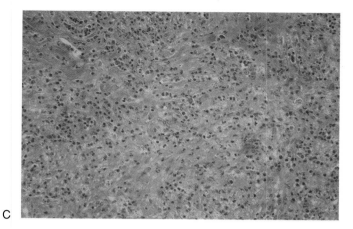
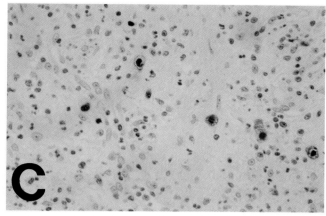

**FIG. 21.** *Continued*

tial simulants of Kaposi's sarcoma and other spindle cell tumors of the skin (31) (Fig. 19).

Other pseudotumors in this generic category may not produce a mass but are nevertheless capable of imitating an infiltrative or in situ neoplasm in biopsy specimens. These lesions are prototypically represented by the cytotoxic effects of cyclophosphamide on the urothelium—potentially simulating in situ transitional cell carcinoma (205) (Fig. 20)—and by florid vaginal adenosis in women whose mothers were given oral diethylstilbestrol during pregnancy (177–180). Without complete and appropriate historical data in either of these settings, there is a risk that the pathologist might misinterpret such lesions as neoplastic.

### Infectious Pseudotumors

One of the most fascinating conceptual developments of the past 20 years has been the elucidation of infectious pathogeneses for tumor-like proliferations that had theretofore been regarded as idiopathic in nature. Particularly because of the advent of the Acquired Immunodeficiency Syndrome (AIDS), tissue reactions to several viruses and bacteria have been characterized that are capable of simulating neoplasms. For example, it is now known that conjointly cytopathic and reparative responses to cytomegalovirus, Epstein–Barr virus (EBV), papovavirus, selected species of mycobacteria, and other bacilli are capable of producing le-

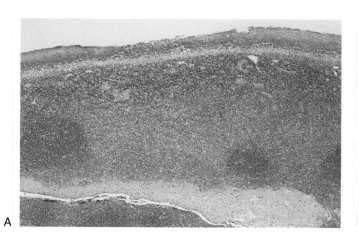
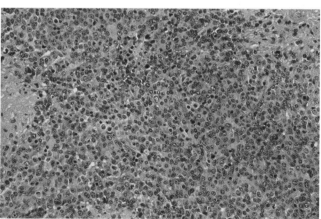

**FIG. 22.** A 15-year-old boy developed rapidly worsening respiratory stridor and was found to have massive enlargement of the left tonsil. There were no systemic complaints. The tonsillectomy specimen **(A–C)** showed a worrisome proliferation of large, atypical, immunoblast-like lymphoid cells, with scattered apoptotic debris and a high mitotic rate. However, positive immunostains for the latent membrane protein (L) of Epstein–Barr virus **(D)** suggested a possible diagnosis of atypical infectious mononucleosis rather than one of malignant lymphoma, and this was subsequently confirmed by serologic studies and an uneventful clinical course.

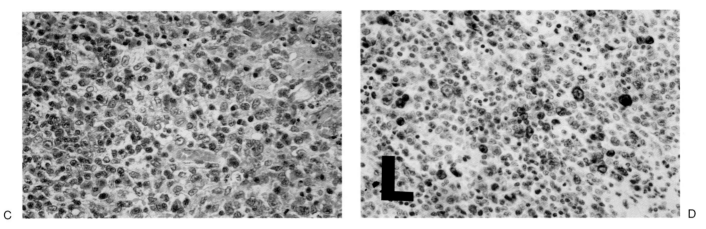

**FIG. 22.** *Continued*

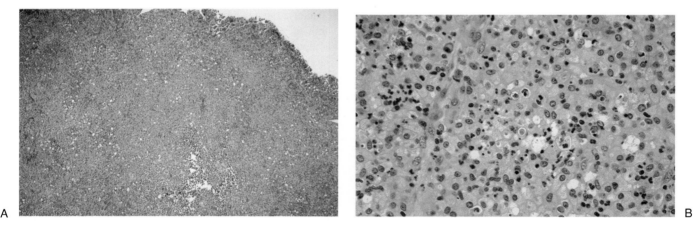

**FIG. 23.** A 77-year-old man had had repeated episodes of acute and chronic prostatitis, and presented with worsening symptoms of urinary obstruction. Transurethral resection of the prostate yielded tissue fragments that were represented by sheets of polygonal eosinophilic cells, with interspersed inflammation **(A, B)**. Although preoperative consideration was given to a potential diagnosis of prostatic carcinoma, the correct interpretation of malakoplakia is derived from the clinical setting and the presence of spherical basophilic inclusions (Michaelis–Gutmann bodies) in the cytoplasm of the lesional cells, which are histiocytes.

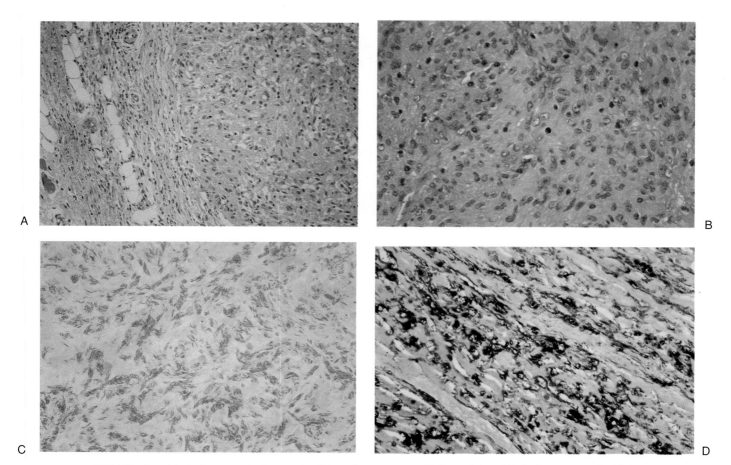

**FIG. 24.** An elderly former missionary to Africa developed multiple nodular skin lesions, one of which was excised. Histologic assessment showed discrete deep dermal and subcuticular aggregates of fusiform and polygonal cells, admixed with some "foamy" histiocytes **(A, B)**. Immunohistochemical evaluation showed that these had a fibroblastic/fibrohistiocytic phenotype, and the diagnosis of "eruptive" fibrous histiocytoma was entertained. However, Fite and Steiner stains of the lesion showed innumerable acid-fast mycobacterial organisms **(C, D)**. The patient subsequently developed other lesions that were typical of leprosy. Therefore, the final diagnosis was that of mycobacterial pseudotumor (so-called histoid leprosy). There was a favorable response to appropriate antibiotic therapy.

sions in several organs showing histologic features that may mirror those of sarcomas, gliomas, or lymphomas (109,206–210) (Figs. 21 and 22).

This general phenomenon is by no means restricted to the context of AIDS. It has also been recognized for a longer period of time as the basic etiology for malakoplakia (Fig. 23) in many organ sites following infection with various bacteria (211–215), "histoid" cutaneous infections with *Mycobacterium leprae* (216) (Fig. 24), and "pseudolymphoma" of the terminal ileum in patients who are infected with *Yersinia* species (218,219). Similarly, the infection-related hemophagocytic syndrome is most often observed in iatrogenically immunosuppressed patients who subsequently become infected with bacteria, viruses, fungi, or parasites (34,35,220–223) (Fig. 25). These conditions are particularly important for physicians to recognize accurately because of the likelihood that they will respond favorably to specific antimicrobial therapy.

## SUMMARY

It is hoped that the foregoing outline will serve as a general framework for an approach by surgical pathologists to the topic of neoplastic mimicry. More specific clinicopathologic details follow, under categorical chapter headings that address particular organ systems and the lesions that potentially may be seen in each location. As a concluding statement, the information introduced here reinforces the constant need for pathologists to ask, "Is this process potentially pseudoneoplastic?" in the process of analyzing a variety of lesions on a daily basis.

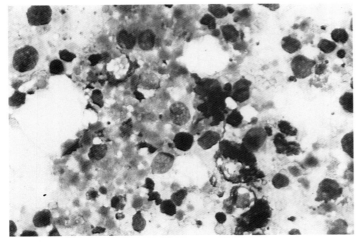

A

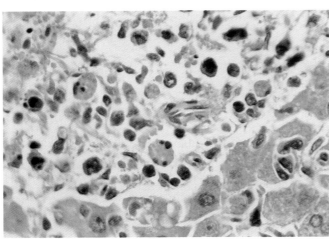

B

**FIG. 25.** A 16-year-old boy developed typical acute myelogenous leukemia and was given several cycles of multiagent chemotherapy. After the fifth course of treatment, he developed rapidly worsening pancytopenia, disseminated intravascular coagulation, and hepatosplenomegaly with biochemical indications of hepatic dysfunction. A bone marrow aspirate **(A)** and a closed liver biopsy **(B)** were obtained, showing numerous histiocytes in each specimen that had ingested erythrocytes and other cellular elements. Possible transformation of the patient's leukemia to the picture of secondary "malignant histiocytosis" (as had been reported in selected literature) was considered. However, subsequent blood cultures were positive for cytomegalovirus and cryptococcus, and the final diagnosis was that of infection-related hemophagocytic syndrome. The patient was successfully treated by aggressive supportive measures and antimicrobial medications, and he survived.

## REFERENCES

1. Ackerman LV. *Surgical pathology.* 3rd ed. St. Louis: CV Mosby, 1964:407–408.
2. Birch-Hirschfeld A. Die Krankheiten der Orbita. In: Graefe A, Saemisch T, eds. *Handbuch der Gesamten Augenheilkunden.* vol. 9, part 1. Berlin: Springer-Verlag, 1930;111–130.
3. Garner A. Pathology of "pseudotumors" of the orbit: a review. *J Clin Pathol* 1973;26:639–648.
4. Umiker WO, Iverson L. Postinflammatory "tumors" of the lung. *J Thorac Surg* 1954;28:55–62.
5. Kuzela DC. Ultrastructural study of a postinflammatory "tumor" of the lung. *Cancer* 1975;36:149–156.
6. Makela V, Mattila S, Makinen J. Plasma cell granuloma (histiocytoma) of the lung and pleura. *Arch Pathol Microbiol Scand (A)* 1972; 80:634–640.
7. Bahadori M, Liebow AA. Plasma cell granulomas of the lung. *Cancer* 1973;31:191–208.
8. Alvarez-Fernandez E, Escalona-Zapata J. Pulmonary plasma cell granuloma: an electron microscopic and tissue culture study. *Histopathology* 1983;7:279–286.
9. Warter A, Satge D, Roeslin N. Angioinvasive plasma cell granulomas of the lung. *Cancer* 1987;59:435–443.
10. Sherwin RP, Kern WH, Jones JC. Solitary mast cell granuloma (histiocytoma) of the lung. *Cancer* 1965;18:634–641.
11. Scott HW, Morrow AG, Payne TPB. Solitary xanthoma of the lung. *Thorac Surg* 1948;17:821–825.
12. Titus JL, Harrison EG Jr, Clagett OT, Anderson MV, Kuaff LY. Xanthomatous and inflammatory pseudotumor of the lung. *Cancer* 1962; 15:522–538.
13. Wentworth P, Lynch MJ, Fallis JC, et al. Xanthomatous pseudotumor of lung. *Cancer* 1968;22:345–355.
14. Buell R, Want N, Seemayer TA, Ahmed MN. Endobronchial plasma cell granuloma (xanthomatous pseudotumor): a light and electron microscopic study. *Hum Pathol* 1976;7:411–426.
15. Alegre JA, Deust J. Xanthogranuloma as a coin lesion of the lung. *Dis Chest* 1958;33:427–431.
16. Spencer H. The pulmonary plasma cell–histiocytoma complex. *Histopathology* 1984;8:903–916.
17. Liebow AA, Hubbel DS. Sclerosing hemangioma (histiocytoma, xanthoma) of the lung. *Cancer* 1956;9:53–75.
18. Jensen PS, Putnam CE. Hemophilic pseudotumor: diagnosis, treatment, and complications. *Am J Dis Child* 1975;129:717–719.
19. Hermann G, Yeh HC, Gilbert MS. Computed tomography and ultrasonography of the hemophilic pseudotumor and their use in surgical planning. *Skel Radiol* 1986;15:123–128.
20. Kelly IM, Lees WR, Russell RC. Tumefactive biliary sludge: a sonographic pseudotumor appearance in the common bile duct. *Clin Radiol* 1993;47:251–254.
21. Coulman CU, Greene I, Archibald RWR. Cutaneous pneumocystosis. *Ann Intern Med* 1987;106:396–398.
22. Bellamy PR. The mucosal rosette: a periampullary pseudotumor within a duodenal diverticulum. *Clin Radiol* 1993;47:117–118.
23. Coenen L, Biltjes I. Pseudotumor of the palm due to an anomalous

flexor digitorum superficialis muscle belly. *J Hand Surg* 1991; 16A:1046–1051.

24. Meier S, Cagle O. Rounded atelectasis. *Surg Rounds* 1986;8:85–90.
25. Inoshita T, Boyd W. Rounded atelectasis shown by computed tomography. *South Med J* 1986;79:764–767.
26. Stark P. Round atelectasis: another pulmonary pseudotumor. *Am Rev Resp Dis* 1982;125:248–250.
27. Tallroth K, Kiviranta K. Round atelectasis. *Respiration* 1984;45:71–77.
28. Wick MR, Swanson PE. *Cutaneous adnexal tumors: a guide to pathologic diagnosis.* Chicago: ASCP Press, 1991;28.
29. Goldstein N. Ephidrosis (local hyperhidrosis): nevus sudoriferus. *Arch Dermatol* 1967;96:67–71.
30. Kin JH, Hur H, Lee CW, Kim YT. Apocrine nevus. *J Am Acad Dermatol* 1988;18:579–581.
31. Amazon K, Robinson MD, Rywlin AM. Ferrugination caused by Monsel's solution: clinical observations and experimentations. *Am J Dermatopathol* 1980;2:197–205.
32. Tschen JA, Fechner RE. The juxtaoral organ of Chievitz. *Am J Surg Pathol* 1979;3:147–154.
33. Danforth RA, Baughman RA. Chievitz's organ: a potential pitfall in oral cancer diagnosis. *Oral Surg* 1979;48:231–235.
34. Risdall RJ, McKenna RW, Nesbit ME, et al. Virus-associated hemophagocytic syndrome: a benign histiocytic proliferation distinct from malignant histiocytosis. *Cancer* 1979;44:993–1002.
35. Risdall RJ, Brunning RD, Hernandez JI, Gordon DH. Bacteria-associated hemophagocytic syndrome. *Cancer* 1984;54:2968–2972.
36. McBroom JM, Ramsay AD. The clinicopathological meeting: a means of auditing diagnostic performance. *Am J Surg Pathol* 1993;17:75–80.
37. Pettinato G, Manivel JC, DeRosa N, Dehner LP. Inflammatory myofibroblastic tumor (plasma cell granuloma): clinicopathologic study of 20 cases with immunohistochemical and ultrastructural observations. *Am J Clin Pathol* 1990;94:538–546.
38. Matsubara O, Tan-Liu NS, Kenney RM, Mark EJ. Inflammatory pseudotumor of the lung: progression from organizing pneumonia to fibrous histiocytoma or to plasma cell granuloma in 32 cases. *Hum Pathol* 1988;19:807–814.
39. Critchley M, Earl CJC. Tuberous sclerosis and allied conditions. *Brain* 1932;55:311–352.
40. Stillwell TJ, Gomez MR, Kelalis PP. Renal lesions in tuberous sclerosis. *J Urol* 1987;138:477–481.
41. Blute ML, Malek RS, Segura JW. Angiomyolipoma: clinical metamorphosis and concepts for management. *J Urol* 1988;139:20–31.
42. Malone MJ, Johnson PR, Jumper BM, et al. Renal angiomyolipoma: six case reports and literature review. *J Urol* 1986;135:349–357.
43. Rhodes AH. Neoplasms: benign neoplasias, hyperplasias, and dysplasias of melanocytes. In: Fitzpatrick TB, et al, eds. *Dermatology in general medicine.* 3rd ed. New York: McGraw-Hill, 1987;877–966.
44. Berardi RS, Lee SS, Chen HP, Stines GJ. Inflammatory pseudotumors of the lung. *Surg Gynecol Obstet* 1983;156:89–96.
45. Chen HP, Lee SS, Berardi RS. Inflammatory pseudotumor of the lung: ultrastructural and light microscopic study of a myxomatous variant. *Cancer* 1984;54:861–865.
46. Barbareschi M, Ferrero S, Aldovini D, et al. Inflammatory pseudotumor of the lung: immunohistochemical analysis on four new cases. *Histol Histopathol* 1990;5:205–211.
47. Cotelingam JD, Jaffe ES. Inflammatory pseudotumor of the spleen. *Am J Surg Pathol* 1984;8:375–380.
48. Monforte-Munoz H, Ro JY, Manning JT Jr, et al. Inflammatory pseudotumor of the spleen: report of two cases with a review of the literature. *Am J Clin Pathol* 1991;96:491–495.
49. Perrone T, DeWolf-Peeters C, Frizzera G. Inflammatory pseudotumor of lymph nodes: a distinctive pattern of nodal reaction. *Am J Surg Pathol* 1988;12:351–361.
50. Kemper CA, David RE, Dereskinski SC, Dorfmann RF. Inflammatory pseudotumor of intraabdominal lymph nodes manifesting as recurrent fever of unknown origin: a case report. *Am J Med* 1991;90:519–523.
51. Isaacson P, Buchanan R, Mepham BL. Plasma cell granuloma of the stomach. *Hum Pathol* 1978;9:355–358.
52. Tada T, Wakabayashi T, Kishimoto H. Plasma cell granuloma of the stomach. *Cancer* 1984;54:541–544.
53. Ohtsuki Y, Akagi T, Moriwaki S, Hatano M. Plasma cell granuloma of the stomach combined with gastric cancer. *Acta Pathol Jpn* 1983;33:1251–1257.

54. Marn CS, Hsu FK. Inflammatory myofibrohistiocytic proliferating presenting as giant gastric pseudotumor. *Gastrointest Radiol* 1992;17:316–318.
55. Abrebanel P, Sarfaty S, Gal R, Chaimoff C, Kessler E. Plasma cell granuloma of the pancreas. *Arch Pathol Lab Med* 1984;108:531–532.
56. Wu JP, Yunis EJ, Fetterman G, et al. Inflammatory pseudotumors of the abdomen: plasma cell granulomas. *J Clin Pathol* 1973;26:943–948.
57. Pisciotto PT, Gray GF, Miller DR. Abdominal plasma cell pseudotumor. *J Pediatrics* 1978;93:628–630.
58. Day DL, Sane S, Dehner LP. Inflammatory pseudotumor of the mesentery and small intestine. *Pediatr Radiol* 1986;16:210–215.
59. Ashfaq R, Timmons CF. Xanthomatous pseudotumor of the small intestine following treatment for Burkitt's lymphoma. *Arch Pathol Lab Med* 1992;116:299–301.
60. Vujanic GM, Milovanovic D, Aleksandrovic S. Aggressive inflammatory pseudotumor of the abdomen 9 years after therapy for Wilms' tumor: a complication, coincidence, or association? *Cancer* 1992;70:2362–2366.
61. Johnston SJ, Beaver BL, Sun CC, et al. Inflammatory pseudotumor of the retroperitoneum. *MD Med J* 1991;40:787–790.
62. Chen KTK. Inflammatory pseudotumor of the liver. *Hum Pathol* 1984;15:694–696.
63. Gough J, Chakrabarti S. Inflammatory pseudotumor of the liver in a patient with chronic sclerosing cholangitis. *Am J Gastroenterol* 1993;88:1452–1453.
64. Henegan MA, Kaplan CG, Priebe CJ, Partin JS. Inflammatory pseudotumor of the liver: a rare cause of obstructive jaundice and portal hypertension in a child. *Pediatr Radiol* 1984;14:433–435.
65. Anthony PP, Telesinghe PU. Inflammatory pseudotumor of the liver. *J Clin Pathol* 1986;39:761–768.
66. Shek TW, Ng IO, Chan KW. Inflammatory pseudotumor of the liver: report of four cases and review of the literature. *Am J Surg Pathol* 1993;17:231–238.
67. Fish AE, Brodey PA. Plasma cell granuloma of the kidney. *Urology* 1976;8:89–91.
68. Vujanic GM, Berry PJ, Frank JD. Inflammatory pseudotumor of the kidney with extensive metaplastic bone. *Pediatr Pathol* 1992;12:557–561.
69. Davides KC, Johnson SH, Marshall M Jr, et al. Plasma cell granuloma of the renal pelvis. *J Urol* 1972;107:938–939.
70. Nochomovitz LE, Orenstein JM. Inflammatory pseudotumor of the urinary bladder: possible relationship to nodular fasciitis. *Am J Surg Pathol* 1985;9:366–373.
71. Dietrick DD, Kabalin JN, Daniels GF Jr, et al. Inflammatory pseudotumor of the bladder. *J Urol* 1992;148:141–144.
72. Lamovec J, Zidar A, Trsinar B, Jancar J. Sclerosing inflammatory pseudotumor of the urinary bladder in a child. *Am J Surg Pathol* 1992;16:1233–1238.
73. Coyne JD, Wilson G, Sandhu D, Young RH. Inflammatory pseudotumor of the urinary bladder. *Histopathology* 1991;18:261–264.
74. Parveen T, Fleischmann J, Petrelli M. Benign fibrous tumor of the tunica vaginalis testis. *Arch Pathol Lab Med* 1992;116:277–280.
75. Yamashima T, Honma T, Uchijima Y. Myofibroblastic pseudotumor mimicking epididymal sarcoma: a clinicopathologic study of three cases. *Pathol Res Pract* 1992;188:1054–1059.
76. Yapp R, Linder J, Schenker JR, Karrer FW. Plasma cell granuloma of the thyroid. *Hum Pathol* 1985;16:848–850.
77. Holck S. Plasma cell granuloma of the thyroid. *Cancer* 1981;48:830–832.
78. Earl PD, Lowry JC, Sloan P. Intraoral inflammatory pseudotumor. *Oral Surg Oral Med Oral Pathol* 1993;76:279–283.
79. Inui M, Tagawa T, Mori A, et al. Inflammatory pseudotumor in the submandibular region: clinicopathologic study and review of the literature. *Oral Surg Oral Med Oral Pathol* 1993;76:333–337.
80. Misselevitch I, Podoshin L, Fradis M, et al. Inflammatory pseudotumor of the neck. *Otolaryngol Head Neck Surg* 1991;105:864–867.
81. Hytiroglou P, Brandwein MS, Strauchen JA, et al. Inflammatory pseudotumor of the parapharyngeal space. *Head and Neck* 1992;14:230–234.
82. Pettinato G, Manivel JC, Insabato L, et al. Plasma cell granuloma (inflammatory pseudotumor) of the breast. *Am J Clin Pathol* 1988;90:627–632.
83. Eimoto T, Yanaka M, Kurosawa M, Ikeya F. Plasma cell granuloma (inflammatory pseudotumor) of the spinal cord and meninges. *Cancer* 1978;41:1929–1936.

84. West SG, Pttman DL, Coggin JT, Intracranial plasma cell granuloma. *Cancer* 1980;46:330–335.

85. Sitton JE, Harkin JC, Gerber MA. Intracranial inflammatory pseudotumor. *Clin Neuropathol* 1992;11:36–40.

86. Olmos PR, Falko JM, Rea GL, et al. Fibrosing pseudotumor of the sella and parasellar area producing hypopituitarism and multiple cranial nerve palsies. *Neurosurgery* 1993;32:1015–1021.

87. Chang Y, Horoupian DS, Lane B, et al. Inflammatory pseudotumor of the choroid plexus in Sjogren's disease. *Neurosurgery* 1991;29:287–290.

88. Yanagihara N, Segoe M, Gyo K, Ueda N. Inflammatory pseudotumor of the facial nerve as a cause of recurrent facial palsy: case report. *Am J Otol* 1991;12:199–202.

89. Fetsch JF, Montgomery EA, Meis JM. Calcifying fibrous pseudotumor. *Am J Surg Pathol* 1993;17:502–508.

90. Dickens P, Lam AK. Sudden death associated with cardiac inflammatory pseudotumor. *Forens Sci Int* 1991;49:89–93.

91. Gal AA, Koss MN, McCarthy WF, Hochholzer L. Prognostic factors in pulmonary fibrohistiocytic lesions. *Cancer* 1994;73:1817–1824.

92. Nishimaki T, Matsuzaki H, Sato Y, et al. Cyclosporin for inflammatory pseudotumor. *Intern Med* 1992;31:404–406.

93. Bastlein C, Burlefinger R, Holzberg E, et al. Common variable immunodeficiency syndrome and nodular lymphoid hyperplasia in the small intestine. *Endoscopy* 1988;20:272–275.

94. Bejaoui M, Guezmir M, Hamdi M, et al. Lymphoid hyperplasia of the intestine in children: 15 cases. *Ann Pediatrics (Paris)* 1992;39:359–364.

95. Yeong ML, Bethwaite PB, Prasad J, Isbister WH. Lymphoid follicular hyperplasia: a distinctive feature of diversion colitis. *Histopathology* 1991;19:55–61.

96. Colarian J, Calzada R, Jaszewski R. Nodular lymphoid hyperplasia of the colon in adults: is it common? *Gastrointest Endosc* 1990;36:421–422.

97. Servois V, Vuillerme MP, Faure C. Iconographic rubric: benign lymphoid hyperplasia of the colon. *Arch Fr Pediatrics* 1988;45:827–828.

98. Scherak O, Kolarz G, Popp W, et al. Lung involvement in rheumatoid factor-negative arthritis. *Scand J Rheumatol* 1993;22:225–228.

99. Franchi LM, Chin TW, Nussbaum E, et al. Familial pulmonary nodular lymphoid hyperplasia. *J Pediatrics* 1992;121:89–92.

100. Grattan-Smith D, Harrison LF, Singleton EB. Radiology of AIDS in the pediatric patient. *Curr Probl Diagn Radiol* 1992;21:79–109.

101. Koss MN, Hochholzer L, Nichols PW, et al. Primary non-Hodgkin's lymphomas and pseudolymphomas of the lung: a study of 161 patients. *Hum Pathol* 1983;14:1024–1038.

102. Brodell RT, Santa Cruz DJ. Cutaneous pseudolymphomas. *Dermatol Clin* 1985;3:719–734.

103. Spina D, Miracco C, Santopietro R, et al. Distinction between diffuse cutaneous malignant follicular center cell lymphoma and lymphoid hyperplasia by computerized nuclear image analysis. *Am J Dermatopathol* 1993;15:415–422.

104. Hammer E, Sangueza O, Suwanjindar P, et al. Immunophenotypic and genotypic analysis in cutaneous lymphoid hyperplasias. *J Am Acad Dermatol* 1993;28:426–433.

105. Fan K, Kelly R, Kendrick V. Nonclonal lymphocytic proliferation in cutaneous lymphoid hyperplasias: a flow-cytometric and morphological analysis. *Dermatology* 1992;185:113–119.

106. Slater DN. Diagnostic difficulties in "non-mycotic" cutaneous lymphoproliferative diseases. *Histopathology* 1992;21:203–213.

107. Takano Y, Kato Y, Sugano H. Histopathological and immunohistochemical study of atypical lymphoid hyperplasia and benign lymphoid hyperplasia of the stomach. *Jpn J Cancer Res* 1992;83:288–293.

108. Mopsik ER, Adrian JC, Klein LE. Follicular lymphoid hyperplasia of the hard palate: report of a case. *J Oral Maxillofac Surg* 1992;50:538–540.

109. Samoszuk M, Ramzi E, Ravel J. Disseminated persistent lymphoid hyperplasia containing Epstein–Barr virus and clonal rearrangements of DNA. *Diagn Mol Pathol* 1993;2:57–60.

110. Slootweg PJ, Panders AK, Nikkels PG. Psammomatoid ossifying fibroma of the paranasal sinuses. *J Craniomaxillofac Surg* 1993;21:294–297.

111. Chan KW, Khoo US, Ho CM. Fibro-osseous pseudotumor of the digits: report of a case with immunohistochemical and ultrastructural studies. *Pathology* 1993;25:193–196.

112. Bosse A, Niesert W, Wuisman P, Roessner A. Fibrous dysplasia versus osteofibrous dysplasia: morphological, differential diagnostic, and clinical aspects. Experiences from the Westfalen bone tumor registry. *Z Orthop Ihre Grenzgeb* 1993;131:42–50.

113. Kearns D, McGill T, Potsic W. Fibrous dysplasia. *Head and Neck* 1992;14:510–512.

114. Steiner MS, Goldman SM, Fishman EK, Marshall FF. The natural history of renal angiomyolipoma. *J Urol* 1993;150:1782–1786.

115. Betts NJ, Stewart JC, Fonseca RJ, Scott RF. Multiple central giant cell lesions with a Noonan-like phenotype. *Oral Surg Oral Med Oral Pathol* 1993;76:601–607.

116. Koury ME, Stella JP, Epker BN. Vascular transformation in cherubism. *Oral Surg Oral Med Oral Pathol* 1993;76:20–27.

117. Wallis MG, Devakumar R, Hosie KB, et al. Complex sclerosing lesions (radial scars) of the breast can be palpable. *Clin Radiol* 1993;48:319–320.

118. Franquet T, DeMiguel C, Cozcolluela R, Donoso L. Spiculated lesions of the breast: mammographic-pathologic correlation. *Radiographics* 1993;13:841–852.

119. Anderson TJ, Battersby S. Radial scars of benign and malignant breasts: comparative features and significance. *J Pathol* 1985;147:23–32.

120. Weiss SW, Tavassoli FA. Multicystic mesothelioma: an analysis of pathologic findings and biologic behavior in 37 cases. *Am J Surg Pathol* 1988;12:737–746.

121. Mennemeyer R, Smith M. Multicystic peritoneal mesothelioma. *Cancer* 1979;44:692–698.

122. Bhandarkar DS, Smith VJ, Evans DA, Taylor TV. Benign cystic peritoneal mesothelioma. *J Clin Pathol* 1993;46:867–868.

123. Walker AN, Fechner RE, Mills SE, Perry JM. Epithelial polyps of the prostatic urethra: a light microscopic and immunohistochemical study. *Am J Surg Pathol* 1983;7:351–356.

124. Frankenthaler R, Batsakis JG, Suarez PA. Tumefactive fibroinflammatory lesions of the head and neck. *Ann Otol Rhinol Laryngol* 1993;102:481–482.

125. Savage PD, Wick MR, Thompson RC, Skubitz KM. Tumefactive fibroinflammatory lesion of the extremity. *Arch Pathol Lab Med* 1991;115:230–232.

126. Klein MH, Rosenberg ZS, Lehman WB. Nonossifying fibroma of bone: a case report. *Bull Hosp Jt Dis Orthop Inst* 1990;50:64–69.

127. Selby S. Metaphyseal cortical defects in the tubular bones of growing children. *J Bone Joint Surg* 1961;43A:395–404.

128. Bertoni F, Bacchini P, Capanna R, et al. Solid variant of aneurysmal bone cyst. *Cancer* 1993;71:729–734.

129. Dahlin DC, McLeod RA. Aneurysmal bone cyst and other non-neoplastic conditions. *Skel Radiol* 1982;8:243–250.

130. Smith J, Yuppa F, Watson RC. Primary tumors and tumor-like conditions of the clavicle. *Skel Radiol* 1988;17:235–246.

131. Dahlin DC, Unni KK. *Bone Tumors.* 4th ed. Springfield, IL: Charles C Thomas, 1986;406–481.

132. Hunter SB, Ballinger WE Jr, Rubin JJ. Multiple sclerosis mimicking primary brain tumor. *Arch Pathol Lab Med* 1987;111:464–468.

133. Woolner LB, McConahey WM, Beahrs OH. Stroma lymphomatosa (Hashimoto's thyroiditis) and related disorders. *J Clin Endocrinol Metab* 1959;19:53–83.

134. LiVolsi VA. The thyroid and parathyroid. In: Sternberg SS, ed. *Diagnostic surgical pathology.* 2nd ed. New York: Raven Press, 1994:523–560.

135. Price SK, Kahn LB, Saxe N. Dermal and intravascular fasciitis: unusual variants of nodular fasciitis. *Am J Dermatopathol* 1993;15:539–543.

136. Stanley MW, Skoog L, Tani EM, Horwitz CA. Nodular fasciitis: spontaneous resolution following diagnosis by fine needle aspiration. *Diagn Cytopathol* 1993;9:322–324.

137. Lundgren L, Kindblom LG, Willems J, et al. Proliferative myositis and fasciitis: a light and electron microscopic, cytologic, DNA–cytometric, and immunohistochemical study. *APMIS* 1992;100:437–448.

138. Flury D, Von Hochstetter AR, Landolt U, Schmid S. Proliferative myositis: a little-known pseudomalignant lesion. *Schweiz Med Wochenschr* 1993;123:29–34.

139. Jaffe HL. Giant cell reparative granuloma, traumatic bone cyst, and fibrous (fibro-osseous) dysplasia of the jawbones. *Oral Surg* 1953;6:159–175.

140. Lorenzo JC, Dorfman HD. Giant cell reparative granuloma of short tubular bones of the hands and feet. *Am J Surg Pathol* 1980;4:551–563.

141. Hillerdal G. Asbestos-related pleural disease. *Semin Respir Med* 1987;9:65–74.

142. Solomon A, Sluis-Cramer GK, Goldstein B. Visceral pleural plaque formation in asbestosis. *Environ Res* 1979;19:258–264.

143. Stephens M, Gibbs AR, Pooley FD, Wagner JC. Asbestos-induced pleural fibrosis: pathology and mineralogy. *Thorax* 1987;42:583–588.

144. Tylen U, Hilsson U. Computed tomography in pulmonary pseudotumors and their relation to asbestos exposure. *J Comp Assist Tomogr* 1982;6:229–237.

145. Solomon A. Radiological features of asbestos-related visceral pleural changes. *Am J Industr Med* 1991;19:339–355.

146. Howard TJ, Bennion RS, Thompson JE Jr. Xanthogranulomatous cholecystitis: a chronic inflammatory pseudotumor of the gallbladder. *Am Surg* 1991;57:821–824.

147. Dao AH, Wong SW, Adkins RB Jr. Xanthogranulomatous cholecystitis: a clinical and pathologic study of twelve cases. *Am Surg* 1989;55: 32–35.

148. Malek RS, Elder JS. Xanthogranulomatous pyelonephritis: a critical analysis of 26 cases and of the literature. *J Urol* 1978;119:589–595.

149. Sommerville J. Pseudoepitheliomatous hyperplasia. *Acta Dermatoven* 1953;33:236–245.

150. Winer LH. Pseudoepitheliomatous hyperplasia. *Arch Dermatol Syphilol* 1940;42:856–863.

151. Barney PL. Histopathologic problems and frozen section diagnoses in diseases of the larynx. *Otolaryngol Clin North Am* 1970;3:493–513.

152. Yi JU, Lee CW. Acroangiodermatitis: a clinical variant of stasis dermatitis. *Int J Dermatol* 1990;29:515–516.

153. Kolde G, Worheide J, Baumgartner R, Brocker EB. Kaposi-like acroangiodermatitis in an above-knee amputation stump. *Br J Dermatol* 1989;120:575–580.

154. Ackerman LV. Extraosseous localized non-neoplastic bone and cartilage formation (so-called myositis ossificans): clinical and pathological confusion with malignant neoplasms. *J Bone Joint Surg* 1958; 40A:279–298.

155. Goldman AB. Myositis ossificans circumscripta: a benign lesion with a malignant differential diagnosis. *AJR* 1976;126:32–40.

156. Scotti TM. The lesion of Morton's metatarsalgia (Morton's toe). *Arch Pathol* 1957;63:91–102.

157. Montgomery EA, Meis JM, Mitchell MS, Enzinger FM. Atypical decubital fibroplasia: a distinctive fibroblastic pseudotumor occurring in debilitated patients. *Am J Surg Pathol* 1992;16:708–715.

158. Murphy FP, Dahlin DC, Sullivan CR. Articular synovial chondromatosis. *J Bone Joint Surg* 1962;44A:77–86.

159. Magno WB, Lee SH, Schmidt J. Chondocalcinosis of the temporomandibular joint: an external ear canal pseudotumor. *Oral Surg Oral Med Oral Pathol* 1992;73:262–265.

160. Ellis R, Greene AG. Ischial apophyseolysis. *Radiology* 1966;87: 646–648.

161. Linscheid RL, Coventry MB. Unrecognized fractures of long bones suggesting primary bone tumors. *Mayo Clin Proc* 1962;37:599–606.

162. Gad A, Willen H, Willen R, et al. Necrotizing sialometaplasia of the lip simulating squamous cell carcinoma. *Histopathology* 1980; 4:111–118.

163. Granich MS, Pilch BZ. Necrotizing sialometaplasia in the setting of acute and chronic sinusitis. *Laryngoscope* 1981;91:1532–1537.

164. Hyams VJ. Unusual tumors and lesions. In: Gnepp DR, ed. *Pathology of the head and neck*. New York: Churchill-Livingstone, 1988; 459–495.

165. Compagno J, Hyams VJ. Nasal polyposis with atypical stroma. *Arch Pathol Lab Med* 1976;100:224–229.

166. Parisi JE, Scheithauer BW. Glial tumors. In: Nelson JS, Parisi JE, Schochet SS, eds. *Principles and practice of neuropathology*. St Louis: CV Mosby, 1993;123–183.

167. Young RH, Scully RE. Nephrogenic adenoma: a report of 15 cases. *Am J Surg Pathol* 1986;10:268–275.

168. Palmer JK, Emmett JL, McDonald JR. Urethral caruncle. *Surg Gynecol Obstet* 1948;87:611–620.

169. Saul SH. Inflammatory cloacogenic polyp. *Hum Pathol* 1987;18: 1120–1125.

170. Herman AH, Nabseth DC. Colitis cystica profunda: localized, segmental, and diffuse. *Arch Surg* 1973;106:337–341.

171. Rosai J, Dehner LP. Nodular mesothelial hyperplasia in hernia sacs: a benign reactive condition simulating a neoplastic process. *Cancer* 1975;35:165–175.

172. Gambill EE. Pancreatitis associated with pancreatic carcinoma: a study of 26 cases. *Mayo Clin Proc* 1971;46:174–177.

173. Bostwick DG, Egbert BM, Fajardo CF. Radiation injury of the normal and neoplastic prostate. *Am J Surg Pathol* 1982;6:541–551.

174. Bonneau R, Brochu P. Neuromuscular choristoma. *Am J Surg Pathol* 1983;7:521–528.

175. Daroca PJ Jr, Reed RJ, Love GL, Kraus SD. Myoid hamartoma of the breast. *Hum Pathol* 1985;16:212–219.

176. McDonald JR, Harrington SW, Clagett OT. Hamartoma (often called chondroma) of the lung. *J Thorac Surg* 1945;14:128–143.

177. Merchant WJ, Gale J. Intestinal metaplasia in stilbestrol-induced vaginal adenosis. *Histopathology* 1993;23:373–376.

178. Maassen V, Lampe B, Untch M, et al. Adenocarcinoma and adenosis of the vagina. *Geburtshilfe Frauenheilkd* 1993;53:308–313.

179. Antonioli DA, Burke L. Vaginal adenosis: analysis of 325 biopsy specimens from 100 patients. *Am J Clin Pathol* 1975;64:625–638.

180. Robboy SJ, Hill EC, Sandberg EC, Czernobilsky B. Vaginal adenosis in women born prior to the diethylstilbestrol era. *Hum Pathol* 1986;17: 488–492.

181. Jones MA, Andrews J, Tarraza HM. Mesonephric remnant hyperplasia of the cervix: a clinicopathologic analysis of 14 cases. *Gynecol Oncol* 1993;49:41–47.

182. Goldman RL. Hamartomatous polyp of Brunner's glands. *Gastroenterology* 1963;44:57–62.

183. Sibley DA, Cooper PH. Rudimentary meningocele: a variant of "primary cutaneous meningioma." *J Cutan Pathol* 1989;16:72–82.

184. Marrogi AJ, Swanson PE, Kyriakos M, Wick MR. Rudimentary meningocele of the skin: clinicopathologic features and differential diagnosis. *J Cutan Pathol* 1991;18:178–188.

185. Karma P, Rasanen O, Karja J. Nasal gliomas: a review and report of two cases. *Laryngoscope* 1977;87:1169–1179.

186. Genut AA, Miranda FG, Garcia JH. Organized cerebral heterotopia in the ethmoid sinus: a case report. *J Neurol Sci* 1976;28:339–344.

187. Pritchard JE. Fibrous dysplasia of the bones. *Am J Med Sci* 1951;222: 313–332.

188. Nezelof C. Thymic pathology in primary and secondary immunodeficiencies. *Histopathology* 1992;21:499–511.

189. Pescarmona E, Rosati S, Pisacane A, et al. Microscopic thymoma: histologic evidence of multifocal cortical and medullary origin. *Histopathology* 1992;20:263–266.

190. Dobbie JW. Adrenal cortical nodular hyperplasia: the aging adrenal. *J Pathol* 1969;99:1–18.

191. Jones EC, Young RH. The differential diagnosis of prostatic carcinoma: its distinction from premalignant and pseudocarcinomatous lesions of the prostate gland. *Am J Clin Pathol* 1994;101:48–64.

192. Jones EC, Clement PB, Young RH. Sclerosing adenosis of the prostate gland: a clinicopathological and immunohistochemical study of 11 cases. *Am J Surg Pathol* 1991;15:1171–1180.

193. Epstein JI, Armas OA. Atypical basal cell hyperplasia of the prostate. *Am J Surg Pathol* 1992;16:1205–1214.

194. Grange JD, Guechot J, Legendre C, et al. Liver adenoma and focal nodular hyperplasia in a man with high endogenous sex steroids. *Gastroenterology* 1987;93:1409–1413.

195. Wanless IR, Mawdsley C, Adams R. The pathogenesis of focal nodular hyperplasia of the liver. *Hepatology* 1985;5:1194–1200.

196. Boss JH, Scully RE, Wegner KH, et al. Structural variations in the adult ovary: clinical significance. *Obstet Gynecol* 1965;25:747–763.

197. Madeido G, Tieu TM, Aiman J. Atypical ovarian hyperthecosis in a virilized postmenopausal woman. *Am J Clin Pathol* 1985;83: 101–107.

198. Arias-Stella J. Atypical endometrial changes produced by chorionic tissue. *Hum Pathol* 1972;3:450–453.

199. Silverberg SG. Arias-Stella phenomenon in spontaneous and therapeutic abortion. *Am J Obstet Gynecol* 1972;112:777–780.

200. Yokota N, Kuribayashi T, Nagamine M, et al. Paraplegia caused by brown tumor in primary hyperparathyroidism: case report. *J Neurosurg* 1989;71:446–448.

201. Bassler T, Wong ET, Brynes RK. Osteitis fibrosa cystica simulating metastatic tumor: an almost-forgotten relationship. *Am J Clin Pathol* 1993;100:697–700.

202. Leslie KO, Silverberg SG. Microglandular hyperplasia of the cervix. *Pathol Annu* 1982;17:95–114.

203. Proppe KH, Scully RE, Rosai J. Postoperative spindle cell nodules of genitourinary tract resembling sarcomas: a report of eight cases. *Am J Surg Pathol* 1984;8:101–108.

204. Young RH. Spindle cell lesions of the urinary bladder. *Histol Histopathol* 1990;5:505–512.

205. Sencer SF, Haake RJ, Weisdorf DJ. Hemorrhagic cystitis after bone marrow transplantation: risk factors and complications. *Transplantation* 1993;56:875–879.

206. Nash G, Said JW, eds. *Pathology of AIDS and HIV infection.* Philadelphia: WB Saunders, 1992.

207. Umlas J, Federman M, Crawford C, et al. Spindle cell pseudotumor due to *Mycobacterium avium-intracellulare* in patients with acquired immunodeficiency syndrome (AIDS). *Am J Surg Pathol* 1991;15:1181–1187.

208. Wood C, Nickoloff BJ, Todes-Taylor NR. Pseudotumor resulting from atypical mycobacterial infection: a "histoid" variety of *Mycobacterium avium-intracellulare* complex infection. *Am J Clin Pathol* 1985;83:524–527.

209. Brandwein M, Choi HH, Stauchen J, et al. Spindle cell reaction to non-tuberculous mycobacteriosis in AIDS mimicking a spindle cell neoplasm: evidence for dual histiocytic and fibroblast-like characteristics of spindle cells. *Virchows Arch A* 1990;416:281–286.

210. Chen KTK. Mycobacterial spindle cell pseudotumor of lymph nodes. *Am J Surg Pathol* 1992;16:276–281.

211. Chalvardjian A, Picard L, Shaw R, et al. Malakoplakia of the female genital tract. *Am J Obstet Gynecol* 1980;138:391–394.

212. Mollo JL, Groussard O, Baldeyrou P, et al. Tracheal malakoplakia. *Chest* 1994;105:608–610.

213. Lioy-Lupis MT, Quintana RM, Monsalve J, Iotti RM. Testicular malakoplakia. *Arch Esp Urol* 1993;46:822–824.

214. Chan AC, Lorentz TG, Ma L, et al. Fine needle aspiration of cutaneous malakoplakia. *Diagn Cytopathol* 1993;9:576–580.

215. Saad AJ, Donovan TM, Truong LD. Malakoplakia of the vagina diagnosed by fine needle aspiration cytology. *Diagn Cytopathol* 1993;9:559–561.

216. Sandmeier D, Guillou L. Malakoplakia and adenocarcinoma of the cecum: a rare association. *J Clin Pathol* 1993;46:959–960.

217. Mansfield RE. Histoid leprosy. *Arch Pathol* 1969;87:580–585.

218. Vantrappen G, Agg HO, Geboes K, Ponette E. Yersinia enteritis. *Med Clin North Am* 1982;66:639–653.

219. Cover TL, Aber RC. Yersinia enterocolitica. *N Engl J Med* 1989;321:16–24.

220. Bessis D, Sotto A, Taib J, Ciurana AJ. Visceral leishmaniasis with hemophagocytic syndrome. *Clin Infect Dis* 1993;17:611.

221. Bourquelot P, Oksenhendler E, Wolff M, et al. Hemophagocytic syndrome in HIV infection. *Presse Med* 1993;22:1217–1220.

222. Kikuta H, Sakiyama Y, Matsumoto S, et al. Fatal Epstein–Barr virus–associated hemophagocytic syndrome. *Blood* 1993;82:3259–3264.

223. Cantero-Hinojosa J, Diez-Ruiz A, Santos-Perez JL, et al. Lyme disease associated with hemophagocytic syndrome. *Clin Invest* 1993;71:620.

*Pathology of Pseudoneoplastic Lesions,*
edited by M. R. Wick, P. A. Humphrey, and J. H. Ritter.
Lippincott-Raven Publishers, Philadelphia © 1997.

CHAPTER 2

# Pseudoneoplastic Lesions of the Central Nervous System

George M. Kleinman and Douglas C. Miller

A variety of individually uncommon nonneoplastic lesions in the central nervous system (CNS) or its coverings present as masses that clinically or morphologically simulate neoplasms, with the latter being far more common. The relatively limited capacity of brain tissue to react to injury virtually ensures such mimicry in some situations. For example, vascular proliferation around an infarct or an abscess can simulate tumor-associated angiogenesis radiologically and occasionally microscopically as well. Most such nonneoplastic conditions are clinically easily separable from true neoplasms, such as infarcts, or they are readily recognizable in the appropriate clinical setting by pathologic analysis (e.g., radionecrosis) (1). Similarly, aneurysms may present as masses but are not often otherwise pseudotumorous. This chapter addresses entities that are not readily identified as nonneoplastic except by thorough pathologic study, as well as other lesions occupying the borderland between neoplasia and malformation, and reactive cellular proliferations.

The entity "pseudotumor cerebri," more properly termed benign intracranial hypertension, refers to a clinical disorder that is characterized by symptoms and signs of increased intracranial pressure, typically in young obese women (1–4). There are no morphologically identifiable changes in gen-

 G. M. Kleinman: Department of Pathology and Laboratory Medicine, Bridgeport Hospital and Department of Pathology, Yale University School of Medicine, New Haven, Connecticut 06610.
 D. C. Miller: Division of Neuropathology, Department of Pathology, New York University School of Medicine, New York, New York 10016.

uine pseudotumor cerebri, although some cases are now shown to be due to gliomas that are detectable only by magnetic resonance imaging (MRI).

Pseudotumors, as we will use that designation, may be grouped into six major categories: malformations, cysts, inflammatory and necrotizing processes, accumulations of extracellular material, nonneural heterotopias and hamartomas, and nonneoplastic cellular proliferations. The significant entities in each group are listed in the outline below and are then discussed along with issues of differential diagnosis in the remainder of this chapter. In writing this review, we have of necessity taken positions as to whether certain entities are in fact neoplastic. The discerning reader will notice that we have included "lipomas" in the discussion; these presumably (in our view) are maldevelopmental accumulations of fat and are not neoplastic; on the other hand, we have chosen to exclude "granular cell tumor" on the grounds that, by and large, these constitute true neoplasms.

## CLASSIFICATION OF PSEUDONEOPLASTIC LESIONS OF THE CNS

### I. Malformative lesions
A. Neuroepithelial parenchymal malformations
1) Heterotopia
   a) Gray matter heterotopia
   b) Leptomeningeal heterotopia
2) Ganglionic hamartoma
3) Dysplastic gangliocytoma of the cerebellum (Lhermitte–Duclos disease)
4) Cortical dysplasia
5) Tuberous sclerosis
B. Vascular malformations
1) Capillary telangiectasia
2) Cavernous hemangioma
3) Arteriovenous malformations
4) Meningioangiomatosis

### II. Cysts
A. Nonneural epithelial cysts
1) Epidermoid cysts (cholesteatomas)
2) Rathke's cleft cysts
3) Endodermal-type cysts ("neurenteric cysts")
   a) Spinal enterogenous cysts
   b) Intracranial respiratory epithelial cysts
B. Neuroepithelial cysts
1) Colloid cysts of the third ventricle
2) Neuroepithelial cysts of the lateral ventricles
3) Neuroepithelial cysts of the fourth ventricle
4) Extraventricular ependymal cysts
5) Pineal cysts
6) Cerebellar astrocytic cysts
C. Cavum septi pellucidi et vergae
D. Meningeal cysts
1) Arachnoid cysts
2) Glial-ependymal cysts
3) Miscellaneous intra-/paraspinal cysts

### III. Inflammatory and necrotizing mass lesions
A. Demyelinative disease
1) Multiple sclerosis
2) Progressive multifocal leukoencephalopathy
B. Inflammatory and lymphoproliferative processes
1) Inflammatory pseudotumors
   a) Plasma cell granuloma
   b) Castleman's disease (angiofollicular lymphoid hyperplasia)
   c) Multifocal fibrosclerosis
   d) Intraparenchymal lymphoid masses of undetermined nature
2) Rosai–Dorfman disease (sinus histiocytosis with massive lymphadenopathy)
3) Rheumatoid nodules
4) Sarcoidosis
5) Xanthogranulomas
   a) Xanthogranulomas of the choroid plexus
   b) Weber–Christian disease
6) Cholesterol granuloma of the petrous apex
C. Infectious lesions
1) Syphilitic gummas
2) Neuroborreliosis
3) Tuberculoma and tuberculous abscess
4) Cryptoccomas
5) Allergic fungal sinusitis

### IV. Depositions of extracellular material
A. Arachnoiditis ossificans
B. Amyloidoma
C. Pseudoamyloid (intraparenchymal colloid pseudocyst)
D. Pseudogout
E. Calcifying pseudoneoplasm
F. Storage disease
G. Mucocele

### V. Nonneural heterotopias and hamartomas
A. Lipoma
B. Ecchordosis physaliphora
C. Adrenal heterotopia
D. Endometriosis and Mullerian Choristoma
E. Salivary gland heterotopia
F. Neuromuscular hamartoma

### VI. Miscellaneous cellular proliferations
A. Gliosis
B. Hyperplasia Pacchionian granulations
C. Extramedullary hematopoiesis
D. Meningeal cellular nevus
E. Tenosynovial giant cell tumor (villonodular synovitis)
F. Localized hypertrophic neuropathy
G. Villous hypertrophy of the choroid plexus (bilateral choroid plexus papilloma)
H. Papillary endothelial hyperplasia

## MALFORMATIONS

### Neuroepithelial Parenchymal Lesions

#### Gray Matter Heterotopia

Isolated discrete nodules of neurons and glial may occasionally occur within the white matter (Fig. 1A) or along the walls of the ventricle (Fig. 1B), representing a malformation that results from abnormal migration of cortical neurons during embryogenesis (5). These may be single or multiple. Their lack of abnormal or multinucleated neurons, and an absence of glial proliferation, usually permits the distinction between heterotopias and gangliocytomas or gangliogliomas. However, some of the large neurons in these lesions exhibit the same perikaryal surface immunoreactivity for synaptophysin that is seen in gangliogliomas (6,7).

#### Hypothalamic Ganglionic Hamartoma

Projecting from the tuber cinereum or mamillary bodies into the suprasellar space (Fig. 2A), nodules of mature neurons and glial in the "ganglionic hamartoma" resemble hypothalamic nuclei (8–11). The masses may be very large (Fig. 2B). Precocious puberty, acromegaly, and diabetes insipidus have been observed in some patients, and hypothalamic-releasing hormones have been demonstrated in these lesions immunocytochemically (10).

Pallister–Hall syndrome involves a constellation of somatic malformations, notably polydactyly, together with hamartomas that are not otherwise distinguishable from isolated hypothalamic hamartomas (12–14).

#### Dysplastic Gangliocytoma of the Cerebellum (Lhermitte–Duclos Disease)

This lesion usually presents in adolescents or young adults, during the second and third decades (15). Occasional recurrences after resection confer on this lesion features that are shared by both neoplasms and malformations. The focal lesions of dysplastic gangliocytoma (Fig. 3A) that markedly enlarge the cerebellar folia are composed of numerous abnormal, large neurons (Fig. 3B). These superficially resemble abnormal Purkinje cells, but are thought to be of granular neuronal origin and are found below a layer of parallel myelinated nerve fibers (15).

#### Postradiation Hypertrophic Cortical Dysplasia

Rare focal hypertrophy of the cerebral cortex 6–13 years after high-dose therapeutic radiation has been reported as a pseudoneoplastic lesion (16). Microscopy discloses giant,

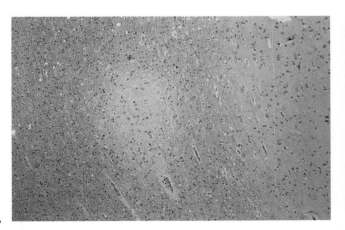

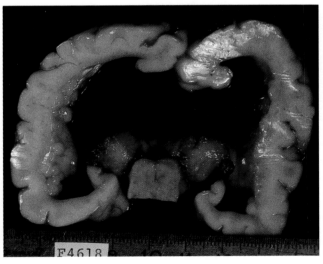

A                                                                                               B

**FIG. 1.** Gray matter heterotopia. **A:** This nodule of large neurons was one of several found in the deep temporal lobe white matter in a young adult with intractable partial complex seizures. The patient underwent a therapeutic temporal lobectomy that revealed focal cortical dysplasia and these heterotopias in the white matter. The gray matter, with its eosinophilic background, stands out against the blue of the myelinated white matter. (Luxol fast blue/hematoxylin and eosin (hereafter, LHE), 25× original magnification.) **B:** This coronal section is from an infant with multiple congenital abnormalities whose brain had hydrocephalus, agenesis of the corpus callosum, and multiple bilateral subependymal/periventricular nodules of heterotopic gray matter.

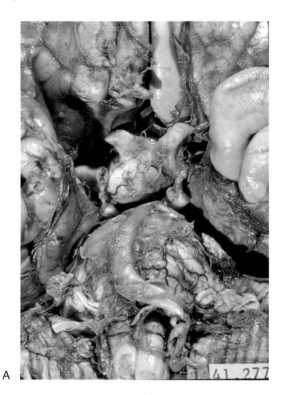

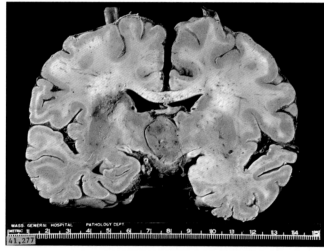

mation, usually the result of neuronal migration abnormalities, that causes seizures, often intractable. In some cases there may be grossly malformed gyri, such as polymicrogyria or pachygyria, but in many cases there are either no grossly visible abnormalities or only a slight thickening of the cortex with blurring of demarcation of the cortex from the white matter (17,18).

### Tuberous Sclerosis

An autosomal dominant condition resulting from defects in one or the other of two distinct genes (19), tuberous sclerosis appears to be sporadic in the majority of cases. Never-

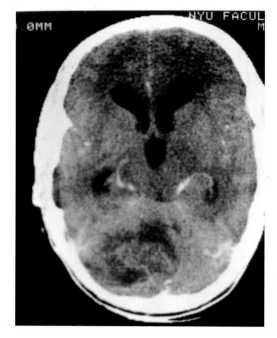

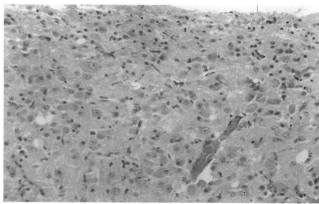

**FIG. 2.** Hypothalamic hamartoma. **A:** This photograph is a close view of the base of the brain in a patient with a ganglionic hamartoma of the hypothalamus. Here the inferior portion of the nodule is apparent as a bulging white tissue just behind the optic chiasm and in front of the brainstem. **B:** A coronal section of the brain from the same case shows the large mass filling the third ventricle. Note that there is no hydrocephalus, indicating the slow growth of the mass along with the brain from infancy.

abnormal neurons, which have a pattern of synaptophysin staining that is usually characteristic of neoplastic ganglion cells. These proliferations are accompanied by more typical sequelae of CNS irradiation, namely, demyelination, telangiectasia, and vascular thickening.

More commonly, cortical dysplasia is a cortical malfor-

**FIG. 3.** Cerebellar dysplastic gangliocytoma. **A:** This CT scan demonstrates the irregular tumor-like enlargement of the cerebellum. **B:** Histologically, the Lhermitte–Duclos lesion is characterized by bizarre large neurons in irregular layers replacing most of the normal foliar elements. (H&E, 100× original magnification.)

theless, unrecognized examples ("forme frustes") may exist among relatives of patients who have the fully expressed syndrome (19–21). In addition to a panoply of other lesions throughout the body, including rhabdomyomas of the heart and angiomyolipomas of the kidney, the brain in tuberous sclerosis is most commonly affected by pale, firm cortical nodules ("tubers") up to 3 cm in diameter. These typically manifest an effacement of the demarcation of cortical gray matter and underlying white matter (Fig. 4A). Microscopy discloses collections of atypical multinucleated astrocytes,

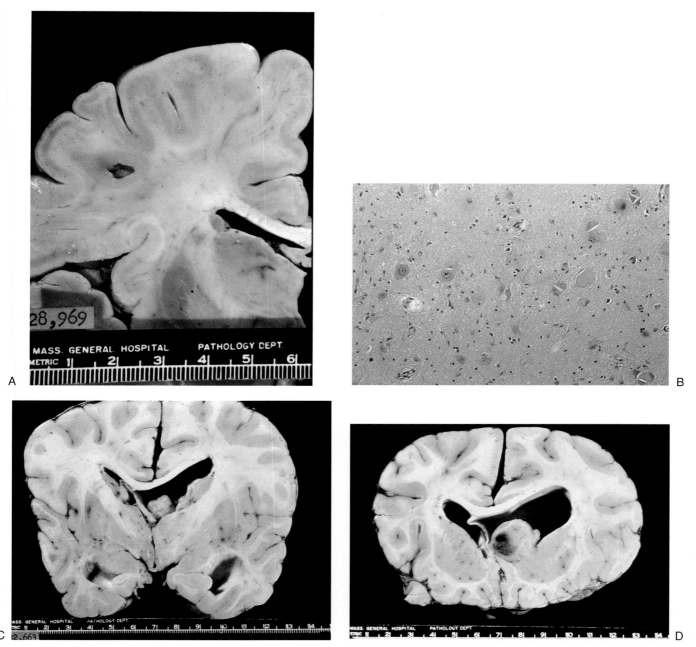

**FIG. 4.** Tuberous sclerosis. **A:** A cortical tuber appears grossly as an ill-defined grayish-white thickening of the cortical ribbon, as shown in this close view of a coronal brain slice in which a tuber occupies the lateral portion of the first frontal gyrus *(arrow)*. **B:** Within a tuber, the cortical architecture is lost, and the disorganized mass consists of a mixture of small neurons, small astrocytes, and large bizarre neuronal cells. (H&E, 63× original magnification.) (Photomicrograph courtesy of Dr. Gleb Budzilovich, NYU Medical Center.) **C:** "Candle gutterings" are heterotopic glioneuronal nodules lining the ventricular spaces, as seen in this gross photograph. **D:** Subependymal giant cell astrocytomas are probably true neoplasms that closely resemble candle gutterings except that they are much larger, grow progressively, and therefore can produce hydrocephalus, as they are characteristically found at the foramen of Monro. Here a large example projects into the right lateral ventricle.

equally bizarre neurons with haphazardly oriented processes, and cell types that are intermediate between these two (Fig. 4B). Heterotopic aggregates of similar cells may be found in the white matter. Additionally, nodules of abnormal neurons and astrocytes often develop along the walls of the ventricles in tuberous sclerosis ("candle gutterings"), particularly the lateral ventricles near the sulcus terminalis (Fig. 4C). These lesions often become heavily calcified. Electron microscopy of the atypical cells in "tuber" has shown both glial and neuronal characteristics, and immunocytochemical studies have demonstrated concomitant expression of GFAP and neurofilament proteins (22,23). True neoplasms may also develop from such lesions, characteristically near the foramen of Monro, and these are known as subependymal giant cell astrocytomas (Fig. 4D).

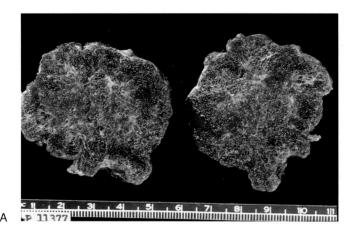

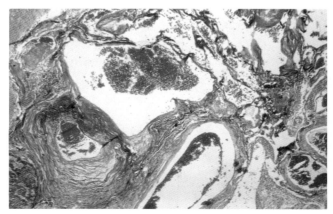

**FIG. 5.** Cavernous hemangioma. **A:** This gross specimen of a surgically resected intracranial dural-based lesion discloses the lobulated outer contour and the numerous vascular spaces on the cut surfaces. **B:** A histologic section of a temporal lobe intraparenchymal brain cavernous angioma reveals the fibrous blue-stained walls of the back-to-back vessels, with no intervening brain parenchyma; note the pink–red brain tissue at the edges). (Azocarmine stain, 12.5× original magnification.)

## Vascular Malformations

### Capillary Telangiectasia

An incidental finding at autopsy, capillary telangiectasias are ill-defined pink and occasionally stippled brown foci composed of thin-walled capillaries, the variable size of which is due to saccular and fusiform dilatations separated by neural tissue (24–27). More than 44% are supratentorial, usually in the cerebral cortex or white matter, and the remainder are infratentorial and most commonly arise in the pons (25). Hemorrhage and neurologic deficits are exceptional in the typical case of capillary telangiectasia. A rare, heavily calcified variant, so-called hemangioma calcificans, usually presents as an epileptogenic temporal lobe lesion (28).

### Cavernous Hemangioma

Cavernous "angiomas" account for approximately 5% of vascular malformations of the CNS (24–27,29). Most occur within the cerebral hemispheres, are up to 1–2 cm in diameter, and are subcortical. Occasionally the basal ganglia, brainstem, and third ventricle may be involved. Cavernous angiomas are rare in the dura, where they may simulate a meningioma.

These sharply demarcated masses have a dark red or purple lobulated surface. Sectioning discloses a sieve of irregular blood-filled spaces (Fig. 5A), with many being back-to-back. Others are separated by fibrous tissue (Fig. 5B). The vessels may be thickened, calcified, or occluded by thrombus. There is little intervening neural tissue (24–27).

Cavernous angiomas may be the source of spontaneous hemorrhage, sometimes repeatedly and occasionally fatally. Cortical examples are often associated with seizures.

### Arteriovenous Malformations Not Further Specified (AVMNOS)

Tangled serpentine coils of arteries and veins that represent idiopathic AVMNOS most commonly occur in the distribution of the middle cerebral artery (Fig. 6A) (24–27). They are A-V shunts with no intervening capillary beds. The largest of all vascular malformations, AVMs usually present during the second to third decades of life with hemorrhage or seizures. Bleeding from such lesions is rarely catastrophic but is frequently recurrent, and the overlying leptomeninges and surrounding brain are often discolored with hemosiderin. Sectioning discloses great variation in both the size of the vessels and the thickness of their walls (Fig. 6B, C). Large dilated draining veins are commonly part of these lesions. Thrombosis, with varying degrees of organization or recanalization, further widens the spectrum of changes in AVMNOS, and spontaneous disappearance of the lesion in imaging studies has been reported (30,31). Microscopically,

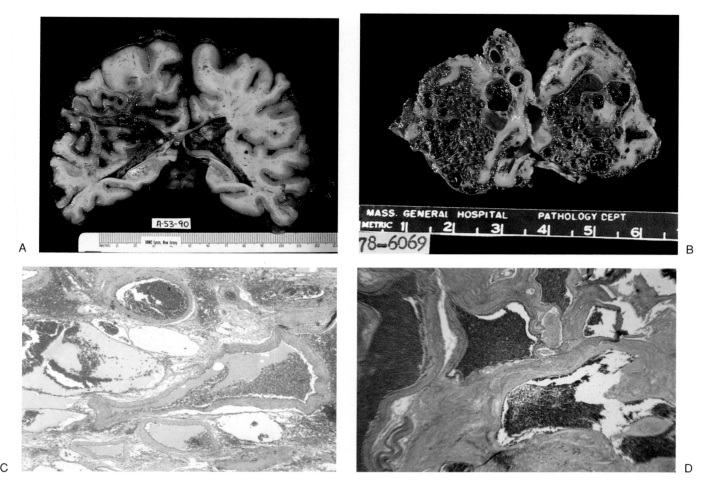

**FIG. 6.** Arteriovenous malformation (AVM). **A:** A coronal slice of brain from a male patient with a large left hemisphere AVM. The lesion, which was associated with a seizure disorder, had been operated on and had undergone therapeutic embolization as well as radiation therapy. At autopsy, the large recurrent lesion is characterized by large irregular vascular channels extending from the pial surfaces both laterally (on the convexity) and medially into the deep white matter. The brain tissue around the vessels of the lesion has brown discoloration from iron pigments left by old hemorrhages and is somewhat degenerate as well. **B:** A surgically resected AVM demonstrates the great variability in the size of the lesion's vascular channels. **C:** Histologically, the AVM contains large thick-walled arterial vessels, complete with smooth muscles, and thinner but often fibrotic veins, with no intervening capillary bed. While some channels are back-to-back, as in cavernous angiomas, many are separated by small portions of gliotic brain tissue. (H&E, 5× original magnification.) **D:** A stain for elastic tissue in a surgically resected AVM demonstrates the continuous serpentine elastic lamina (black surrounding an arterial portion of the lesion, and the lack of any elastic lamina in the adjacent venous channels). (Voerhoff–Van Giesen, 12× original magnification.)

there may be irregular subintimal proliferation of fibrous tissue in AVMNOS. The elastica may be discontinuous or reduplicated (Fig. 6D), and the media are either attenuated or greatly hypertrophied. Calcification and atheroma formation add to the varied histology of this lesion. The vessels are surrounded to varying degrees by gliotic neural tissues often with macrophages containing lipid debris or heme pigment. The gliosis may be sufficiently cellular with atypia or with numerous Rosenthal fibers and eosinophilic granular bodies as to be mistaken for astrocytic neoplasia. Many reports of angioglioma in fact represent misdiagnosed gliosis in asso-

ciation with an AVM. Alternatively, some true neoplasms contain clusters of abnormal vessels simulating AVM or cavernous angioma. One may also see patchy, perivascular infiltrates of lymphocytes in AVMNOS.

### Meningioangiomatosis

Patients with the rare benign lesion termed "meningioangiomatosis" usually present in the second and third decades of life with seizures or headaches. Nearly half of all reported

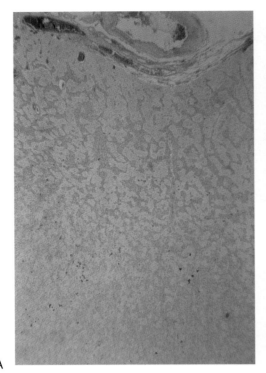

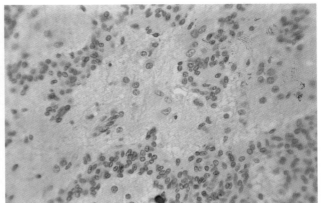

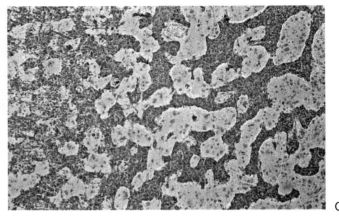

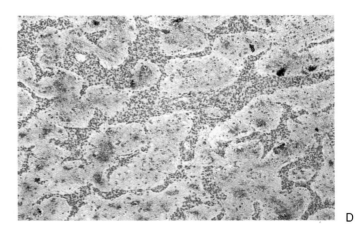

**FIG. 7.** Meningioangiomatosis. **A:** The lesion characteristically consists of cells proliferating along blood vessels penetrating the brain from the surface. (LHE, 6× original magnification.) **B:** A close view of the deep portion of the lesion shows the round and spindly cells filling the perivascular spaces, with intervening gliotic brain tissue containing some residual blue-stained myelinated fibers. (LHE, 100× original magnification.) **C:** The nature of the proliferating cells is less than clear; characteristically, they have strong immunoreactivity for S-100 protein, as shown here, which is not characteristic of meningothelial cells. Anti-S-100 immunoperoxidase [avidin–biotin complex (ABC method) with diaminobenzidine (DAB) for final localization, counterstained with hematoxylin, 25× original magnification]. **D:** The gliosis of the intervening brain tissue is demonstrated here by an immunoperoxidase stain for glial fibrillary acidic protein (GFAP; note that the tumor cells have no immunoreactivity. [Anti-GFAP immunoperoxidase (PAP, DAB), counterstained with hematoxylin, 25× original magnification.]

cases have occurred in patients with neurofibromatosis (32,33). Probably malformative in nature, this lesion involves the cerebral cortex and frequently the overlying meninges, as well as forming firm, well-demarcated gray–tan plaques that are composed of small blood vessels cuffed by fibroblasts and cells resembling meningothelial cells (Fig. 7). Scattered psammoma bodies and sparsely admixed lymphocytes may be present in meningioangiomatosis. At presentation, the diagnosis of a tumor usually follows the detection of a focal mass by radiographic imaging. Proper interpretation depends solely on pathologic examination of the excised lesion. The true nature of the cells in these lesions remains uncertain; the cases in which the cells are meningothelial-like may express epithelial membrane antigen (EMA), which is usually found in normal arachnoidal cells and in meningiomas, but those in which the cells are more fibroblastic do not (33). Meningioangiomatosis often has neurons with neurofibrillary tangles in the abnormal islands of cortex (32).

# CYSTS

## Nonneural Epithelial Cysts

### *Epidermoid Cysts*

Putatively derived from ectodermal elements that are trapped within the developing CNS, epidermoid cysts are most common within the cerebellopontine angle, but they are also found in the parapituitary region and adjacent temporal lobe, the fourth ventricle, and the spinal canal (34–38). The lateral and third ventricles, as well as the interhemispheric fissure, have also been recorded as sites of origin for these lesions (Fig. 8A). The smooth bosselated surfaces of epidermoid cysts are typically pearly gray, and the lumen is filled with grumous, soft white material (keratin) or, on oc-

casion, thick dark brown fluid. The lining of these lesions is simple stratified squamous epithelium (Fig. 8B) identical to that of follicular keratinous cysts of soft tissues.

Forty-eight cases of intramedullary spinal epidermoid cysts have been documented (37). The affected patients ranged from 3 to 71 years of age (average 34). Two thirds of them had cysts in the thoracic region; the remaining lesions involved the lumbar region and the conus medullaris.

Leakage of the contents from epidermoid cysts may elicit a severe chemical meningitis (39–41). Malignant transformation of previously benign epidermoid cysts is rare, but this complication is well recognized in the literature (35). Epidermoid cysts themselves are not usually defined as neoplastic, in contrast to the rather similar "dermoid" cysts (Fig. 8C). The latter lesions are more rare than epidermoid cysts in the cranial cavity, but they outnumber epidermoid cysts in

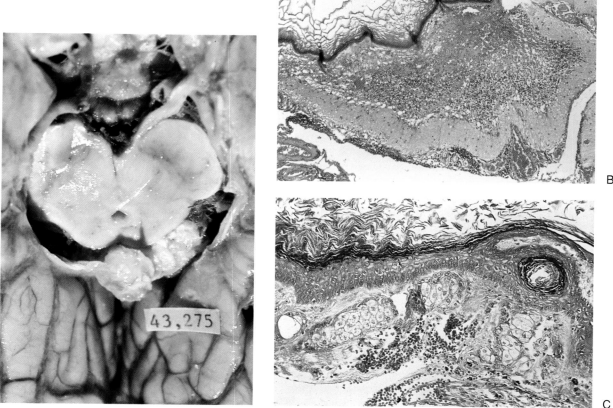

**FIG. 8.** Epidermoid and dermoid cysts. **A:** A pineal region epidermoid cyst, discovered incidentally at autopsy, is seen here in a view of the base of the brain (with the stem and cerebellum removed just above and behind the quadrigeminal plate). **B:** Histologically, an epidermoid cyst (such as this cerebellar example) consists of a thin fibrous wall, and a stratified squamous epithelium with "basket-weave" keratin desquamating off into the cyst lumen. There are no other elements in the wall. These cysts are histologically identical to follicular cysts of the epidermis and can include a granular layer just as follicular cysts do. Here the cyst rests directly on a cerebellar folium; the densely packed small round nuclei are neurons of the cerebellar cortex granular layer. (H&E, 25× original magnification.) **C:** The histologic appearance of a dermoid cyst includes most of the elements of the epidermoid cyst but has additional elements, notably sebaceous glands with cells with pale cytoplasm and hair follicles. (H&E, 25× original magnification.)

the spinal canal. Most intracranial dermoid cysts become manifest during childhood and typically involve the cerebellar vermis or fourth ventricle; they only rarely arise in the pineal region. Congenital subgaleal dermoid cysts typically involve the anterior fontanel (34–36). Most spinal dermoids are lumbosacral and may be either intramedullary or extramedullary. In both the lumbar region and the occiput, a dermal sinus in the skin may overlie the cyst within the nervous system and serve as a route for meningeal infection.

The circumscribed masses representing dermoids, which may be focally calcified, are usually filled with friable yellow material (keratin plus sebaceous secretions) and varying quantities of hair. In addition to stratified squamous epithelium, microscopic examination typically discloses hair follicles, sebaceous glands, and sweat glands in these lesions as with mature cystic teratomas of other body sites (Fig. 8C). There may also be arrector pili muscle bundles, and occasional examples also include other elements such as nodules of cartilage. As with true epidermoid cysts, leakage of contents from a dermoid cyst may produce striking meningitis. Malignant transformation is rare.

### Rathke's Cleft Cyst

Rathke's pouch may persist as a space between the adenohypophysis and neurohypophysis that is lined by cuboidal or columnar epithelium. The latter is sometimes ciliated or may contain goblet cells (Fig. 9) (42,43). Occasionally, symptomatic Rathke's cleft cysts may fill the sella turcica, flattening the pituitary; they may also extend into the suprasellar space. Some reported examples have been exclusively suprasellar. The cysts may be partially devoid of epithelium or they may contain foci of squamous metaplasia. Elements resembling those of typical Rathke's cleft cysts may also be found as part of a craniopharyngioma, i.e., in true neoplasms.

### Endodermal Type Cysts

#### Spinal Neurenteric Cysts

Found typically in the cervical and upper thoracic regions (Fig. 10A), but sometimes at lumbar levels, neurenteric cysts are lined by mucinous columnar epithelium, occasionally showing ciliated or squamous metaplasia (Fig. 10B). Individual examples of such cysts may be connected with a mediastinal endodermal cyst or a gastrointestinal tract duplication through a vertebral defect, which is sometimes located at a level caudal to that of the cyst proper (44–46).

#### Intracranial Neurenteric Cysts

Malcolm et al. reviewed 13 published cases of intracranial neurenteric cysts (47). Patients with those lesions ranged between <1 month and 66 years old (average 32); 10 were women. The cysts occurred in the posterior fossa anterior to the brainstem. No abnormalities of the adjacent bone were present.

### Neuroepithelial Cysts

#### Colloid Cysts of the Third Ventricle

Typically presenting in patients between 20 and 50 years of age, sometimes with sudden death, colloid cysts of the third ventricle constitute 0.5% of all cerebral "tumors" (47–52). These smooth, spherical masses range from 0.3 to 4

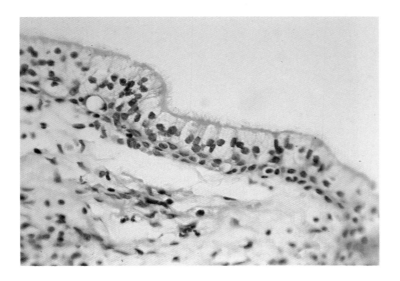

**FIG. 9.** Rathke's cleft cyst. These sellar and suprasellar cysts are lined by a single layer of cuboidal to low columnar epithelial cells. The cells sometimes have prominent ciliated apical surfaces, producing a brush border. (H&E, 100× original magnification.)

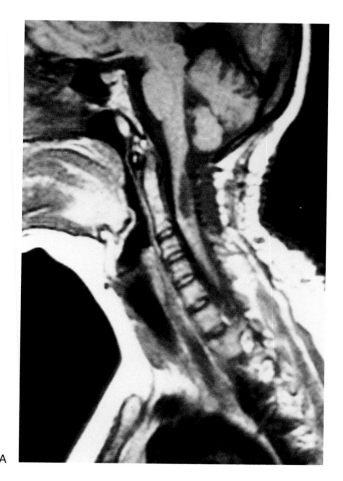

A

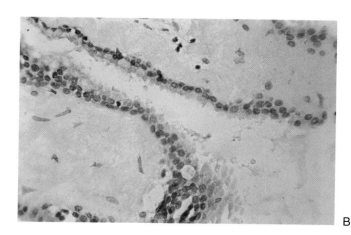

B

**FIG. 10.** Spinal neurenteric cyst. **A:** Sagittal T1-weighted MRI scan revealing a cyst in the upper cervical spinal cord. **B:** Histologic examination of such a cyst reveals a lining of pseudostratified cuboidal cells with a ciliated brush border at the surface, i.e., a respiratory-type epithelium. (H&E, 100× original magnification.)

cm in diameter and are situated in the anterior third ventricle abutting the columns of the fornix, strategically positioned to obstruct the foramen of Monro (Fig. 11A). The thin fibrous connective tissue capsules of colloid cysts are lined by a single layer of cuboidal to columnar cells, which are frequently ciliated or mucinous in nature (Fig. 11B). The translucent or turbid contents of these lesions—representing the product of secretion and desquamation of the lining cells—are often amorphous but may contain precipitates of phospholipids and nucleoproteins that form filamentous aggregates. These may simulate colonies of *Actinomyces* microscopically (Fig. 11C) (52).

The histogenesis of colloid cysts continues to be debated, with the paraphysis (a diverticulum of the telencephalon arising in early embryonic life), diencephalic ependyma, choroid plexus, and ectopic respiratory epithelium (i.e., neurenteric elements) having been suggested as possible tissues of origin (48,51).

### Neuroepithelial Cysts of the Lateral Ventricles

Eight cases of symptomatic neuroepithelial cysts of the choroid plexus have been reported. All arose in the lateral ventricles and six were located in the trigone (53,54). These lesions were lined by a single layer of cuboidal or columnar epithelium, and they were filled with clear liquid resembling cerebrospinal fluid.

### Neuroepithelial Cysts of the Fourth Ventricle

Neuroepithelial cysts of the fourth ventricle are rare. They appear to develop from choroid plexus epithelium (55–57). The lesions are lined by a mixture of cuboidal epithelium and ciliated cells, and they lack the goblet cells that are often found in colloid cysts of the third ventricle. Fourth ventricular cysts must be distinguished from those of cysticercosis. The latter are more common and are characterized by a triple-layered wall consisting of a cuticle, musculature, and radial tegmental cells, with scattered calcareous corpuscles. The protoscolex of the parasite is diagnostic but it may be absent in a sterile cyst, which is the form most frequently encountered in the brain (58).

### Extraventricular Ependymal Cysts

Ependymal cysts lined by a single layer of ciliated, usually columnar cells have been recorded within the cerebral hemi-

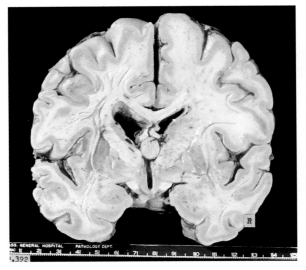

A

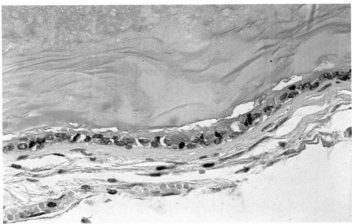

B

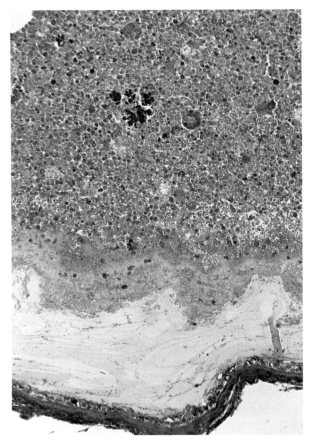

C

FIG. 11. Colloid cyst. **A:** This coronal brain slice reveals a typical 1.0- to 1.5-cm diameter colloid cyst lying between the columns of the fornix at the apex of the third ventricle. This was an incidental finding at autopsy in this case. **B:** Histologic examination reveals that the cyst contains a mucin-like colloid content, within a lining composed of a single layer of cuboidal epithelial cells resting on a thin outer fibrous capsule. (Mucicarmine, 100× original magnification.) **C:** The colloid content, while usually appearing smooth and amorphous in H&E and mucicarmine, can be somewhat granular and may contain precipitates that closely mimic the "sulfur granules" in *Actinomyces* infections. (Phosphotungstic acid-hematoxylin, 100× original magnification.)

spheres and in the subarachnoid space over the cerebral convexities, the cerebellum ("glial-ependymal cysts"), and the spinal leptomeninges (59–69). Thirty-four reported patients with intracranial cysts were between 9 and 73 years old (average 40), although this type of cyst is also recognized in infants (see "Arachnoid Cysts"). Large interhemispheric ependymal cysts, some of which may communicate with the lumina of the ventricles, are often associated with agenesis of the corpus callosum and are usually seen in childhood.

### Pineal Cysts

Small cysts within the pineal gland lined by glia and filled with gelatinous material are commonly encountered as incidental findings at autopsy (Fig. 12A). Occasionally, however, they may be symptomatic (70–72). In the reported cases that have been associated with clinical abnormalities the patients ranged in age from 5 to 56 years (average 28); two thirds were women. Some had a long clinical history of

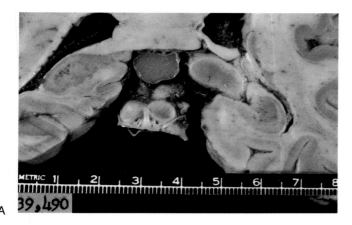

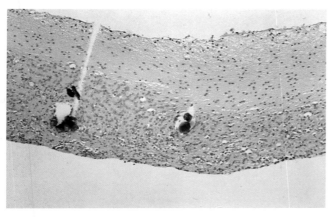

**FIG. 12.** Pineal cyst. **A:** Most pineal cysts are asymptomatic and are discovered only by neuroimaging or incidentally at autopsy, as was the one depicted in this coronal brain slice. The cyst content is typically gelatinous. **B:** The rare symptomatic examples may be surgically resected. Here one such cyst is seen to be lined by astrocytic tissue, which is sharply demarcated from the more cellular residual compressed pineal tissue. (H&E, 25× original magnification.)

visual disturbances, hydrocephalus, or hypothalamic syndromes; almost all had headaches. Pineal cysts range from 1 to 2 cm in maximum diameter are filled with a gelatinous, clear fluid; they are lined by fibrillary astrocytes (Fig. 12B).

### Nonepithelial-lined Cysts

Five intraparenchymal cysts in the cerebral hemispheres and 14 in the cerebellum have been reported to lack an epithelial lining (73,74). These lesions were lined by astrocytes, sometimes with numerous Rosenthal fibers, and they occurred in patients in the fifth to seventh decades of life. The histogenesis of such cysts is speculative. Those in the cerebral hemispheres may arise from buds of the ependymal lining of the ventricles with subsequent destruction of the lining or possibly by rupture of the ependyma with dissection of CSF into the brain. It has been suggested that some

nonepithelial cysts of the cerebellum may represent spontaneous involution of a juvenile pilocytic astrocytoma.

### Cavum Septi Pellucidi et Vergae

Between the two membranous leaves of the developing septum pellucidum there is a space, the cavum septi pellucidi, that is lined by ependyma-like cells (75). Present in 97% of infants, this space usually closes rapidly after 2 months, but it may persist in some individuals into adulthood (Fig. 13) (75–80). The resulting cysts are typically incidental discoveries on imaging studies done for other reasons or are found at autopsy. A second space, the cavum vergae, may occur between the splenium of the corpus callosum and the commissure of the fornix, forming a separate cavity or a single space that is in continuity with the cavum septi pellucidi (75,76). Symptomatic cases have been reported in two boys and a girl, ages 2–8, wherein the lesions were successfully treated by placement of shunts (77–79). The cavum veli interpositi, a diverticulum of the subarachnoid space above the third ventricle, may also become enlarged in association with malformations of the adjacent brain.

### Meningeal Cysts

#### Arachnoid Cysts

Intracranial arachnoid cysts are often asymptomatic, but occasionally they produce acutely or chronically increased intracranial pressure (81–84). Usually, these lesions are filled with clear, colorless liquid resembling cerebrospinal fluid. Electron microscopy has demonstrated the splitting of

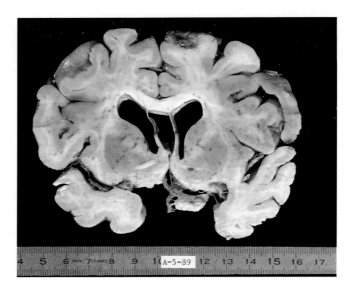

**FIG. 13.** Cavum septi pellucidi. This large example extended the full extent of the septum pellucidum from just behind the genu of the corpus callosum to just in front of its splenium. The cyst contains clear fluid, presumably cerebrospinal fluid.

the arachnoid to enclose the lumina of arachnoid cysts, with the pia remaining separate and intact. Rengachary and Watanabe found that of 208 reported cases, 103 (49%) arose in the Sylvian fissure, 21 (10%) were found in the quadrigeminal cistern, 22 (11%) in the cerebellopontine angle, 19 (9%) in the vermis, 18 (9%) in the sellar region, 10 (5%) in the interhemispheric fissure, 9 (4%) over the cerebral convexities, and 6 (3%) over the clivus (84). Intraventricular arachnoid cysts likewise have been documented (85).

### Glial-Ependymal Cysts

As already alluded to, some clinically diagnosed arachnoid cysts are found histologically to represent a composite of delicate glial fibrillary tissue and a single layer of cuboidal ependymal cells (Fig. 14). These lesions may be discovered in infants, sometimes as a cause of symptomatically raised intracranial pressure, or in older children or adults as an incidental finding (86).

### Miscellaneous Intra-/Paraspinal Cysts

#### Extradural Spinal Meningeal Cysts (Arachnoid Diverticula)

Extradural meningeal cysts may appear at any age and typically involve the thoracic spinal levels. Average patient age at diagnosis is 33 years. Less often, the lesions may occur in the lumbar regions (average age 56) (87–90). These cysts arise from herniation of arachnoid through a congenital defect in the dura in the midline or along the dural sleeve of the nerve roots. In approximately 50% of cases, a communication with the subarachnoid space can be demonstrated.

#### Perineurial Cysts

Most symptomatic perineurial cysts arise on the sacral nerve roots and rarely affect other nerves at other spinal lev-

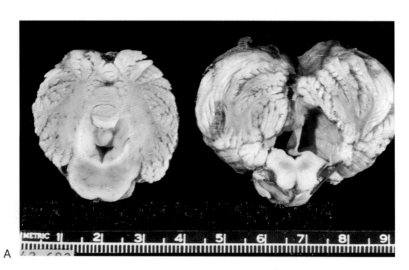

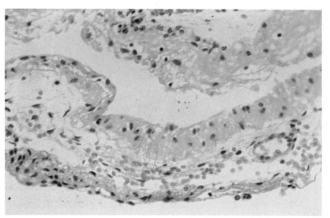

**FIG. 14.** Glial-ependymal cyst. **A:** These cysts, as stated in the text, are grossly and clinically not separable from arachnoid cysts. Here a newborn full-term infant was found incidentally at autopsy to have a cyst apparently in the leptomeninges of the medial surface of the right cerebellar hemisphere (viewed in the photograph from below). **B:** A histologic specimen from a surgically resected "arachnoid cyst" shows that the (now collapsed) lining is composed of thin layers of finely fibrillar eosinophilic tissue, i.e., glial tissue, with an attenuated flattened cuboidal epithelium facing the cyst lumen—ependyma. (H&E, 100× original magnification.)

els (90,91). Patients with these lesions are between 30 and 80 years of age and present with pain or paresthesia. Some individuals have reported antecedent trauma. Bony erosion may be present radiographically. The cysts occur along the nerve roots at or distal to the dorsal root ganglion; they are sometimes multiple and may be as large as 3 cm in diameter. Perineurial cyst may arise between the pia and the perineurium, and their walls contain axons and sometimes ganglion cells.

### Spinal Juxtaarticular Facet Cysts

Clinically apparent cysts developing from the synovium-lined capsules of the vertebral facet joints in the spinal canal are well documented in the literature, but the terminology used to describe them is inconsistent (92–99). The terms "synovial cyst" and "ganglion cyst" are used interchangeably by some authors, but these two entities are distinguished by other observers. A synovial cyst is lined by synovium and is filled with clear, xanthochromic, or bloody fluid, in contrast with the ganglion cyst, which has no lining (Fig. 15) and is filled with gelatinous material. Most patients with generic cysts of this type are in the fifth to seventh decades, and the lower lumbar region is the site that is most commonly affected. The cysts are in continuity with the articular facets and impinge on the lumbar ligamentum flavum. Nine reported cases occurred at the L3–4 level.

### Ligamentum Flavum Cysts

Abdullah et al. and Vernet et al. reported a total of 10 cases of clinically evident cysts that developed in the ligamentum flavum in patients who were between the ages of 43 and 72 (average 55) (100,101). These cysts arose from, and were partially embedded within, the ligamentum flavum, in contrast to cysts of the articular facets. The walls of ligamentum flavum cysts are composed of dense fibrous connective tissue, and these lesions may develop subsequent to myxoid changes in the ligament, along with liquefaction or necrosis.

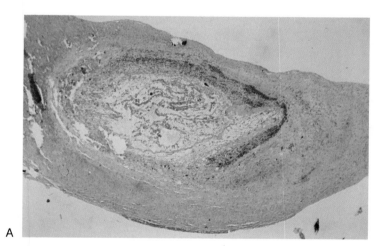

A

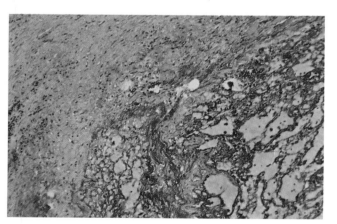

B

**FIG. 15.** Spinal juxtaarticular facet cyst. **A:** This example is of the "ganglion cyst" type, i.e., it is a cyst enclosed by a collagenous capsule without any epithelial or synovial lining. (H&E, 2.5× original magnification.) **B:** At higher power, the loose lamellar arrangements of connective tissue without any lining cells, surrounding a mucinous or gelatinous content, is more apparent. (Movat's Pentachrome stain, 100× original magnification.)

## INFLAMMATORY AND NECROTIZING MASS LESIONS OF THE CNS PARENCHYMA

### Demyelinating Disease

#### Multiple Sclerosis

Multiple sclerosis (MS) and other demyelinating syndromes usually do not present as pseudotumorous lesions. However, there are well-documented instances in which single or multiple mass lesions when biopsied were shown to represent a demyelinating process and not a neoplastic one (102–104). In two recent series, there were a total of 48 patients between 8 and 72 years old (average 39) who presented with symptoms and imaging data mimicking those of a brain or spinal cord tumor (Fig. 16A). In some patients the

lesions occurred at sites other than those usually associated with MS and lacked the characteristic progression or recurrences of typical MS. Therefore, they may have been other forms of demyelinating disease (104). When they are intensely inflammatory, these lesions may simulate primary CNS lymphoma microscopically (Fig. 16B); in contrast, more gliotic lesions can be confused with high-grade astrocytomas. The hypercellularity imparted by an admixture of histiocytes and reactive astrocytes in the active demyelinating lesions, the presence of pleomorphic reactive astrocytes (such as multinucleated Creuztfeldt astrocytes), and the observation of mitotic figures may lead to the misinterpretation as high-grade glioma (Fig. 16C). An aqueous-mounted frozen section may provide a clue to the correct diagnosis. Brightly refractile droplets of lipid in the lesional histiocytes

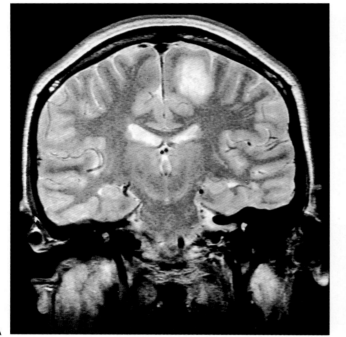

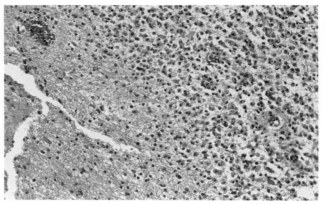

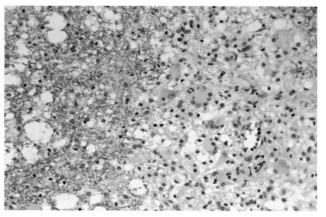

**FIG. 16.** Tumefactive multiple sclerosis or other demyelinating syndrome. **A:** A T2-weighted coronal MRI scan reveals a bright mass lesion in the white matter of the first frontal gyrus and adjacent anterior parietal lobe. This was operated on as a presumptive glioma but was histologically a demyelinating lesion. **B:** Some active and inflamed demyelinating lesions, at biopsy, are no cellular that they mimic and can be misdiagnosed as primary CNS non-Hodgkin's lymphoma. Of note here is the relatively sharp border between the hypercellular lesion and the adjacent brain. A close inspection (or cell marker immunohistochemistry) reveals that some of the cells are not lymphocytes but macrophages, and that the infiltrate is a mixture of B and T cells with no monoclonal population. (H&E, 50× original magnification.) **C:** More chronic examples can mimic astrocytomas. Here, at the border of the lesion, there are highly pleomorphic astrocytes, including a multinucleated example. Clues to the correct diagnosis are the sharp edge against well-myelinated white matter and the presence in the lesion of numerous macrophages, some of which retain blue-stained LFB-positive myelin debris. (LHE, 100× original magnification.)

help to identify the latter population of cells in demyelinating plaques. Demonstration of demyelination with relative sparing of axons is the ultimate diagnostic feature (103).

### Progressive Multifocal Leukoencephalopathy

Once seen most often as a terminal complication of lymphoproliferative diseases or therapeutic immunosuppression, progressive multifocal leukoencephalopathy (PML) is an opportunistic CNS infection produced by the JC virus and now is encountered frequently in neurosurgical specimens in patients with AIDS (105–107). The radiologic characteristics of the lesions, which are usually multiple and restricted to white matter, and do not produce mass effects, often suggest the diagnosis (107).

The lesions consist of relatively small (2–5 mm) discrete foci that may enlarge and coalesce (Fig. 17A, B). Microscopically, myelin sheaths are destroyed but axons are rela-

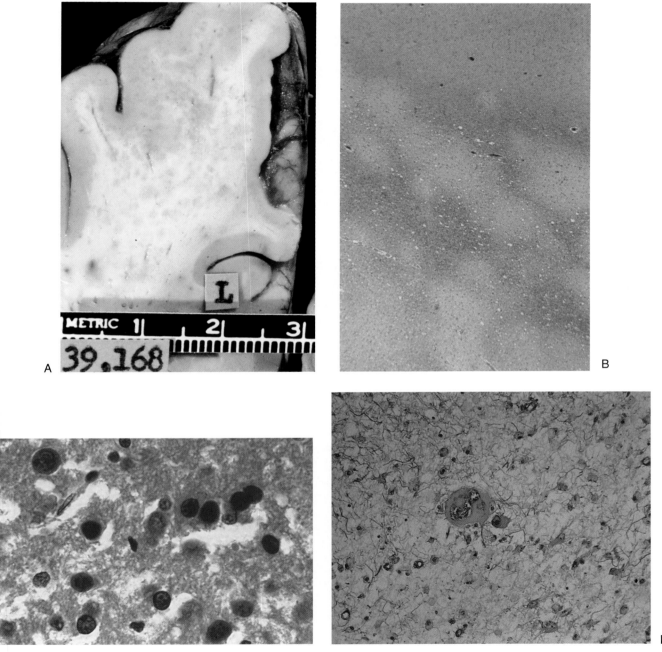

**FIG. 17.** Progressive multifocal leukoencephalopathy. **A:** Section through the cerebral hemisphere shows numerous small lesions in the white matter. **B:** Multiple, coalescing foci of myelin are present in the subcortical white matter. (LHE, 25× original magnification.) **C:** At the periphery of the lesion, enlarged hyperchromatic and homogeneous oligodendrocyte nuclei. (HE, 400× original magnification.) **D:** Giant, pleomorphic astrocytes are found in the majority of cases. (HE, 400× original magnification.)

tively spared. A characteristic feature is the alteration of the oligodendrocytes at the periphery of the lesions: the virus-filled nuclei are enlarged and the normal chromatin pattern is effaced (Fig. 17C). In most cases, abnormally hypertrophied astrocytes with pleomorphic nuclei are present (Fig. 17D) (105–107). The intermingling of astrocytes and macrophages and altered oligodendrocytes distinguishes PML from a neoplasm.

**Inflammatory and Lymphoproliferative Processes**

*Inflammatory Pseudotumors*

No fewer than 34 cases have been described of intradural masses with varying proportions of lymphoid cells, plasma cells, and fibrous connective tissue in the cerebral parenchyma. They were attached to the dura (including the falx and tentorium) or the choroid plexus (108–130). Some "inflammatory pseudotumors" are largely composed of lymphoid cells and as such resemble either low-grade follicular lymphoma, Castleman's disease (angiofollicular [giant] lymph node hyperplasia), or related entities (128–130). Others are largely sclerotic, simulating focal pachymeningitis (120–123). Approximately one third have been associated with systemic multifocal fibrosclerosis or multiple "tumefactive fibroinflammatory lesions." This group of disorders includes mediastinal fibrosis, retroperitoneal fibrosis, sclerosing cholangitis, Riedel's thyroiditis, orbital pseudotumors, and fibroinflammatory soft tissue masses (124–127).

*Plasma Cell Granuloma (Hyalinizing Granuloma)*

Sixteen mass lesions composed of inflammatory cells and connective tissue (sometimes clinically mimicking meningioma) have been reported in patients between the ages of 11 and 80 years (average 36) (108–119). Sites of origin have included the frontal convexity, the sella turcica and floor of the anterior fossa, the tentorium, falx, and glomus of the choroid plexus, the cervical spinal meninges, the hypothalamus, and the fourth ventricle. These plasma cell granulomas are circumscribed, firm masses that usually consist of a polyclonal mixture of T and B lymphocytes, plasma cells, and histiocytes, with varying numbers of fibroblasts and collagen fibers.

This variant of "inflammatory pseudotumors" must be distinguished from histologic variants of meningioma that exhibit extensive tumoral infiltration by inflammatory cells (131,132). Some of the latter, such as "chordoid" meningioma, have also been associated with systemic illness, including fever or anemia (131).

*Castleman's Disease*

Five intracranial masses resembling Castleman's disease (angiofollicular lymph node hyperplasia) have been docu-

mented (Fig. 17) (128–130). Three cases were of the hyaline vascular type; these occurred in the right parietal meninges of a 28-year-old man and an 82-year-old woman, and in the right frontal meninges of a 63-year-old woman. One case of the plasma cell type arose in the left occipital meninges in a 63-year-old woman. Another lesion showed histologic features of both variants and involved the posterior fossa dura in a 30-year-old woman.

*Multifocal Fibrosclerosis*

Twelve patients between the ages of 16 and 71 years (average 48) have been described with orbital or multifocal fibrosclerosis and fibroinflammatory intracranial mass lesions (124–127). Nine had concurrent orbital pseudotumors, two had retroperitoneal fibrosis, and one had mediastinal fibrosis.

*Intracerebral Lymphoid Masses of Undetermined Nature*

Primary CNS lymphoma is virtually always high grade histologically. However, a few examples of allegedly low-grade small lymphocytic lymphoma have been described in this context. We have encountered eight similar lesions in which the neoplastic character of the infiltrate was uncertain. Each case concerned a single tumor-like focus (Fig. 18A) composed of small lymphocytes that infiltrated the brain (Fig. 18B). In all but two examples there was a long survival after no therapy other than surgery and the use of perioperative steroids.

**Sinus Histiocytosis with Massive Lymphadenopathy (SHML) (Rosai–Dorfman Disease)**

Patients usually present with SHML at a median age of 20 years with massive cervical lymphadenopathy (more than 87% of cases) (133–135). In the lymph nodes, the sinusoids are distended by aggregates of large histiocytes and smaller numbers of lymphocytes, plasma cells, and neutrophils. The nonhistiocytic cells are observed both free in the sinusoids and within the cytoplasm of the histiocytes. Rosai–Dorfman disease is not restricted to lymph nodes, and at least one extranodal site of involvement has been found in 43% of cases. These include the skin, upper respiratory tract, and bones (135). Only 50% of patients with CNS involvement, however, have nodal disease. The most common locations for SHML in the nervous system are the spinal or cranial epidural space or dura, sometimes with infiltration of the overlying bone (Fig. 19A, B). The optic nerve, cerebellar vermis, and suprasellar space have also been affected. Two thirds of SHML patients with CNS disease have additional extranodal involvement, most often in the bones or salivary glands (135). Extralymphatic lesions, including those in the cra-

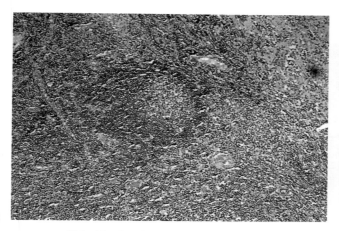
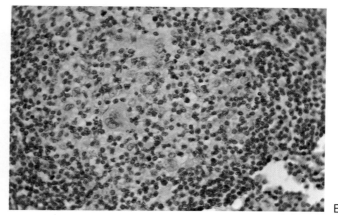

**FIG. 18.** Castleman's disease. This intracranial dura-based mass clinically, radiographically, and surgically resembled a meningioma. **A:** Histologically, however, it is a lymphoid mass with well-formed follicles. (H&E, 25× original magnification.) **B:** At higher power, the follicle center contains some hyperplastic and hyalinized blood vessels; these were also present in some interfollicular zones. (H&E, 100× original magnification.)

nium, consist of masses of histiocytes with glassy eosinophilic cytoplasm and intracellular lymphocytes, as well as intervening zones filled with lymphocytes and plasma cells (Fig. 20).

### Rheumatoid Arthritis

Dural rheumatoid nodules composed of necrobiotic collagen and palisading histiocytes have been observed over the cerebral convexities and in the clivus (Fig. 21) (136–138). In addition, cervical myelopathy caused by subluxation of the first cervical vertebra has been reported in patients with longstanding rheumatoid disease (136). In florid examples of rheumatoid granulomas, groups of lesional histiocytes may be mistaken for neoplastic elements. However, the low-power microscopic image of the process is usually sufficient to suggest the correct diagnosis.

### Sarcoidosis

In roughly 5% of cases, sarcoidosis involves the CNS, where it usually affects the cranial nerves, meninges, or hy-

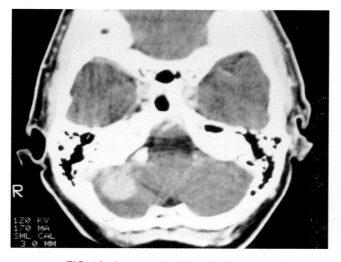
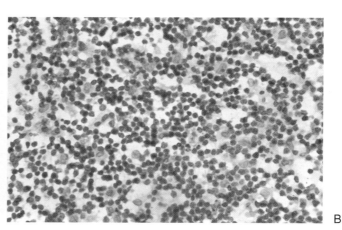

**FIG. 19.** Intracerebral lymphoid masses of undetermined nature. **A:** A CT scan in this previously healthy 68-year-old woman who presented with headache and ataxia showed a solitary right cerebellar hemisphere mass. This was resected. **B:** The histologic examination revealed a sheet of small, reactive-appearing lymphocytes with scattered macrophages and a background gliosis. Immunophenotype studies revealed that most of the cells were T lymphocytes.

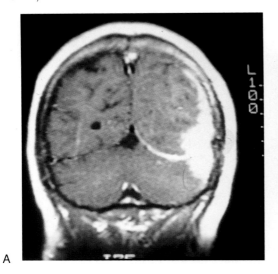

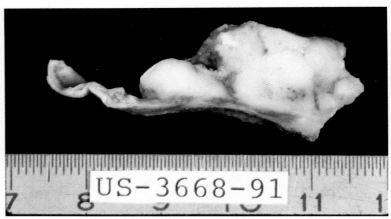

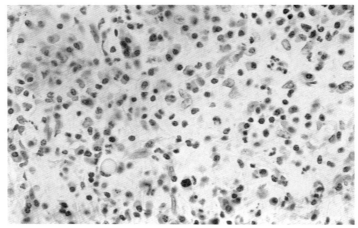

**FIG. 20.** Rosai–Dorfman disease. **A:** A coronal T1-weighted MRI scan in this previously healthy 69-year-old woman with a diagnosis of "tentorial meningioma" shows the full extent of a large dural-based mass with supratentorial, infratentorial, and transtentorial components. **B:** When resected, the specimen showed a close attachment to the dura and was composed of a firm, fleshy lobulated tissue. **C:** Histologic examination revealed no meningiomatous tissue but only fibrous tissue with sheets of histiocytes (some showing emperipolesis of lymphocytes) and zones with many plasma cells and some lymphocytes, as seen here. (H&E, 100× original magnification.)

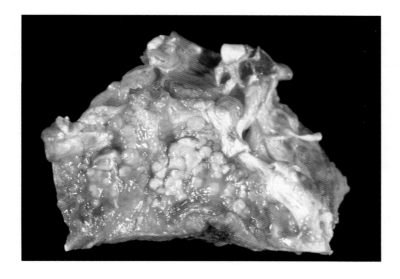

**FIG. 21.** Rheumatoid nodule. This example was a mass projecting back from the clivus, impinging on the ventral pons and medulla. (Courtesy of Dr. William C. Schoene, Boston, MA.)

pothalamus. Occasionally, the lesions form intracranial masses (140). The patients range in age from 13 to 72 years (average 32), and only 60% are known to have systemic sarcoidosis. Thus, isolated CNS sarcoidosis is well recognized. CNS lesions of the nervous system may be the initial presenting manifestation of subsequent widespread disease. In patients with intracranial sarcoidal lesions, 85% of the masses involve the cerebral hemispheres, and headaches or seizures are the most common presenting symptoms. Microscopy discloses characteristic noncaseating granulomas (Fig. 22), which, again, may be so floridly cellular that concern over a neoplasm is engendered.

## Xanthogranulomas

### Xanthogranulomas of the Choroid Plexus

Choroid plexus xanthogranulomas (XGs) are usually incidental findings in 1.6–7% of autopsies, typically in older individuals. Twenty-six cases of symptomatic XG have been described, 5 in children (141–148). Twelve cases involved the lateral ventricles and 14 cases involved the third ventricle. Of the 5 children, 4 had large, bilateral masses; the largest was an 8 × 3 × 2.5-cm, 30-g lesion. The lesions vary from gray–white flecked with yellow to diffusely yellow–tan. Microscopy typically discloses foamy macrophages, lymphocytes, plasma cells, acicular clefts of cholesterol, and multinucleate giant cells (Fig. 23).

A putative origin for XGs is desquamated choroid epithelial cells that have become trapped with the stroma, and degenerate, accumulating lipid within their cytoplasm (145). Disintegration of the cells releases the accumulated lipid, eliciting an inflammatory reaction. Three cases of XG arising in association with neuroepithelial cysts have been reported (149–151). We have seen one case (shown to us by Dr. Marius Valsamis) that clinically mimicked a colloid cyst.

### Weber–Christian Disease

Rarely, Weber–Christian disease (relapsing febrile, nodular, nonsuppurative panniculitis) may involve the dura, with lesions composed of foamy macrophages, inflammatory cells, and fibrosis (152).

### Cholesterol Granuloma of the Petrous Apex

Cholesterol granuloma is possibly the result of obstruction of the petrous apex air cells by hemorrhage; it is a cystic lesion filled with brown fluid or semisolid material flecked with cholesterol crystals (153). Microscopy shows fibrous tissue, a lack of epithelial and glial tissue, chronic inflammation, and hemosiderin in macrophages.

## Infectious Lesions

### Syphilitic Masses (Gummas)

Treponema pallidum, the spirochete that is the etiologic agent of syphilis, is well known as a pathogen in the nervous system (154–157). In the preantibiotic era, syphilitic infection was thought to be the etiology of an enormous array of neurologic and psychiatric syndromes, including, most classically, subacute to chronic meningitis; multiple infarcts due to obliterative meningeal endarteritis ("meningovascular syphilis"); dementia ("general paresis"); locomotor ataxia with loss of a sense of joint position, leading to severe arthropathies ("Charcot joints"); and lightning-like pain in the lower extremities (tabes dorsalis). None of these disorders is associated with mass lesions, except in rare instances in which parenchymal infarcts are large enough. Rarely, a granulomatous reaction to the infection may also produce macroscopically tumefactive masses that are identical to those termed gummas in other somatic tissues. Gummas tend

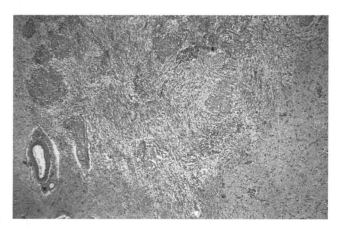
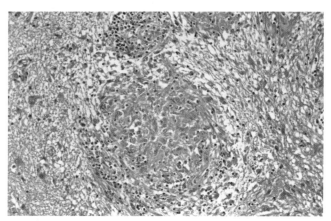

A                                                                                                                                    B

**FIG. 22.** Sarcoidosis. **A, B:** The sharply delimited granulomas of sarcoidosis are often surrounded by a less-organized lymphocytic and mononuclear infiltrate. Usually, as here, the granulomas are not necrotizing. (Both H&E, A: 5× original magnification; B: 25× original magnification.)

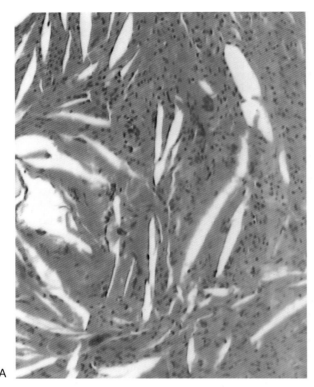 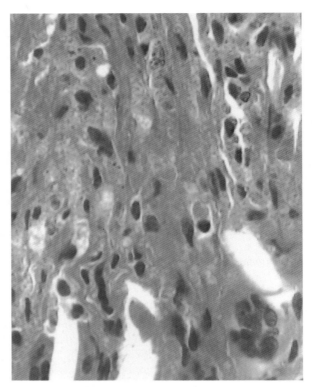

A                                                                                                          B

**FIG. 23.** Xanthogranuloma of choroid plexus. **A, B:** Histologically these lesions consist of masses of fat-filled macrophages (xanthoma cells) with scattered hemosiderin-filled cells, some chronic inflammation with lymphocytes, and fibrous tissue obliterating the architecture of the choroid plexus. There are often, as here, some multinucleated foreign body–type giant cells. (H&E original magnification, A: 33×, B: 125×.) (Case courtesy of Dr. David Louis, Boston, MA.)

to be superficial in the brain, but they are potentially observed in the cortex, the hypothalamus, the surfaces of the brainstem, and the spinal cord. These lesions consist of confluent agglomerations of granulomas (Fig. 24) with central zones of necrosis. Well-developed gummas also exhibit a peripheral fibrous capsule, outside of which there is a zone of gliosis and chronic inflammation similar to that seen around ordinary bacterial abscesses (154–157).

Neurosyphilis, along with other manifestations of lues, became so uncommon in developed countries that at least one entire generation of neuropathologists has had essentially no experience with that disease. The AIDS epidemic has been accompanied by a resurgence in the incidence of syphilis, and it has become apparent that coinfection with HIV-1 and *Treponema pallidum* results in accelerated growth of the latter organisms (155). Thus, neurosyphilis has been reported with a higher frequency in AIDS patients than would have been expected from the pre-AIDS experience. In at least one instance, multiple gummas with numerous spirochetes were reported in the context of AIDS as a manifestation of "quaternary" syphilis, i.e., aggressive disseminated neurosyphilis with a plethora of organisms in the affected tissue (156).

The diagnosis of gummatous syphilis can be strongly suspected if a large tumor-like mass represented by multiple

caseating granulomas is found in the appropriate clinical setting. Proof depends on demonstration of the organisms, traditionally accomplished by application of silver stains (Warthin–Starry or others) but more reliably accomplished at present with immunostaining techniques (157). The density of organisms in gummas is usually said to be low, making their localization and identification difficult, but in AIDS patients the load of treponemes is much higher than that seen in other cases.

### Neuroborreliosis (Lyme Disease)

Spirochetes of the genus *Borrelia* have been implicated as the etiologic agents of chronic relapsing fever and Lyme disease (158,159). There may be cerebral infection in these diseases, with meningoencephalitis or cranial neuropathies. No gummas have been reported; however, some patients have had focal brain lesions on MRI scans (158). These lesions have been interpreted as demyelinative in nature.

### Tuberculoma and Tuberculous Masses

Human diseases caused by *Mycobacterium tuberculosis*, like those linked with *T. pallidum*, had markedly decreased

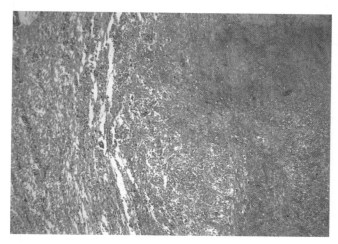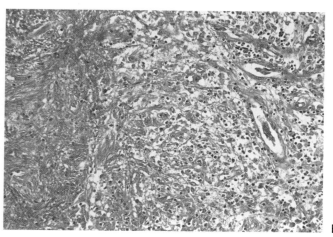

A    B

**FIG. 24.** Gumma. **A:** The gumma has a rounded contour with an extensive central necrotic zone; this zone is often larger than the usual necrotic area in a tuberculous granuloma. (H&E, 5× original magnification.) **B:** The lipid-filled epithelioid histiocytes are tightly organized with intervening vessels into the individual abutting granulomas adjacent to the necrotic zone. (H&E, 25× original magnification.)

in incidence in the years prior to the onset of the AIDS epidemic (154–155,160). This, and the decreasing frequency with which autopsy examinations were performed, led to a lessened experience with the pathologic patterns of tuberculous infections of the CNS. Most such infections, as described classically, were basal meningitides with a subacute to chronic course, often complicated by infarction caused by mycobacterial vasculitis in meningeal vessels. A well-recognized variant was manifested by the occurrence of solitary or multiple tumor-like masses that, when excised, were shown to be inflammatory granulomatous masses with central caseation necrosis (Fig. 25A) (160). Acid-fast bacilli were

demonstrable with standard stains (e.g., Ziehl–Nielsen) (Fig. 25B) or with the auramine-rhodamine fluorescent technique in more than 90% of cases.

True abscesses, without granulomas, have always been much rarer in tuberculous brain disease. However, the AIDS epidemic has again altered that landscape; true abscesses with suppurative and necrotic centers have been described in AIDS patients in several instances (107). At New York University Medical Center–Bellevue Hospital at least three such lesions have necessitated surgical management and neuropathologic diagnosis in the last 3 years. The density of organisms has varied greatly from case to case in that setting.

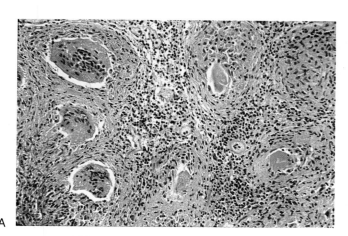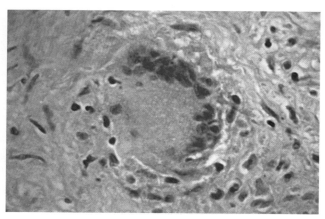

A    B

**FIG. 25.** Tuberculoma. **A:** This photomicrograph of a cerebral mass from a patient with longstanding tuberculous meningitis shows the multilobulated granulomatous tissue, with necrotic central zones in some granulomas. (H&E, 10× original magnification.) **B:** Acid-fast bacilli (mycobacteria) in the necrotic center of a granulomatous nodule. (Ziehl–Nielsen stain, 250× original magnification.)

### Cryptococcomas

Cryptococcus neoformans is the most common fungal pathogen in patients with AIDS. It usually causes meningoencephalitis, in which an inflammatory infiltrate is minimal or often completely absent (107, 156–158). In some instances, organisms collect and proliferate in loculated spaces, either in the brain parenchyma proper (especially the basal ganglia) or the meninges (especially deep recesses and sulci such as the Sylvian fissure) (Fig. 26). These foci can closely simulate tumors in imaging studies, and pathologic examination is necessary to establish the correct diagnosis in such cases.

### Allergic Fungal Sinusitis

Thought to represent an allergic reaction to various fungi in persons whose immunity is not suppressed, allergic fungal sinusitis forming a destructive mass involving the anterior and middle cranial fossa, the orbit, cavernous sinus, clivus, and nasopharynx in a 38-year-old woman has been reported. Cultures grew Aspergillus fumigatus and Aspergillus flavus (161).

## DEPOSITIONS OF EXTRACELLULAR MATERIAL

### Arachnoiditis Ossificans (Arachnoid Ossification)

Arachnoid ossifications (AOs) range from small flecks to large sheets of firm, white tissue; they are very common and usually asymptomatic, even when extensive (162). One patient recorded with an AO had signs of spinal cord compression that responded to excision of the ossified tissue (163). This condition is typically found on the posterior surface of the lower thoracic cord (Fig. 27) but may occur in the lumbosacral or cervical regions, or anteriorly. Microscopy characteristically discloses a thin plaque of lamellar bone, in which psammoma bodies or clusters of arachnoid cells may occasionally be found. This constellation of findings may engender concern over the diagnosis of metastatic "psammocarcinoma" from the thyroid or Mullerian tract. However, attention to the entire clinicopathologic picture is distinctive for AO and usually obviates the need for additional special diagnostic studies.

### Amyloidoma

At least six examples of mass-like deposits of amyloid in the cerebral hemispheres, four of which occurred in the occipital lobes, have been reported in patients from 28 to 60 years old (average 47) (164–169). These gray to yellow, firm, waxy lesions involve the white matter of the centrum semiovale or subependymal tissue. Microscopy shows amorphous, eosinophilic, and congophilic material, often arranged in relation to the walls of cerebral blood vessels, which may also be involved (Fig. 28). Varying numbers of lymphocytes, plasma cells, and macrophages may be present. In addition to intraparenchymal locations, amyloidomas have been reported in the Gasserian ganglion, within the sella, the cerebellopontine angle and jugular foramen, and in the choroid plexus.

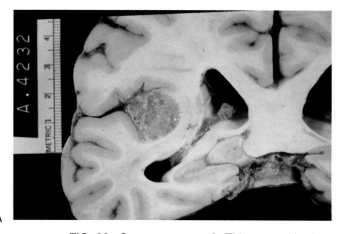
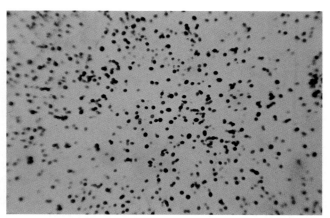

A

B

**FIG. 26.** Cryptococcoma. **A:** This coronal brain slice is from a hemophiliac patient who acquired AIDS from contaminated clotting factors in the early years of the AIDS epidemic. He had a protracted course with cryptococcal meningitis, responsive to antibiotics but relapsing whenever they were stopped. At autopsy, he had several similar soft gelatinous macroscopic masses, of which this left Sylvian fissure example was the largest. **B:** Microscopic examination revealed that each mass was an agglomerate of myriad cryptococci with minimal fibrosis and no inflammatory response. (Grocott Methenamine silver stain, 100× original magnification.)

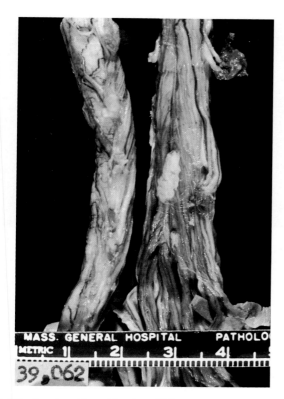

**FIG. 27.** Arachnoid ossification. This gross photograph of a portion of spinal cord (from a patient with amyotrophic lateral sclerosis) has a typical broad area of white ossification in the meninges of the lower thoracic cord.

## Pseudoamyloid (Intraparenchymal Colloid Pseudocysts)

Bentalanffy et al. reported a case of a loculated accumulation of colloid-like material in the centrum semiovale and adjacent body of the lateral ventricle in a 32-year-old woman (170). At the 32nd Annual Diagnostic Slide Session at the American Association of Neuropathologists Meeting in Baltimore in 1991, Herrick and Forno presented a case of a 54-year-old woman with a history of seizures since childhood and insulin-dependent diabetes, who had multiple, circumscribed, waxy yellow lesions measuring 0.3–12.3 cm in the cerebral hemispheres, brainstem, and cerebellum (171). In our surgical accessions we have seen a similar case involving the temporal lobe in a 46-year-old woman (Fig. 29A). The multiloculated spaces contained waxy, gelatinous material (Fig. 29B, C), lacked an epithelial lining, and were bordered by fibrous or glial tissue infiltrated by plasma cells, lymphocytes, and macrophages (Fig. 29D, E). The amorphous material was strongly PAS-positive and diastase-resistant, but it was Alcian blue–negative and noncongophilic.

## Pseudogout

Myelopathy due to deposition of calcium pyrophosphate in the cervical ligamentum flavum has been reported in five women and three men between the ages of 61 and 80 years (average 69) and in the atlantooccipital ligament in three women from 76 to 85 years old (average 82) (172–178). This condition is sometimes associated with a variable inflammatory infiltrate of lymphocytes and foreign body giant cells and features the presence of the rectangular or rhomboidal crystals that stain blue with hematoxylin and eosin (H&E) (Fig. 30A). They are birefringent, and polarization with a quartz retardation filter shows the characteristics of pyrophosphate (Fig. 30B). Most cases involving the cervical ligamentum flavum have occurred in Japan, where there is a high but unexplained incidence of calcification of the posterior longitudinal ligament (176).

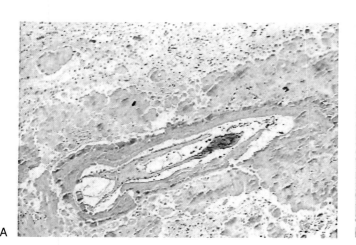

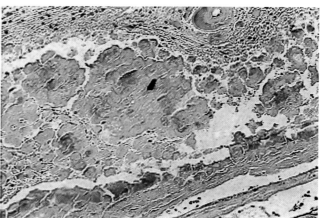

**FIG. 28.** Amyloidoma. **A:** This intracerebral mass, when resected and examined histologically, is seen to consist of amorphous hyaline eosinophilic material, often as confluent rounded masses. (H&E, 6× original magnification.) **B:** The amyloid nature of the material is suggested by its strong staining with Congo red (33× original magnification).

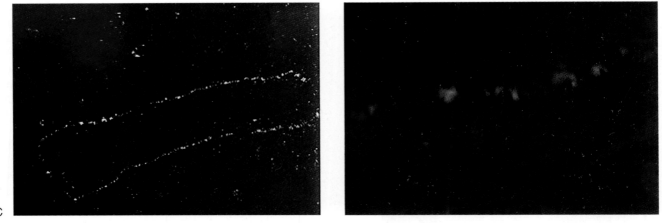

C

D

**FIG. 28.** *Continued* **C:** The amyloid exhibits the appropriate dichroic birefringence when examined with cross-polarized light. (Congo red 6× original magnification.) **D:** At high power, the typical apple-green birefringence is apparent. (Congo red, 125× original magnification.)

### Calcifying Pseudotumor

At least 17 cases of calcifying fibrous lesions have been reported in the spinal meninges, foramen magnum, cerebellopontine angle, skull base, cerebellar tonsils, and frontal lobes (179–182). Two thirds of cases involved men who complained of pain for 1–5 months. The masses are yellow–gray, 1–10 cm in diameter, and predominantly calcified. Histologic examination shows epithelioid histiocytes and giant cells, which are focally arranged around amorphous calcific material, forming granulomatous nodules. Fine particles of calcium salt are present along with varying quantities of fibrovascular stroma, occasionally with scattered lymphocytes or macrophages (Fig. 31). This lesion may represent a form of "tumoral calcinosis." We have recently seen a similar lesion in a lumbar dorsal root ganglion in a 63-year-old woman.

### Storage Disease

Myelopathy secondary to marked thickening of the spinal dura has been reported in a patient with Maroteaux–Lamy mucopolysaccharidosis (183–186).

### Mucocele

Mucoceles are common lesions of the frontal and ethmoid sinuses, and they usually result from obstruction of the sinus ostia (184). Because it is distended with retained secretions, the bony confines of the expanding sinus may be eroded resulting in communications with the orbits, frontal lobes, or pituitary (187–190). The clinical and radiologic signs are usually more important to diagnosis than the histologic findings. The latter are nondescript, consisting of fibrous connective tissue with a lining of columnar epithelium.

### NONNEURAL HETEROTOPIAS AND HAMARTOMAS

### Lipoma

Intracranial "lipomas" are typically incidental findings, most often arising in the region of the corpus callosum and often accompanying agenesis of that structure (191–194). Symptoms are most commonly represented by seizures or mental retardation, and are usually more related to associated cerebral malformations than to the lipoma itself. The tu-

**FIG. 29.** Pseudoamyloid. **A:** This T1-weighted coronal brain MRI scan reveals a low-signal mass in the right temporal lobe. **B:** An intraoperative photograph shows the gray gelatinous material emerging from the white matter. (Courtesy of Dr. Paul Cooper, Department of Neurosurgery, NYU Medical Center.) **C:** Gross photograph from an autopsy of another patient showing a mass of pseudoamyloid material in the right cerebellar hemisphere. **D:** Histologic examination reveals that the pseudoamyloid material consists of hyaline globules, closely mimicking true amyloid (cf Fig. 28A: PAS, 12× original magnification.) **E:** A higher-power view shows the absence of any lining for the cysts and the blandly gliotic bordering tissue, although considerable chronic inflammation can be seen in some areas (not shown). PAS, 125× original magnification. (Courtesy of Dr. Lysia S. Forno, Palo Alto, CA and Dr. Maie K. Herrick, San Jose, CA).

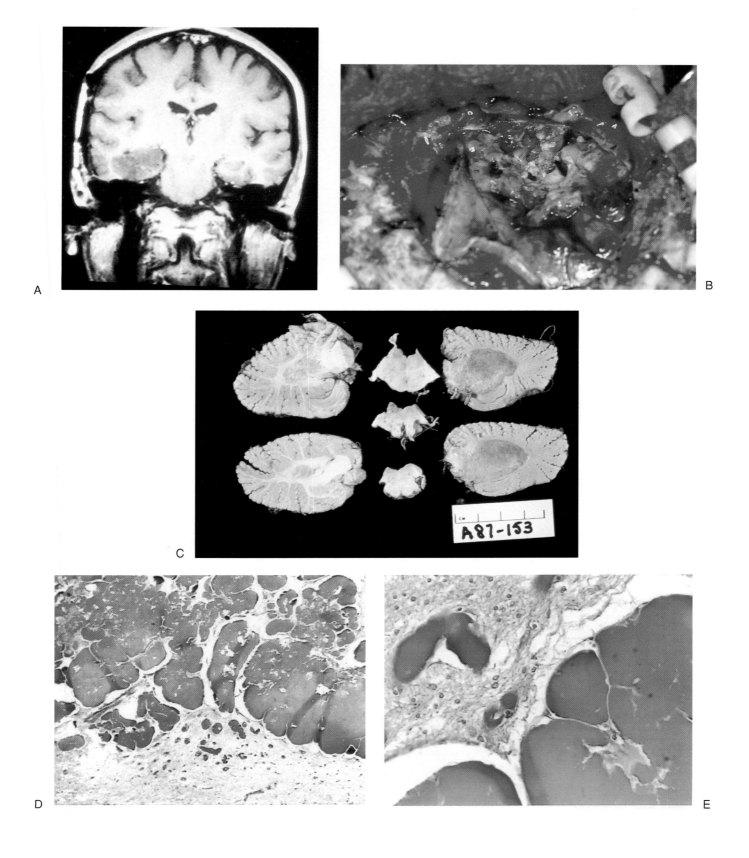

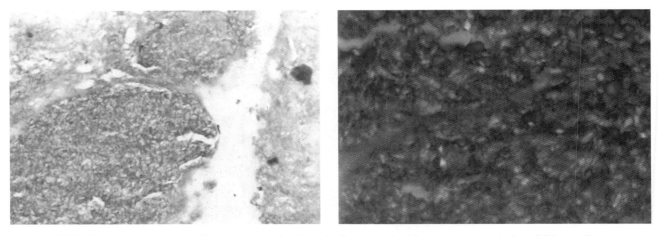

**FIG. 30.** Pseudogout. **A:** Histologic examination of affected spinal ligaments reveals, in addition to the focal inflammatory reaction, deposits of irregular crystalline basophilic material. (H&E, 70× original magnification.) **B:** Polarization reveals that the crystals are dichroic, with a characteristic pattern for pyrophosphate using a quartz retardation filter. (H&E, 125× original magnification.)

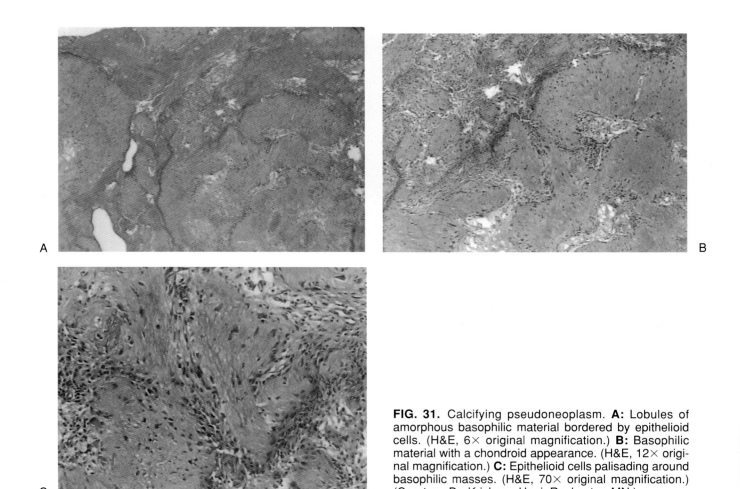

**FIG. 31.** Calcifying pseudoneoplasm. **A:** Lobules of amorphous basophilic material bordered by epithelioid cells. (H&E, 6× original magnification.) **B:** Basophilic material with a chondroid appearance. (H&E, 12× original magnification.) **C:** Epithelioid cells palisading around basophilic masses. (H&E, 70× original magnification.) (Courtesy Dr. Krishnan Unni, Rochester, MN.)

*Pathology of Pseudoneoplastic Lesions,*
edited by M. R. Wick, P. A. Humphrey, and J. H. Ritter.
Lippincott-Raven Publishers, Philadelphia © 1997.

# CHAPTER 3

# Pseudoneoplastic Lesions of the Head and Neck

Samir K. El-Mofty

The head and neck constitute a relatively small area of the human body. However, its anatomic diversity and pathologic complexity are unparalleled. The intricacy of this region is illustrated by the multitudinous disciplines of surgical pathology under which the lesions of that topographic area may be classified. These subspecialties include neuropathology, dermatopathology, bone and soft tissue pathology, endocrine pathology, gastrointestinal pathology, otolaryngologic pathology, and oral pathology.

Many lesions of the head and neck are morphologically identical to their counterparts in other anatomic sites. However, some are unique, as exemplified by proliferations relating to the intimate anatomic relationship of the sinonasal tract to the brain, the presence of the odontogenic apparatus in the maxillofacial skeleton, or the singular attributes of the major salivary glands. In this chapter, emphasis is placed on those entities that are exclusive to this site. A few others that are either very rare or have a special predilection for this location are also described. Lesions are listed under three main headings: oral and maxillofacial structures, salivary glands, and sinonasal tract and larynx. Pseudotumors occurring in the head and neck as frequently as in other anatomic sites are amply discussed in the remaining chapters of this monograph and are generally considered only briefly here.

 S. K. El-Mofty: Lauren V. Ackerman Laboratory of Surgical Pathology, Department of Pathology, Washington University School of Medicine, St. Louis, Missouri 63110.

## PSEUDOTUMORS OF THE ORAL AND MAXILLOFACIAL STRUCTURES

### Juxtaoral Organ of Chievitz

Microscopic observation of embryonic epithelial structures in the mouths and jaws of adults is not an uncommon event. These residues include nests of the dental lamina and the epithelial sheath of Hertwig, remnants of the nasopalatine duct, and the juxtaoral organ of Chievitz (1). The microscopic presentation of the latter structure as epithelial nests with an intimate association with peripheral nerves is of particular significance. Lack of familiarity with this normal structure by pathologists may lead to an erroneous diagnosis of intraneural or perineural invasion by a carcinoma (1–3). In particular, misinterpretation of this structure in frozen sections can result in unnecessary and extensive surgical procedures. The odontogenic epithelial remnants and those of the nasopalatine duct are present in the bones of the jaws and are readily identified. On the other hand, the juxtaoral organ of Chievitz is found in the soft tissues of the retromolar trigone and ascending ramus area, a site that is commonly the focus of oral cancer surgery and therefore lends itself to diagnostic "traps" in the context being discussed.

In 1885, Chievitz, a Danish histologist, described cords of epithelium that were associated with the buccal sulcus in embryos (4). It was later found that this tissue is separate from the parotid anlage and that it becomes detached from the surface epithelium (5). In postnatal life, the organ of Chievitz (OC) lies deep to the internal pterygoid muscle near the pterygomandibular raphe, and it is associated with small branches of the buccal nerve. The function of this structure, if any, is unknown. The proximity of the epithelial cells of the OC to nonmyelinated nerves, and the electron microscopic demonstration of neurosecretory-like granules in their cytoplasm, suggests a possible neurosecretory function (6). So far, however, there has been no confirmation of such a hypothesis, and the OC is more likely a "passive, non-functional, epithelial remnant" (7).

Microscopically, the OC is composed of rounded epithelial nests. Serial sectioning indicates that these masses are in continuity with one another (7). The constituent cells show variable morphologic features. They may be polygonal, resembling squamous epithelium (Fig. 1), or columnar with clear cytoplasm. These elements are usually palisaded at the periphery of the cell nests, with their long axes aligned perpendicularly to the basement membrane. Some cells have a basaloid appearance with elongated dense nuclei, little cytoplasm, and indistinct cell membranes. No frank keratinization or keratohyaline granules are present in such cells. On rare occasions, the epithelial nests of the OC may show duct-like structures with central lumina, containing mucin-negative secretions (6). The cell groups of the OC are associated with one or more nerve fibers. These may be present at the periphery of the inclusion (Fig. 1) or between the epithelial nests. Uncommonly, the nerves may be wrapped around the OC.

It is important for surgical pathologists to recognize the juxtaoral OC as a normal anatomic structure to prevent its misdiagnosis as squamous cell carcinoma. Because occasional examples of this structure may show glandular foci in the squamous epithelium, a distinction from mucoepidermoid carcinoma could also be difficult in selected instances; in that regard, it is pertinent that the retromolar trigone, where the OC is situated, is a common site for mucoepidermoid carcinoma of the oral minor salivary glands. Lastly, the chance of inclusion of the OC in the margins of a surgical resection could lead to the misinterpretation that the margins of a cancer specimen were positive for tumor.

Manifestation of the juxtaoral OC as an intraoral mass is extremely rare, but this eventuality has indeed been reported in a 5-year-old girl (8). The lesion in that case presented as a hard, fixed mass measuring 1.5 cm in diameter in the retromolar area along the ascending ramus of the mandible. Microscopic analysis showed the typical features of an OC, and the clinical course was uneventful thereafter.

### Pseudoepitheliomatous Hyperplasia

Pseudoepitheliomatous hyperplasia (PEH), also known as pseudocarcinomatous hyperplasia, denotes the reactive, non-

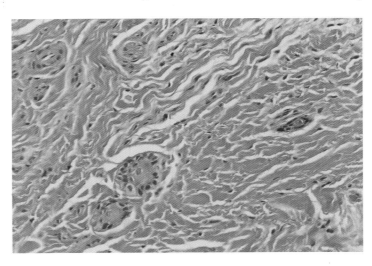

**FIG. 1.** Organ of Chievitz. Squamous epithelial nests in close proximity to nerve fibers. (Courtesy of Dr. Susan Zant, Department of Pathology, Indiana University School of Dentistry, Indianapolis, IN.)

neoplastic growth of mucosal surface epithelium into the underlying connective tissue. The downward proliferation of the squamous mucosa may be marked and it may appear in selected sections as isolated islands with focal keratinization. This finding makes the distinction from squamous cell carcinoma extremely difficult in selected cases. Some degree of epithelial hyperplasia is commonly present at the edges of all chronic nonspecific (usually traumatic) ulcers of the oral cavity. Marked PEH is, however, characteristically associated with specific mucosal lesions of the mouth, particularly with inflammatory papillary hyperplasia ("palatal papillomatosis"), granular cell tumor, and oral lesions of discoid lupus erythematosus. These conditions are considered further in the following sections.

*1. PEH in inflammatory papillary hyperplasia (palatal papillomatosis [PP]).* This constellation of findings is a peculiar presentation of "fibrous hyperplasia" of the oral mucosa. It occurs predominantly, but not exclusively, in the hard palate under a full maxillary denture. Old, ill-fitting dentures and poor oral hygiene contribute to the development of this lesion (9,10).

The condition manifests itself clinically as juxtaposed papillary projections that can involve a large part of the palatal surface. They may be edematous, erythematous, or normal in color. Microscopically, PP is composed of numerous small, usually uniform papillary projections (Fig. 2A), constituted by parakeratotic and occasionally orthokeratotic stratified squamous epithelium. The supporting fibrous connective tissue cores usually contain an inflammatory cell infiltrate. Elongated mucosal ridges in PP often show pseudoepitheliomatous hyperplasia (9,10) (Fig. 2B); however, the epithelial islands do not extend deeply into the underlying tissue and there is no significant atypia, hyperchromasia, or keratin pearl formation. Furthermore, intraepithelial exocytosis of inflammatory cells and degeneration of some individual squamous cells are regularly seen in pseudoepitheliomatous hyperplasia. These features are important in distinguishing this lesion from well-differentiated squamous cell carcinoma. Inflammatory papillary mucosal hyperplasia should also be distinguished from oral verrucous carcinoma (OVC). In the latter condition, the epithelial proliferation and keratinization are much more marked. Usually, keratin plugging of the surface epithelium is also present in OVC, and papillary projections are irregular, with epithelial cords extending deeply into the underlying submucosa. Inflammatory papillary hyperplasia has no known preneoplastic po-

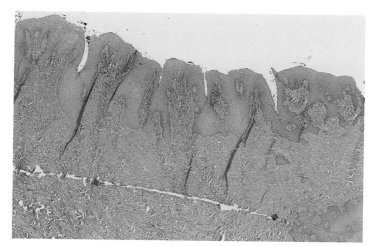

A

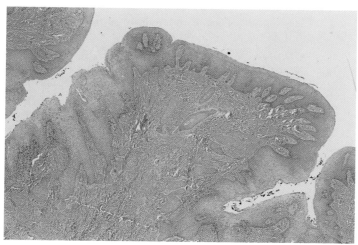

B

**FIG. 2. A:** Small uniform papillary projections seen in inflammatory papillary hyperplasia of the palate. **B:** Higher magnification; elongated mucosal ridges produce a pseudoepitheliomatous pattern.

tential, and an etiologic relationship between that lesion and infection with *Candida albicans* has been suggested. However, such organisms are not commonly identified in this context (10,11).

*2. PEH associated with granular cell tumor.* Granular cell tumors (GCT) may originate in a variety of tissues, especially the skin and mucous membranes. Roughly 30% arise in the tongue (9,10,12,13). There appears to be no age preference for this lesion in adults, but it is rare in children. In the oral cavity and the mucosa of the upper aerodigestive tract in general, GCT presents itself as a firm submucosal nodule. Microscopically, one observes masses of large polyhedral cells with acidophilic granular cytoplasm. Nuclei are small, vesicular, and centrally placed (13). The granular cells extend deeply into the submucosa. Pseudoepitheliomatous hyperplasia is commonly present in the surface mucosa over the tumor mass (Fig. 3). In fact, PEH may be so pronounced in this setting that a diagnosis of squamous cell carcinoma may be made erroneously (9,10,12,13). Such serious mistakes are more likely to occur in small biopsies that show little, if anything, of the underlying GCT. Thus, it is obvious that a definitive diagnosis of carcinoma should be made only with extreme circumspection and caution in the evaluation of those specimens.

*3. PEH in oral lesions of discoid lupus erythematosus.* The reported prevalence of oral involvement in patients with cutaneous discoid lupus erythematosus (DLE) varies from 4% to 25% (14,15). The former of these lesions usually fol-

lows the appearance of the skin eruption, but it may occur simultaneously (15). In addition, oral lesions of DLE may present themselves at the vermilion border of the lower lip in the absence of cutaneous disease (15). The majority of oral lesions of DLE affect the buccal and labial mucosa, frequently bilaterally (16,17). On clinical examination, they are erythematous plaques with dispersed white papules or macules and peripherally radiating white striae, surrounded by telangiectasias (14,15,18). Microscopically, the mucosal lesions show hyperorthokeratosis or parakeratinization and keratotic plugging and atrophy, alternating with hyperplasia of the surface epithelium. Hydropic degeneration of the basal epithelium and keratinocytic loss with formation of colloid (Civatte) bodies are common. PEH is frequently seen in the hyperplastic mucosal foci and is occasionally so marked that a diagnosis of squamous cell carcinoma is considered (Fig. 4). Nevertheless, a dense inflammatory cell infiltrate forms a band beneath the oral epithelium in DLE, and intraepithelial leukocytic migration is a common feature as well. The deeper connective tissue shows focal, usually perivascular, patchy inflammatory cell infiltrates that are composed predominantly of lymphocytes (14–18). Edema of the lamina propria and thick PAS-positive subepithelial deposits are additional characteristic features.

The distinction of pseudoepitheliomatous hyperplasia associated with DLE from oral squamous cell carcinoma may be established by noting a lack of nuclear or architectural atypia and nuclear hyperchromatism in the epithelial islands of PEH. Invasion of the hyperplastic epithelial nests by leukocytes and degeneration of some of the keratinocytes as seen in DLE are usually absent in squamous cell carcinoma. Finally, immunofluorescent studies show immunoglobulin and complement deposition in the epithelial basement membrane in DLE but not carcinoma (19). Table 1 shows the main histopathologic differences between PEH and squamous cell carcinoma in the oral cavity.

## Eosinophilic Ulcer of the Oral Mucosa (Traumatic Eosinophilic Granuloma)

Eosinophilic ulcer of the oral mucosa (EUOM) is a benign, self-healing lesion that is most commonly represented by an ulcer on the lateral or ventral surface of the tongue that clinically resembles squamous cell carcinoma. On the other hand, it is often misdiagnosed as a lymphoreticular malignancy at a histologic level. The lesion may initially appear as a raised white or red area of induration before it ulcerates. It is painless and usually affects adults in their sixth and seventh decades (20–22). Microscopically, a polymorphous inflammatory cell infiltrate is seen that extends deeply into the submucosa and between muscle fibers (Fig. 5A). Eosinophils and large mononuclear cells usually dominate the picture (Fig. 5B). The latter elements have pale nuclei and often show brisk mitotic activity. Lymphocytes, plasma cells, macrophages, neutrophils, and plasma cells are usually

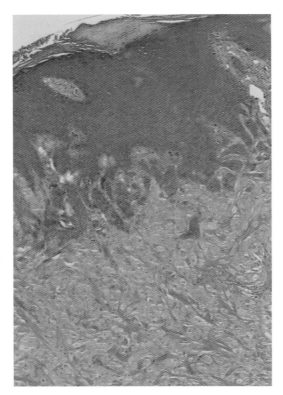

**FIG. 3.** Pseudoepitheliomatous hyperplasia in surface mucosa covering granular cell tumor of the tongue.

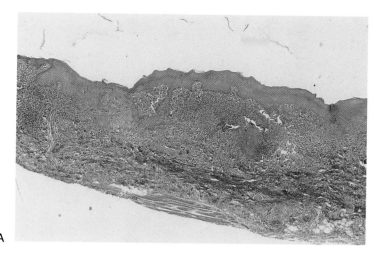

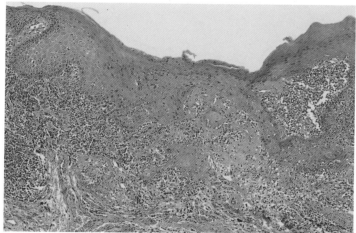

**FIG. 4. A:** Oral lesion of discoid lupus erythematosus. Epithelial atrophy alternating with hypertrophy. **B:** Higher magnification showing intense lymphocytic infiltrate and pseudoepitheliomatous hyperplasia.

present in variable numbers in different lesions. The large mononuclear cells with pale nuclei are thought to be derived from myofibroblasts (22). The polymorphic nature of the cellular infiltrate and immunophenotype of the large atypical cells help to distinguish eosinophilic ulcer from primary malignant lymphoma of the oral mucosa.

Based on clinical and experimental evidence (21), it has been suggested that trauma may have an etiologic role in the

genesis of EUOM. More recent immunohistochemical observations (22) suggest a role for T-cell immunity in the origination of the lesion as well.

Eosinophilic ulcer of the oral mucosa resolves spontaneously, even without surgical intervention. Multiple synchronous and metachronous lesions at different sites in the mouth have been reported (20,22,23), and multifocality therefore should not be confused with recurrence.

**TABLE 1.** *Comparison of histopathologic features of PEH and squamous cell carcinoma in the oral cavity*

| Feature | PEH | Carcinoma |
|---|---|---|
| Depth of extension | Superficial | Deep |
| Architecture of deep front | Even | Irregular |
| Cellular pleomorphism | Usually absent | Present |
| Nuclear hyperchromatism | Absent | Present |
| N:C ratio | Not changed | Increased |
| Keratin pearl formation | Usually none | Common |
| Intraepithelial inflammatory cell exocytosis | Common | Uncommon |
| Keratinocytic degeneration | Common | Uncommon |

PEH, Pseudoepitheliomatous hyperplasia.

## Fibroosseous Cementifying Lesions of the Jaws

The term "benign fibro-osseous lesion" is widely applied to a group of proliferations involving the craniofacial skeleton that are characterized by a fibrous stroma containing various combinations of bone and "cementum-like" material. A wide variety of lesions—including developmental and dysplastic conditions, as well as neoplastic ones—have been included under this general rubric. The distinction between neoplastic and nonneoplastic entities in this category requires correlation of historical, clinical, and radiographic findings with the histopathologic features. Two nonneoplastic cemento-osseous lesions are commonly encountered in

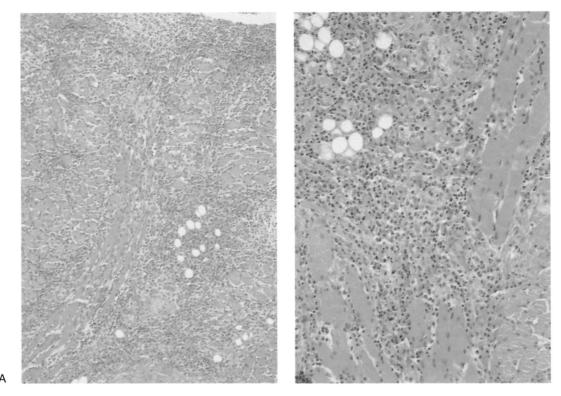

**FIG. 5.** Eosinophilic ulcer of the oral mucosa (traumatic eosinophilic granuloma). **A:** Polymorphous inflammatory cell infiltrate extending deeply into the musculature of the tongue. **B:** Eosinophils and large mononuclear cells in between muscle fibers.

the jaws; *periapical cemental dysplasia (cementoma)* and *florid cemento-osseous dysplasia*. These two entities should ideally be identified clinically and radiographically, and it should be uncommon to receive surgical specimens of them. Indeed, operative intervention is contraindicated in the case of florid cemento-osseous dysplasia because even a simple biopsy or dental extraction may result in local infection, pain, and a complicated clinical course (24).

Periapical cemental dysplasia (periapical cementoma) is a relatively common condition, particularly in middle-aged black women. It is a nonneoplastic, presumably dysplastic disorder. The anterior mandibular teeth are most often involved by asymptomatic periapical radiolucencies, which in older lesions become heavily calcified. In their early stages, the lesions are radiolucent and may be confused with periapical inflammatory disease. Treatment is not required (5).

Florid cemento-osseous dysplasia is infrequently seen and has been reported under various alternative designations. This condition is usually seen in middle-aged or elderly black women and radiographically is characterized by extensive sclerotic areas (Fig. 6), often symmetrically involving the posterior quadrants of the mandible and maxilla (24,25).

Periapical cemental dysplasia and florid cemento-osseous

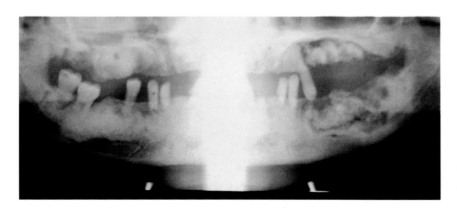

**FIG. 6.** Panoramic radiograph showing florid cemento-osseous dysplasia of the jaws. Radiopaque masses are present bilaterally in both the mandible and maxilla.

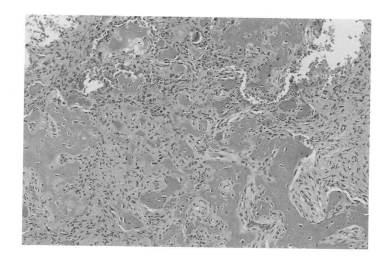

**FIG. 7.** Florid cemento-osseous dysplasia, showing fibrous connective tissue with bone and cementum-like calcified structures.

dysplasia are microscopically analogous to one another and are composed of proliferating fibrous connective tissue stroma containing foci of cementum. Osteoid or bone are invariably present as well (Fig. 7). More advanced lesions show an increase in mineralization. In florid cemento-osseous dysplasia, large sclerotic masses are formed that are hypocellular and extremely dense, with little marrow space and few Haversian systems (24,25).

Ossifying fibroma of the jaws is regarded as a true neoplasm. Like the cemento-osseous dysplasias, it affects the tooth-bearing areas of the jaws. It differs from those diseases, however, in that it is usually solitary and expansive. Cementum-like large sclerotic masses are not formed in ossifying fibromas (24).

It is of importance to note that metastases to the jaws of some carcinomas, particularly those of the breast and prostate, may show radiographic features that are very similar to those of the cemento-osseous dysplasia. However, unlike the latter condition, metastatic jaw lesions are commonly associated with pain, bone expansion, looseness of teeth, and paresthesia of the lip. Past medical history of breast or prostate carcinoma should prompt a biopsy of suspicious jaw lesions.

## Hyperplastic Dental Follicular Tissue and Dental Papilla

The tooth follicle and dental papilla are normal components of the ectomesenchyme of the tooth germ (26,27). Nevertheless, they are commonly misdiagnosed microscopically as odontogenic tumors. The dental papilla forms dentin and matures into pulp tissue, whereas the tooth follicle develops into the periodontal membrane and its attachments. These structures anchor the tooth roots into their sockets in the alveolar bone of the jaws (28). The tooth follicle normally is apparent in radiographs as a thin circular radiolucency around unerupted or impacted teeth. Enlarge-

ment or asymmetry of that structure is not uncommon around impacted third molars and canines, but these eventualities are frequently confused with the attributes of neoplastic processes by clinicians. Dental papillae and tooth follicles are commonly encountered by the pathologist in patients during their first and second decades of life, usually in association with impacted molar teeth and, less frequently, impacted canines or supernumerary teeth (29). Microscopically, the tooth follicle is composed predominantly of collagenous fibrous connective tissue, with variable myxomatous components (Fig. 8A). Areas of calcification and small islands of odontogenic epithelium cells are invariably present as well. Occasionally, the fibrous follicular tissue may be lined by a thin layer of epithelial cells that may be columnar, cuboidal, or squamous in nature. They are derived from the enamel organ and are termed the "reduced enamel epithelium" (Fig. 8B).

The dental papilla is a well-circumscribed elliptical or oval piece of immature mesenchymal tissue composed of loose myxoid stroma and small stellate or fusiform cells that are evenly spaced (Fig. 9). The surface of the papilla may be mantled by a layer of elongated palisaded odontoblasts (Fig. 9B).

Tooth follicles and dental papillae are normal components of odontogenesis that are ubiquitous in the jaws during the early phases of dental development. Nonetheless, as mentioned above, they are frequently misdiagnosed as odontogenic tumors by pathologists with limited experience in head and neck pathology. In order to avoid this error and the attending clinical ramifications, special attention should be paid to correlating the histologic findings with complete historical, clinical, and radiographic information. This is not only helpful but in many cases essential to ensuring accurate diagnosis.

In particular, the detection of odontogenic epithelial rests in the follicles may lead to erroneous diagnoses of ameloblastoma or ameloblastic fibroma (29). The epithelium

**FIG. 8. A:** Hyperplastic dental follicle, represented by collagenous fibrous connective tissue containing small nests and strands of odontogenic epithelial rests. **B:** Dental follicle with myxoid change and a lining of reduced enamel epithelium superiorly.

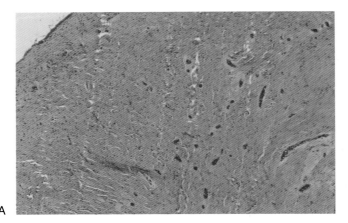

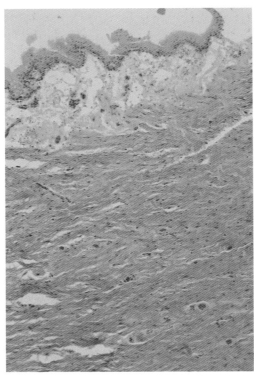

A

B

in those neoplasms, however, typically shows ameloblastic differentiation with aggregates of tall, columnar, peripheral cells manifesting reversed nuclear polarity. More central cells form a loose stellate reticulum. In contrast, the diminutive odontogenic rests present in the dental follicles are com-

posed only of small cuboidal cells that may show focal squamous metaplasia.

Frequently, dental follicles and, even more commonly, dental papillae are misdiagnosed as myxomas or odontogenic fibromas (29). These two true mesenchymal odonto-

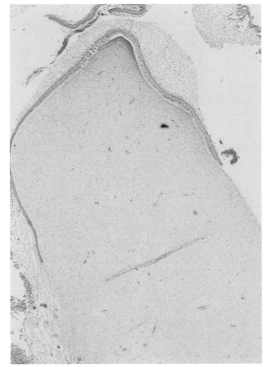

A

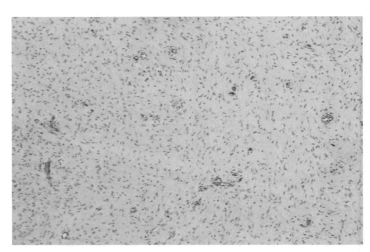

B

**FIG. 9. A and B:** Dental papilla associated with enamel organ in an early formative stage. The subjacent homogeneous matrix is composed of predentin. The enamel organ is present superiorly. A layer of palisaded odontoblasts is seen below the predentin **(B). C:** Higher magnification showing loose myxoid stroma and small stellate and fusiform cells. No epithelial rests are present in the surface of the dental papilla.

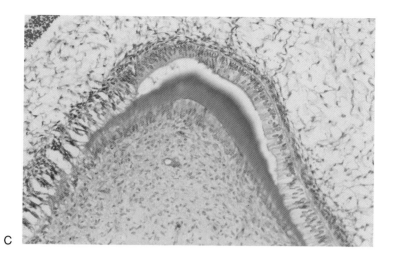

C

**FIG. 9.** *Continued*

genic tumors are expansive and locally destructive lesions (30–32), whereas vestigial odontogenic tissues, both follicular and papillary, are confined, well circumscribed, and symmetrical, and never cause osseous destruction. Microscopically at high-power magnification, isolated foci in dental papillae are indistinguishable from the image of odontogenic myxoma. Unlike the latter lesion, the surfaces of papillae are lined with palisaded cuboidal or columnar odontoblasts. Also, the dental papilla is entirely devoid of epithelium, whereas odontogenic myxoma not uncommonly contains epithelial islands. Likewise, odontogenic fibromas tend to contain more numerous epithelial islands than do dental follicles, and the latter structures commonly show an attenuated epithelial lining that represents the reduced enamel epithelium.

Calcified structures that are occasionally present in the dental follicles may suggest a diagnosis of calcifying epithelial odontogenic tumor (Pindborg's tumor) (29). In that neoplasm, however, the epithelial cells are polygonal and form sheets, frequently with nuclear and cytologic pleomorphism. In addition, calcifying epithelial odontogenic tumors typically show amyloid deposits and characteristic calcified lamellar structures known as Liesegang rings (32). None of those secondary features is observed in dental follicles.

## PSEUDOTUMORS OF THE SALIVARY GLANDS

Salivary glands are exocrine glands whose purpose is to secrete saliva into the oral cavity. There are three pairs of major glands located outside the mouth: parotid, submandibular, and sublingual. In addition, numerous minor, mostly mucus-secreting glands are distributed throughout the oral mucosa, as well as a multitude of mucoserous glands found in the upper aerodigestive tract. Though these are not strictly salivary in nature, they are subject to similar pathologic processes. Tumor-like conditions of the salivary glands are, in general, nonneoplastic lesions that manifest themselves clinically as masses, indurations, or ulcers that mimic neoplasms, not only clinically but, on occasion, microscopically.

### Polycystic (Dysgenetic) Disease of the Parotid

Polycystic disease of the salivary glands is an extremely rare condition that predominantly affects the parotid gland. It resembles polycystic disorders of other organs, such as the kidney, pancreas, and lungs (33,34). It may occur in one salivary gland, but it usually affects both glands and is believed to be a developmental malformation of the ductal system (34–36). The presence of this condition is usually appreciated during childhood but occasionally is first noted in adult life. It is seen in females almost exclusively (35,37). A recurrent, fluctuant, painless swelling of the affected gland, which may be longstanding, is the typical clinical scenario. There is no significant change in salivary flow.

On microscopic examination, the overall architecture of the affected glands appears to be preserved; nevertheless, the lobules are distended and largely replaced by epithelial-lined cystic spaces that may contain short septal projections (Fig. 10). The lining cells vary from flat and cuboidal to columnar. Occasionally, such cells show rounded snout-like luminal borders similar to those of apocrine cells. Cytoplasmic vacuolization is common. The vacuoles may label positively with fat stains (34). Remnants of glandular acini may be found between the cysts (Fig. 10), and ducts sometime communicate directly with the cystic cavities. The lumina of the cysts may contain secretions and, occasionally, eosinophilic bodies with concentric radial patterns similar to those of spheroliths and microliths (Fig. 10C). With the exception of a few scattered macrophages, inflammatory cells are generally absent (34,36).

Although dysgenesis of the parotid is extremely rare, it is nevertheless important to be familiar with this entity in order to avoid misdiagnosis of a cystic neoplasm. The light microscopic appearance of polycystic disease of the parotid is distinctive, but it could be confused with that of cystadenoma or low-grade mucoepidermoid carcinoma. The former of these two neoplasms is frequently well circumscribed and has a thick capsule (38), whereas in polycystic parotids the gland is diffusely cystified and its overall lobular architecture preserved. The lining of the cystic structures in cystadenoma is composed of cuboidal, columnar, oncocytic, or mucous cells

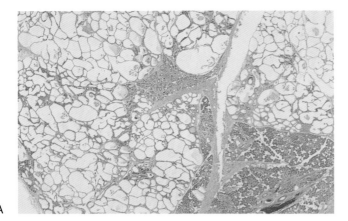

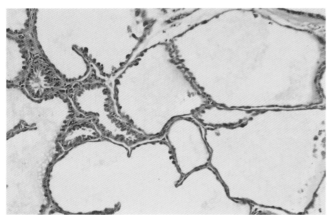

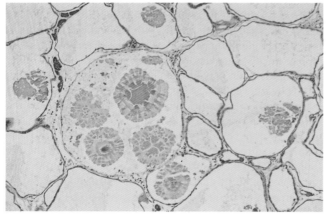

**FIG. 10.** Polycystic disease of the parotid gland. The salivary gland lobules are distended and largely replaced by cystic spaces. **A:** Parenchymal remnants are seen between the cysts. **B:** Intraluminal septal projections are seen. The epithelial cells lining the cysts are cuboidal or columnar, and some show snout-like luminal borders. **C:** Intraluminal microlith-like bodies are present.

that tend to show focal stratification and may form ramifying papillary projections. The lining of the cystic spaces in polycystic parotid disease is one cell layer thick, and, as stated above, often the cells are vacuolated with luminal decapitation profiles. The spheroliths and microliths that are characteristic of polycystic parotid disease are lacking in both cys-

tadenoma and mucoepidermoid carcinoma. In addition, low-grade cystic mucoepidermoid tumors are distinguished from polycystic parotid disease by their infiltrative growth pattern. The lining of the cysts in mucoepidermoid carcinoma commonly includes mucous cells, as well as overtly epidermoid and intermediate cells (38). Extracellular mucin is often abundant in mucoepidermoid carcinoma as well, but it is inconspicuous or absent in polycystic disease.

Polycystic dysgenetic disease of the parotid gland is an innocuous condition. Surgery should be done only for diagnostic or cosmetic purposes.

### Adenomatoid Hyperplasia of the Minor Salivary Glands

Adenomatoid hyperplasia of the palatal minor salivary glands was first described in 1971 (39) as a lesion of the oral mucous glands that presented clinically as a tumor. Although the condition has a wide age distribution, it is most common during the fourth to sixth decades of life, affecting males slightly more frequently than females (40,41). The lesions become evident as localized painless sessile masses. The covering mucosa is intact and has a normal color or, less frequently, it may be erythematous or bluish. The majority of the lesions of adenomatoid hyperplasia range in size from 1 to 1.5 cm. The palate is the most frequent site of incidence; the retromolar pad, lip, and buccal mucosa are affected more rarely (41). The duration of growth is usually described as "months." Histologic evaluation shows dense aggregates of unremarkable mucous acini and ducts (Fig. 11). In most in-

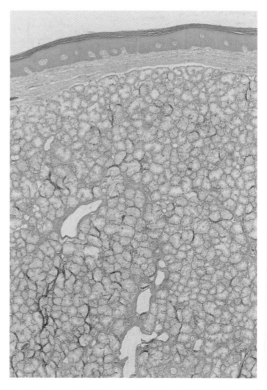

**FIG. 11.** Adenomatoid hyperplasia of the minor salivary glands. Unremarkable mucous acini and ducts are present in the hyperplastic palatal salivary glands.

stances, the glands are separated from the surface epithelium by a band of fibrous or fibroadipose tissue, but occasionally the glandular structures encroach on the surface. Inflammation is usually absent.

Adenomatoid hyperplasia should be distinguished histologically from neoplastic conditions. The former of these disorders shows normal cytologic and architectural features of mucous minor salivary glands. The pathogenesis of the hyperplasia is not known. It is a harmless condition and its proper identification is important merely to avoid misinterpretation as another process. It should be mentioned, however, that a case was reported in which a mucoepidermoid carcinoma developed 12 years after the diagnosis of adenomatoid hyperplasia of mucous glands (40). This association is, in the author's opinion, probably coincidental.

## Necrotizing Sialometaplasia

Necrotizing sialometaplasia (NSM) is a condition that predominantly affects the minor salivary glands, most commonly in the palate. This lesion can be easily misdiagnosed as a malignant neoplasm, both clinically and microscopically. The histologic hallmark of the condition is acinar necrosis and ductal squamous metaplasia. Local ischemia is

believed to play an etiologic role and the term "salivary gland infarction" has been used to describe NSM by some authors (42). Prior to its identification in 1973 (43), some cases of necrotizing sialometaplasia were treated as malignant tumors (usually thought to be squamous carcinomas) with aggressive surgery. This approach is now known to be contraindicated.

Necrotizing sialometaplasia may affect children as well as adults of various ages. However, the mean age of incidence is 45.5 years (44). Males are almost twice as commonly affected as females. The lesions occur predominantly in the palate, but they have been observed in other sites in the mouth, as well as extraoral locations in the upper aerodigestive tract (45,46) and in the major salivary glands (47). In the palate, NSM usually presents itself as a deep, crater-like ulcer, but it occasionally takes the form of a nonulcerating submucosal nodule (43). The ulcer is usually relatively small, measuring 1–3 cm in maximum dimension. Bilateral lesions may be encountered. Most cases are asymptomatic, although a few patients complain of numbness or a burning sensation. The lesions develop rapidly and heal spontaneously in a few weeks.

Microscopically, the salivary gland lobules in NSM show either complete or partial coagulative necrosis of the mucous

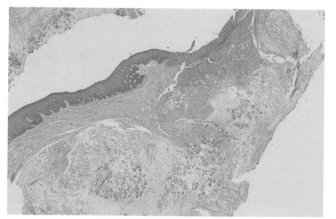
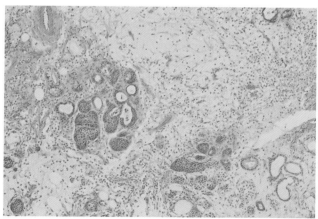

**FIG. 12.** Necrotizing sialometaplasia of the palate. **A, B:** Lobular distribution of acinar necrosis and squamous metaplasia of the ducts. **B, C:** Residual luminal spaces are seen in the squamous nests.

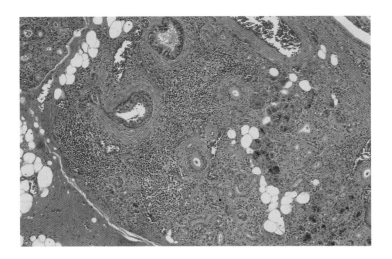

**FIG. 13.** Chronic sclerosing sialadenitis, or Kuttner's tumor, showing an inflammatory cell infiltrate and early periductal fibrosis.

acini. Squamous metaplasia of the ducts produces scattered squamous epithelial islands (Fig. 12). The intralobular septa commonly show degenerative changes. Acute inflammatory cells and foam cell macrophages are usually present. Pools of mucin occasionally form in the lobules. Granulation tissue is usually present near the base of the ulcerated epithelium. The metaplastic squamous cells may show reactive atypia, but their distribution generally follows the lobular architecture of the salivary glands. The squamoid nests may occasionally show residual luminal spaces as well (Fig. 12B, C). Mucous cells may be present within the squamous epithelial islands, potentially simulating the appearance of mucoepidermoid carcinoma. However, the lobular nature of the proliferation and the clinical history militate against a diagnosis of malignancy.

As stated above, an ischemic basis for necrotizing sialometaplasia is the most accepted etiology. This is supported by an inability to culture any specific microorganisms from the lesions, their appearance after surgical procedures, and experimental evidence (44,47–49).

As also indicated previously, NSM should be distinguished from neoplastic mucosal diseases, particularly squamous cell carcinoma and mucoepidermoid carcinoma, both of which show a predilection for the palate. In this regard, the presence of mucous acinar necrosis and the preservation of the overall lobular architecture are the most important features in separating NSM from the specified neoplastic conditions. Metaplastic squamous cells in NSM demonstrate no invasiveness into the surrounding structures. The squamoid islands are cytologically bland and may show residual ductal lumina. Once the lesions of NSM are properly diagnosed, there is no need for active intervention and they usually heal spontaneously in 5–6 weeks (44).

## Chronic Sclerosing Sialadenitis of the Submandibular Gland ("Kuttner's Tumor")

Chronic sclerosing sialadenitis (CSS) is a chronic inflammatory process that affects the submandibular gland and produces a large indurated mass that is indistinguishable from a neoplasm on clinical examination. The pathogenesis of this condition is believed to be related to salivary duct obstruction and subsequent ascending infection and/or an autoimmune response to the altered ductal epithelium (42,50). Roughly 50% of patients with CSS also have sialolithiasis

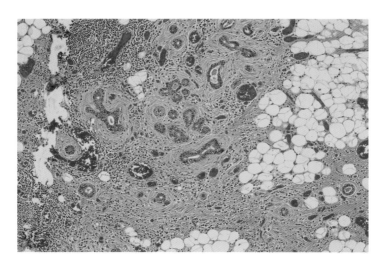

**FIG. 14.** Massive fibrosis and effacement of lobular architecture in advanced chronic sclerosing sialadenitis of the submandibular gland.

(42,52). The peak age of incidence is in the fourth and fifth decades, and males are more commonly affected. The diagnosis is usually histologically made after the gland has been removed for presumptive neoplasia.

Histologically, the disease is characterized by chronic inflammation and scarring. In its early stages only, a periductal lymphocytosis is present. The inflammatory cell infiltrate becomes more diffuse with time, concomitant with the appearance of periductal fibrosis (Fig. 13). In the late phase of the disease, massive fibrosis of the gland takes place and the lobular architecture is effaced (42,52) (Fig. 14), with marked loss of the secretory glandular parenchyma. Secondary lymphoid follicles with reactive germinal centers may appear as well (42,51,52). The distinction of Kuttner's tumor from myoepithelial sialadenitis (MESA) and inflammatory pseudotumor of the salivary glands is outlined below and in Table 2.

## Myoepithelial Sialadenitis (MESA)

MESA is a form of lymphocytic sialadenitis that exhibits characteristic metaplastic changes of the ductal epithelium and myoepithelial cells. This condition is also known as "benign lymphoepithelial lesion" (BLEL) of the salivary glands. MESA of the parotid gland is characteristically seen in Sjogren's syndrome, but it may also occur outside of that condition (53,54). The pathogenesis of sporadic MESA is not known. This condition was first reported by Johann Mikulicz in 1892 (55) in a 42-year-old man who presented with bilateral enlargement and firmness of the lacrimal glands and the major salivary glands. Unilateral parotid swelling due to MESA also may occur and may clinically resemble a neoplasm. Parotid BLEL is less likely to be misdiagnosed as another condition if it is associated with the clinical manifestations of Sjogren's syndrome. It is of importance to note that there is an increased risk for the development of primary salivary glandular lymphoma in association with MESA (56,57).

With or without Sjögren's syndrome, MESA commonly affects middle-aged women. Diffuse swelling and/or induration of the parotid gland and, less frequently, the submandibular gland represents the classical presentation of this disease, which may be unilateral or bilateral. The latter changes are usually painless but may be associated with slight tenderness in some cases. MESA shows a spectrum of microscopic alterations that parallel its clinical progression. Histologic changes range from focal lymphocytic infiltration with mild acinar atrophy and preservation of the lobular architecture in the early phases, to dense confluent lymphocytosis with formation of germinal centers and accompanying destruction of the glandular parenchyma in the later stages (Fig. 15). Damage to the glandular tissue is proportionate to the intensity of the lymphocytic infiltrate. Cyclical degeneration and reactive proliferation of salivary ducts results in the formation of characteristic "epimyoepithelial islands" (Fig. 15B). Apart from these structures, dilated ducts that are infiltrated with lymphocytes are present in the majority of cases (58,59). Some ducts also may show intraluminal calcifications. In addition to the typical lymphocytic infiltrate of MESA, which is composed of sheets of mature small lymphocytes with focal germinal centers, interspersed groups of monocytoid B cells also may be present. The latter cells have distinct borders and abundant, clear, or pale amphophilic cytoplasm, and clusters of them are found in the parafollicular and intrafollicular locations with a tendency to surround the epimyoepithelial islands (58,59).

The detection of malignant lymphoma superimposed on a background of fully developed MESA is not an easy task. In this setting, lymphomas are usually focal and histologically deceptive (57). A morphologic and immunologic continuum from areas of polyclonal reactive hyperplasia to monoclonal B-cell lymphoma has been documented in several cases of MESA (58,59). This progression from inflammatory to neoplastic disease implies that salivary gland lymphoma may be part of the spectrum of lymphomas arising in mucosa-asso-

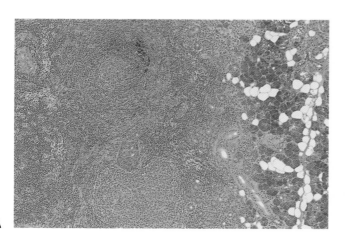 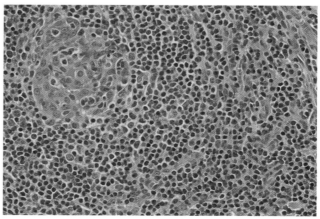

A                                                                                                          B

**FIG. 15.** Myoepithelial sialadenitis of the parotid gland, showing a dense and confluent lymphocytic infiltrate with germinal centers and epimyoepithelial islands. **A:** Remnants of the lobular parenchyma are seen on the right. **B:** Higher magnification of an epimyoepithelial island.

ciated lymphoid tissue (MALT). In further consonance with that supposition, salivary gland lymphomas are frequently monocytoid B cell in type (60,61). Confluence of "proliferation areas" of monocytoid B cells, when associated with nuclear atypia and a brisk mitotic rate, signals the onset of neoplastic change in this context (58,59).

Immunologic and molecular studies can be employed to verify the monoclonal lineage of lymphomas. Malignant lymphomas of salivary glands developing in association with MESA (including monocytoid B-cell lymphomas) are usually low grade and localized, and they are relatively indolent (58,60,61).

### Human Immunodeficiency Virus Infection–Associated Cystic Lymphoid Hyperplasia

Cystic lymphoid hyperplasia of the parotid gland accompanies the persistent generalized lymphadenopathy (PGL) phase of HIV infection. The salivary changes are analogous to those seen in MESA, but with more prominent dilatation and squamous metaplasia of the salivary ducts. Clinically, unilateral or bilateral enlargement of the affected gland occurs and may last for several months or longer (62,63). The

pathologic changes start in the intraglandular lymphoid tissue and in the paraparotid lymph nodes. Florid follicular hyperplasia is associated with squamous epithelial cysts filled with keratin (Fig. 16) and scattered epimyoepithelial islands (62–64). Immunoblastic hyperplasia may be so marked that it simulates malignant lymphoma. Again, special studies may be required to distinguish between these possibilities.

### Inflammatory Pseudotumor of the Salivary Glands

"Inflammatory pseudotumors "are interesting and enigmatic lesions that have been reported in virtually all organs and tissues in the body. These lesions have only recently been reported for the first time in the major salivary glands (65). The authors of the cited report reviewed six cases from the files of the Armed Forces Institute of Pathology (AFIP). The parotid was the site of the lesion in all cases. Males and females were equally affected and their ages ranged from 46 to 87 years with a mean age of 70 years. Clinically, the patients presented with a swelling of the parotid gland of several months duration. All of the lesions were treated surgically without subsequent recurrence (33).

Grossly, inflammatory pseudotumor of the parotid gland ranges from 1 to 2.7 cm in greatest dimension. It is lobulated,

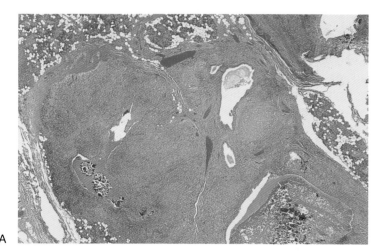

A

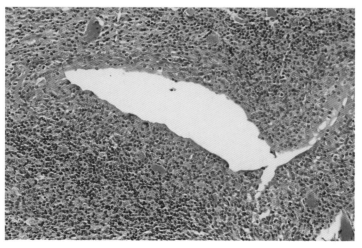

B

**FIG. 16. A:** Follicular hyperplasia of lymphoid tissue and squamous epithelial cysts seen in the parotid gland of a human immunodeficiency virus–positive patient. **B:** Higher magnification showing squamous epithelial lining within a solid lymphocytic infiltrate.

**TABLE 2.** *Comparison of inflammatory pseudoneoplastic lesions of the salivary glands*

| | Kuttner's tumor | MESA | Inflammatory pseudotumor |
|---|---|---|---|
| Site | Submandibular | Parotid > submandibular | Parotid |
| Age in decades | 5–6 | 6–7 | 7–8 |
| Sex | M > F | F > M | M = F |
| Histologic features | Periductal lymphocytic infiltrate, progressive scarring | Diffuse lymphocytes with myoepithelial islands | Circumscribed fibrohistiocytic proliferation with plasma cells |

MESA, myoepithelial sialadenitis.

yellow–gray–tan, firm, and nodular. The lesion tends to be circumscribed but not encapsulated. All except one of these masses have been confined within the parotid capsule (65).

Microscopically, the lesion is composed of multiple confluent nodules. The predominant cells are round or spindle-shaped with morphologic appearances like those of histiocytes or myofibroblasts. The spindle cells are haphazardly arranged in poorly formed fascicles or vaguely storiform configurations (Fig. 17). The nuclear chromatin of the cells is fine and evenly distributed. No nuclear atypia is noted and mitotic activity is inconspicuous. Lymphocytic and plasmocytic infiltrates are usually dense, with a plasma cell predominance. The latter feature is characteristic of many inflammatory pseudotumors in general, and the term "plasma cell granuloma" is sometimes used synonymously. Occasional eosinophils and neutrophils are seen as well in some cases. Focal aggregates of foamy cell macrophages may also be present in some lesions. Vascularity is not conspicuous and extracellular collagen is scant. Increased fibrosis may be evident as the lesion progresses (65).

Immunohistochemical staining of the lesions discloses a biphasic cell population composed of myofibroblasts and histiocytes with variable staining for CD68, smooth muscle actin, muscle-specific actin, and vimentin (65).

Because of histologic similarities between inflammatory pseudotumors and fibrous histiocytomas, it has been suggested that the lesions are related and that inflammatory pseudotumor might be a low-grade fibrohistiocytic tumor that has elicited a marked lymphoplasmocytic reaction (66). The term "inflammatory fibrohistiocytic proliferation" has

been proposed (67) to replace the conventional designations of inflammatory pseudotumor or plasma cell granuloma.

Inflammatory pseudotumor should be distinguished from chronic sclerosing sialadenitis and myoepithelial sialadenitis. Chronic sclerosing sialadenitis (Kuttner's tumor) is much more likely to be seen in the submandibular gland in association with sialolithiasis. Histologically, that condition is characterized by progressive periductal lymphocytic infiltrates and scarring, which can eventually lead to diffuse parenchymal destruction. In contrast, inflammatory pseudotumor is a localized, well-defined fibrohistiocytic proliferation with abundant plasma cells. A comparison of the clinicopathologic features of inflammatory pseudotumor, chronic sclerosing sialadenitis, and MESA is presented in Table 2.

## Oncocytosis and Oncocytic Nodular Hyperplasia

The term "oncocytosis" is used to indicate multifocal oncocytic metaplasia (and occasionally hyperplasia) in the salivary glands. Glandular swelling may accompany florid oncocytosis, suggesting the presence of a neoplasm and prompting an incisional or excisional biopsy. However, the majority of examples of oncocytosis are secondary or incidental findings seen in specimens removed for other reasons. About 60% of cases of oncocytosis in the AFIP files were associated with well-defined salivary tumors, including oncocytoma, Warthin's tumor, pleomorphic adenoma, and acinic cell carcinoma (68).

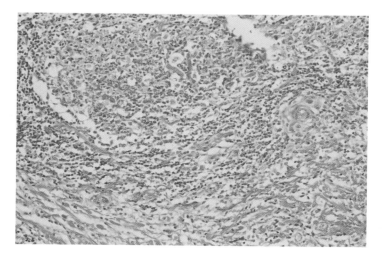

**FIG. 17.** Inflammatory pseudotumor of the parotid gland. Irregular fascicles of spindle cells are admixed with a diffuse inflammatory cell infiltrate. Some fibrosis is also evident. (Courtesy of Dr. Doug Gnepp, Department of Pathology, Rhode Island Hospital, Providence, RI.)

In a review of 3500 salivary tumors submitted to the British Salivary Gland Tumor Panel, Palmer et al. (69) identified 26 cases that were either oncocytomas or benign lesions showing extensive oncocytic changes. Five of these were characterized as examples of oncocytosis, three were multinodular oncocytic hyperplasia, and two showed diffuse oncocytosis. In an additional four cases, multinodular oncocytic hyperplasia was associated with overt oncocytoma.

Clinically, the patients' ages at the time of diagnosis ranged from 28 to 87 years (42,68,69). Males and females were affected equally. However, in another study all of the patients were female (42). The parotid gland is the most common site (42,68,69). The submandibular gland and the minor glands of the mouth are much less frequently affected.

Microscopically, oncocytosis may be represented by scattered foci of enlarged polygonal cells with eosinophilic granular cytoplasm and centrally placed nuclei. The cells may form ductal and acinar structures or sheets and trabeculae. Fine fibrous septa may separate clusters of cells. The overall lobular architecture of the gland is preserved. Rarely, complete oncocytic metaplasia of the lobules produces the diffuse pattern of oncocytosis involving ducts and acini (42,69,70). Clear cell changes are not uncommon in oncocytosis (Fig. 18) and are believed to be due to the accumulation of intracytoplasmic glycogen (71). Oncocytes stain positively with phosphotungstic acid hematoxylin (PTAH). Ultrastructurally, the cytoplasm of such cells is packed with pleomorphic mitochondria that have vesicular and aberrant cristae (68).

Oncocytoma can be distinguished from oncocytosis because it is a well-defined, solitary, commonly encapsulated neoplasm. In contrast, oncocytosis is a multifocal, metaplastic change that does not disrupt the lobular architecture of the glandular parenchyma.

The term "nodular oncocytosis" or "nodular oncocytic hyperplasia" refers to two or more tumor-like nodules that

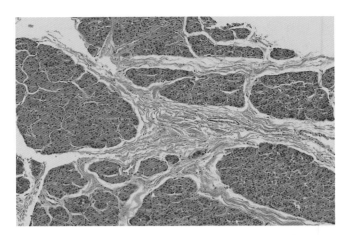

**FIG. 19.** Nodular oncocytic hyperplasia. Hyperplastic oncocytes form tumor-like multinodular structures.

show hyperplasia of metaplastic oncocytes (42,69) (Fig. 19). It has been suggested that oncocytomas may develop from some examples of nodular oncocytic hyperplasia by progressive enlargement of the latter (42,69–71). The presence of focal ductal and acinar oncocytic metaplasia in other parts of the glands in addition to the occasional presence of normal acini at the periphery of the large nodules in oncocytic nodular hyperplasia may be useful in distinguishing this lesion from true oncocytoma (69).

The multiple scattered clear cell foci that are seen occasionally in cases of oncocytosis (Fig. 18) can lead to an erroneous diagnosis of metastatic clear cell carcinoma, most notably of renal origin. In contradistinction to metastatic neoplastic disease, oncocytosis lacks an invasive growth pattern and typical eosinophilic oncocytes are commonly present. The clear cell groups of metastatic renal cell carcinoma demonstrate more cellular and nuclear pleomorphism and show more prominent vascularity. If this distinction is difficult, it may be prudent to evaluate the kidneys radiographically.

### Salivary Gland Hamartoma of the Nasopharynx (Salivary Gland Anlage Tumor; "Congenital Pleomorphic Adenoma")

Salivary gland hamartoma of the nasopharynx is a recently defined lesion that affects newborn infants (72). It presents as a polypoid mass that measures up to 3 cm in diameter. Respiratory distress at birth or within the first few days of life is a common manifestation. Of nine cases reviewed (72), seven of the infants were males. The masses were attached to the posterior pharyngeal wall at the midline by a delicate pedicle.

Microscopically, the mucosal surface of the lesion is composed of nonkeratinizing stratified squamous epithelium with focal projections of squamous nests and duct-like structures extending into an underlying myxedematous superficial spindle cell stroma (Fig. 20A, B). This zone is interposed between the mucosal surface and more central densely

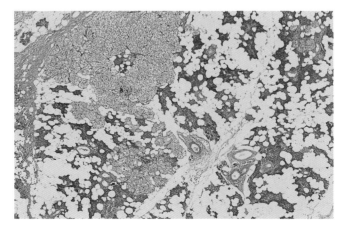

**FIG. 18.** Parotid gland showing oncocytosis with clear cell changes. The overall lobular architecture of the gland is preserved.

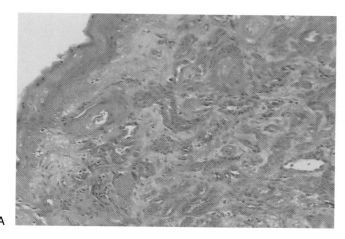

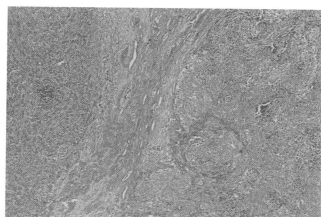

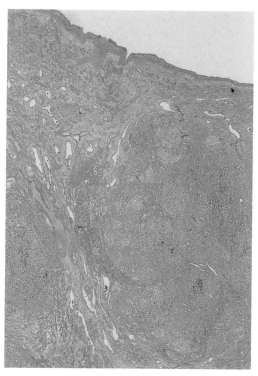

**FIG. 20.** Salivary gland hamartoma. **A:** Squamous nests and duct-like structures extend from the squamous epithelial surface into superficial myxoid stroma. **B:** Densely cellular deeper stromal nodules composed of spindle cells. **C:** Duct-like structures are present between deep stromal nodules.

cellular stromal nodules that are composed of spindle cells. The latter contain duct-like structures and keratinizing and nonkeratinizing epithelial nests (Fig. 20B, C).

Immunohistochemical staining shows reactivity for cytokeratin and epithelial membrane antigen in the peripheral epithelial components. The cells of the central stromal nodules show variable immunoreactivity for cytokeratin, vimentin, and muscle-specific actin. Both components are reactive for salivary gland amylase. The histologic and immunophenotypic features of the proliferation are similar in some respects to those of developing salivary gland.

The hamartomatous nature of this congenital salivary lesion is suggested by its limited growth potential, location in the midline, and histologic similarity to salivary anlage. There is, however, some histologic similarity to pleomorphic adenoma as well. The latter is extremely rare as a congenital lesion in the midline of the nasopharynx. Growth of epithelial buds from the surface mucosa is not observed in pleomorphic adenomas. On the other hand, salivary gland hamartoma lacks the chondroid or myxoid stroma that is commonly present in mixed tumors. Teratomas can present very early in life, often as a mass that is apparent at birth. Nevertheless, they are composed of complex mixtures of mature and immature tissue, notably neuroepithelium, cartilage, respiratory epithelium, and enteric elements (72,73).

"Sialoblastoma" is another congenital salivary gland tumor (74,75). It presents at birth as a very large mass occurring exclusively in the parotid gland and shows a rapid growth rate. Microscopically, this lesion is composed predominantly of solid epithelial nests. The cells are large and polygonal with hyperchromatic nuclei and one or two prominent nucleoli. Mitotic activity may be brisk.

The duality of salivary gland hamartoma of the nasopharynx, with epithelial and spindle cell components, may recall the biphasic histology of synovial sarcoma, which is known to occur in the head and neck (76). Synovial sarcoma is, however, extremely rare as a congenital lesion. Budding of epithelium from the mucosa, as seen in salivary gland hamartoma, is not observed in synovial sarcoma. Moreover, the spindle cells in synovial sarcoma are arranged in fascicles rather than nodules.

## PSEUDOTUMORS OF THE SINONASAL TRACT AND LARYNX

### Cerebral Heterotopia (Nasal Glioma) and Encephalocele

The term "glial heterotopia" has been used to indicate the presence of cerebral tissue outside the cranium. When the heterotopic tissue maintains its connection to the brain, the condition is known as an encephalocele. Distinction between these two pathologic entities is of the utmost importance because of the risk of an infected encephalocele producing secondary meningitis (77). Herniation of brain tissue outside the cranium exists in three anatomic locations (78), occipital (accounting for 75% of the cases), sincipital, and basal. Basal lesions present as masses in the nasal cavity, paranasal sinuses, pharynx, or palate. Both occipital and sincipital forms may be visible externally, the former at the back of the skull in the suboccipital area and the latter on the bridge of the nose and glabella. In 15–20% of cases of cerebral heterotopia, the closure of cranial sutures is incomplete and a fibrous or glial connection persists (79). These cases are difficult to distinguish from true encephaloceles.

The term "nasal glioma" has, in the past, been used inaccurately to describe cerebral heterotopia in the nose. The neoplastic implication of the term is erroneous. Most of these lesions only exhibit a growth rate that is commensurate with that of surrounding host tissue (80). They are congenital and are usually discovered during the first few years of life, although cases detected in adults have been reported (81). The condition is more common in males by a ratio of 3:1 (82). Nasal cerebral heterotopia is not usually associated with other developmental malformations, whereas true encephaloceles do show such linkage in 30% of cases. Two thirds of cases of glial heterotopia are located outside the nasal cavity. Some examples have both intranasal and extranasal components (83). Extranasal lesions usually present as smooth, nonpulsatile subcutaneous masses on either side of the nasal bridge. The overlying skin may acquire a bluish or red discoloration (84). Intranasal lesions may fill one side of the nose and may cause septal deviation. The attachment of the masses is usually high on the lateral wall of the nose in the region of the middle turbinate. They are firm and non-pulsatile and do not transilluminate (84). The surface mucosa is glistening and may be red, yellow, or gray. Other clinical findings are variable but may include respiratory obstruction, epistaxis, anosmia, or cosmetic facial deformity (84).

True nasal encephaloceles usually manifest as soft pulsatile masses that can be transilluminated. The patients may additionally present with meningitis or cerebrospinal rhinorrhea. When intranasal encephaloceles are mistaken for nasal polyps and surgically removed, the clinical outcome can be disastrous.

Microscopically, cerebral heterotopia shows large aggregates or small islands of glial tissue that is composed of astrocytes and fine fibrillary material, scattered haphazardly in fibrovascular connective tissue (Fig. 21). No capsule or plane of demarcation is evident and the glial tissue may extend to the nasal mucosal surface and may be interspersed with mucous glands in the submucosa (Fig. 21A). The astrocytes are usually evenly spaced and may be multinucleated. Their nuclei are usually enlarged (Fig. 21B). Mitosis is usually not detectable and, if present, it may be a consequence of ischemia or inflammation. Rarely, oligodendroglial cells and ependyma may be found (85). Neurons are present in a minority of cases and usually are sparse. Their identification may require special studies (86). Immunohistochemical

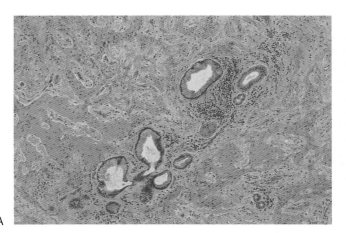
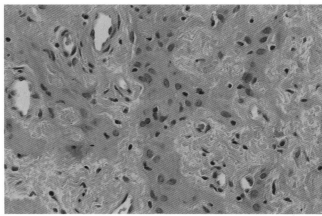

A                                                                                                                                B

**FIG. 21.** Cerebral heterotopia of the nose. **A:** Nests and strands of glial tissue composed of astrocytes and fine fibrillary material scattered in fibrovascular connective tissue and between mucoserous glands of the nose. **B:** Higher magnification showing astrocytic cells in fibrillary material.

stains for glial fibrillary acidic protein (GFAP) and neuron-specific enolase (NSE) are used for the delineation of astrocytes and neurons, respectively. PTAH stains could also be used to identify glial tissue in collagenized stroma. Because of the occasional presence of neurons as well as glia, the term "cerebral" has been preferred to glial in describing the heterotopia.

The admixture of glial tissue with normal mucous glands of the nose and its presence in abundant collagenous fibrovascular stroma distinguish central neural heterotopia from true encephalocele (84). In the latter condition, the brain tissue is devoid of extraneous components. The neural tissue in encephalocele shows various degrees of organization (87); dura and leptomeninges may be recognizable. The histologic distinction between heterotopia and true encephalocele is not always possible. Ideally, microscopic examination should not be used as the primary means of achieving this goal. It is essential that clinical and radiographic information should also be garnered prior to any attempt at corrective surgical intervention. The presence of mature neural tissue in a sinonasal biopsy, particularly in a child, should also raise the possibility of a teratoma, in which case thorough sampling of the specimen will show tissue from other germ layers (87).

## Antrochoanal Polyps

Antrochoanal polyps are nonneoplastic inflammatory lesions of the upper respiratory tract. The majority are large, solitary, unilateral polyps that arise from the maxillary sinus, usually on the posterior, inferior, medial, or lateral walls. They extend in an hourglass fashion through the ostium of the sinus into the middle nasal meatus and then through the choana into the nasopharynx (88,89). Polyps arising from the sphenoid or ethmoid sinuses are rare (90). Antrochoanal polyps may be large enough to fill the entire nasopharynx and extend below the soft palate into the oropharynx (90). They are more common in males, usually between the ages

of 10 and 39 years (91). A minority of the patients have an atopic background. Twenty-five percent show multicompartmental sinusitis (90). In general, only 3–6% of adult patients are found to have synchronous, conventional nasal polyps at the time of diagnosis (92,93). Some series, however, have found a higher incidence of this association [as much as 22.3% (91) in selected studies]. In the pediatric population (94), up to 28% of children with antrochoanal polyps also have conventional nasal polyps.

Typically, the condition presents clinically with a unilateral nasal obstruction and a mass. Radiographic examination shows a posterior choanal and nasopharyngeal soft tissue density, associated with unilateral mucosal thickening and partial opacification of the antrum. There is no erosion or destruction of contiguous bone. The anterior bowing of the posterior wall of the maxillary sinus that is so characteristic of nasopharyngeal angiofibroma is not evident. On gross examination, antrochoanal polyps have smooth shiny surfaces and are nonlobulated.

Microscopically, these lesions resemble common nasal polyps, with well-vascularized edematous stroma and scattered inflammatory cells (Fig. 22). Unlike classical polyps of the nose, however, antrochoanal polyps lack marked tissue eosinophilia, and entrapped mucous glands are uncommon. Due to their configurations and anatomic relationships, antrochoanal polyps, particularly longstanding ones, are vulnerable to vascular compromise (90). Compression of the vascular supply of the polyp may lead to vascular dilatation, stasis, edema, infarction, neovascularization, and, eventually, stromal fibrosis and scarring. Excessively vascularized polyps are termed "angiomatous polyps" (90,95). These can be confused radiologically and pathologically with angiofibroma (95). Reactive stromal cell atypia, which may erroneously give the impression of a sarcoma, is often evident in angiomatous polyps (90,96).

As just mentioned, antrochoanal polyps bear considerable clinical and microscopic resemblance to nasopharyngeal angiofibromas. Like the latter lesions, antrochoanal polyps may present as polypoid nasopharyngeal masses in adoles-

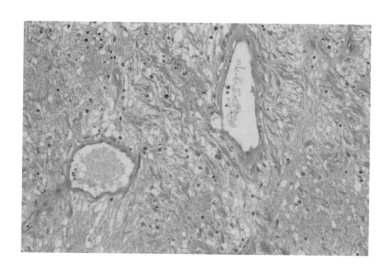

**FIG. 22.** Antrachoanal polyp composed of well-vascularized edematous stroma and scattered inflammatory cells.

cent males. However, antrochoanal polyps rarely cause significant epistaxis or distortion of the posterior wall of the maxillary sinus on radiographic examination. Their external surfaces are smooth, shiny, and typically free of nodularity, whereas those of angiofibroma are commonly coarsely nodular. On microscopic examination, fibrosed polyps, in contrast to angiofibromas, are less vascular. The former may contain mucous glands and inflammatory cells, even in the absence of ulceration. In angiofibromas, inflammation is usually limited to zones near the mucosal surface in association with epithelial disintegrity. The vessels in polyps are not gaping and do not show a staghorn appearance. They tend to have more muscular walls of uniform thickness. In contrast, blood vessels in angiofibroma are commonly devoid of smooth muscle or show walls those are irregular in thickness with characteristic pad-like thickening (97). The stromata of angiofibromas are more cellular than those of fibrous polyps. They contain coarse and thin bundles of collagen fibers and are rarely myxoid. Constituent cells are plump and may be stellate in shape.

### Stromal Cell Atypia in Nasal Polyps and in Vocal Cord Nodules

The microscopic appearance of the majority of nasal polyps, including antrochoanal polyps, is typically bland and banal. Essentially, they show edematous connective tissue, telangiectatic blood vessels, and inflammatory cells. On occasion, however, the mesenchymal stromal cells show reactive morphologic alterations that could be misinterpreted as malignant in character. These changes have been variously called mesenchymal cell atypia, stromal atypia, and pseudosarcomatous change (98–101). Stromal cell atypia is believed to occur in inflammatory polyps that are subject to vascular compromise and secondary degeneration, as well as necrosis and neovascularization (101). Nonetheless, these lesions are usually clinically and grossly indistinguishable from usual sinonasal polyps, and this statement also pertains to their low-power microscopic images. However, on closer inspection, atypical cells are seen distributed unevenly in the edematous stroma. They are large and may be strikingly pleomorphic, rounded, spindle-shaped, or stellate with dark nuclei and prominent nucleoli (Fig. 23). Some cells contain two or more nuclei. Very few mitotic figures are seen (102). The cytoplasm varies from eosinophilic to amphophilic and is coarsely vacuolated or foamy in appearance (101,102). Immunohistochemical and electron microscopic analysis of the atypical cells has suggested fibrohistiocytic differentiation (102).

The clinical presentation and gross appearance of the lesions, in addition to the focal nature of the atypical cells, should allow for a proper interpretation. A malignant diagnosis may be wrongly entertained if only selected fields are examined under high-power magnification (99,101).

Stromal cell atypia is also seen—but much less frequently—in laryngeal polyps (103,104). Clinically, these are

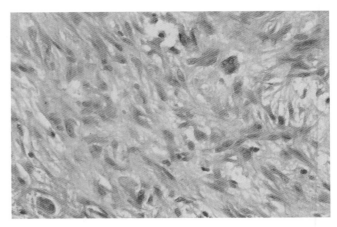

**FIG. 23.** Nasal polyp with stromal cell atypia, showing large pleomorphic cells with hyperchromatic nuclei.

indistinguishable from usual true vocal cord nodules. However, pathologists who are not familiar with the occurrence of stromal atypia in benign laryngeal nodules may confuse such lesions with polypoid malignant neoplasms of the larynx. In particular, botryoid rhabdomyosarcoma and spindle cell carcinoma are potential misinterpretations in this context. The absence of surface epithelial dysplasia, carcinoma in situ, or invasive squamous cell carcinoma distinguishes stromal atypia from spindle cell carcinoma. Similarly, rhabdomyosarcoma shows a density of overtly atypical cells with marked mitotic activity and a roughly lamellar disposition under the surface epithelium that yields a characteristic "cambium layer." In selected instances, immunostains may be necessary to address these differential diagnoses. Such studies demonstrate reactivity for keratin in spindle cell carcinoma and positivity for desmon in rhabdomyosarcoma, whereas neither of these determinants is expected in atypical laryngeal polyps.

As in the case of usual vocal cord nodules, those with stromal atypia are adequately treated by simple excision.

### Contact Ulcers of the Larynx

Contact ulcers of the larynx (CULs) are exophytic ulcerated lesions that usually affect the posterior surface of the larynx. They are believed to be caused by mechanical, chemical, or traumatic injury. Vocal abuse, persistent coughing, acidic reflux, and prior endotracheal intubation represent recognized etiologic factors (105–107). CULs occur in adults, more commonly in males. However, post-intubation contact ulcers are—for unknown reasons—more likely to be seen in females (106,107).

Presenting symptoms are variable, the most frequent of which is hoarseness. Other manifestations include dysphagia, dysphonia, choking, and pain. The duration of symptoms varies widely, from weeks to years. Laryngoscopic examination reveals small ulcerated nodular or polypoid le-

**TABLE 2.** *Summary of clinical and pathologic features of inflammatory pseudotumors of the lung*

| | Bahadori and Liebow (1973) | Spencer (1984) | Matsubara et al. (1987) | Pettinato et al. (1990) |
|---|---|---|---|---|
| Number of cases | 40 | 27 | 32 | 19[a] |
| Mean age (y) | 29 | 36 | 50 | 27 |
| Age range (y) | 1–68 | 4–76 | 2–77 | 2–72 |
| Male/female | 15:25 | 16:11 | 14:15 | 9:10 |
| Symptoms present (%) | 40 | 56 | 40 | 60 |
| Previous respiratory infection (%) | 5 | 37 | 25 | 21 |
| Right/left lung | 21/18 | 13/12 | 9/18 | 1/19 |
| Size (cm) | 0.8–1.2 | ND | 1–15 | 1.2–15 |
| Follow-up: | | | | |
|   Well (%) | 90 | ND | 100 | 91 |
|   Recurrence (%) | 5 | ND | 7 | 9 |

ND; not described.

[a] Original reports described 20 cases, but 1 case was of esophageal origin.

tion. Occasionally, they may assume the form of sessile intrabronchial lesions; they may also extend through the pleura or along bronchi to involve the mediastinal soft tissue (28,35,36) or the thoracic vertebrae (37).

### Histopathologic Characteristics

"Typical" pulmonary IPT is a discrete lesion in which the microscopic architecture of the lung has been destroyed and replaced, to a variable extent, by inflammatory cells and a (myo-)fibroblastic proliferation. The histologic appearance of the lesion demonstrates a considerable spectrum, with variations in the number of plasma cells, lymphocytes, fibroblasts and myofibroblasts, macrophages, foam cells, and other leukocytes. Depending on the dominant cellular constituents and the major growth pattern, IPTs have been classified into three broad types (30). These include the "orga-

nizing pneumonia," "fibrous histiocytoma," and "lymphoplasmocytic" variants of the lesion. They may well simply represent different stages in the evolution or progression of IPT, when defined in a generic sense.

The "organizing pneumonia-like" form of IPT is characterized by intraalveolar lymphohistiocytic inflammation and peripheral fibrosis (Figs. 5–7), as well as a central fibrous zone (Fig. 8). Fibroblasts proliferate into areas of fibrinoinflammatory exudate in alveoli, alveolar ducts, and bronchioles, and gradually replace them (Fig. 9). The alveolar architecture in early lesions (as well as the peripheral aspects of more well-developed IPTs) is preserved, but it is obscured by superimposed fibrous tissue with a whorled configuration (Fig. 10). Intact alveolar walls are always the most discernible at the "advancing edge" of the mass (Fig. 11). Neutrophils, which are sometimes admixed with lymphocytes and plasma cells, may form microabscesses in the central ar-

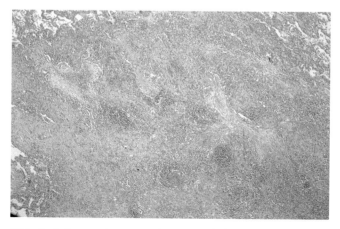

**FIG. 5.** Inflammatory pseudotumor of the lung, organizing pneumonia type. The periphery demonstrates intraalveolar lymphohistiocytic infiltration and fibrosis.

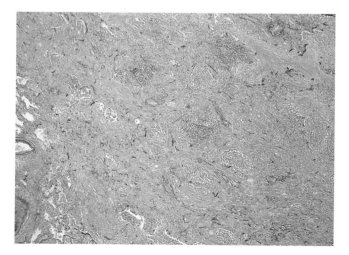

**FIG. 6.** An elastic van Gieson stain demonstrates prominent intraalveolar fibrosis.

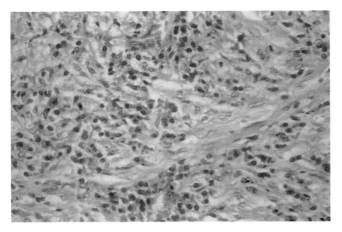

**FIG. 7.** High-power examination shows an infiltrate of lymphocytes, plasma cells, histiocytes, and fibroblasts in this lesion.

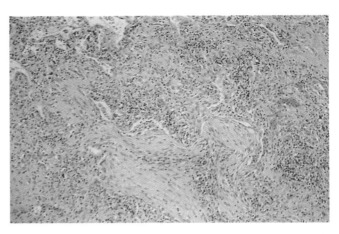

**FIG. 9.** High-power view of the lesion in Fig. 5. Organizing fibroblastic tissue proliferates within alveoli, alveolar ducts, and bronchioles.

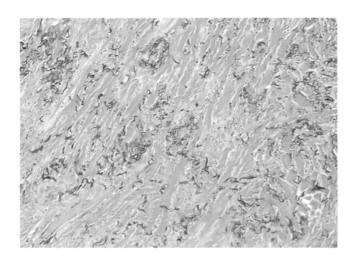

**FIG. 8.** This example of pulmonary inflammatory pseudotumor demonstrates marked central scirrhous reaction.

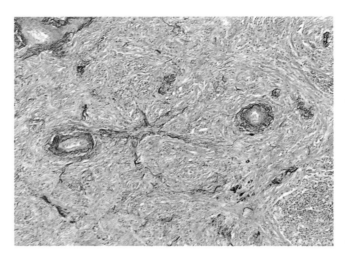

**FIG. 10.** Although partially preserved, alveolar structures in this inflammatory pseudotumor are becoming obscured by intraalveolar plugs of fibrous tissue (elastic van Gieson).

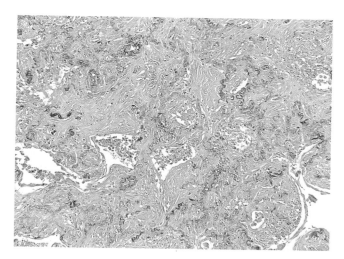

**FIG. 11.** Branching plugs of fibrous tissue fill a bronchiole and alveolar ducts in this lesion (elastic van Gieson).

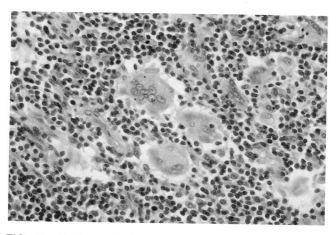

**FIG. 13.** Multinucleated giant cells, of the Touton type, are present in a dense infiltrate of chronic inflammatory cells in this inflammatory pseudotumor.

eas and peripheral portions of the lesions (Fig. 12). This may result in small foci of cavitation. The alveoli surrounding the lesion are filled with foamy macrophages and lined by hyperplastic pneumocytes. Multinucleated cells of the Touton type are sometimes apparent (Fig. 13), as are foci of dystrophic calcification, osteoid metaplasia, and myxomatous change (Fig. 14). Purulent and granulomatous inflammation suggestive of active infectious pneumonitis are not part of the typical morphotype of IPT, but lipoid pneumonia may develop distal to points of bronchial obstruction in cases where the lesion has filled a major airway. Late in the evolution of IPTs and in their central aspects, alveolar architecture tends to be effaced and the parenchyma is replaced by mature collagen. This matrical component may be present in broad bundles that transect the lesion, and it may assume a keloidal appearance as well (Fig. 15).

The "fibrous histiocytoma" variant of pulmonary IPT is characterized by the proliferation of spindle cells that are arranged in whorls, interlacing fascicles, and storiform patterns (Figs. 16 and 17). The nuclei of the fusiform cells contain dispersed chromatin that is only occasionally hyperdense; mitoses are generally rare or absent altogether. The lesional stroma is again collagenous, but its density is variable. In some cases, matrical collagen may be confluent, yielding the configuration of a discrete "scar" (Fig. 18).

In the "lymphoplasmocytic" subtype of IPT, plasma cells and lymphocytes comprise the majority of the lesion (Fig. 19). Aggregates of lymphoid cells may become confluent, and large germinal centers can be seen therein (Figs. 20 and 21). On the other hand, fibroblasts and xanthoma cells are usually inconspicuous. Lymphocytes, plasma cells, macrophages, and collections of neutrophils infiltrate around bronchioles and may fill alveolar septae at the advancing edge of the lesion (Figs. 22 and 23).

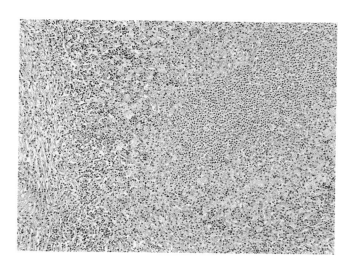

**FIG. 12.** Microabscess within a pulmonary inflammatory pseudotumor.

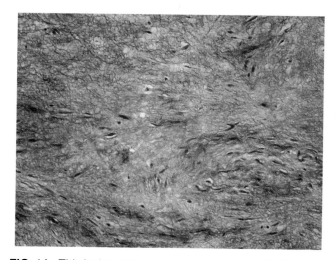

**FIG. 14.** This lesion demonstrates marked myxoid change in the stroma.

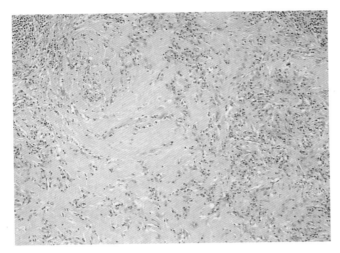

**FIG. 15.** Central hyalinization is present in this pulmonary pseudotumor.

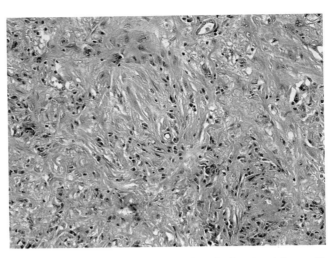

**FIG. 17.** Spindle-shaped cells in interlacing fascicles, with admixed plasma cells and histiocytes.

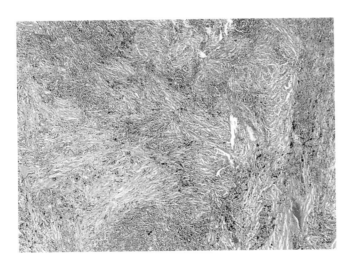

**FIG. 16.** Pulmonary inflammatory pseudotumor, of the "fibrous histiocytoma type." Spindle-shaped cells are arranged in interlacing fascicles, with a partial storiform pattern.

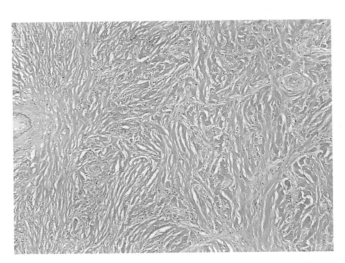

**FIG. 18.** This example of inflammatory pseudotumor demonstrates thick collagen bundles, in a swirling or storiform pattern.

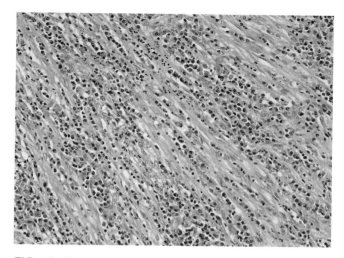

**FIG. 19.** Pulmonary inflammatory pseudotumor of the "lymphoplasmocytic type." Plasma cells and lymphocytes compose the majority of this proliferation.

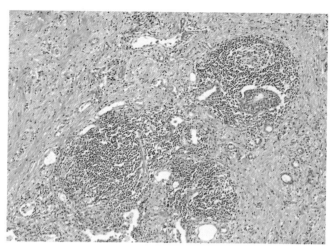

**FIG. 21.** This example of inflammatory pseudotumor demonstrates confluent lymphoid aggregates, without any evidence of lymphocyte atypia.

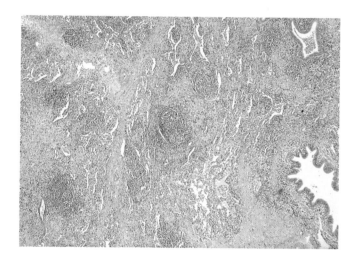

**FIG. 20.** A low-power view demonstrates lymphoid aggregates in this lymphohistiocytic pseudotumor.

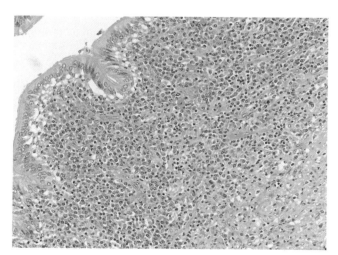

**FIG. 22.** Plasma cells and lymphocytes infiltrate a bronchial wall.

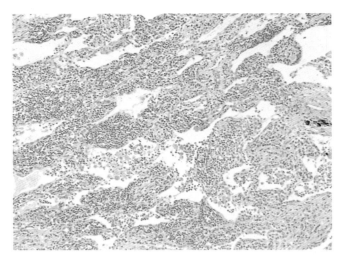

FIG. 23. Lymphoid cells expand alveolar septa at the periphery of this pulmonary pseudotumor.

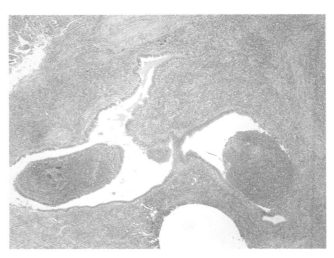

FIG. 25. An example of endobronchial growth in a pulmonary inflammatory pseudotumor.

The three histologic variants of IPT cited above often overlap, and it is therefore relatively uncommon to find absolutely "pure" examples of any one of them. None is composed of solid sheets of lymphocytes or plasma cells, thus tending to obviate confusion with lymphoma or plasmacytoma of the lung. It has been well documented that IPT of the lung may permeate into the lumina of bronchi or pulmonary blood vessels (Fig. 24), and roughly 10% demonstrate endobronchial growth (Fig. 25). Vascular inflammation—potentially simulating that seen in angiocentric immunoproliferative lesions—is observed at least focally in 50–75% of cases (30,38) (Fig. 26). Matsubara et al. (30) found lymphocytic infiltration and scarring of vascular walls in several examples, often in association with organizing thrombi. As implied above, these vascular changes are thought to be sec-

ondary rather than a reflection of a primary vasculitic process or a neoplastic infiltrate.

Electron microscopy of pulmonary IPT has shown a polymorphous cellular population, composed of fibroblasts, myofibroblasts, pericytes, endothelial cells, lymphocytes, plasma cells, macrophages, and primitive mesenchymal cells with few distinguishing cytoplasmic organelles (1,39–47). Microorganisms are not found. Tomita et al. (48) reported a single case of a well-circumscribed intrapulmonary IPT measuring 4 cm in diameter. Ultrastructural attributes of this lesion were such that the author felt that endothelial cells of intratumoral blood vessels arose in continuity from more nondescript spindle cells that were as-

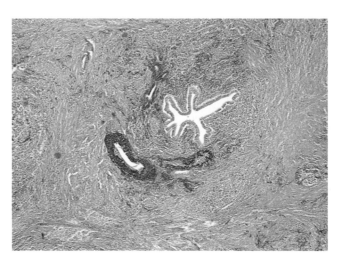

FIG. 24. A bronchiole and blood vessel are invaded by fibrosis and an inflammatory infiltrate.

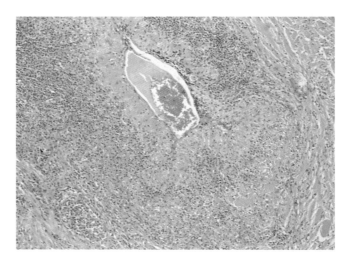

FIG. 26. A typical vascular lesion in pulmonary inflammatory pseudotumor, with lymphocytic infiltration, fibrous scarring, and narrowing of the lumen. Such a process may mimic angiocentric immunoproliferative lesions.

sociated with inflammatory cell aggregates. Those authors proposed the term "sclerosing vascular plasma cell granuloma" to encompass such observations, which have not been reproduced by other investigators to date.

Immunohistologic evaluations of pulmonary IPT have revealed reactivity for vimentin, smooth muscle actin isoforms, and desmin within the spindle cells of the lesion (1,32,38,45,47,49,50) (Fig. 27), supporting the contention that these represent fibroblasts and myofibroblasts. "Histiocytic" markers such as CD68 are also present in a minority of intralesional cells. Both kappa and lambda light chain immunoglobulins (LCIs) are detectable in the plasma cells, supporting a polytypic population (1,32,38); lymphocyte subset markers likewise demonstrate an admixture of B cells and T cells. Mutant p53 protein has not been detected in pulmonary IPT to date, as it has in a variety of carcinomas of the lung.

## Etiologic Considerations

The etiologic factors underlying the development of IPT of the lung are presently unknown. As stated above, this lesion is generally felt to be nonneoplastic and of a probable inflammatory "reactive" origin. This premise is bolstered by the pattern of intraalveolar organization and polymorphous inflammation seen in IPT at a microscopic level, and it also has support from the commonly obtained history of a previous febrile illness, with respiratory complaints, which is attached to many cases. Moreover, the lack of atypia in constituent cells, the polyclonality of infiltrating hematopoietic elements, and the indolent, generally static clinical nature of the lesions represent additionally corroborating pathogenetic information.

Occasional cases have resolved completely after nonexcisional biopsies or treatment with corticosteroids; these features are much more consistent with an inflammatory process than with a neoplasm. Previous respiratory infections have been recorded in 5–37% of cases, as shown in Table 2. Some case reports on IPT have suggested that there is an overlap in appearance between that lesion and tumefactive pulmonary infections with *Aspergillus* (51), *Rickettsia* (52,53), *Mycoplasma* (54), various viruses (55), *Mycobacterium* (56,57), *Cryptococcus* (58), *Corynebacterium* (59), and other microorganisms (60). Ozaki et al. (61) found that the number of neutrophils and levels of neutrophil-related chemotactic activity were markedly increased in bronchoalveolar lavage fluid taken from patients with pulmonary IPT. These observations also suggest that the latter condition is basically a chronic inflammatory process. Finally, rare examples have been documented after trauma to the lung (62).

As alluded to earlier, some physicians believe that IPT of the lung is in fact neoplastic. In a few instances it has exhibited aggressive biological behavior with infiltration of adjacent bones, soft tissues, blood vessels, and other vital structures (28,35,37,45,63,64). In addition to this uncommon manifestation of the disease, a limited potential for recurrence and a histologic resemblance between some forms of IPT and fibrous histiocytomas represent supplementary evidence for a possible neoplastic etiology. However, this may simply reflect our imperfect ability to separate inflammatory conditions that mimic true neoplasms from the latter proliferations themselves.

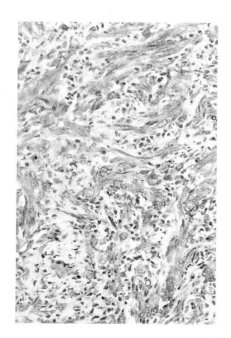 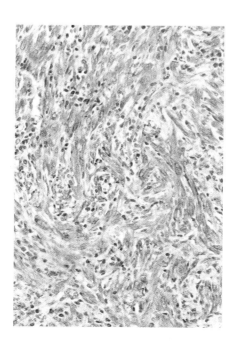

**FIG. 27.** Pulmonary inflammatory pseudotumor, demonstrating conjoint immunoreactivity for vimentin *(left)* and smooth muscle actin *(right)* (avidin-biotin-peroxidase complex technique). Such findings are in keeping with a myofibroblastic process.

## Involvement of Other Tissues

As exemplified by entries in most other chapters in this book, IPT is by no means confined to the lung although that organ is the principal seat of its development. Because of the uncertainties attached to the pathogenesis of IPT, it is not known whether histologically similar proliferations in the lung and elsewhere differ in their causative mechanisms. Further study will be required to address this point.

## Differential Diagnosis

The differential diagnosis of inflammatory pseudotumor is multifaceted because of its variable histologic appearance. The "lymphoplasmocytic" variant of IPT may resemble primary or secondary pulmonary plasmacytoma, malignant lymphoma, or lymphoid hyperplasia ("lymphoid interstitial pneumonia"). Among the latter conditions, plasmacytomas are distinguished by their monotypism for cytoplasmic LCIs (65), and selected lymphomas also may demonstrate that characteristic. Moreover, malignant lymphomas are generally less well circumscribed than IPTs and appear as more cytologically monotonous infiltrates of obviously atypical lymphoid elements (66,67). The presence of occasional giant cells and polymorphous inflammation may recall the characteristics of Hodgkin's disease, but it should be remembered that the latter process extremely rarely involves the lung as a primary extranodal lesion. Furthermore, the Reed–Sternberg cells of Hodgkin's lymphoma express the CD15 and CD30 antigens immunophenotypically, whereas these determinants are not apparent in the large hematopoietic cells of IPT (68). Localized and diffuse forms of pulmonary lymphoid hyperplasia are composed predominantly of mature lymphocytes (66), in contrast to the heterogeneous cellular composition of IPT.

The "fibrous histiocytoma" subtype of pulmonary IPT resembles some examples of primary or secondary malignant fibrous histiocytoma (MFH) or sarcomatoid carcinoma of the lung. In addition, it may simulate various benign mesenchymal tumors and so-called pulmonary sclerosing hemangioma. The presence of marked cellular atypia, necrosis, or mitotic activity should skew differential diagnostic opinion toward MFH or carcinoma and away from IPT (69,70). In addition, immunoreactivity for mutant p53 protein is a potential feature of MFH but not IPT (71); similar comments apply to the restriction of keratin immunoreactivity to sarcomatoid carcinomas. The endobronchial growth of IPTs may recapitulate the presenting symptom complexes of endoluminal fibromas, nerve sheath tumors, and other benign mesenchymal neoplasms, none of which contain a mixture of inflammatory cells as seen in the first-cited proliferations (46,72).

There is some minor difference of opinion as to whether or not "pulmonary hyalinizing granuloma" is a part of the spectrum of IPT in the lung. For those observers who prefer to conceptually separate the two, it is felt that the former of these lesions shows more lamellar hyalinized collagen than that seen in classical IPT. Hyalinizing granulomas of the lung are also rather commonly multiple, whereas "usual" IPT is not (73). Sclerosing hemangiomas were once considered synonymous with IPTs, but they are now appreciated as probably pneumocytic epithelial proliferations (74). These lesions may demonstrate focal matrical sclerosis but they also show characteristic aggregates of small bland cuboidal cells together with micropapillary and angiomatoid foci. Moreover, inflammation is absent or scanty in sclerosing hemangiomas, and their constituent cells express epithelial markers—such as keratin (74)—where IPT does not.

## Treatment and Prognosis

There are some examples of pulmonary IPT that have been observed for extended periods before surgical excision or autopsy examination. These cases have shown that the lesions tended to remain stable or increased in size very slowly. Spontaneous complete resolution also has been recorded (64). As mentioned above, a few lesions have diminished in size after small biopsies were taken or corticosteroids (75,76) or irradiation (77) were administered. Surgical removal is usually necessary to establish a firm diagnosis of IPT and if the lesion has been completely excised no further intervention is required. On the other hand, it is logical to expect that incomplete removal—particularly if invasion of adjacent extrapulmonary tissues is present—will be followed by continued growth, justifying adjuvant therapy. In particular, involvement of the pleura, pulmonary hilum, diaphragm, or mediastinum is associated with morbidity from IPTs of the lung (35–38), and they may even exceptionally prove fatal if they are massive and infiltrate the mediastinum extensively. Long-term surveillance of patients who have had uncomplicated pulmonary IPTs demonstrates no untoward clinical events in such cases.

## MYCOBACTERIAL SPINDLE CELL PSEUDOTUMOR

Spindle cell pseudotumors arising as a reaction to mycobacterial infection have been described in the skin, bone marrow, and lymph nodes in immunosuppressed subjects (78–81). These lesions closely resemble the histoid variant of leprosy (82), and the majority of recent reports on them have documented the presence of atypical mycobacteria (78–81). Mycobacterial pseudotumors are discussed in other chapters in this book, including those on the hematolymphoid system and skin. A single case has been reported in the lung (83). The subject was a 32-year-old black man, with diabetes, who had received a kidney and pancreas transplant. This was complicated by multiple episodes of acute rejection, requiring aggressive immunomodulatory chemotherapy. He developed respiratory failure and disseminated granular infiltrates on chest radiographs. Sputum cultures grew *Mycobacterium tuberculosis,* and despite multidrug therapy the patient died shortly after presentation.

At autopsy, the lungs contained numerous firm yellow–gray nodules, some of which were centered on small bronchi. Histologic sections showed that these consisted of rather uniform spindle cells with a fascicular pattern. Significant atypia and mitotic activity were not appreciated. There were scattered lymphocytes and plasma cells, without formation of overt granulomas. The cytoplasm of the fusiform elements was described as "foamy," and some hemosiderin was present. These features are similar to those of mycobacterial pseudotumors as reported in other locations, as illustrated in Figs. 28 and 29. The proliferating cells were immunopositive for lysozyme, without reactivity for S-100 protein, keratin, actin, desmin, or von Willebrand factor. A Ziehl–Neelsen stain revealed abundant acid-fast bacilli. Other organs were not involved by the process.

Most examples of this entity in other anatomic sites have been associated with *Mycobacterium avium-intracellulare* or *M. kansasii* (80). The above-cited pulmonary case is unusual in that it was associated with *M. tuberculosis,* as proven by culture (83). Whether this is a characteristic of pulmonary lesions of this type is obviously unclear, based on the study of only a single case.

Another reported feature in these lesions in other sites represents a potential source of diagnostic confusion. That is, there has been reproducible cross reaction of certain desmin antibodies with mycobacteria, erroneously suggesting the presence of a myogenic lesion (80). This is particularly problematic in the context under discussion here because myogenic tumors may figure prominently in the differential diagnosis of mycobacterial pseudotumors. However, the

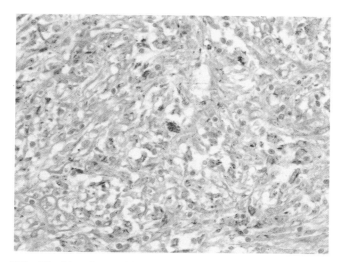

**FIG. 29.** Mycobacterial pseudotumor, with abundant acid-fast bacilli identified in the constituent cells (Ziehl–Neelsen stain).

documented lack of immunostaining for actin and ultrastructural features supporting histiocytic differentiation argue against a myogenous derivation (83). Other processes that potentially must be distinguished from pulmonary mycobacterial pseudotumors include Kaposi's sarcoma, MFH, spindle cell melanoma, and neural lesions (83). Obviously, familiarity with peculiar tissue reactions to mycobacteria and a clinical history of immunosuppression should suggest the diagnosis in most cases, and an acid-fast stain will be confirmatory. In some cases, the nature of the lesion is more obvious because of overtly granulomatous foci therein. Features of malignancy, such as tumoral necrosis, marked nuclear atypia, and a high mitotic rate, are absent. The lack of those findings should dissuade one from rendering a diagnosis of pulmonary sarcomatoid carcinoma, MFH, or other sarcomas. The pattern of immunostaining—with the exception of the above-described cross-reaction with certain desmin antibodies—is typical of histiocytic cells in mycobacterial pseudotumors.

## PULMONARY LYMPHOID HYPERPLASIA

Considerable controversy still surrounds lymphoid infiltrates in the lungs, and the use of such diagnostic terms as "lymphoid interstitial pneumonia (LIP)," "lymphoplasmocytic pneumonia," "plasmocytic interstitial pneumonia," and "pseudolymphoma." Our view is that some of the latter entities—in particular, selected examples of LIP and most cases of "pseudolymphoma"—are, in fact, low-grade malignant lymphomas of the bronchus-associated lymphoid tissue (84,85). Accordingly, these entities are not discussed further here. We focus on those examples of LIP that appear to lack evidence of clonality by immunohistologic and genotypic analysis, and therefore qualify as peculiar tumefactive hy-

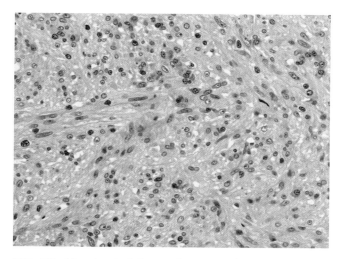

**FIG. 28.** Mycobacterial pseudotumor, with bland spindle cells, arranged in intersecting fascicles. Such arrangements mimic true spindle cell neoplasms, particularly smooth muscle tumors.

perplasias. In accord with that approach, we agree entirely with Koss (86) in his statement that LIP (and, perhaps, other forms of pulmonary lymphoid hyperplasia) "is not a single etiological or pathogenetic entity, but rather a morphological expression in the lung of a variety of diseases."

## Clinical Features

As summarized by Koss (86), the potential clinical manifestations of LIP are manifold. They include cough, dyspnea, weight loss, fever, hemoptysis, chest pain, and joint pain. The last of these symptoms may be associated with other physical abnormalities and laboratory manifestations of an autoimmune disorder in the context of collagen vascular diseases, including rheumatoid arthritis and its variants, lupus erythematosus, or myasthenia gravis. Other conditions in which immunity is disturbed—such as primary biliary cirrhosis, Blackfan–Diamond syndrome, lupoid chronic hepatitis, and the acquired immunodeficiency syndrome (AIDS)—also have been associated with pulmonary lymphoid hyperplasia (86–88). Paraproteinemias are common in patients with LIP, particularly featuring the presence of polyclonal hypergammaglobulinemia (89). In a distinct minority of cases, however, hypogammaglobulinemia may be evident (87). Results of spirometric testing are usually noncontributory.

Radiographic abnormalities on chest roentgenograms are likewise inconstant. They potentially include diffuse interstitial densities throughout one or both lung fields; randomly dispersed nodular lesions of variable sizes; or a combination of these findings (87,90–91). Interestingly, roughly 50% of

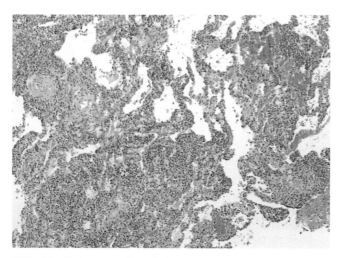

**FIG. 30.** Pulmonary lymphoid interstitial pneumonia (LIP), with a dense lymphoid infiltrate, centered around bronchovascular structures, with extension into adjacent alveolar septal tissue.

cases present with a localized single mass (86), raising the suspicion of a carcinoma on radiologic grounds. As indicated by Liebow and Carrington (90), mediastinal lymphadenopathy and pleural effusions are rare in cases of LIP and should suggest another diagnosis.

The biological behavior of pulmonary lymphoid hyperplasias is difficult to predict. Most observers have found that there were as many patients who died with this condition as those who had stable disease or improvement, and overall mortality approximates 50% at 5 years after diagnosis (87,88). Exogenous steroids or alkylating antineoplastic drugs have been employed to treat LIP, with more or less random success (86,92). Using current technologies (see below), it should be possible to define those lymphoid infiltrates of the lung that show evidence of monotypism and therefore have the attributes of malignant lymphoma. It remains to be seen whether prospective identification of such cases and their exclusion from series of LIP will narrow the behavioral spectrum of that disorder. In that regard, it is pertinent to note that approximately 5–10% of patients with LIP have developed disseminated lymphoma on long-term follow-up (93,94).

## Pathologic Characteristics

Lymphoid cells in LIP and other forms of pulmonary lymphocytic infiltration tend to follow the routes of lymphatic drainage in the lung. Accordingly, they are centered around blood vessels and tubular airways in a "coat sleeve" distribution or as nodular aggregates (86,87,90,91,93). In most cases, diffuse permeation outward into the interalveolar septa is also seen in this condition (Fig. 30). The population of constituent cells is polymorphous, but it is principally composed of small mature lymphocytes. "Transformed" lymphocytes with larger, more irregular nuclear contours as well as immunoblast-like elements are also regularly present, and a scattering of plasma cells, macrophages, and neutrophils completes the histologic picture (86) (Figs. 31 and 32). Germinal centers are evident in approximately 20–30% of cases, in our experience, and primarily arise in those cases where the lymphoid infiltrate is nodular (89,90). Unlike neoplastic follicles, the germinal centers contain a heterogeneous population of immunoblasts, together with phagocytic "tingible body" macrophages (Fig. 33). The central aspects of these structures may contain amorphous hyalinized matrical material that is deposited around blood vessels, in a fashion recalling the features of Castleman's disease (see discussion below, as well as the chapter in this book on hematolymphoid proliferations). Stromal amyloid has been observed focally in pulmonary lymphoid hyperplasia, as have epithelioid granulomas (86). Neither of the latter two features is reliable in separating LIP from low-grade lymphoid neoplasia. However, striking monomorphism, subendothelial aggregates of lymphocytes in pulmonary blood

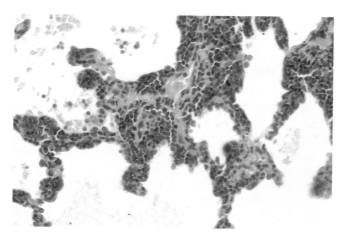

FIG. 31. Pulmonary LIP, with a alveolar septal infiltrate of small lymphocytes and plasmacytoid cells.

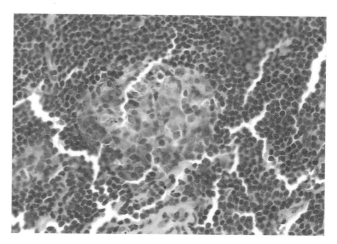

FIG. 33. A germinal center in pulmonary LIP, with surrounding dense lymphoid infiltrate.

vessels, abundant apoptosis, mitotic activity, or nuclear irregularity in the constituent cells should skew diagnostic opinion toward an interpretation of lymphoma (92,93).

Malignant lymphoproliferative diseases are characterized either by their aberrant immunophenotypes—with monotypism for LCIs or deletion of "pan-B" or "pan-T" cell antigens (84,85)—or by rearrangement of immunoglobulin genes or T-cell receptor genes using Southern blot methodology or the polymerase chain reaction (94,95). The most suitable substrate for immunohistology or genotyping analyses is that of frozen tissue. Thus, it is best to cryopreserve a representative portion of any wedge biopsy of the lung with this point in mind, if lymphoproliferative disease is considered in differential diagnosis. If only formalin-fixed, paraffin-embedded specimens are available for immunohistochemical evaluation, it has been our experience that a dominance (>70%)

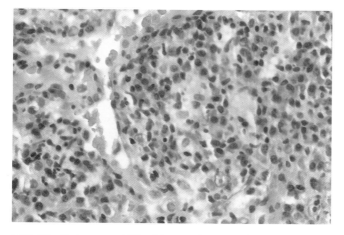

FIG. 32. Pulmonary LIP, with constituent cells including lymphocytes, rare eosinophils, and histiocytes.

of CD20− lymphocytes would argue in favor of a neoplastic infiltrate, in extrapolation from results obtained in the skin (96). However, specific examination of this premise in the lung—in correlation with genotyping studies or clinical follow-up—has, admittedly, not been undertaken to date.

### Etiologic Factors

Several theories have focused on the potential causes for pulmonary lymphoid hyperplasia. These principally concern two major pathogenetic mechanisms: dysregulation of immunity and virally driven reactive lymphoproliferation (86,87,91,97–99). It should be noted that these are not necessarily mutually exclusive. In favor of the former explanation, many patients with LIP have clear-cut clinical and serologic evidence of an autoimmune disease, as outlined above. Regarding the potential contribution of viral infection, it is similarly salient that genomic segments of the Epstein–Barr virus have been identified in constituent lymphocytes in some examples of LIP (97,98); moreover, that agent may exert a mitogenic effect in concert with the human immunodeficiency virus in the context of AIDS-related LIP (99). Regardless of whether or not these postulates are valid, they unfortunately do not hold promise in distinguishing LIP from low-grade malignant lymphoma. Examples of the latter disorder in the lungs and elsewhere have also demonstrated an association with the specified viruses, which may represent commensals or epiphenomenal infectious agents.

### Differential Diagnosis

As stated repeatedly in the foregoing discussion, the principal differential diagnostic consideration in cases of LIP is that of low-grade malignant lymphoma of the bronchus-associated lymphoid tissue (BALT) (84–86,93). To reiterate, the demonstration of lymphoid monotypism by immunohistologic evaluation or genotyping analyses is the best method for separation of these disorders with certainty, in a prospective fashion. Short of applying those techniques, there are, unfortunately, no conventional morphologic features of either disease group that allow for its definitive identification.

Rarely, Castleman's disease (angiofollicular lymph node hyperplasia [ALNH]) does involve the pulmonary parenchyma and might be confused with the multinodular form of LIP on cursory microscopic inspection (100). Nevertheless, detailed inspection of such cases will reveal the prototypic "onion skinning" of lymphocytes around distorted germinal centers in "hyaline-vascular" ALNH, or sheets of plasma cells in its plasmacellular subtype (86,100). Neither of these architectural features is expected in LIP. Also, it should be emphasized that ALNH is extraordinarily uncommon as a primary intrapulmonary lesion.

Isolated examples of acute viral pneumonia are typified by exuberant interstitial lymphoid infiltrates. Nevertheless, the clinical context of that disorder—featuring a rapidly evolving course and symptoms of an infectious disease—should allow for its accurate recognition in the absence of special pathologic studies. It is more difficult to distinguish LIP from extrinsic allergic alveolitis (hypersensitivity pneumonitis [HP]) pathologically because both of those disorders potentially feature the presence of exuberant lymphoid inflammation and epithelioid granulomas. Usually, clinical information regarding hypersensitivity to certain fungi and other organic antigens is necessary to identify HP definitively; conversely, the presence of histologic bronchiolitis obliterans would shift diagnostic preference towards LIP (86).

## PSEUDONEOPLASTIC CHANGES AS A CONSEQUENCE OF LUNG INJURY

Exfoliative cytology of the respiratory tract has been employed as a useful clinical tool in the diagnosis of pulmonary neoplasms for more than 50 years (101). However, as is true of any technique, inherent pitfalls in the method have been recognized and well documented, and some of these concern the potential for the over diagnosis of benign reparative or inflammatory conditions in the lung as neoplastic disorders. The incidence of this eventuality should be no greater than 0.25% of all cytologic specimens, according to established guidelines (102). To a lesser extent, the same pitfalls attend the interpretation of small transbronchial biopsy specimens of the lung parenchyma in surgical pathology.

There are several possible explanations for erroneous cytologic diagnoses of malignancy in the context of benign diseases. The pathologist or the screening technologist may simply misinterpret reparative processes or inflammatory epithelial atypia as carcinoma; this should be a rare event indeed in competent hands (103,104). Another potential source of error is the shedding of malignant cells from the oropharynx or nasopharynx into a "respiratory" cytology specimen (105,106). Both of these scenarios are problematic only if there are concomitant abnormalities on chest radiographs that might cause clinicians to consider a neoplasm diagnostically, and therefore knowledge of the radiologic findings is an essential piece of information for cytopathologists to have.

Along the same lines, however, there are particular mass lesions that are capable of inciting benign but atypical epithelial proliferations in the surrounding lung parenchyma, such that exfoliated cells in those cases may be mistaken as carcinomatous in nature (Fig. 34). These disorders include symptomatically "occult" pulmonary infarcts, granulomatous agglomerations, and foci of bronchiectasis with surrounding pneumonitis, which are typically associated with atypical squamous metaplasia of bronchial epithelium (107–112) (Fig. 35). Consequently, a misdiagnosis of squamous carcinoma is the usual error in such instances.

Another more diverse group of diseases that may simulate adenocarcinoma in cytologic or small biopsy specimens includes radiation pneumonitis, postchemotherapy atypia in alveolar lining cells, bronchiectasis, pulmonary infarction, viral pneumonias of various types, pulmonary vasculitides, inhalation of toxic chemicals, noninfectious interstitial pneumonitides, and diffuse alveolar damage (113–120) (Fig. 36). Again, these conditions are most vexing to the cytopathologist in the concurrent presence of a localized radiographic abnormality in the lungs. Nevertheless, because of the broad spectrum of roentgenographic appearances that bronchioalveolar adenocarcinoma is capable of assuming—including that of uncomplicated pneumonia (121)—scrutiny

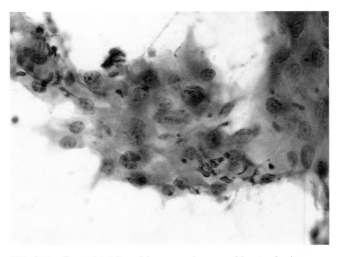

**FIG. 34.** Bronchial brushing specimen, with atypical squamous metaplasia. Constituent cells have irregular, hyperchromatic nuclei and visible nucleoli, and are arranged in cohesive sheets. Inflammatory cells are admixed. Cytopathology specimen was misinterpreted by multiple observers as squamous carcinoma (see Fig. 35).

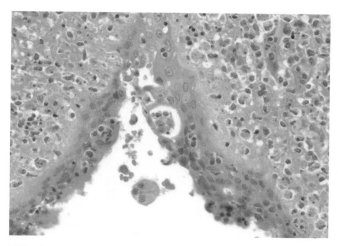

**FIG. 35.** Atypical squamous metaplasia; resection specimen from Fig. 34. An angioinvasive lymphoma is present, infiltrating the peribronchial tissue. Extensive infarction was identified. In this specimen, atypical squamous epithelium is present, with enlarged, irregular nuclei, hyperchromasia, and prominent nucleoli. A clue to the benign nature of this process, also present in Fig. 34, is a relatively normal N/C ratio.

of chest X-ray films is, unfortunately, less a safeguard in this specific setting. As summarized by Stanley et al. (122), pseudomalignant glandular pulmonary metaplasias may be recognized by their greater cellular heterogeneity than that seen in true adenocarcinomas, lower nuclear-to-cytoplasmic ratios than those of malignant tumors, "scalloping" of cell borders in metaplastic aggregates, and focal intercellular "windows" in pseudoneoplastic gland-like proliferations. It is also pertinent to emphasize that special techniques—such as immunostaining for tumor-associated glycoprotein-72—are not capable of making the distinction in question and may even contribute further to misdiagnosis (123). In fact, there are no absolutely effective methods whereby mistaken cytologic or biopsy diagnoses of pulmonary malignancy can

be avoided in selected cases. Pathologists and clinicians must be apprised of that fact, while at the same time striving to maximize diagnostic accuracy by all possible means.

## THYMIC AND MEDIASTINAL LESIONS

Relatively few pseudoneoplastic proliferations of the mediastinum and thymus gland have been reported. These are principally represented by "inflammatory pseudotumors" (IPT) and tumefactive fibroinflammatory lesions such as fibrosing mediastinitis.

### Inflammatory Pseudotumors

Only anecdotal reports of "plasma cell granuloma," "inflammatory pseudotumor (IPT)", or "inflammatory myofibroblastic tumor" have been recorded in the literature thus far. Marchevsky (124) illustrated such a lesion in an adult patient of unstated age and gender, and he related that the clinical, radiologic, and macroscopic features of this mass closely simulated those of an invasive thymoma. We have seen another similar example, in a 36-year-old man who presented with a 3-month history of progressive cough and who is well 2 years after subsequent thymectomy. The resected specimen demonstrated only the fascicular proliferation of bland myofibroblasts that characterizes IPT in other sites, and a mixture of bland chronic inflammatory cells was also dispersed throughout the mass. The immunohistochemical characteristics of thymic IPT were not addressed by Marchevsky (124). However, our case showed an absence of keratin and epithelial membrane antigen, and vimentin and actin isoforms were instead detectable in the proliferating spindle cells. The lymphocytes contained in IPTs have a T-cell immunophenotype, and constituent plasma cells express polytypic light chain immunoglobulins.

These features aid in excluding the primary differential di-

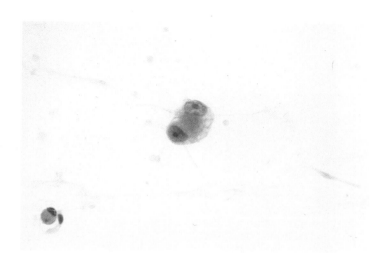

**FIG. 36.** Atypical epithelial cells in a bronchial brushing specimen, with cellular enlargement, prominent nucleoli, and irregular nuclear contours. A diagnosis of adenocarcinoma was rendered; subsequent lobectomy demonstrated only organizing pneumonitis. Clues to the benign nature of this process include degenerative vacuolization and a relatively low N/C ratio.

agnostic alternatives to thymic IPT, namely, spindle cell thymoma and sclerosing non-Hodgkin's lymphoma (125). Both of the latter conditions are, of course, true neoplasms. Thymomas are typically definable on the basis of their conventional morphologic attributes alone. However, sclerosing lymphomas may show a high density of variably collagenized stromal connective tissue, and careful examination is sometimes necessary to detect the atypical lymphocytes in those neoplasms (126). In contrast to the lymphoid population in IPT, the tumor cells of sclerosing mediastinal lymphomas are B lymphocytes (127).

Coffin et al. (128) and Kaplan and colleagues (129) have also described several examples of IPT that apparently arose in the extrathymic soft tissues of the mediastinum. An additional case of mediastinal IPT was reported by Tong and coworkers (130) in a patient with a complicated history including myelodysplasia and azacytidine therapy. The latter case showed the typical histologic features of IPT, with bland spindle cells and abundant plasma cells; immunostains disclosed positivity for vimentin and α-isoform actin positivity, as well as CD68. Constituent plasma cells were immunopolytypic. Microscopically similar lesions—but with a greater degree of nuclear atypia in the proliferating spindle cells—have been documented by Meis and Enzinger under the rubric "inflammatory fibrosarcoma" (131).

### Idiopathic Fibrosing Mediastinitis (Tumefactive Fibroinflammatory Lesion)

Reports on idiopathic fibrosing mediastinitis (IFM) have been made under a plethora of diagnostic synonyms, including "desmoid retraction," "lipogranuloma," "sclerosing xanthogranuloma," "isolated lipodystrophy," "inflammatory pseudotumor," and "fibrosing Weber–Christian disease." These diverse terms reflect the fact that the pathogenesis of IFM has been linked by sundry authors to that of many other conditions. It is certainly true that the most common cause of mediastinal fibrosis is an idiosyncratic reaction to infections of the lungs and mediastinal lymph nodes by mycobacterial or fungal organisms (132–141). Hence, one is obliged to exclude the presence of these agents before offering the conclusion that the process in question is indeed idiopathic.

The most common clinical presentation of IFM is that of progressive dyspnea or cough. In addition, the superior vena caval syndrome—with suffusion of the soft tissues of the head and neck and dilatation of accessory thoracic subcutaneous veins—is a distinct possibility. Unlike mediastinal fibrosis associated with infection, as cited above, fever and sweats are typically absent in IFM. Patients are generally adults over the age of 40 years, and IFM has no apparent predilection for either gender. In unusual cases, a mass may be felt on deep palpation of the infraclavicular fossae; however, most examples of IFM are made manifest only through the results of radiologic studies. These show irregular widening and density of the mediastinal soft tissue on plain films of the thorax (140). Computed tomography (CT) or magnetic

resonance imaging (MRI) are more specific in delineating the presence of a mass (or multiple masses) containing variable quantities of entrapped fat and fibrous tissue (141); internal calcification may also be evident.

Histologically, one observes densely hyalinized tumefactive fibrous tissue in the mediastinum, with a haphazard pattern of involvement of anatomic subcompartments. The fibrosis may extend into the lungs and great vessels, and may markedly compromise the luminal diameter of mediastinal or hilar pulmonary vasculature. The latter finding probably secondarily explains the fat necrosis that may accompany the above-cited changes as well. Scattered throughout the mass in a regional fashion, one finds aggregates of mature lymphocytes, plasma cells, histiocytes, foam cells, and occasional eosinophils (132–141) (Fig. 37). Importantly, none of these hematopoietic elements should show any cytologic atypia or monomorphism; likewise, there must be no hint of epithelial cell nests or cellular spindle cell proliferation in the fibroinflammatory matrix of bona fide IFM.

The last-named caveats relate to the previously mentioned fact that occasional examples of metastatic carcinoma or malignant lymphoma may involve the mediastinal soft tissue in a fashion that grossly and microscopically simulates the profile of IFM. This differential diagnosis also applies to tumefactive fibrosing entities at other topographic sites. Thus, it goes without saying that extensive sampling and scrupulous inspection of histologic sections should be undertaken to exclude an occult malignancy.

Because of its morphologic features, one may also confuse IFM with IPT or aggressive fibromatosis (desmoid tumor) (142,143). Nonetheless, these conditions are quite separate and are unrelated to one another. IFM is extremely hypocellular and uniformly collagenous with regional inflammation. The attributes of IPT have been described above

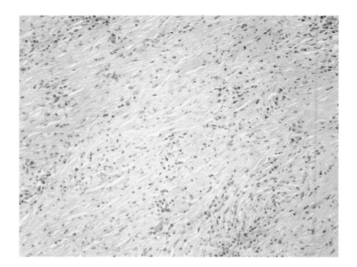

**FIG. 37.** Sclerosing mediastinitis, with dense bands of collagen, and lymphocytes, infiltrating between the collagen bands. There is no atypia of the lymphocytes, nor is there any evidence of a proliferation of the stromal cells.

in reference to lesions of the lungs and thymus, and are not repeated here. Fibromatosis is characterized by a distinctive fusiform and stellate cell proliferation that is regularly punctuated by thick-walled small blood vessels; it is accompanied by deposition of a myxoid stroma and a relative absence of lymphocytes and plasma cells (142,143).

Following the seminal description of the concept of "tumefactive fibroinflammatory lesions" (TFILs) by Wold and Weiland (144), in reference to masses of the head and neck, other authors have embraced that terminology and the paradigm attached to it (145,146). This model groups several histologically similar diseases mechanistically and suggests that they are all probably autoimmune in nature. Such disorders include IFM, Riedel's thyroiditis (and possibly also sclerosing Hashimoto's thyroiditis), retroperitoneal fibrosis (Ormond's disease), primary sclerosing cholangitis, and "retractile mesenteritis" (147–154). It is therefore of pathobiological interest that several patients have been described who suffered from more than one of these conditions synchronously or metachronously. Importantly, one must distinguish between TFILs, and inflammatory myofibroblastic "pseudotumors" and "inflammatory fibrosarcomas." At least the latter of these two entities is thought to be a true neoplasm, and cellular density and nuclear atypia in both lesions are notably higher than those seen in TFILs.

Treatment for mediastinal fibrosis is individualized and usually conservative in nature, and it is tailored to relieving the symptoms and signs of any given patient. Only rare cases necessitate surgical debulking of the fibrous mass. Potential complications of this condition primarily relate to the entrapment of mediastinal and hilar pulmonary structures in the tumefactive mass, and include such problems as pulmonary hemorrhage or infarction. However, the general outlook for affected individuals is said to be favorable if these secondary problems can be treated successfully. Some patients with TFILs have had beneficial results from the administration of exogenous steroids (146).

## Mesothelial Inclusions In Mediastinal Lymph Nodes

A final mediastinal lesion that is worthy of brief discussion is that of mesothelial cell inclusions. Rutty and Lauder (155) reported a case of a 23-year-old man with a mediastinal T-cell lymphoma. An incidental histologic finding was the subcapsular presence of small nests of bland cells in several mediastinal lymph nodes. These cells were polygonal with eosinophilic cytoplasm and bland, oval nuclei. No mitoses, pleomorphism, or glandular differentiation were present. An absence of these findings should dissuade one from a diagnostic interpretation of metastatic carcinoma. The lesional cells co-expressed keratin and vimentin, and ultrastructural examination showed features of mesothelial cells including slender microvilli and desmosomes. Similar lesions have also been described by other investigators (156,157).

## Pleural Lesions

Pseudoneoplastic processes in the pleural spaces, as in the lungs, are represented by a limited number of lesions. Perhaps the most common of these is mainly a cytopathologic entity, namely, mesothelial hyperplasia as seen in pleural effusion specimens. As mentioned in the introduction to this book, cytologic mimics of malignancy encompass such a wide variety of entities that they cannot be addressed completely in this text. We focus on some facets of this topic, but for a more complete discussion the reader may consult comprehensive treatises (158–160). Also, one can see extension into the pleura of pulmonary or mediastinal lesions such as hyalinizing granuloma or inflammatory pseudotumor of the lung. Nonetheless, several distinct pseudoneoplastic pleural lesions account for a significant number of clinical cases, and thus, familiarity and facility with the nuances of these proliferations are important for most pathologists. Also, because several of the entities are associated with asbestos exposure, they may often be part of a legal action in which both the diagnosis and pathologist come under scrutiny.

## Reactive Mesothelial Proliferations

The correct microscopic classification of mesothelial lesions can be quite challenging (161). This is most often true in the context of pleural fluid cytology but also may be a diagnostic dilemma in pleural biopsies (161,162). Several problems arise in this setting, including the distinction of reactive proliferations from mesothelioma or from metastatic carcinoma, and the separation of benign and malignant lymphocytic effusions. Several of these problems can be rightly considered within the realm of "pseudoneoplasia."

Reactive mesothelial cell proliferations have often been dispatched with the descriptive but vague label of "atypical mesothelial cells" in older cytologic parlance (163). Because such terminology implies a possible connection to malignancy or at least premalignancy, its use is not advocated. Instead, one can and should simply indicate that mesothelial cells are hyperplastic or reactive (164). Such mesothelial cell proliferations can be seen in a variety of pathologic conditions, including cirrhosis, anemia, viral infections, collagen vascular diseases, radiation pleuritis, responses to pleural metastases, or a variety of chronic pleural infections (165). Thus, an accurate and adequate clinical history is an absolute necessity when evaluating pleural fluid specimens or pleural biopsies (166).

In both contexts, features that favor malignancy include the presence of papillae or other complex architectural structures, striking nuclear atypia, necrosis, and pathologically shaped mitotic figures (166). Similarly, as summarized by Bedrossian and co-workers, there are contrasting criteria for diagnosing reactive or hyperplastic mesothelial lesions in biopsy specimens, to the exclusion of malignant mesothelial

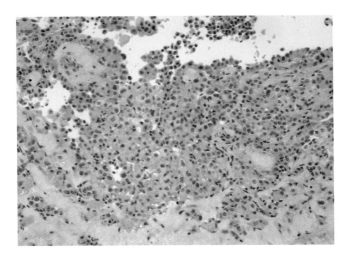

**FIG. 38.** Marked pleural mesothelial hyperplasia. Despite small papillary projections, there is no evidence of invasion, and the constituent mesothelial cells are bland, without atypical mitoses or cellular necrosis.

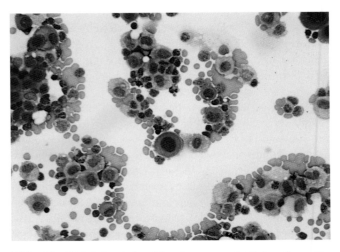

**FIG. 39.** Wright's stained benign mesothelial cells, with characteristic variation in size, low N/C ratios, "double-layered" cytoplasm, and brush-border-like appearance.

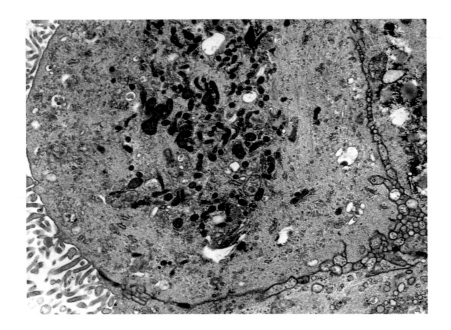

**FIG. 40.** Ultrastructural features of mesothelial cells, including almost circumferential, elongated, thin microvilli, and desmosomes, are identified in this electron micrograph of epithelioid mesothelioma.

neoplasms (167). The former benign lesions are characterized by only superficial entrapment of cellular nests in the stroma; an intense inflammatory infiltrate that is heaviest near the mesothelial surface; abundant vascular proliferation with only scanty spindle cells; the lack of overtly malignant cytologic features; and an absence of atypical mitotic figures (Fig. 38). In contrast, mesothelioma demonstrates convincingly invasive growth, with or without a dense spindle cell proliferation; inflammation in mesothelioma is scant or is heaviest in areas that are farthest away from the pleural surface. Moreover, obviously atypical nuclear details may be present and abnormal mitoses can often be appreciated.

Despite the almost universal reference to cytologic atypia in the literature on mesotheliomas, experience with examination of pleural biopsies suggests that this finding is often unimpressive in some well-differentiated forms of those tumors. On the other hand, it can be quite impressive in reactive mesothelium (168). In general, the cytologic criteria for malignant mesothelioma include an elevated nucleocytoplasmic ratio, irregularity of the nuclear membranes, and coarse abnormally clumped chromatin. However, even by morphometric analysis, conflicting results have been obtained. Studies by Marchevsky et al. (169), Kwee and colleagues (170), and Oberholzer and co-workers (171) all suggest that nuclear morphometry—including such details as mean nuclear profile diameter, nuclear/cytoplasmic area, and "nuclear texture"—can discriminate benign from malignant mesothelial cells. In contrast, other evaluations have suggested that such features are not useful in this context (172).

Several attributes of mesothelial cells can be observed in both benign and malignant proliferations in cytologic specimens. These include cytoplasmic vacuolization, binucleation or multinucleation, and a brush-border pattern over the entire free surface of the cells that is said to correspond to the ultrastructural finding of elongated microvilli (Figs. 39 and 40) (173). In general, reactive cells tend to exfoliate singly or in small clusters (158). Large formations, including morular structures with knobby cellular outlines or papillary structures, should raise the index of suspicion for a diagnosis of mesothelioma, as should the presence of uniformly dense hypercellularity in an effusion specimen (Fig. 41) (174). It should also be understood that this discussion applies only to epithelial or biphasic varieties of malignant mesothelioma because sarcomatoid subtypes rarely shed diagnostic malignant cells into body cavities. If effusions are present in the latter instance, they often contain only inflammatory cells and reactive but cytologically benign mesothelial cells (175). Recently, the concept of mesothelioma *in situ* has been introduced for some flat or microscopic lesions of the serous cavities (Fig. 42) (176). However, criteria for the prospective distinction of reactive proliferations from such early lesions in small biopsies or cytologic specimens are lacking, and this is thus, at the present time, an uncharted area of anatomic pathology.

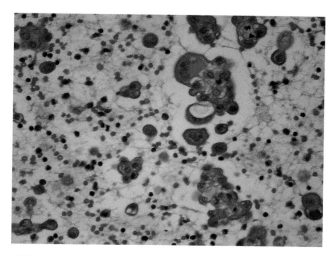

**FIG. 41.** Cell block preparation of epithelioid malignant mesothelioma. The specimen is hypercellular, with complex architectural aggregates, including glandular structures. The nuclei are markedly hyperchromatic, with irregular nuclear contours.

Immunohistochemistry has little value in the distinction between reactive and malignant mesothelium. Both types of cells express a broad spectrum of keratin types (177). Some studies have suggested that purely epithelioid mesotheliomas express plasmalemmal epithelial membrane antigen (EMA) and vimentin, whereas benign mesothelial cells are negative for both markers (178). However, our experience has shown the latter determinants to be shared liberally by both pathologic processes. As expected, both cell types are reproducibly negative for carcinoembryonic antigen (CEA),

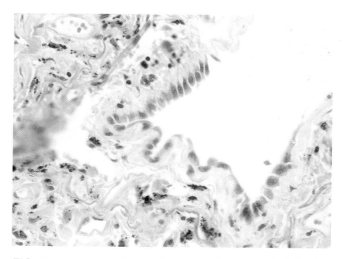

**FIG. 42.** This case demonstrates atypical mesothelial cells, with an adjacent classic epithelioid mesothelioma, outside of this field. These mesothelial cells demonstrate enlarged, hyperchromatic nuclei, with prominent nucleoli. Whether this represents "mesothelioma *in situ*" or simply reactive atypia is unclear by current criteria.

TAG-72 (the target of B72.3), and CD15. Thus, whereas a panel of antibodies against vimentin, keratin, EMA, CEA, CD15, and TAG-72 is helpful in distinguishing adenocarcinoma from mesothelioma, it cannot reliably separate benign and malignant mesothelial proliferations (179). We have encountered several cases where an incorrect diagnosis of pleural mesothelioma was made using cytology specimens, in part based on a failure of the cellular constituents to label for CEA, TAG-72, and CD15. In fact, however, the cells in question were simply reactive mesothelium, as borne out by a lack of clinical disease progression over extended follow-up periods (Fig. 43).

Interest is also intense with respect to immunostaining for other gene products that might suggest malignancy. Markers of cellular proliferation, such as proliferating cell nuclear antigen, have been suggested to possible utility in this context (180). In recent history, proteins translated from mutant p53 genes have received considerable attention (181–184). It has been suggested that p53 is often aberrant (with correspondingly detectable protein products) in malignant mesothelioma but is rarely so in benign or reactive mesothelial proliferations (181,182). When they are immunopositive for p53 protein, reactive mesothelia are often described as showing either weak staining, or both cytoplasmic and nuclear labeling that raises the suspicion of a spurious result (183). Although it may provide adjunctive interpretative support, immunostaining for mutant p53 protein should surely not be used in isolation. It must always be integrated with histologic and cytologic findings, as well as clinical and radiographic details (184).

In view of the generally dismal outcome in mesothelioma cases and the lack of effective therapy for that tumor, diagnostic caution is generally appropriate in this context. With those facts in mind, it would be much more disastrous to la-

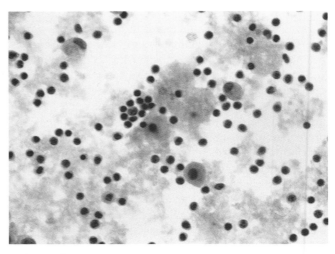

FIG. 44. Small lymphocytic effusion, with mainly small round lymphocytes, and a few mesothelial cells and histiocytes. This effusion, which may mimic small lymphocytic malignancies, was from a patient subsequently demonstrated to have pulmonary tuberculosis (Papanicolaou stain).

bel a patient with a reactive proliferation as having a mesothelioma than it would be to undercall an abnormal but less than totally diagnostic specimen as "suspicious for mesothelioma." With the "tincture of time," such cases will declare themselves as mesothelioma if that is what they truly represent.

In regard to the distinction of reactive mesothelial cells from metastatic carcinoma, more clear-cut criteria exist (167). The cytologic attributes of benign mesothelial cells include relative cellular monomorphism (Fig. 45) (158). In contrast, carcinomatous effusions often feature a distinctly dimorphic cellular population, although this may be subtle in cases of mammary or gastric carcinoma (Fig. 46) (158). Periodic acid–Schiff (PAS) stains, done with and without diastase digestion, will identify neutral mucins in a substantial number of metastatic adenocarcinomas but not in mesothe-

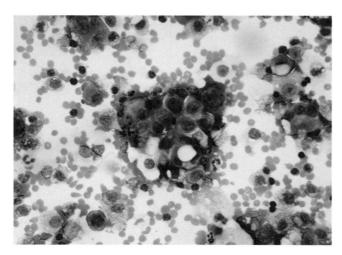

FIG. 43. Adenocarcinoma in pleural effusion. Unlike reactive mesothelial proliferations, which show a single cell population, there is clearly a background of mesothelial and inflammatory cells, and a second population of malignant cells, in complex clusters.

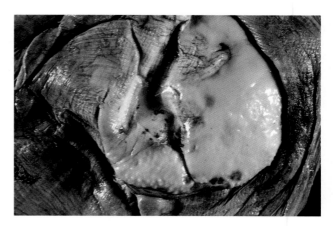

FIG. 45. Hyalinized pleural plaque, with a raised, tan–pink, irregular-shaped lesion, on the diaphragmatic pleura.

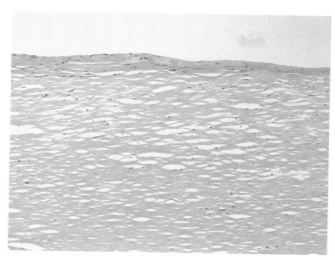

**FIG. 46.** Typical pleural hyaline plaque. The lesion is almost acellular and shows dense collagen bundles, with a characteristic "basket-weave"-pattern.

lial proliferations (173,185). In contrast, the latter generally contain only glycogen. Some intracytoplasmic vacuoles in mesothelial cells will also contain hyaluronic acid that is stainable with Alcian blue at pH 2.5 and digestible with hyaluronidase. These inclusions may show weak cross-reactivity with mucicarmine stains, potentially prompting an erroneous diagnosis of carcinoma; nonetheless, such staining will disappear following hyaluronidase treatment, unlike the mucicarmine reactivity of adenocarcinomas (185). Lastly, as documented above, a selected panel of immunostains will detect the majority of carcinomas but will not label either reactive or malignant mesothelial cells (158–160,163, 164,167,173,185–189). Also, stains for oncogenic markers, including protein products of c-erb-B2, p53, and H-ras (190), may also be useful in selected instances in this specific context.

**Small Lymphocytic Effusions**

Another common problem of pseudoneoplastic lesions in the pleural space concerns the ability of various conditions to induce a lymphocytic effusion that closely mimics malignant lymphoid processes. This conundrum almost never involves a question of large-cell or high-grade lymphoma, but rather revolves around the differential diagnosis of small, relatively mature lymphocytic proliferations (small lymphocytic lymphoma [SLL] or chronic lymphocytic leukemia versus benign lymphoid infiltrates) (Fig. 44). A short list of conditions that may produce striking pleural lymphocytic effusions, in addition to lymphomas, includes tuberculosis, reaction to pleural malignancies (thought to represent lymphatic obstruction by tumor), effusions due to laceration of the intrathoracic lymphatic vessels, or other nonspecific chronic effusions (160). The cytologic features of benign and malig-

nant small lymphocytic lesions can be remarkably similar; both may be composed almost exclusively of compact, round, uniform lymphocytes, admixed with a few mesothelial cells. Although it is rare as a presenting manifestation of SLL, pleural effusion may be seen in a sizable number of patients later in the evolution of the disease. When presented with such an effusion, a history of known SLL is obviously valuable, but it does not in and of itself exclude one or another of the infectious diseases that may produce a lymphocytic effusion and that may complicate the course of a malignant lesion. Adjunctive pathologic techniques may also be useful. Because the great majority of cases of SLL are B-lymphocytic in nature (158,160), one can simply perform immunostains or *in situ* hybridization studies to look for the presence of monotypism for light chain immunoglobulins (LCIs) in aspirate smears. Also, conjoint expression of CD20 (a pan-B-cell marker) and CD43 (a pan-T-cell marker) may provide similarly helpful information in paraffin-embedded cell blocks (see above). One expects reactive processes to be composed mainly of T cells, whereas most cases of SLL will be almost exclusively B cell in nature (158,160). Other studies have also suggested that polymerase chain reaction techniques for immunoglobulin heavy chain gene rearrangements can be applied successfully to cytologic material, in order to document monoclonality (191).

In a pragmatic sense, this is another clinical situation in which it is important to remember that malignant effusions typically reaccumulate over a short time. If initial immunostains and clinical information are not sufficient for a definitive diagnosis, more cell-rich fluid can be readily reobtained by pleurocentesis and more thoroughly evaluated by flow cytometry and other special techniques. In the long run, this is probably the most logical approach, and it is certainly more cost-effective than immediate application of several adjunctive pathologic procedures to each and every lymphocytic effusion.

**Hyaline Pleural Plaques**

Hyaline pleural plaques (HPPs) constitute important lesions, because of their association with occupational dust exposures and the necessity to distinguish these benign proliferations from mesothelial neoplasms. HPPs were first described more 60 years ago in association with asbestos exposure (192,193). Thereafter, these lesions have also been documented in talc workers (194).

*Pathogenesis and Association with Asbestos Exposure*

As just stated, many studies have linked asbestos exposure to the development of hyaline plaques (192,193,195–212). A large review of multiple autopsy studies by Schwartz (211) revealed a widely variable incidence of pleural plaques in routine necropsies, with an average of 12.2%. Most studies have failed to demonstrate the presence of asbestos fibers in the plaques themselves but instead have examined subjacent pulmonary parenchyma. Asbestos bodies are typically found only in that location. Warnock and co-workers (210) reported an association of all types of asbestos with plaque development, although there were significantly increased numbers of amosite and crocidolite fibers. Studies by Churg (195,196) and others (199,200,203,210) have also suggested that there is an increase in commercial amphibole fibers in the lungs in association with HPPs. The number of fibers detected is generally above that seen in a control group of non-exposed patients but less than that found in individuals with documented asbestosis (203,210).

At this point it should be stressed that the foregoing comments apply principally to those individuals with bilateral, parietal pleural plaques. On the other hand, unilateral plaques or visceral pleural fibrous thickening may occur whenever there is chronic pleural irritation from any cause. Other conditions associated with unilateral plaques or visceral fibrosis include infections such as tuberculosis or empyema, chronic or recurrent pleural hemorrhage, or chest wall trauma (200,207,208).

### Clinical and Gross Features

Plaques are most often detected in older individuals (in the seventh and eighth decades of life) (195,207). Those associated with asbestos exposure show an average latency of approximately 20 years from the time of initial dust inhalation to diagnosis (195–210). HPPs tend to occur in the lower thorax and involve the parietal surfaces, and often have a parallel orientation to the ribs (201). The diaphragm is another favored location (Fig. 45). Less often, there is involvement of the visceral pleura, and, rarely, lesions will occur on the pericardial surfaces as well (198,209). The affected individuals have few if any symptoms that are directly related to the presence of the plaques. It has been stated that most pulmonary function abnormalities are likely due to superimposed chronic obstructive pulmonary disease or coexisting pulmonary asbestosis (195,196). Plain film radiographs have limited sensitivity for the detection of uncomplicated HPPs, but the rate of detection increases markedly when the plaques are calcified (201,203). Likewise, the advent of computed tomography has improved the recognition of these lesions (212).

### Histologic Features

The classic pattern of HPPs features hypocellular, dense bundles of collagen, often with a basket-weave pattern (Fig. 46). There may be associated chronic inflammation and in some cases acute inflammation or fibrin may be noted on the luminal surface. The latter changes may reflect the proposed mechanism of formation of the lesion, namely, that of recurrent organizing pleuritis. As one might assume from the radiographic findings, calcification is often evident pathologically.

### Differential Diagnosis

The chief differential diagnostic consideration in cases of HPP is that of mesothelioma and, more specifically, its desmoplastic variant. Desmoplastic mesothelioma (DM) shares many of the histologic attributes of HPP in that it can be composed of relatively bland cells that are separated by dense bands of collagen (213). Afflicted patients may also share a history of asbestos exposure. Nonetheless, although both lesions may be hypocellular, there will be greater cellularity in DM, at least focally, as compared with HPP (213) (Fig. 47). The cells of DM may also exhibit a greater degree of pleomorphism than HPP. The growth patterns in these lesions can provide valuable diagnostic clues as well. Involvement of the visceral pleura or diffuse involvement of the pleural space is a feature of DM and should argue strongly against an interpretation of HPP (214).

Special studies may be helpful in this differential diagnostic context. When stained with antibodies to low-molecular-weight keratin, HPP demonstrates no more than a rare entrapped mesothelial cell, with conversely diffuse, strong vimentin reactivity (215). On the other hand, DM typically shows strong, diffuse reactivity in the spindled cells for both markers (215) (Fig. 48). Caution should be exercised, however, in that activated submesothelial fibroblasts may show some keratin positivity (177). Thus, organizing pleuritis often demonstrates focal keratin reactivity, but the reactivity in DM is typically much more intense and global. Antibodies

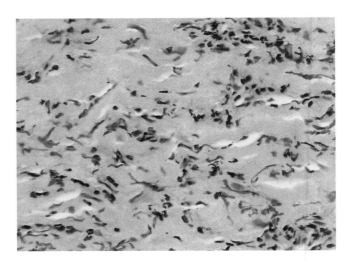

**FIG. 47.** Subtle desmoplastic mesothelioma, with dense collagen, resembling a hyaline plaque. There is modestly increased cellularity, and some of the stromal cells show hyperchromatic, atypical nuclei. Scattered chronic inflammatory cells are also present. This case was initially misdiagnosed as a hyaline plaque but clinically evolved as a diffuse malignant mesothelioma.

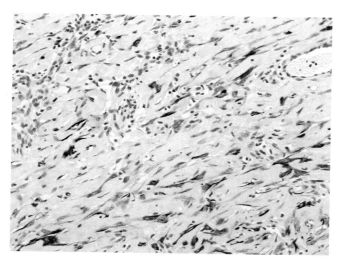

**FIG. 48.** Immunostaining of lesion from Fig. 49 confirms the presence of cytokeratin in the atypical stroma cells, confirming the diagnosis of desmoplastic mesothelioma (avidin-biotin-peroxidase complex technique).

typically used to compare epithelioid mesothelioma and carcinoma, such as those against CD15, TAG-72, or CEA, have no particular value in the analysis of spindle cell lesions (216). Electron microscopy may also not be helpful in this setting because the cells of DM, in analogy to those of HPP, most often resemble fibroblasts or myofibroblasts. Unlike epithelial mesothelioma, the cells of DM lack elongated microvilli and complex cellular junctions (217).

Although some areas in solitary fibrous tumors of the pleura (FTPs) may contain the sort of keloidal collagen seen in HPPs, FTPs show greater cellularity and dissimilar histologic patterns, such as storiform, hemangiopericytoma-like, or "pattern-less" configurations (218). Moreover, FTPs typically present as localized, often polypoid masses rather than as plaques. Solitary fibrous tumors also have no known relationship to asbestos exposure (218).

*Clinical Implications*

The great majority of patients with HPPs have few if any symptoms that are directly attributable to the plaques themselves (196,219). Thus, there is no indication for surgical removal of such lesions. The possible relationship of HPPs that are associated with asbestos exposure to bronchogenic carcinoma or mesothelioma has been the subject of many studies, which have been reviewed in other texts (220). In summary, it seems fair to say that plaques themselves are not precursor lesions for malignancies but merely reflect an underlying exposure to mineral dusts. Quantitation of that exposure by objective means such as tissue digestion and fiber counting, procurement of other pertinent clinical facts (such as a history of cigarette smoking), and examination of the lung for asbestosis must be done to further estimate the magnitude of risk for an associated malignancy (220).

## DIFFUSE PLEURAL FIBROSIS

A related pathologic process is that of diffuse pleural fibrosis (DPF). It may be associated with connective tissue disorders such as lupus erythematosus or rheumatoid arthritis, as well as chronic infections; however, like hyaline plaques, there is also a strong link to asbestos exposure (221–225). Some studies have suggested that in cases of DPF there is a greater level of dust exposure than that seen with hyaline plaques, and patients are more likely to have some degree of functional pulmonary impairment (222,224). Unlike pleural plaques, DPF often involves the visceral pleura and there may be apical pulmonary involvement. In severe cases, obliteration of the pleural space is possible with fusion of the visceral and parietal pleural layers (224).

Histologically, one sees bland fibrous tissue, generally without the basket weave–like nature of hyaline plaques (221–225). There is often hypervascularity as well as scattered foci of chronic inflammation, with plasma cells, lymphocytes, and histiocytes. Associated inflammatory exudate may be evident on the free lesional surface. As with HPPs, differential diagnosis largely centers on the exclusion of a desmoplastic mesothelioma (214,214). The foregoing statements concerning the immunohistochemical characteristics of HPP also apply to DPF. There is also certainly overlap of the clinical presentation of DPF and DM, in that both have the ability to encase the lung in a rind of fibrosis of variable thickness.

## MULTICYSTIC MESOTHELIOMA

The lesion known as multicystic mesothelioma (MCM) is a relatively recent addition to the pathologic literature (226–236). Most cases have been reported in the peritoneum rather than the pleura, and often involve the pelvis in women (229). There is controversy over whether the lesions are reactive proliferations or low-grade neoplasms (233). Those observers who believe that the lesions are nonneoplastic have coined the alternative term "peritoneal inclusion cyst" (234,235). Peritoneal MCMs often present in subjects with endometriosis or other conditions that might cause peritoneal irritation. It has been suggested that this relationship supports the interpretation of a "reactive" lesion (235). Multiple lesions are sometimes observed metachronously; those who conversely favor these lesions as neoplastic argue that this phenomenon represents recurrence (233), whereas others preferring a reactive condition suggest that multiplicity simply represents multifocality or incomplete removal of the initial lesion (234). No cases have metastasized, although Weiss and Tavasolli have described several cases with putatively invasive or destructive growth (233).

There has also been one report of this entity in the pleural cavity (236). This case occurred in a 37-year-old woman who presented with pleuritic chest symptoms. She was a

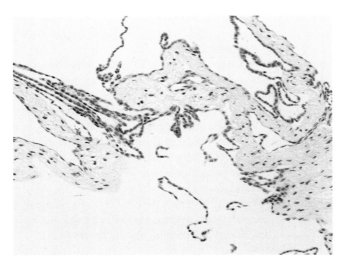

**FIG. 49.** Multicystic mesothelioma, with multiple cysts lined by a flattened to cuboidal single layer of mesothelial cells. Some examples contain an extensive stromal lymphoid infiltrate, although that feature is not prominent in this case.

cigarette smoker and, interestingly, had a childhood history of asbestos exposure. Radiographs demonstrated several pleural-based masses; at thoracotomy, four multicystic lesions were removed. No recurrences developed over 8 months of follow-up. Microscopically, the multicystic lesions were lined by flattened to cuboidal cells, with edema in the intervening stroma, in identity with the above-described peritoneal lesions (Figs. 49–50). The cellular lining was continuous with the adjacent pleural mesothelium. Cytologic atypia and mitoses were lacking. The lining cells showed immunoreactivity for keratin, EMA, and vimentin, and bound *Ulex europeaus* lectin. Ultrastructural features of mesothelial cells, including long, slender microvilli, desmosomes, and perinuclear filament bundles, were evident.

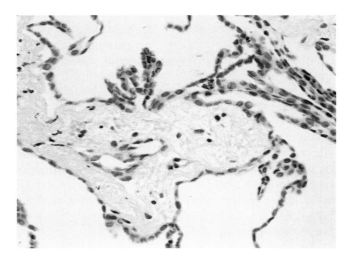

**FIG. 50.** Higher-power view of the lesion from Fig. 51 demonstrates the benign appearance of the constituent mesothelial cells.

## CALCIFYING FIBROUS PSEUDOTUMOR

The unique entity known as calcifying fibrous pseudotumor (CFPT) has been recently described in the pleura by Pinkard et al. (237). This lesion is histologically similar, if not identical, to calcifying fibrous pseudotumors of the soft tissue, as defined by Fetsch and co-workers (238).

The three described cases of pleural CFPT all occurred in young adults (age range 23–34 years); two were female and one was male (237). Two patients manifested with chest pain whereas the third was asymptomatic. Pleural-based masses were seen by chest radiographs in all cases and CT scans also demonstrated partially calcified nodular lesions. Only one subject had multiple masses.

Histologically, all patients had circumscribed but non-encapsulated fibrous lesions that were composed of dense, hyalinized, collagenous tissue, with interspersed bland spindle cells (Figs. 51 and 52). The masses were generally hypocellular, particularly at their peripheries, and no nuclear atypia of the fusiform cells was present. A scant chronic inflammatory infiltrate was seen, without lymphoid aggregates, giant cells, or necrosis. All lesions also featured calcifications of the psammomatous as well as dystrophic types (226). These histologic features are identical to those of calcifying fibrous pseudotumors of the soft tissue. Electron microscopy of one pleural case showed fibroblast-like cells, without evidence of mesothelial or epithelial features. Entities that were mentioned as differential diagnostic considerations included HPP, DPF, inflammatory pseudotumor, calcified or hyalinizing granulomas, and amyloidosis. The clinical presentation, gross features, and microscopic features argue against any of these considerations. Follow-up

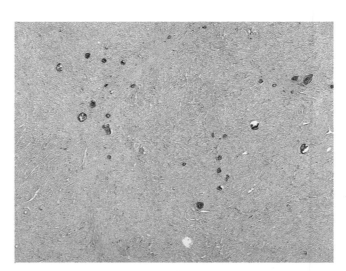

**FIG. 51.** Haphazardly organized, hypocellular fibrous tissue, with clusters of psammoma-like calcifications, are characteristic of calcifying fibrous pseudotumor of the pleura. (Photomicrograph generously provided by Dr. Nanette Ballard Pinkard, Division of Anatomic Pathology, University of Alabama at Birmingham.)

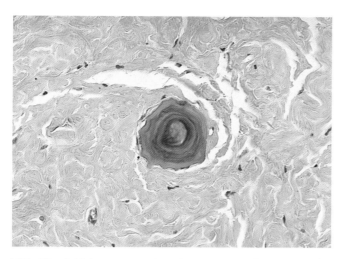

**FIG. 52.** A higher-power view demonstrates the concentric, laminated calcifications, and the bland cytologic features of the stroma cell component. (Photomicrograph generously provided by Dr. Nanette Ballard Pinkard, Division of Anatomic Pathology, University of Alabama at Birmingham.)

was short in these cases; the authors speculated that, in analogy to soft tissue CFPT, one might expect rare local recurrences but no instances of aggressive behavior.

## REFERENCES
### Lung

1. Koss MN. Unusual tumor-like conditions of the lung. *Adv Pathol Lab Med* 1994;7:123–150.
2. Albrecht E. Uber Harmartome. *Verh Dtsch Ges Pathol* 1904; 7:153–157.
3. McDonald JR, Harrington SW, Clagett OT. Hamartoma (often called chondroma) of the lung. *J Thorac Cardiovasc Surg* 1945;14:128-143.
4. Tomashefski JF Jr. Benign endobronchial mesenchymal tumors: their relationship to parenchymal pulmonary hamartomas. *Am J Surg Pathol* 1982;6:531–540.
5. Koutras P, Urschel HC, Paulson DL. Hamartoma of the lung. *J Thorac Cardiovasc Surg* 1971;61:768–776.
6. Carter D, Eggleston JC. Tumors of the lower respiratory tract. In: *Atlas of tumor pathology*. Series 2. Washington, DC: Armed Forces Institute of Pathology, 1980;221–231.
7. Carney JA. The triad of gastric epithelioid leiomyosarcoma, functioning extra-adrenal paraganglioma, and pulmonary chondroma. *Cancer* 1979;43:374–382.
8. Wick MR, Ruebner BH, Carney JA. Gastric tumors in patients with pulmonary chondroma or extra-adrenal paraganglioma: an ultrastructural study. *Arch Pathol Lab Med* 1981;105:527–531.
9. Van Den Bosch JMM, Wagenaar SS, Corrin B, et al. Mesenchymoma of the lung (so called hamartoma): a review of 154 parenchymal and endobronchial cases. *Thorax* 1987;42:790–793.
10. Salminen US. Pulmonary hamartoma: a clinical study of 77 cases in a 21 year period and review of the literature. *Eur J Cardiothorac Surg* 1990;4:15–18.
11. Hansen CP, Holtveg H, Francis D, Raasch L, Bertelsen S. Pulmonary hamartoma. *J Thorac Cardiovasc Surg* 1992;104:674–678.
12. Wang SC. Lung hamartoma: a report of 30 cases and review of 477 cases. *Chung Hua Wai Ko Tsa Chih* 1992;30:540–542.
13. Hamper UM, Khouri NF, Stitik FP, Siegelman SS. Pulmonary hamartoma: diagnosis by transthoracic needle aspiration biopsy. *Radiology* 1985;155:15–18.
14. Bateson EM. Histogenesis of intrapulmonary and endobronchial hamartomas and chondromas (cartilage-containing tumors): a hypothesis. *J Pathol* 1970;101:77–83.
15. Bateson EM. So-called hamartoma of the lung: a true neoplasm of fibrous connective tissue of the bronchi. *Cancer* 1973;31:1458–1467.
16. Bateson EM. Relationship between intrapulmonary and endobronchial cartilage-containing tumors (so-called hamartoma). *Thorax* 1965;20:447–461.
17. Incze JS, Lui PS. Morphology of the epithelial component of human lung hamartomas. *Hum Pathol* 1977;8:411–419.
18. Stone FJ, Churg AM. The ultrastructure of pulmonary hamartoma. *Cancer* 1977;39:1064–1070.
19. Perez-Atayde AR, Seiler MW. Pulmonary hamartoma: an ultrastructural study. *Cancer* 1984;53:485–492.
20. Johansson M, Dietrich C, Mandahl N, et al. Recombinations of chromosomal bands 6p21 and 14q24 characterize pulmonary hamartomas. *Br J Cancer* 1993;67:1236–1241.
21. Fletcher JA, Pinkus GS, Donovan K, et al. Clonal rearrangement of chromosome band 6p21 in the mesenchymal component of pulmonary chondroid hamartoma. *Cancer Res* 1992;52:6224–6228.
22. Nappi O, Glasner SD, Swanson PE, Wick MR. Biphasic and monophasic sarcomatoid carcinomas of the lung. *Am J Clin Pathol* 1994;102:331–340.
23. Liebow AA. Tumors of the lower respiratory tract. In: *Atlas of tumor pathology*. Series 1. Washington, DC: Armed Forces Institute of Pathology, 1952;139–141.
24. Landreneau RJ, Hazelrigg SR, Ferson PF, et al. Thoracoscopic resection of 85 pulmonary lesions. *Ann Thorac Surg* 1992;54:415–420.
25. Nakano M, Fukuda M, Sasayama K, et al. Nd-YAG laser treatment for central airway lesions. *Nippon Kyoubu Shikkan Gakkai Zasshi* 1992; 30:1007–1015.
26. Pettinato G, Manivel JC, Rosa ND, Dehner LP. Inflammatory myofibroblastic tumor (plasma cell granuloma): clinicopathologic study of 20 cases with immunohistochemical and ultrastructural observations. *Am J Clin Pathol* 1990;94:538–546.
27. Umiker WO, Iverson L. Post-inflammatory tumors of the lung: report of four cases simulating xanthoma, fibroma, or plasma cell tumor. *J Thorac Surg* 1954;28:55–62.
28. Bahadori M, Liebow AA. Plasma cell granulomas of the lung. *Cancer* 1973;31:191–208.
29. Spencer H. The pulmonary plasma cell/histiocytoma complex. *Histopathology* 1984;8:903–916.
30. Matsubara O, Tan-Liu NS, Kenney RM, Mark EJ. Inflammatory pseudotumors of the lung: progression from organizing pneumonia to fibrous histiocytoma or to plasma cell granuloma in 32 cases. *Hum Pathol* 1988;19:807–814.
31. Carter D, Eggleston JC. Inflammatory pseudotumor. In: *Atlas of tumor pathology*. Series 2. Washington, DC: Armed Forces Institute of Pathology, 1980;300–307.
32. Monzon CM, Gilchrist GS, Burgert EO, et al. Plasma cell granuloma of the lung in children. *Pediatrics* 1982;70:268–274.
33. Berardi RS, Lee SS, Chen HP, Stines GJ. Inflammatory pseudotumors of the lung. *Surg Gynecol Obstet* 1983;156:89–96.
34. Shirakawa T, Fukuda K, Takenaka S, et al. Two cases of inflammatory pseudotumor of the lung with a review of 46 cases reported in the Japanese literature. *Nippon Kyoubu Shikkan Gakkai Zasshi* 1989;27: 1342–1348.
35. Sweetman WR, Hartley LJ, Bauer AJ, Salyer JM. Postinflammatory tumor of the lung: report of a case simulating malignant thymoma. *J Thorac Surg* 1958;35:802–806.
36. Ishiguro M, Miura N, Ota M, et al. A case of inflammatory pseudotumor of the lung that extended to involve the mediastinum. *Nippon Kyoubu Shikkan Gakkai Zasshi* 1991;29:606–610.
37. Hong HY, Castelli MJ, Walloch JL. Pulmonary plasma cell granuloma (inflammatory pseudotumor) with invasion of thoracic vertebrae. *Mt Sinai J Med* 1990;57:117–121.
38. Warter A, Satge D, Roeslin N. Angioinvasive plasma cell granuloma of the lung. *Cancer* 1987;59:435–443.
39. Kuzela DC. Ultrastructural study of a post-inflammatory "tumor" of the lung. *Cancer* 1975;36:149–156.
40. Buell R, Wang NS, Seemayer TA, Ahmed MN. Endobronchial plasma cell granuloma (xanthomatous pseudotumor): a light and electron microscopic study. *Hum Pathol* 1976;7:411–426.
41. Shirakusa T, Miyazaki N, Kitagawa T, Sugiyama K. Ultrastructural study of plasma cell granuloma: report of a case. *Br J Dis Chest* 1979; 73:289–296.
42. Alvarez-Fernandez E, Escalona-Zapata J. Pulmonary plasma cell

granuloma: an electron microscopic and tissue culture study. *Histopathology* 1983;7:279–286.

43. Chen HP, Lee SS, Berardi RS. Inflammatory pseudotumor of the lung: ultrastructural and light microscopic study of a myxomatous variant. *Cancer* 1984;54:861–865.

44. Keen PE, Weutzner S. Inflammatory pseudotumor of mesentery: a complication of ventriculoperitoneal shunt. *J Neurosurg* 1973;38: 371–373.

45. Muraoka S, Sato T, Takahashi T, Ando M, Shimoda H. Plasma cell granuloma of the lung witih extrapulmonary extension. *Acta Pathol Jpn* 1985;35:933–944.

46. Sajjad SM, Begin LR, Dail DH, Lukeman JM. Fibrous histiocytoma of lung: a clinicopathologic study of two cases. *Histopathology* 1981; 5:325–334.

47. Facchetti F, Peeters CDW, Wever ID, Frizzera G. Inflammatory pseudotumor of lymph nodes: immunohistochemical evidence for its fibrohistiocytic nature. *Am J Pathol* 1990;137:281–289.

48. Tomita T, Dixon A, Watanabe I, Mantz F, Richany S. Sclerosing vascular variant of plasma cell granuloma. *Hum Pathol* 1980;11: 197–202.

49. Toccanier MF, Exquis B, Groebli Y. Granulome plasmocytaire du poumon. Neuf observations avec etude immunohistochemique. *Ann Pathol* 1982;2:21–28.

50. Barbareschi M, Ferrero S, Aldovini D, et al. Inflammatory pseudotumor of the lung: immunohistochemical analysis of four new cases. *Histol Histopathol* 1990;5:205–211.

51. Mohsenifar Z, Bein ME, Mott LJM, Tashkin DP. Cystic organizing pneumonia with elements of plasma cell granuloma. *Arch Pathol Lab Med* 1979;103;600–601.

52. Janigan DJ, Marrie TJ. An inflammatory pseudotumor of the lung in Q fever pneumonia. *N Engl J Med* 1983;308:86–88.

53. Lipton JH, Fong TC, Gill MJ, Burgess K, Elliot PD. Q fever inflammatory pseudotumor of the lung. *Chest* 1987;92:756–757.

54. Park SH, Choe GY, Kim CW, Chi JG, Sung SH. Inflammatory pseudotumor of the lung in a child with Mycoplasma pneumonia. *J Korean Med Sci* 1990;5:213–223.

55. Harjula A, Mattila S, Kyoesola K, Heikkilae L, Maekinen J. Plasma cell granuloma of lung and pleura. *Scand J Thorac Cardiovasc Surg* 1986;20:119–121.

56. Loo KT, Seneviratne S, Chan JKC. Mycobacterial infection mimicking inflammatory pseudotumor of the lung. *Histopathology* 1989;14: 217–219.

57. Kim I, Kim WS, Yeon KM, Chi JG. Inflammatory pseudotumor of the lung manifesting as a posterior mediastinal mass. *Pediatr Radiol* 1992;22:467–468.

58. Kuhr H, Svane S. Pulmonary pseudotumor caused by Cryptococcus neoformans. *Tidsskr Norweg Laegeforen* 1991;111:3288–3290.

59. Bishopric GA, D'Agay MF, Schlemmer B, Sarfati E, Brocheriou C. Pulmonary pseudotumor due to *Corynebacterium equi* in a patient with the acquired immunodeficiency syndrome. *Thorax* 1988;43: 486–487.

60. Yanagisawa K, Traquina DN. Inflammatory pseudotumor:an unusual case of recurrent pneumonia in childhood. *Int J Pediatr Otorhinolaryngol* 1993;25:261–268.

61. Ozaki T, Haku T, Kawano T, Yasuoka S, Ogura T. Neutrophil recruitment in the respiratory tract of a patient with plasma cell granuloma of the lung. *Chest* 1990;98:770–772.

62. Freschi P, Pocecco M, Carini C, Silvestri F, Alcaro P. Pseudotumor inflammatorio polmonare post-traumatico: descrizione di un caso. *Ped Med e Chir* 1989;11:93–96.

63. Hutchins GM, Eggleston JC. Unusual presentation of pulmonary inflammatory pseudotumor (plasma cell granuloma) as esophageal obstruction. *Am J Gastroenterol* 1979;71:501–504.

64. Mandelbaum I, Brashear RE, Hull MT. Surgical treatment and course of pulmonary pseudotumor (plasma cell granuloma). *J Thorac Cardiovasc Surg* 1981;82:77–82.

65. Roikjaer O, Thomsen JK. Plasmacytoma of the lung. *Cancer* 1986;58: 2671–2674.

66. Colby TV. Lymphoproliferative diseases. In: Dail DH, Hammar SP, eds. *Pulmonary pathology.* 2nd ed. New York: Springer-Verlag, 1994; 1097–1122.

67. Weiss LM, Yousem SA, Warnke RA. Non-Hodgkin's lymphomas of the lung. *Am J Surg Pathol* 1985;9:480–490.

68. Yousem SA, Weiss LM, Colby TV. Primary pulmonary Hodgkin's disease: a clinicopathologic study of 15 cases. *Cancer* 1985;57: 1217–1224.

69. Lee JT, Shelburne JD, Linder J. Primary malignant fibrous histiocytoma of the lung: a clinicopathologic and ultrastructural study of five cases. *Cancer* 1984;53:1124–1130.

70. Yousem SA, Hochholzer L. Malignant fibrous histiocytoma of the lung. *Cancer* 1987;60:2532–2541.

71. Calamari S, Brown RW, Cagle PT. p53 immunostaining in the differentiation of inflammatory pseudotumor of the lung from sarcoma (abstracted). *Lab Invest* 1994;70:149A.

72. Tan-Liu N, Matsubara O, Grillo HC, Mark EJ. Invasive fibrous tumor of the tracheobronchial tree: clinical and pathologic study of seven cases. *Hum Pathol* 1989;20:180–184.

73. Yousem SA, Hochholzer L. Pulmonary hyalinizing granuloma. *Am J Clin Pathol* 1987;87:1–6.

74. Alvarez-Fernandez E, Carretero-Albinana L, Menarguez-Palance J. Sclerosing hemangioma of the lung: an immunohistochemical study of intermediate filaments and endothelial markers. *Arch Pathol Lab Med* 1989;113:121–124.

75. Doski JJ, Priebe CJ Jr, Driessnack M, et al. Corticosteroids in the management of unresected plasma cell granuloma (inflammatory pseudotumor) of the lung. *J Ped Surg* 1991;26:1064–1066.

76. Umeki S. A case of plasma cell granuloma which resolved after steroid therapy. *Nippon Kyoubu Shikkan Gakkai Zasshi* 1993;31: 123–126.

77. Imperato JP, Folkman J, Sagerman RH. Cassady JR. Treatment of plasma cell granuloma of the lung with radiation therapy: a report of two cases and a review of the literature. *Cancer* 1986;57:2127–2129.

78. Wood C, Nickoloff BJ, Todes-Taylor NR. Pseudotumor resulting from atypical mycobacterial infection: a "histoid" variety of mycobacteria avium intracellulare complex infection. *Am J Clin Pathol* 1985;83:524–527.

79. Brandwein M, Choid H-SH, Strauchen J, Stroler M, Jagirdar J. Spindle cell reaction to nontuberculous mycobacteriosis in AIDS mimicking a spindle cell neoplasm: evidence for dual histiocytic and fibroblast-like characteristics of cells. *Virchows Arch Pathol Anat* 1990;416: 281–286.

80. Umlas J, Federman M, Crawford C, O'Hara BAC, Fitzgibbons J, Modeste A. Spindle cell pseudotumor due to *Mycobacterium avium-intracellulare* in patients with acquired immunodeficiency syndrome (AIDS): positive staining of mycobacteria for cytoskeleton filaments. *Am J Surg Pathol* 1991;15(12):1181–1187.

81. Chen KT. Mycobacterial spindle cell pseudotumor of lymph nodes. *Am J Surg Pathol* 1992;16(3):276–281.

82. Wade HW. The histoid variety of lepromatous leprosy. *Int Lepr* 1963; 31:129–142.

83. Sekosan M, Cleto M, Senseng C, Farolan M, Sekosan J. Spindle cell pseudotumors in the lungs due to *Mycobacterium* tuberculosis in a transplant patient. *Am J Surg Pathol* 1992;18:1065–1068.

84. Isaacson PG, Spencer J. Malignant lymphoma of mucosa-associated lymphoid tissue. *Histopathology* 1987;11:445–462.

85. Addis BJ, Hyjek E, Isaacson PG. Primary pulmonary lymphoma: a reappraisal of its histogenesis and its relationship to pseudolymphoma and lymphoid interstitial pneumonia. *Histopathology* 1988;13;1–7.

86. Koss MN. Lymphoproliferative disorders of the lung. In: Marchevsky AM, ed. *Surgical pathology of lung neoplasms.* New York: Marcel Dekker, 1990;433–486.

87. Koss MN, Hochholzer L, Langloss JM, Wehunt WD, Lazarus AA. Lymphoid interstitial pneumonia: clinicopathological and immunopathological findings in 18 cases. *Pathology* 1987;19:178–185.

88. Morris JC, Rosen MJ, Marchevsky AM, Teirstein AS. Lymphocytic interstitial pneumonia in patients at risk for the acquired immune deficiency syndrome. *Chest* 1987;91:63–67.

89. Strimlan CV, Rosenow EC III, Divertie MB, Harrison EG Jr. Pulmonary manifestations of Sjogren's syndrome. *Chest* 1976;70: 354–361.

90. Liebow AA, Carrington CB. Diffuse pulmonary lymphoreticular infiltration association with dysproteinemia. *Med Clin North Am* 1973; 57:809–843.

91. Kradin RL, Mark EJ. Benign lymphoid disorders of the lung with a theory regarding their development. *Hum Pathol* 1983;14:857–867.

92. Vath RR, Alexander CB, Fulmer JD. The lymphocytic infiltrative lung diseases. *Clin Chest Med* 1982;3:619–634.

93. Koss MN, Hochholzer L, Nichols PW, Wehunt WD, Lazarus AA. Pri-

mary non-Hodgkin's lymphomas and pseudolymphomas of the lung: a study of 161 patients. *Hum Pathol* 1983;14:1024–1038.

94. Banerjee D, Dildar A. Malignant lymphomas complicating lymphoid interstitial pneumonia. *Hum Pathol* 1982;13:780–782.

95. Salhany KE, Pietra GG. Extranodal lymphoid disorders. *Am J Clin Pathol* 1993;99:472–485.

96. Ritter JH, Adesokan PN, Fitzgibbon JF, Wick MR. Paraffin section immunohistochemistry as an adjunct to morphologic analysis in the diagnosis of cutaneous lymphoid infiltrates. *J Cutan Pathol.* 1994;21:481–493.

97. Andiman WA, Eastman R, Martin K, et al. Opportunistic lymphoproliferations associated with Epstein–Barr viral DNA in infants and children with AIDS. *Lancet* 1985;2:1390–1393.

98. Schooley RT, Carey RW, Miller G, et al. Chronic Epstein–Barr virus infection associated with fever and interstitial pneumonitis. *Ann Intern Med* 1986;104:636–646.

99. Resnick L, Pitchenik AE, Fisher E, Croney R. Detection of HTLV-III/LAV-specific IgG and antigen in bronchoalveolar lavage fluid from two patients with lymphocytic interstitial pneumonia associated with AIDS-related complex. *Am J Med* 1987;82:553–556.

100. Keller AR, Hochholzer L, Castleman B. Hyaline-vascular and plasma cell types of giant lymph node hyperplasia of the mediastinum and other locations. *Cancer* 1972;29:670–676.

101. Wandall HH. A study on neoplastic cells in sputum as a contribution to the diagnosis of primary lung cancer. *Acta Chir Scand* 1944;91 (Suppl 93):1–143.

102. Koss LG. *Diagnostic cytology and its histologic basis.* 4th ed. Philadelphia: JB Lippincott, 1992;849–864.

103. Erozan YS. Cytopathologic diagnosis of pulmonary neoplasms in sputum and bronchoscopic specimens. *Semin Diagn Pathol* 1986; 3:188–195.

104. Jay SJ, Wehr K, Nicholson DP, Smith AL. Diagnostic sensitivity and specificity of pulmonary cytology. *Acta Cytol* 1980;24:304–312.

105. Pearson FG, Thompson DW, Delarue NC. Experience with the cytologic detection, localization, and treatment of radiographically undemonstrable bronchial carcinoma. *J Thorac Cardiovasc Surg* 1967; 54:371–382.

106. Zavala DC. Diagnostic fiberoptic bronchoscopy: techniques and results of biopsy in 600 patients. *Chest* 1975;68:12–19.

107. Truong LD, Underwood RD, Greenberg SD, McLarty JW. Diagnosis and typing of lung carcinomas by cytopathologic methods: a review of 108 cases. *Acta Cytol* 1985;29:379–384.

108. Berkheiser JW. Bronchiolar proliferation and metaplasia associated with bronchiectasis, pulmonary infarct, and anthracosis. *Cancer* 1959; 12:499–508.

109. Berkheiser JW. Bronchiolar proliferation and metaplasia associated with thromboembolism: a pathological and experimental study. *Cancer* 1963;16:205–211.

110. Kawecka M. Cytological evaluation of the sputum in patients with bronchiectasis and the possibility of erroneous diagnosis of carcinoma. *Acta Union Int Cancer* 1959;15:469–473.

111. Marchevsky AM, Nieburgs HE, Olenko F, et al. Pulmonary tumorlets in cases of "tuberculoma" of the lung with malignant cells in brush biopsy. *Acta Cytol* 1982;26:491–494.

112. Johnston WW, Frable WJ. Cytopathology of the respiratory tract: a review. *Am J Pathol* 1976;84:371–424.

113. Saccomanno G, Archer VE, Saunders RD, et al. Development of carcinoma of the lung as reflected in exfoliated cells. *Cancer* 1974;33: 256–270.

114. Koss LG, Richardson HI. Some pitfalls of cytological diagnosis of lung cancer. *Cancer* 1955;8:937–947.

115. Plamenac P, Nikulin A, Pikula B. Cytologic changes of the respiratory tract in young adults as a consequence of high levels of air pollution exposure. *Acta Cytol* 1973;17:241–244.

116. Kern WH. Cytology of hyperplastic and neoplastic lesions of terminal bronchioles and alveoli. *Acta Cytol* 1965;9:372–379.

117. McKee G, Parums DV. False positive cytodiagnosis in fibrosing alveolitis. *Acta Cytol* 1990;34:105–107.

118. Meyer EC, Liebow AA. Relationship of interstitial pneumonia and honey-combing and typical epithelial proliferation to cancer of the lung. *Cancer* 1965;18:322–351.

119. Williams JW. Alveolar metaplasia: its relationship to pulmonary fibrosis in industry and development of lung cancer. *Br J Cancer* 1957: 11:30–42.

120. Johnston WW. Type II pneumocytes in cytologic specimens: a diag-

121. Clayton F. The spectrum and significance of bronchioloalveolar carcinoma. *Pathol Annu* 1988;23(2):361–394.

122. Stanley MW, Henry-Stanley MJ, Gajl-Peczackska KJ, Bitterman PB. Hyperplasia of type II pneumocytes in acute lung injury. *Am J Clin Pathol* 1992;97:669–677.

123. Grotte D, Stanley MW, Swanson PE, Henry-Stanley MJ, Davies S. Reactive type II pneumocytes in bronchoalveolar lavage fluid from acute respiratory distress syndrome can be mistaken for cells of adenocarcinoma. *Diagn Cytopathol* 1990;6:317–322.

## Mediastinum and Thymus

124. Marchevsky AM. Mediastinal tumor-like conditions and tumors that can simulate thymic neoplasms. In: Givel J-C, ed. *Surgery of the thymus.* Berlin: Springer-Verlag, 1990;151–162.

125. Wick MR, Rosai J. Epithelial tumors; neuroendocrine, germ cell, and nonepithelial tumors. In: Givel J-C, ed. *Surgery of the thymus.* Berlin: Springer-Verlag, 1990;79–150.

126. Miller JB, Variakojis D, Bitran JD, et al. Diffuse histiocytic lymphoma with sclerosis: a clinicopathologic entity frequently causing superior vena caval obstruction. *Cancer* 1981;47:748–756.

127. Perrone TA, Frizzera G, Rosai J. Mediastinal diffuse large-cell lymphoma with sclerosis: a clinicopathologic study of 60 cases. *Am J Surg Pathol* 1986;10:176–191.

128. Coffin CM, Watterson J, Priest JR, Dehner LP. Extrapulmonary inflammatory myofibroblastic tumor (inflammatory pseudotumor): a clinicopathologic and immunohistochemical study of 84 cases. *Am J Surg Pathol* 1995;19:859-872.

129. Kaplan G, Sarino EF, Principato DJ. Pseudotumor of the mediastinum. *Chest* 1973;63:620–621.

130. Tong TR, Gil J, Batheja N, et al. Inflammatory pseudotumor of the mediastinum associated with azacytidine therapy, acute myeloid leukemia, and previous chemotherapy for astrocytoma. *Int J Surg Pathol* 1995;3:49–58.

131. Meis JM, Enzinger FM. Inflammatory fibrosarcoma of the mesentery and retroperitoneum: a tumor closely simulating inflammatory pseudotumor. *Am J Surg Pathol* 1991;15:1146–1156.

132. Baum GL, Green RA, Schwarz J. Enlarging pulmonary histoplasmoma. *Am Rev Respir Dis* 1960;82:721–726.

133. Schowwengerdt CG, Suyemoto R, Main FB. Granulomatous and fibrous mediastinitis: a review and analysis of 180 cases. *J Thorac Cardiovasc Surg* 1969;57:365–379.

134. Light AM. Idiopathic fibrosis of the mediastinum: a discussion of three cases and review of the literature. *J Clin Pathol* 1978;31:78–88.

135. Dines DE, Payne WS, Bernatz PE, Pairolero PC. Mediastinal granulomas and fibrosing mediastinitis. *Chest* 1979;75:320–324.

136. Strimlan CV, Dines DE, Payne WS. Mediastinal granuloma. *Mayo Clin Proc* 1975;50:702–705.

137. Ferguson TB, Burford TH. Mediastinal granuloma: a 15 year experience. *Ann Thorac Surg* 1965;1:125–141.

138. Kunkel WM Jr, Clagett OT, McDonald JR. Mediastinal granulomas. *J Thorac Surg* 1954;27:565–574.

139. Salyer JM, Harrison HN, Winn DF Jr, Taylor RR. Chronic fibrous mediastinitis and superior vena caval obstruction due to histoplasmosis. *Dis Chest* 1959;35:364–377.

140. Wieder S, Rabinowitz JG. Fibrous mediastinitis: a late manifestation of mediastinal histoplasmosis. *Radiology* 1977;125:305–312.

141. Tecce PM, Fishman EK, Kuhlman JE. CT evaluation of the anterior mediastinum: spectrum of disease. *Radiographics* 1994;14:973–990.

142. DasGupta TK, Brasfield RD, O'Hara J. Extra-abdominal desmoids: a clinicopathological study. *Ann Surg* 1969;170:k109–117.

143. Yokoyama R, Tsuneyoshi M, Enjoji M, et al. Extra-abdominal desmoid tumors: correlations between histologic features and biologic behavior. *Surg Pathol* 1989;2:29–42.

144. Wold LE, Weiland LH. Tumefactive fibroinflammatory lesions of the head and neck. *Am J Surg Pathol* 1983;7:477–482.

145. Olsen KD, DeSanto LW, Wold LE, Weiland LH. Tumefactive fibroinflammatory lesions of the head and neck. *Laryngoscope* 1986; 96:940–944.

146. Savage PD, Wick MR, Thompson RC, Skubitz KM. Tumefactive fibroinflammatory lesion of the extremity. *Arch Pathol Lab Med* 1991; 115:230–232.

147. DeBoer WA. Riedel's thyroiditis, retroperitoneal fibrosis, and sclerosing cholangitis: diseases with one pathogenesis? *Gut* 1993;34:714.

148. Kelly JK, Hwang WS. Idiopathic retractile (sclerosing) mesenteritis and its differential diagnosis. *Am J Surg Pathol* 1989;13:513–521.

149. Ormond JK. Bilateral ureteral obstruction due to envelopment and compression by an inflammatory retroperitoneal process. *J Urol* 1948; 59:1072–1079.

150. Osborne BM, Butler JJ, Bloustein P, Sumner G. Idiopathic retroperitoneal fibrosis (sclerosing retroperitonitis). *Hum Pathol* 1987;18: 735–739.

151. Ross DS, Daniels GH. Riedel's thyroiditis associated with Hashimoto's thyroiditis. *J Endocrinol Invest* 1992;107:591–595.

152. Turner-Warwick R, Nabarro JDN, Domach D. Riedel's thyroiditis and retroperitoneal fibrosis. *Proc R Soc Med* 1966;59:596–598.

153. Zimmerman-Belsing T, Feldt-Rasmussen U. Riedel's thyroiditis: an autoimmune or primary fibrotic disease? *J Intern Med* 1994;235: 271–274.

154. Mitchinson MJ. The pathology of idiopathic retroperitoneal fibrosis. *J Clin Pathol* 1970;23:681–689.

155. Rutty GN, Lauder I. Mesothelial inclusions within mediastinal lymph nodes. *Histopathology* 1994;25:483–487.

156. Brooks JSJ, LiVolsi VA, Pietra GG. Mesothelial cell inclusions in mediastinal lymph nodes mimicking metastatic carcinoma. *Am J Clin Pathol* 1990;93:741–748.

157. Chen KTK. Benign glandular inclusions of the peritoneum and periaortic lymph nodes. *Diagn Gynecol Obstet* 1981;3:265–268.

## Pleura

158. Cibas ES. Effusions (pleural, pericardial, and peritoneal) and peritoneal washings. In: Atkinson B, ed. *Atlas of diagnostic cytopathology*. Philadelphia: WB Saunders, 1990.

159. Bibbo M. *Comprehensive cytopathology*, Philadelphia: WB Saunders, 1991.

160. Koss LG. *Diagnostic cytology and its histopathologic bases*. 4th ed. Philadelphia: JB Lippincott, 1994.

161. McCaughey WTE, Al-Jabi M. Differentiation of serosal hyperplasia and neoplasia in biopsies. *Pathol Annu* 1986;21(1):271–293.

162. Sears D, Hajdu SI. The cytologic diagnosis of malignant neoplasms in pleural and peritoneal effusions. *Acta Cytol* 1987;31:85–97.

163. Kobayashi TK, Gotoh T, Nakano K, et al. Atypical mesothelial cells associated with eosinophilic pleural effusions: nuclear DNA content and immunocytochemical staining reaction with epithelial markers. *Cytopathology* 1993;4:37–46.

164. Chen CJ, Chang SC, Tseng HH. Assessment of immunocytochemical and histochemical staining in the distinction between reactive mesothelial cells and adenocarcinoma in body effusions. *Chinese Med J* 1994;54:149–155.

165. Schultenover SJ. Body cavity fluids. In: Ramzi I, ed. *Clinical cytopathology and aspiration biopsy*. East Norwalk, CT: Appleton-Lange, 1990;165–180.

166. Leong AS-Y, Stevens MW, Mukherjee TM. Malignant mesothelioma: cytologic diagnosis with histologic, immunohistochemical, and ultrastructural correlation. *Semin Diagn Pathol* 1992;9:141–150.

167. Bedrossian CWM, Bonsib S, Moran C. Differential diagnosis between mesothelioma and adenocarcinoma: a multimodal approach based on ultrastructure and immunocytochemistry. *Semin Diagn Pathol* 1992; 9:91–96.

168. Kutty CPK, Remeniuk E, Varkey B. Malignant-appearing cells in pleural effusion due to pancreatitis. *Acta Cytol* 1981;25:412–416.

169. Marchevsky AM, Hauptman E, Gil J, Watson C. Computerized interactive morphometry as an aid in the diagnosis of pleural effusions. *Acta Cytol* 1987;31:131–136.

170. Kwee WS, Veldhuizen RW, Alons CA, et al. Quantitative and qualitative differences between benign and malignant mesothelial cells in pleural fluid. *Acta Cytol* 1982;26:401–406.

171. Oberholzer M, Ettlin R, Christen H, et al. The significance of morphometric methods in cytologic diagnostics: differentiation between mesothelial cells, mesothelioma cells, and metastatic adenocarcinoma cells in pleural effusions with special emphasis on chromatin texture. *Analyt Cell Pathol* 1991;3:25–42.

172. Ranaldi R, Marinelli F, Barbatelli G, et al. Benign and malignant mesothelial lesions of the pleura: quantitative study. *Appl Pathol* 1986;4:55–64.

173. Battifora H. The pleura. In: Sternberg SS, ed. *Diagnostic surgical pathology*. 2nd ed. New York: Raven Press, 1994.

174. Roberts GH, Campbell GH. Exfoliative cytology of diffuse mesothelioma. *J Clin Pathol* 1972;25:557–582.

175. Bolen JW. Tumors of serosal tissue origin. *Clin Lab Med* 1987; 7:31–50.

176. Whitaker D, Henderson DW, Shilkin KB. The concept of mesothelioma in situ: implications for diagnosis and histogenesis. *Semin Diagn Pathol* 1992;9:151–161.

177. Bolen JW, Hammar SP, McNutt MA. Reactive and neoplastic serosal tissue: a light-microscopic, ultrastructural, and immunocytochemical study. *Am J Surg Pathol* 1986;10:34–47.

178. Singh HK, Silverman JF, Berns L, Haddad MG, Park HK. Significance of epithelial membrane antigen in the workup of problematic serous effusions. *Diagn Cytopathol* 1995;13:3–7.

179. Lidang-Jensen M, Johansen P. Immunocytochemical staining of serous effusions: an additional method in routine cytology practice? *Cytopathology* 1994;5:93–103.

180. Bethwaite PB, Delahunt B, Holloway LJ, Thornton A. Comparison of silver-staining nucleolar organizer region (AgNOR) counts and proliferating cell nuclear antigen (PCNA) expression in reactive mesothelial hyperplasia and malignant mesothelioma. *Pathology* 1995;27:1–4.

181. Kafiri G, Thomas DM, Shepherd NA, Krasz T, Lane DP, Hall PA. p53 expression is common in malignant mesothelioma. *Histopathology* 1992;21:331–334.

182. Cagle PT, Brown RW, Lebovitz RM. p53 immunostaining in the differentiation of reactive processes from malignancy in pleural biopsy specimens. *Hum Pathol* 1994;25:443–448.

183. Walts AE, Said JW, Koeffler HP. Is immunoreactivity for p53 useful in distinguishing benign from malignant effusions? Localization of p53 gene product in benign mesothelial and adenocarcinoma cells. *Mod Pathol* 1994;7:462–468.

184. Humphrey PA. p53: mutations and immunohistochemical detection, with a focus on alterations in urologic malignancies. *Adv Pathol Lab Med* 1994;7:579–596.

185. Hammar SP. Pleural diseases. In: Dail DH, Hammar SP, eds. *Pulmonary pathology*, 2nd ed. New York: Springer-Verlag, 1994.

186. Athanassiadou P, Athanassiades P, Lazaeris D, et al. Immunocytochemical differentiation of reactive mesothelial cells and adenocarcinoma cells in serous effusions with the use of carcinoembryonic antigen and fibronectin. *Acta Cytol* 1994;38:718–722.

187. Nance KV, Silverman JF. Immunocytochemical panel for the identification of malignant cells in serous effusions. *Am J Clin Pathol* 1991; 95:867–874.

188. Mottolese M, Salzano M, Vincenzoni C, et al. The use of a panel of monoclonal antibodies can lower false negative diagnoses of peritoneal washings in ovarian tumors. *Cancer* 1991;68:1803–1807.

189. Johnston WW, Szpak CA, Lottich SC, et al. Use of monoclonal antibody (B72.3) as an immunocytochemical adjunct to diagnosis of adenocarcinoma in human effusions. *Cancer Res* 1985;45:1894–1900.

190. el-Habashi A, el-Morsi B, Freeman SM, el-Didi M, Marrogi AJ. Tumor oncogenic expression in malignant effusions as a possible method to enhance cytologic diagnostic sensitivity. An immunocytochemical study of 87 cases. *Am J Clin Pathol* 1995;103:206–214.

191. Alkan S, Lehman C, Sarago C, Sidawy MK, Karcher DS, Garrett CT. Polymerase chain reaction detection of immunoglobulin gene rearrangement and bcl-2 translocation in archival glass slides of cytologic material. *Diagn Mol Pathol* 1995;4:25–31.

192. Sparks JW. Pulmonary asbestosis. *Radiology* 1931;17:1249–1257.

193. Smith AR. Pleural calcification resulting from exposure to certain dusts. *AJR* 1952;69:375–382.

194. Porro FW, Patten JR, Hobbs AA. Pneumoconiosis in the talc industry. *AJR* 1942;47:507–524.

195. Churg A. Asbestos fibers and pleural plaques in a general autopsy population. *Am J Pathol* 1982;109:88–96.

196. Churg A, dePaoli L. Environmental pleural plaques in residents of a Quebec chrysotile mining town. *Chest* 1988;94:58–60.

197. Craighead JE. Report of the pneumoconiosis committee of the College of American Pathologists and the National Institute for Occupational Safety and Health. *Arch Pathol Lab Med* 1982;106:544–96.

198. Fondimare A, Duwoos H, Desbordes J, et al. Plaques fibroyalines calcifiees du foie dans l asbestose. *Nouv Presse Med* 1973;3:893.

199. Hillerdal G. Pleural plaques in a health survey material: frequency, development and exposure to asbestos. *Scand J Respir Dis* 1978;59: 257–263.

200. Hillerdal G. The pathogenesis of pleural plaques and pulmonary asbestosis: possibilities and impossibilities. *Eur J Respir Dis* 1980;61: 129–138.

201. Hourihane DO, Lessof L, Richardson PC. Hyaline and calcified pleural plaques as an index of exposure to asbestos: a study of radiological and pathological features of 100 cases with a consideration of epidemiology. *Br Med J* 1966;1:1069–1074.

202. Kishimoto T, Ono T, Okada K, Ito H, Relationship between numbers of asbestos bodies in autopsy lung and pleural plaques on chest x-ray film. *Chest* 1989;95:549–552.

203. Kiviluoto R. Pleural calcification as a roentgenologic sign of nonoccupational endemic anthophyllite asbestosis. *Acta Radiol* 1960;194:1–67.

204. LeBouffant L, Martin JC, Durif S, Daniel H. Structure and composition of pleural plaques. In: Bogovski P, Gilson JC, Timbrell V, Wagner JC, eds. *Biological effects of asbestos*. Lyon, France: International Agency for Research on Cancer, 1973;249–257.

205. Mattson S, Ringqvist T. Pleural plaques and exposure to asbestos. *Scand J Respir Dis* 1970;75:1–41.

206. Meurman L. Asbestos bodies and pleural plaques in a Finnish series of autopsy cases. *Acta Pathol Microbiol Scand* 1966;181:7–107.

207. Roberts GH. The pathology of parietal pleural plaques. *J Clin Pathol* 1961:348–353.

208. Solomon A. Radiologic features of asbestos-related visceral pleural changes. *Am J Indust Med* 1991;19:339–355.

209. Wain SL, Roggli VL, Foster WL Jr. Parietal pleural plaques, asbestos bodies and neoplasia: a clinical, pathologic and roentgenographic correlation of 25 consecutive cases. *Chest* 1985;86:707–713.

210. Warnock ML, Prescott BT, Kuwahara TJ. Numbers and types of asbestos fibers in subjects with pleural plaques. *Am J Pathol* 1982;109:37–46.

211. Schwartz DA. New developements in asbestos-induced pleural disease. *Chest* 1991;99:91–98.

212. Ameille J, Brochard P, Brechot JM, et al. Pleural thickening: a comparison of oblique chest radiographs and high resolution computed tomography in in subjects exposed to low levels of asbestos pollution. *Int Arch Occup Environ Health* 1993;64:545–548.

213. Wilson GE, Haselton PS, Chatterjee AK. Desmoplastic mesothelioma: a review of 17 cases. *J Clin Pathol* 1992;45:295–298.

214. Cantin R, Al-Jabi M, McCaughey WT. Desmoplastic diffuse mesothelioma. *Am J Surg Pathol* 1982;6:215–222.

215. Epstein JI, Budin RE. Keratin and epithelial membrane antigen immunoreactivity in non-neoplastic fibrous pleural lesions: implications for the diagnosis of desmoplastic mesothelioma. *Hum Pathol* 1986;17:566–571.

216. Cagle PT, Truong LD, Spencer EJ, Greenberg SD. Immunohistochemical differentiation of sarcomatoid mesotheliomas from other spindle cell neoplasms. *Am J Clin Pathol* 1989;92:566–571.

217. Dardick I, Srigley JR, McCaughey WT, van Nostrand AW, Richie AC. Ultrastructural aspects of the histogenesis of diffuse and localized mesothelioma. *Virchows Arch A Path Anat* 1984;402:373–378.

218. Moran CA, Suster S, Koss M. The spectrum of histologic growth patterns in benign and malignant fibrous tumors of the pleura. *Semin Diagn Pathol* 1992;9:169–180.

219. Kilburn KH, Warshaw R. Pulmonary functional impairment associated with pleural asbestos disease: circumscribed and diffuse thickening. *Chest* 1990;98:965–972.

220. Greenberg SD. Benign asbestos-related pleural diseases. In: Roggli VL, Greenberd SD, Pratt SD, eds. *Pathology of asbestos-associated diseases*. Boston: Little, Brown.

221. Epler GR, McCloud TC, Gaensler EA. Prevalence and incidence of benign asbestos pleural effusion in a working population. *JAMA* 1982;247:617–622.

222. Gibbs Ar, Stephens M, Griffiths DM, Blight BJN, Pooley FD. Fiber distribution in the lungs and pleura of subjects with asbestos-related diffuse pleural fibrosis. *Br J Indust Med* 1991;48:762–770.

223. Moalli PA, Mac Donald JL, Goodglick LA, Kane AB. Acute injury and regeneration of the mesothelium in response to asbestos fibers. *Am J Pathol* 1987;128:426–445.

224. Stephens M, Gibbs Ar, Pooley Fd, Wagner JC. Asbestos-induced diffuse pleural fibrosis: pathology and mineralogy. *Thorax* 1987;42:583–588.

225. Taskinen E, Ahlmon K, Wukeri M. A current hypothesis of the lymphatic transport of inspired dust to the parietal pleura. *Chest* 1973;193–196.

226. Krieger JS, Fisher ER, Richards MR. Multiple mesothelial cysts of the peritoneum. *Am J Surg* 1952;84:328–330.

227. Mennemeyer R, Smith M. Multicystic peritoneal mesothelioma: a report with electron microscopy of a case mimicking intra-abdominal cystic hygroma (lymphangioma). *Cancer* 1979;44:692–698.

228. Miles AJM, Hart WR, McMahan JT. Cystic mesothelioma of the peritoneum: report of a case with multiple recurrences and review of the literature. *Clev Clin Quart* 1986;53:109–114.

229. Nirodi NS, Lowry DS, Wallace RJ. Cystic mesothelioma of the pelvic peritoneum: two case reports. *Br J Obstet Gynecol* 1984;91:201–204.

230. Philip G. Benign cystic mesothelioma. Case reports. *Br J Obstet Gynecol* 1984;91:932–938.

231. Schneider V, Partridge JR, Gutierrez F, Hurt WG, Maizels MS, Demay RM. Benign cystic mesothelioma involving the female genital tract: report of four cases. *Am J Obstet Gynecol* 1983;145:355–359.

232. Villaschi S, Autelitano F, Santeusanio G, Balistreri P. Cystic mesothelioma of the peritoneum. A report of three cases. *Am J Clin Pathol* 1990;94:758–761.

233. Weiss SW, Tavassoli FA. Multicystic mesothelioma. An analysis of pathologic findings and biologic behavior in 37 cases. *Am J Surg Pathol* 1988;12:737–746.

234. Ross MJ, Welch WR, Scully RE. Multilocular peritoneal inclusion cysts (so-called cystic mesotheliomas). *Cancer* 1989;64:1336–1346.

235. McFadden DE, Clement PB. Peritoneal inclusion cysts with mural mesothelial proliferation. *Am J Surg Pathol* 1986;10:844–854.

236. Ball NJ, Urbanski SJ, Green FH, Kieser T. Pleural multicystic mesothelial proliferation. The so-called multicystic mesothelioma. *Am J Surg Pathol* 1990;14:375–378.

237. Pinkard NB, Wilson RW, Lawless N, Dodd LG, Mcadams HP, Koss MN, Travis WD. Calcifying fibrous pseudotumor of the pleura: a report of three cases of a newly described entity involving the pleura. *Am J Clin Pathol* 1996;105:189–194.

238. Fetsch JF, Montgomery EA, Meis JM. Calcifying fibrous pseudotumor. *Am J Surg Pathol* 1993;17:502–508.

## ADDENDUM REFERENCES

### *Pulmonary Hamartomas and Differential Diagnostic Considerations*

Belikova TP, Yashunskaya NI, Kogan EA. Computer-aided differential diagnosis of small solitary pulmonary nodules. *Comput Biomed Res* 1996;29:48–62.

Boshnakova T, Michallova V. Multipe endobronchial chondromatous hamartomas in a child. *Eur J Pediatr Surg* 1995;5:377–379.

Chadwick SL, Corrin B, Hansell DM, Geddes DM. Fatal hemorrhage from mesenchymal cystic hamartoma of the lung. *Eur Resp J* 1995;8:2182-2184.

Gabka CJ, Muller C, Baretton G, Dienemann H, Schildberg FW. Recurrent multiple leiomyomatous hamartomas of the lung. *Chirugie* 1995;66:530-533.

Gjevre JA, Myers JL, Prakash UB. Pulmonary hamartomas. *Mayo Clin Proc* 1996;71:14–20.

Joshi JM, Rege JD, Badhe VP. Pulmonary hamartoma. *J Assoc Phys India* 1995;43:712–713.

Kasmierczak B, Rosigkeit J, Wanschura S, Meyer-Bolte K, Van de Ven WJ, Kayser K, Krieghoff B, Kastendiek H, Barnitzke S, Bullerdiek J. HMGI-C rerrangements as the molecular basis for the majority of pulmonary chondroid hamartomas: a survey of 30 tumors. *Oncogene* 1996;12:515–521.

King TC, Myers J. Isolated metastasis to a pulmonary hamartoma. *Am J Surg Pathol* 1995;19:472–475.

Leroyer C, Quiot JJ, Dewitte JD, Briere J, Clavier J. Mesenchymal cystic hamartoma of the lung. *Respiration* 1993;60:305–306.

Minoletti F, Sozzi G, Calderone C, DePalma S, Pilotti S, Azzarelli A, Periotti MA. Varient translocation t (6;10) (p21; q22) in pulmonary chondroid hamartoma. *Genes Chromosomes & Cancer* 1996;15:246–248.

Suster S, Primary sarcomas of the lung. *Semin Diagn Pathol* 1995;12:140–157.

Suster S, Moran CA. Pulmonary adenofibroma: report of two cases of an unusual type of famartomatous lesion of the lung. *Histopathology* 1993;23:547–551.

Suzuki N, Ohno S, Ishili Y, Kitamura S. Peripheral intrapulmonary hamartoma accompanied by a similar endotracheal lesion. *Chest* 1994;106:1291–1293.

Taniyama K, Sasaki N, Yamaguchi K, Motohiro K, Tahara E. Fibrolipomatous hamartoma of the lung: a case report and review of the literature. *Jpn J Clin Oncol* 1995;25:159-163.

Umemori Y, Ando A, Okabe K, Uno K, Aoe M, Date H, Moriyama S, Shimizu N. Clinical analysis of lung cancer in patients with chondromatous hamartoma. *Jpn J Thorac Surg* 1995; 48:1061-1064.

Van Klaveren RJ, Hassing HH, Wiersma-van Tilburg JM, Lacquet LK, Cox AL. Mesenchymal cystic hamartoma of the lung: a rare cause of relapsing pneumothorax. *Thorax* 1994;499:1175-1176.

Wanschura S, Kazmierczak B, Pohnke Y, Meyer-Bolte K, Barnitzke S, Van de Ven WJ, Bullerdiek J. Transcriptional activation of HMGI-C in three pulmonary hamartomas each with a der (14) t (12; 14) as the sole cytogentic abnormality. *Cancer Letters* 1996;102:17-21.

Wiatrowska BA, Yazdi HM, Matzinger FR, MacDonald LL. Fine needle aspiration biopsy of pulmonary hamartomas: radiologic, cytologic, and immunocytochemical study of 15 cases. *Acta Cytol* 1995;39:1167-1174.

### *Inflammatory Pseudotumor and Plasma Cell Granuloma of the Lung*

Ahn JM, Kim WS, Yeon KM, Kim IO, Im JG, Han MC. Plasma cell granuloma involving the tracheobronchial angle in a child: a case report. *Pediatr Radiol* 1995;25:204-205.

Anthony PP. Inflammatory pseudotumor (plasma cell granuloma) of lung, liver and other organs. *Histopathology* 1993;23:501-503.

Boman F, Champigneulle J, Boccon-Gibod L, Merlin JL, DeMiscault G, Schmitt C, Sommelet D, Floquet J. Inflammatory myofibroblastic tumor of the lung with endobronchial, infiltrating, moltifocal, and recurrent forms. *Ann Pathol* 1995;15:207-210.

Chan YF, White J, Brash H. Metachronous pulmonary and cerebral inflammatory pseudotumor in a child. *Ped Pathol* 1994;14:805-815.

Copin MC, Gosselin BH, Ribet ME. Plasma cell granuloma of the lung: fifficulties in diagnosis and prognosis. *Ann Thorac Surg* 196;61:1477-1482.

Gelmetti W, Eschenbach C, Kohler M, Grunder HG. Inflammatory pseudotumor (plasma cell granuloma) of the lung in childhood: a case report. *Forschr Gebiete Rontgenstr Neuen Bildg Verf* 1996;164:85-87.

Ledet SC, Brown RW, Cagle PT. p53 immunoreactivity in the differentiation of the inflammatory pseudotumor from sarcoma involving the lung. *Mod Pathol* 1995;8:282-286.

Mas Estelles F, Andres V, Vallcanera A, Muro D, Cortina H. Plasma cell granuloma of the lung in childhood: atypical radiologic findings and association with hypertrophic osteoarthropathy. *Pediatr Radiol* 1995;25:369-372.

Rohrilch P, Peuchmaur M, Cocci SN, Gasselin ID, Garel C, Aigrain Y, Galanaud P, Vilmer E, Emillie D. Interleukin-6 and interleukin-1 beta production in a pediatric plasma cell granuloma of the lung. *Am J Surg Pathol* 1995;19:590-595.

Snyder CS, Dell Aquila, M, Haghighi P, Baergen RN, Suh YS, Yi ES. Clonal changes in inflammatory pseudotumor of the lung: a case report. *Cancer* 1995;76:1545-1549.

Wick MR, Ritter JH, Nappi O. Inflammatory sarcomatoid carcinoma of the lung: report of three cases and comparison with inflammatory pseudotumors in adult patients. *Hum Pathol* 1995;26:1014-1021.

### *Mycobacterial Spindle Cell Pseudotumor*

Corkill M, Stephens J, Bitter M. Fine needle aspiration biopsy of mycobacterial spindle cell pseudotumor: a case report. *Acta Cytol* 1995;39:125-128.

### *Pulmonary Lymphoid Hyperplasia & Differential Diagnostic Alternatives*

Bragg DG, Chor PJ, Muray KA, Kjeldsberg CR. Lymphoproliferative disorders of the lung: histopathology, clinical manifestations, and imaging features. *Am J Roentgenol* 1994;163:273-281.

Franchi LM, Chin TW, Nussbaum E, Riker J, robert M, Talbert WM. Familial pulmonary nodular lymphoid hyperplasma. *J Pediatr* 1992;121:89-92.

Koss MN. Pulmonary lymphoid disorders. *Semin Diagn Pathol* 1995;12:158-171.

Kossakowska AE, Eyton-Jones S. Urbanski SJ. Immunoglobulin and T-cell receptor qene rearrangements in lesions of mucosa-associated lymphoid tissue. *Diagn Molec Pathol* 1993;2:233-240.

Scherak O, Kolarz G, Popp W, Wottawa A, Ritschka L, Braun O. Lung involvement in rheumatoid factor-negative arthritis. *Scand J Rheumatol* 1993;22:225-228.

Teruya-Feldstein J, Temeck BK, Slas MM, Kingma DW, Raffeld M, Pass HI, Mueller B, Jaffe ES. Pulmonary malignant lymphoma of mucosa-associated lymphoid tissue (MALT) arising in a pediatric HIV-positive patient. *Am J Surg Pathol* 1995;19:357-363.

### *False-Positive Respiratory Cytology Specimens*

Ritter JH, Wick MR, Reyes A, Coffin CM, Dehner LP. Flase-positive interpretations of carcinoma in exfoliative respiratory cytology. *Am J Clin Pathol* 1995;104:133-140.

### *Mediastinal Inflammatory Pseudotumor and Fibrosing Mediastinitis*

Bittner RC, Kaiser D, Felix R. Invasive plasma cell granuloma of the mediastinum. *Fortschr Gebiete Rontgen Neuen Bildg Verf* 1994;160:94-95.

Lagerstrom CF, Mitchell HG, Graham BS, Hammon JW Jr. Chronic fibrosing mediastinitis and superior vena caval obstruction from blastomycosis. *Ann Thorac Surg* 1992;54:764-765.

Otto HF. Differential diagnostic problems in fibrosing mediastinitis. *Pathologe* 1992;13:90-94.

Sherrick AD, Brown LR, Harms GF, Myers JL. The radiographic findings of fibrosings mediastinitis. *Chest* 1994;106:484-489.

Suzuki T, Hori G. Fibrosing mediastinitis, sclerosing mediastinitis. *Jpn J Clin Med* 1994;4 (Suppl);442-444.

### *Pleural Mesothelial Hyperlasia and Differential Diagnostic Alternatives*

Mayall FG, Goddard H, Gibbs AR. p53 immunostaining in the distinction between benign and malignant mesothelial proliferations using formalin-fixed paraffin sections. *J Pathol* 1992;168:377-381.

### *Lymphocyte-Rich Pleural Effusions*

Dhodapkar M, Yale SH, Hoagland HC. Hemorrhagic pleural effusion and pleural thicking as a complication of chronic lymphocytic leukemia. *Am J Hematol* 1993;42:221-224.

Miyahara M, Shimamoto Y, Sano M, Nakano H, Shibata K, Matsuzaki M. Immunoglobulin gene rearrangement in T-cell reactive pleural effusion of a patient with B-cell chronic lymphocytic leukemia. *Acta Haematol* 1996;96:41-44.

Morrone N, Gama E, Silva-Volpe VL, Dourado AM, Mitre F, Coletta EN. Bilateral pleural effusion due to mediastinal fibrosis induced by radiotherapy. *Chest* 1993;104:1276-1278.

### *Mesothelioma-like Diffuse Pleural Fibrosis*

Scott EM, Marshall TJ, Flower CD, Steward S. Steward S. diffuse pleural thickening: percutaneous CT-guided cutting needle biopsy. *Radiology* 1995;194:867-870.

### *Pseudoneoplastic Pleural Fibrous Plaques*

Takahashi K, Sera Y, Okubo T.A. A descriptive epidemiological study on pleural plaque cases identified from the workers periodical health examinations in Kitakyushu, Japan. *Jpn J Industr Health* 1993;35:302-313.

## Multicystic Mesothelioma

Devaney K, Kragel PJ, Devaney EJ. Fine-needle aspiration cytology of multicystic mesothelioma. *Diagm Cytopathol* 1992;8:68-72.

## Calcifying Pleural Fibrous Pseudotumor

Eramus JJ, McAdams HP, Patz EF Jr. Murray JG, Pinkard NB. Calcifying fibrous pseudotumor of pleura: radiologic features in three cases. *J Comput Asst Tomogr* 1996;20:763-765.
Reed MK, Margraf LR, Nikaidoh H, Cleveland DC. Calcifying fibrous pseudotumor of the chest wall. *Ann Thorac Surg* 1996;62:873-874.

*Pathology of Pseudoneoplastic Lesions,*
edited by M. R. Wick, P. A. Humphrey, and J. H. Ritter.
Lippincott-Raven Publishers, Philadelphia © 1997.

CHAPTER 5

# Pseudoneoplastic Lesions of the Alimentary Tract

Patrick L. Fitzgibbons

**Pseudoneoplastic Lesions Common to the Entire Gut**
  Inflammatory Fibroid Polyp
  Inflammatory Myofibroblastic Tumor
  Pseudosarcomatous Inflammatory Conditions and
    Hyperplastic Polyps
  Gastrointestinal Xanthomas
  Lipoma-like Lesions
  Ectopias and Heterotopias
  Infections of the Gut Presenting as Pseudotumors
**Pseudotumors of the Esophagus**
  Fibrovascular Polyp
**Pseudoneoplastic Lesions of the Stomach**
  Focal Lymphoid Hyperplasia of the Stomach (Gastric
    Pseudolymphoma)
**Pseudoneoplastic Vascular Lesions**

**Pseudoneoplastic Lesions of the Intestines**
  Pseudotumors Associated with Mucosal Prolapse
  Colitis Cystica Profunda
  Inflammatory Cloacogenic Polyp
  Malakoplakia
  Tumefactive Endometriosis
  Pseudotumors Associated with Diverticular Disease
  Polypoid Prolapsing Mucosal Folds of Diverticular
    Disease
  Solitary Cecal Diverticulitis
  Hypertrophic Anal Papilla
  Pseudoneoplastic Conditions in the Retrorectal Space
  Elastofibromatous Lesions
  Smooth Muscle Pseudotumors
**References**

There are many different types of pseudoneoplastic lesions that involve the gastrointestinal tract, but most are uncommon. The gross appearances of gastrointestinal pseudotumors vary widely. Some lesions present as small mucosal plaques or pedunculated polyps, whereas others are diffusely infiltrative lesions that imitate linitis plastica. Remaining pseudoneoplastic conditions may take the form of ulcers or cystic masses, and some are extrinsic lesions that only secondarily involve the gut. Many disorders in this generic category can be found throughout the entirety of the gastrointestinal tract, whereas a few demonstrate a more restricted anatomic distribution. As is true of other chapters in this book, primary attention is directed at those proliferations that might be confused with neoplasms by pathologists because of morphologic mimicry. Accordingly, such lesions as amyloidosis, selected heterotopias, tumefactive infections, foreign body reactions, and various cysts of the alimentary

tract are not discussed here, despite the fact that they may represent "pseudotumors" at a clinical level.

## PSEUDONEOPLASTIC LESIONS COMMON TO THE ENTIRE GUT

### Inflammatory Fibroid Polyp

There are diverse, seemingly related fibroinflammatory lesions that are histologically, immunologically, and ultrastructurally similar and that occur in the gastrointestinal tract as localized polypoid masses. The most common of these is the *inflammatory fibroid polyp*. First reported by Vanek in 1949 as "eosinophilic granuloma with eosinophils" (1), this lesion has subsequently been called by a variety of names including *inflammatory pseudotumor, inflammatory fibrous polyp,* and *eosinophilic granuloma.* In 1953, Helwig and Ranier proposed the term "inflammatory fibroid polyp" and this is now the preferred designation (2). Recently, another category of fibroinflammatory lesions that may involve the

P.L. Fitzgibbons: Department of Pathology, St. Jude Medical Center, 101 E. Valencia Mesa Drive, Fullerton, California 92635.

gastrointestinal tract—so-called *inflammatory myofibroblastic tumors*—has received increased attention; these proliferations are discussed in detail below. It is important to recognize, however, that although the aforementioned entities are felt to be clinically distinct and are discussed separately here, there is considerable overlap in their histology, immunoreactivity, and possible histogenesis. It is hoped that improved diagnostic classifications will be developed as additional studies of these uncommon disorders evolve.

Inflammatory fibroid polyps (IFPs) are most often found in the gastric antrum or distal ileum, but they have been reported in all parts of the gut (2–9). These localized inflammatory proliferations closely mimic gastrointestinal neoplasms both radiographically and clinically, and they are rarely identified correctly preoperatively. IFP has been reported in all age groups but it is primarily a disease of adults with an average age of 50–60 years at diagnosis. The lesion may be slightly more common in men but there is no significant sex predilection.

Presenting symptoms are dependent on size and location. Most inflammatory fibroid polyps are small (<3.0 cm), polypoid, submucosal masses, but examples as large as 19 cm have been reported. Ileal lesions tend to be larger on average than those in the stomach, and patients with IFP in the small intestine are more likely to present with bowel obstruction or intussusception. Although individuals with large gastric IFPs may also experience disturbed emptying of the stomach, lesions arising at that site are more likely to be discovered incidentally during surgery or endoscopic examination for an unrelated problem. These patients do not have peripheral eosinophilia or an increased prevalence of atopic disorders (10).

IFP is represented by a localized proliferation of inflammatory and mesenchymal elements that arises in the submucosa (11). It begins as a small, sessile growth that gradually enlarges to become a polypoid, exophytic mass, but the gross appearance varies depending upon the exact site of origin. Gastric IFPs are often small, sessile polypoid excrescences that are usually well demarcated from the adjacent gastric wall. Ileal lesions, in contrast, are typically described as pedunculated or dumbbell-shaped, with the masses projecting outward into the muscularis externa and subserosa, as well as the lumen. The mucosa over the surface of the mass often shows extensive ulceration, especially in polyps that are associated with obstruction (Fig. 1). In this situation, the surface of the polyp is often bright red and granular. IFP may be soft and fleshy or firm and rubbery, depending on the quantity of fibrous stroma. Accordingly, it is easily mistaken both grossly and histologically for leiomyoma or another gastrointestinal stromal tumor. The cut surfaces of IFPs are usually homogeneous and gray–white, and may assume a "whorled" configuration.

Despite its circumscribed macroscopic appearance, microscopic examination of IFP reveals an unencapsulated infiltrative process. In many cases, particularly those arising in the ileum, the junction between the mass and the adjacent in-

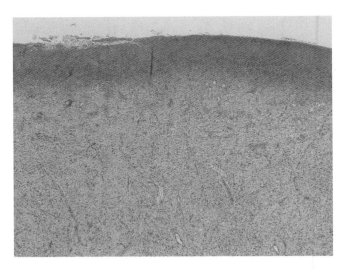

**FIG. 1.** Inflammatory fibroid polyp of the ileum. The mucosal surface is extensively ulcerated.

testinal wall is difficult to discern with precision and the cellular proliferation can extend through the muscularis externa and into the mesentery (Fig. 2). In contrast to ileal lesions, gastric IFPs are usually more well demarcated from the adjacent muscularis, but they show extension of the cellular infiltrate into the overlying mucosa. Histologic features include a proliferation of uniform, fibroblastic-type spindle cells and mixed acute and chronic inflammatory cells in a richly vascularized stroma. This pattern has often been described as resembling organizing granulation tissue (Figs. 3 and 4). The inflammatory infiltrate in IFPs consists of neutrophils, eosinophils, lymphocytes, and plasma cells, with scattered small lymphoid follicles. The number of eosinophils is variable, but it is often striking and may prompt diagnostic consideration of eosinophilic enteritis or the tumefactive hypereosinophilic syndrome. In the early stages of this lesion, its stroma has a myxoid appearance;

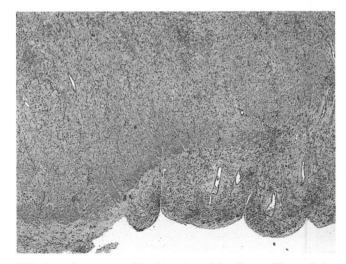

**FIG. 2.** Inflammatory fibroid polyp of the ileum. The cellular infiltrate diffusely involves the muscularis externa and extends to the serosal surface at the bottom of the figure.

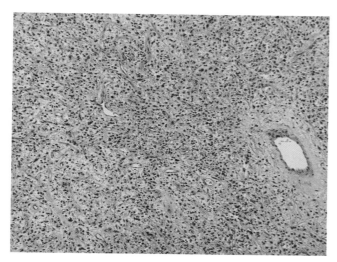

**FIG. 3.** Inflammatory fibroid polyp of the ileum. There is a mixed inflammatory cell infiltrate and numerous small blood vessels within a myxoid stroma.

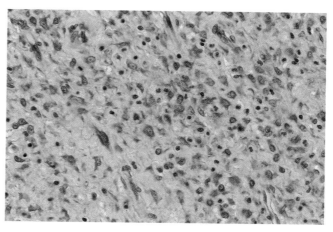

**FIG. 5.** Inflammatory fibroid polyp of the ileum stained with antivimentin antibody. The spindle cells are weakly reactive for vimentin.

with evolution, the matrix becomes more heavily collagenized and a marked resemblance to gastrointestinal stromal tumors may eventuate (8). Pseudosarcomatous changes in the matrical components of IFPs have been well described, with some cases manifesting hypercellular stroma, numerous mitotic figures, and marked atypia of the proliferating spindle cells (6). Similar stromal cells have, of course, been described in many benign polypoid lesions of the respiratory and genitourinary tracts and should not be assumed to indicate the presence of malignancy (see below, as well as corresponding chapters on those tissue sites). Osteoclast-like giant cells are not a documented feature of IFP.

Based on histologic examination alone, some investigators initially believed that IFP was a true neoplasm of either neural or vascular origin. Nevertheless, this conclusion has not been supported by immunohistochemical analysis or clinical observation (7,12–17). The stromal spindle cells of IFP consistently express vimentin but do not label with antibodies to S-100 protein, neuron-specific enolase, or factor VIII–related antigen (Figs. 5 and 6). Although these elements may react with antibodies to muscle-specific actin (HHF-35) or $\alpha$-smooth muscle actin, they do not express desmin (Fig. 7). A recent evaluation of 46 IFPs revealed focally positive staining of the proliferating spindle cells for the "histiocytic" markers CD68 and MAC-387 in roughly one third of cases (17). The latter study identified four immunophenotypic patterns: lesions expressing vimentin alone; others labeling for vimentin and actin; IFPs expressing vimentin and a "histiocytic" marker; and lesions expressing all three of these categories of determinants. Electron microscopic analyses have also shown heterogeneity among IFPs, with evidence that the proliferating spindle

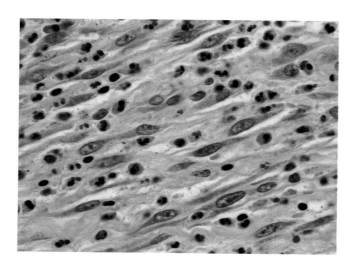

**FIG. 4.** Inflammatory fibroid polyp of the ileum. Note eosinophils, plasma cells, neutrophils, and fibroblasts.

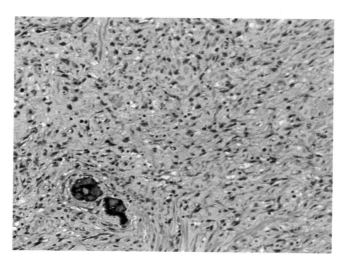

**FIG. 6.** Inflammatory fibroid polyp of the ileum stained with anti-S-100 protein. Except for the entrapped ganglion, there is no staining for S-100 protein.

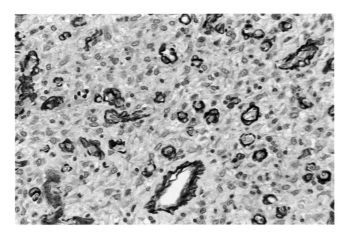

**FIG. 7.** Inflammatory fibroid polyp of the ileum stained with anti–muscle-specific actin (HHF-35). In addition to small blood vessels, some of the spindle cells also stain with muscle-specific actin, and these cells probably represent myofibroblasts.

cells probably show both myofibroblastic (7,12) and "fibrohistiocytic" differentiation (15).

Because many of these lesions contain a dominant population of eosinophils, IFP was at one time thought to be part of a disease spectrum with eosinophilic gastroenteritis (18,19). Both of these lesions have been called "eosinophilic granuloma." Although eosinophilic gastroenteritis can also present with mass lesions and cause obstruction (20), it is now well accepted that there is no relationship between that disease and IFP. Eosinophilic gastroenteritis has been defined by the presence of gastrointestinal symptoms in patients with eosinophilic infiltration of the gut and no evidence of a systemic or parasitic disease that would explain that finding (21). An alternative definition includes symptomatic patients who have characteristic radiographic findings and peripheral eosinophilia (22). The disorder most commonly affects the gastric antrum and proximal small intestine but can involve other parts of the gut. Eosinophilic gastroenteritis is seen in all age groups, and most patients have a history of associated allergic disorders (10). In contrast to IFP, which is a localized fibroinflammatory lesion, eosinophilic gastroenteritis is also a poorly circumscribed process that is characterized by diffuse infiltration of the gut wall by eosinophils, without a coexistent fibrovascular component (20–24) (Fig. 8). There is usually preferential involvement of one of the layers of the gastric or intestinal wall (e.g., yielding so-called mucosal, mural, and serosal variants) (22).

We would also hasten to add that designating IFP "eosinophilic granuloma" invokes unnecessary confusion with Langerhan's cell disease affecting the gastrointestinal tract. The latter process has a typical constellation of clinical and morphologic features that do not overlap with those of IFP.

Another lesion, called *pseudotumoral enterocolitis,* may also enter the differential diagnosis. Two patients have been

reported who presented with peripheral eosinophilia and massive, tumor-like eosinophilic infiltrates that at least partially involved the gastrointestinal tract (25,26). In both cases, no specific cause of the eosinophilia could be found, and administration of corticosteroids proved ineffective in treating the disorder. The masses in one patient were associated with intestinal ulceration and intussusception, and both affected individuals ultimately died of the disorder. Whether pseudotumoral enterocolitis represents a truly neoplastic proliferation of eosinophilic leukocytes—in similarity to granulocytic sarcoma—is unknown at the present time.

Despite its occasional resemblance to neural, vascular, or smooth muscle tumors, IFP has long been considered a nonneoplastic, tumefactive inflammatory lesion. This conclusion was initially based on the overall microscopic appearance of the condition and on the fact that the histologic features appear to change over time (8). Several authors have drawn attention to similarities between IFP and nodular fasciitis (12,17). The concept that IFP is fibroinflammatory and "reactive," rather than a neoplastic process, has been strongly supported by immunohistologic and ultrastructural analysis as detailed above. The immunophenotypic variability of this condition is closely mirrored by that seen in the cellular constituents of healing wounds (27,28). Moreover, it is perfectly consonant with the inconstant expression of actin and mesenchymal intermediate filament proteins by myofibroblasts (29). Again in likeness to nodular fasciitis, it has been speculated that IFP represents an exaggerated and idiosyncratic host response to mucosal injury in the gut (13,30).

## Inflammatory Myofibroblastic Tumor

Inflammatory fibroid polyp must be distinguished from the abdominal inflammatory myofibroblastic tumor (IMT), a

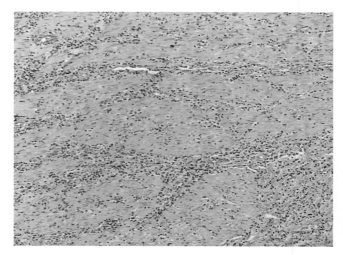

**FIG. 8.** Eosinophilic gastroenteritis. The muscularis externa of the stomach is diffusely infiltrated by eosinophils, and there is little accompanying fibrosis or vascular proliferation.

lesion with distinctive clinical features that has also been classified as *cellular inflammatory pseudotumor, plasma cell granuloma, myxoid hamartoma,* and *inflammatory fibrosarcoma.* Although it perhaps does not represent a homogeneous clinicopathologic entity, the term "plasma cell granuloma" is well recognized and has long been used to refer to localized inflammatory masses, usually involving the lungs (31). Many extrapulmonary examples have been documented as well, and the abdomen is the second most common site for this group of lesions. We have included a discussion of this lesion here, in full recognition of the fact that some observers believe IMT to be a true neoplasm, because in our opinion this point has not been definitively settled.

Abdominal IMT exhibits significant clinical differences from the attributes of inflammatory fibroid polyps (Table 1). The former of these two lesions usually occurs in children between the ages of 2 and 16 years, although a small percentage of cases does occur in adults. The condition most commonly presents in the small or large bowel mesentery (32–37), but cases have been reported in the stomach (38–42), colon (43), and esophagus (44,45). Patients with mesenteric IMT are often clinically ill with systemic complaints including fever and weight loss. These symptoms usually disappear after resection of the mass (33,41). There are characteristic laboratory findings as well, including hypochromic-microcytic anemia, thrombocytosis, hypergammaglobulinemia, and an elevated sedimentation rate. Such signs also typically resolve after surgical extirpation. Radiographic studies may reveal an infiltrative, "aggressive" appearance that closely simulates that of a malignancy (38).

Mesenteric IMTs may be solitary or multicentric. Unifocal examples are large, well-circumscribed, lobular masses that are tightly adherent to surrounding structures such as the bladder and abdominal wall, and they often require extensive surgical resection. Although these lesions probably do not arise *de novo* in the gut, they may invade through the intestinal wall, extend to the luminal surface, and present as polypoid masses that simulate the macroscopic features of sarcoma botryoides (Dr. C. M. Coffin, personal communication).

Initial descriptions of the microscopic features of abdominal IMTs stressed a highly cellular plasma cell infiltrate. In that respect, plasmacytoma is often included in the differential diagnosis. Unlike the latter, it should be remembered that "plasma cell granuloma" demonstrates polytypism for intracellular light chain immunoglobulins and therefore does not

represent a neoplastic infiltrate (39,40,45,46). Coffin and associates (47) recently described three major histologic patterns in abdominal IMTs: (a) spindle cell lesions with intermingled inflammatory cells resembling fibrous histiocytomas; (b) myxoid, vascular, and inflammatory proliferations simulating nodular fasciitis; and (c) dense plate-like aggregations of collagen mimicking scars or desmoid tumors. Most of the fusiform cells in IMTs are cytologically uniform, with oval to elongated hyperchromatic nuclei, small nucleoli, and moderate amounts of eosinophilic cytoplasm. They are arranged in a fascicular or storiform growth pattern (Figs. 9 to 12). There is usually no significant mitotic activity in abdominal IMTs; cytologic atypia is similarly lacking in most examples but some lesions do contain bizarre stromal giant cells.

As is true of the inflammatory fibroid polyp, immunohistochemical and ultrastructural findings in IMTs provide strong evidence that the predominant cell type is the myofibroblast (34,42,43,45,48). The spindle cells in IMT are consistently reactive with antibodies to vimentin, smooth muscle actin, muscle-specific actin, and the "histiocytic" markers CD68 and $\alpha_1$-antitrypsin, but they are negative for S-100 protein and factor VIII–related antigen. An interesting finding in one study was the unexplained presence of keratin immunoreactivity (34), which has not been reproduced in the experience of other observers (Dr. Mark R. Wick, personal communication).

As stated earlier, it remains uncertain whether abdominal IMT is a true neoplasm. Initial reports stressed the inflammatory histologic appearance of this proliferation and the dramatic resolution of signs and symptoms after resection of the mass, and cautioned that this was a benign, nonneoplastic disease for which radical surgery was not indicated. More recent reports, however, have suggested that the prognosis is more uncertain. Even after apparently complete resection of their lesions, some patients may have recurrences with concomitant reappearance of constitutional symptoms (34,45,47,49). In addition, there is some evidence that some of these masses may represent monoclonal neoplastic proliferations (50). Meis and Enzinger reported several patients with seeming metastasis and tumor-related fatality, and concluded that IMT was a malignant neoplasm composed of fibroblasts. Consequently, those authors favored the designation *inflammatory fibrosarcoma* (34). Although it is unclear whether IMTs and the cases reported by Meis and Enzinger are analogous, there have been suggestions that histologic

**TABLE 1.** *Comparison of inflammatory fibroid polyp with inflammatory myofibroblastic tumor*

|  | Inflammatory fibroid polyp | Inflammatory myofibroblastic tumor |
|---|---|---|
| Peak age range | 50–60 | 2–16 |
| Male/female ratio | 1.3:1.0 | 1:1 |
| Predominant site | Stomach, ileum | Small and large bowel mesentery |
| Typical gross appearance | Sessile or pedunculated polyp | Infiltrative mass |
| Constitutional signs and symptoms | Usually absent | Fever, weight loss, anemia |

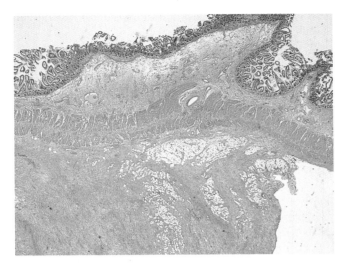

**FIG. 9.** Inflammatory myofibroblastic tumor of the ileum. Spindle cell proliferation involving the external surfaces of the ileum in an 8-year-old boy. (Case courtesy of Dr. Cheryl Coffin, Department of Pathology, Washington University Medical Center, St. Louis, MO.)

examination may allow one to identify those cases that have a higher risk of untoward behavior (51).

It is interesting that despite significant clinical differences the immunohistochemical and ultrastructural findings in IMT are so similar to those of inflammatory fibroid polyp. Regardless of exact histogenesis, it appears that patients with IMT should be treated by complete surgical removal of their masses with close clinical follow-up and surgical extirpation of any recurrences.

## Pseudosarcomatous Inflammatory Conditions and Hyperplastic Polyps

Benign, inflammatory polypoid lesions with atypical stromal cells are found in many different organ systems includ-

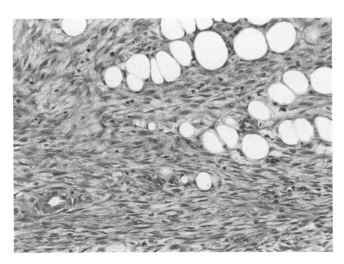

**FIG. 10.** Inflammatory myofibroblastic tumor of the ileum. Uniformly hypercellular spindle cell proliferation surrounds adipocytes.

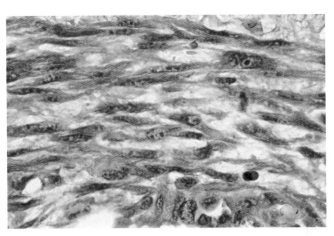

**FIG. 11.** Inflammatory myofibroblastic tumor of the ileum. Uniform fibroblastic cells with only rare plasma cells.

ing the upper respiratory tract, urinary bladder, and digestive tract. Although these cells are thought to represent "reactive" mesenchymal elements, such lesions can be easily mistaken for malignancy due to alarming degrees of cellularity and bizarre cytologic atypia. In the gastrointestinal tract, sarcomatoid stromal cells have been described in biopsies from the distal esophagus in patients with reflux esophagitis, as well as in gastric ulcers and eroded hyperplastic gastric polyps, pseudopolyps from patients with inflammatory bowel disease, granulation tissue adjacent to surgical anastomoses, and hypertrophic anal papillae (52–57). The atypical cells range from widely scattered dendritic-shaped elements in a variably myxoinflammatory background to closely packed groups of atypical spindle cells that are clustered along the base of an ulcerated mucosal surface. The cells often have a "ganglion-like" appearance with large, vesicular nuclei and macronucleoli (Figs. 13–15).

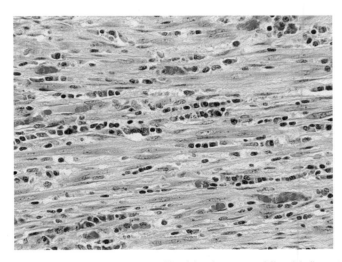

**FIG. 12.** Inflammatory myofibroblastic tumor. Mixed inflammatory and spindle cell proliferation involving the colon of a 10-year-old girl. This patient presented with fever, which resolved after surgery. Note the compact layers of fibroblasts and large number of plasma cells.

Immunohistochemical studies have shown consistent immunoreactivity for vimentin and an absence of staining for epithelial, endothelial, and neural markers, and, as such, these results offer little help in making a diagnostic distinction between pseudosarcomatous proliferations and true gastrointestinal stromal neoplasms. Ultrastructural findings are similarly indeterminate. The correct interpretation is most surely reached by integrating clinical, radiographic, and histologic observations.

### Gastrointestinal Xanthomas

Xanthomas are localized accumulations of lipid-laden macrophages. Most gastrointestinal lesions of this type are small gastric xanthomas (xanthelasmas) that are unassociated with any signs or symptoms and have no clinical significance. On occasion, however, xanthomas may be found in other parts of the gastrointestinal system as large, tumefactive masses that may clinically simulate alimentary tract neoplasms such as poorly differentiated carcinomas, stromal tumors, or metastatic melanoma or carcinoma (58–60). Though they were previously identified most often at autopsy, the increased recognition of gastric xanthomas probably is attributable to the wider use of upper gastrointestinal endoscopy. Xanthomas of the stomach are characteristically observed in elderly individuals and are not found in children. These lesions occur most often in the gastric fundus and usually present as yellow or tan, plaque-like nodules that rarely

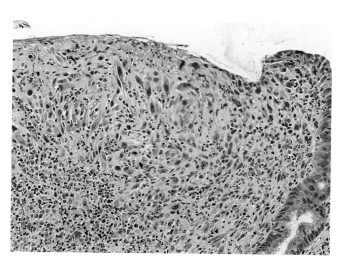

**FIG. 14.** Atypical stromal cells in an inflammatory pseudopolyp. There is a proliferation of hyperchromatic spindle cells beneath the ulcerated surface.

measure more than a few millimeters in diameter. They are composed of intramucosal collections of foamy, lipid-laden macrophages that are often localized to the superficial part of the mucosa (Figs. 16 and 17). A number of diverse gastric lesions may present as mucosal histiocytic infiltrates (Table 2) but the most important differential diagnostic consideration is that of signet ring cell carcinoma of the stomach (Fig. 18). In both instances, gastric glands are displaced by an infiltrate of large cells with abundant, vacuolated cytoplasm; nonetheless, application of histochemical stains allows for ready distinction of epithelial and xanthomatous proliferations. The cells in mucosal xanthomas contain neutral lipid and stain positively with the oil red O or Sudan black methods; they do not stain with Alcian blue, mucicarmine, or periodic acid–Schiff (PAS) techniques, as expected in primary or secondary carcinomas.

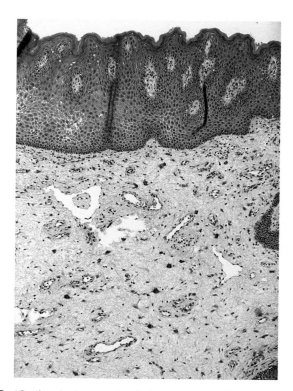

**FIG. 13.** Atypical stromal cells in a hypertrophic anal papilla. Enlarged, dendritic-shaped fibroblasts are scattered throughout the stroma.

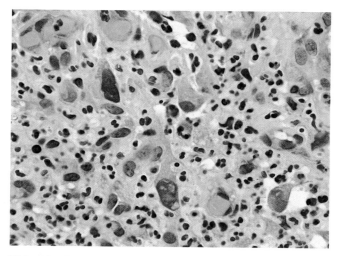

**FIG. 15.** Atypical stromal cells in an inflammatory pseudopolyp. Higher magnification showing marked nuclear pleomorphism.

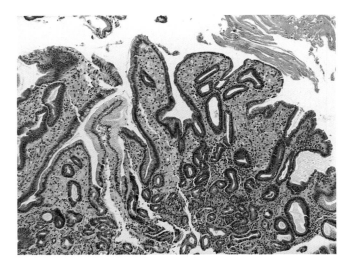

**FIG. 16.** Gastric xanthoma. The superficial portion of the mucosa is expanded by histiocytes.

Cutaneous xanthomas are most common in patients with disturbances of lipid metabolism such as diabetes mellitus, hypercholesterolemia, or liver disease, but no such correlation between dyslipidemia and gastrointestinal xanthomas has been found. Whereas the pathogenesis is uncertain in most cases, there does appear to be an association with prior mucosal injury. Gastric xanthomas have been reported in patients with concomitant chronic gastritis, intestinal metaplasia, and gastric ulcers, and the incidence is markedly increased after partial gastrectomy (63–65). Large xanthomatous masses have also been reported in individuals who have received chemotherapy for intestinal lymphoma (66). This association has led to speculation that mucosal xanthomas reflect a localized impairment of lipid metabolism that occurs in injured epithelium. According to this hypothesis, a mucosal insult results in focal cellular necrosis with the sub-

**TABLE 2.** *Localized infiltrative histiocytic diseases of the gastrointestinal tract*

Malakoplakia
Mycobacterium avium-intracellulare complex
Rosai–Dorfman disease (61,62)
Whipple's disease
Wolman's disease
Xanthoma

sequent influx of phagocytic histiocytes. The latter elements then persist in the lamina propria as foam cells. One of the problems with such theories is that gastric xanthomas can be found in as many as 60% of all autopsies, most of which do not manifest any evidence of mucosal abnormalities.

## Lipoma-like Lesions

A submucosal lipoma is a localized fatty mass that presents itself as a discrete polypoid nodule and is assumed to be a benign neoplasm of adipocytes. Lipomas are relatively common in the gut and can be found anywhere in the gastrointestinal tract (67). They usually take the form of solitary excrescences that measure <2 cm and are rarely associated with clinical symptoms. Nonetheless, there are several lesions that should be distinguished from true submucosal lipoma, including *mucosal pseudolipomatosis* and *lipomatous hypertrophy of the ileocecal valve*.

### Mucosal Pseudolipomatosis

"Mucosal pseudolipomatosis" is a term used to refer to a characteristic histologic change that is most often identified in rectal biopsies. This change is represented by a cluster of regular-appearing empty spaces in the lamina propria that closely simulate fat cells (Fig. 19). The lesion has been previously reported as "lipomatosis," but in a histochemical and

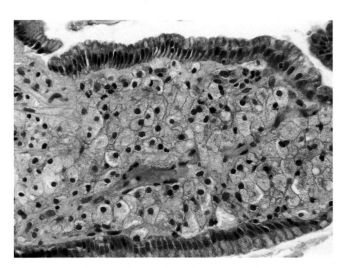

**FIG. 17.** Gastric xanthoma. A uniform population of foamy macrophages distends the mucosa.

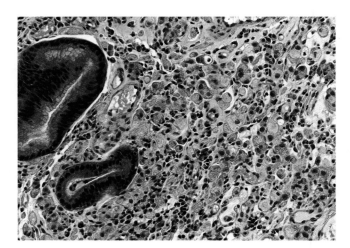

**FIG. 18.** Signet ring carcinoma of the stomach. Individual cells have a striking resemblance to xanthoma cells.

ultrastructural study, Snover et al. (68) showed that the spaces in question were not adipocytes. Instead, they appear to represent microscopic pockets of entrapped gas, perhaps introduced during endoscopy. Mucosal pseudolipomatosis is most often an incidental histologic finding but it may also present as an irregular, white or yellow, slightly elevated mucosal plaque measuring several millimeters to centimeters in maximal dimension. As stated, histochemical analysis with the oil red O or Sudan black techniques is necessary to make the distinction between the latter condition—which is negative with both methods—and true lipomatosis, which yields positive results.

### Lipomatous Hypertrophy of the Ileocecal Valve

The ileocecal valve is that segment of the terminal ileum that projects into the colon at the junction between the cecum and ascending colon (69). The valve is composed of all layers of the gut wall, and it exhibits a gradual merging of small bowel mucosa with colonic mucosa. Although the submucosa of the ileocecal valve characteristically contains some fat, one may occasionally find excessive deposits of adipose tissue that then invoke the designations of "lipomatous hypertrophy," *lipomatosis,* or *lipohyperplasia.* Lipomatous hypertrophy of the ileocecal valve (LHIV) is more common in women and may be associated with increased body weight and fatty deposits elsewhere (70). Although autopsy studies have suggested that this is a common finding that may, to some extent, represent a normal anatomic variation, some patients with LHIV have presented with right lower quadrant abdominal pain and were found to have a mass in the cecum by radiographic or endoscopic examination.

Excessive deposits of adipose tissue may involve the entire valve, resulting in a diffuse enlargement ("pouting ileum"). Alternatively, they may present focally as a discrete, polypoid mass (71,72). In either case, histologic examination reveals lobules of unremarkable adipose tissue

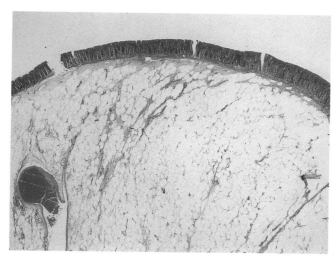

**FIG. 20.** Lipomatous hypertrophy of the ileocecal valve. A large polypoid excrescence composed of adipose tissue projects from the ileocecal valve and is covered by unremarkable colonic mucosa.

within the submucosa (Fig. 20), which is unencapsulated in contrast to true lipoma. There is no real clinical significance to the former of these lesions, and no relationship with other intestinal disease has been demonstrated. In general, LHIV is considered a common, incidental finding in surgical specimens; admittedly, a distinction from true lipoma of the gut may not be possible in selected cases.

## Ectopias and Heterotopias

### Pancreatic Heterotopia

*Pancreatic heterotopia* is said to be the most common form of gastrointestinal ectopy. Nests of misplaced pancreatic tissue can be found in almost any part of the alimentary tract. Nonetheless, they are usually seen in the stomach, proximal small intestine, and Meckel's diverticula, in which sites a histologic resemblance to neoplastic proliferations may occasionally be assumed (73–75). There appear to be two major patterns of pancreatic heterotopia. In the first, nests of pancreatic acinar tissue with scattered endocrine islets are identified in the submucosa of the stomach or intestine; the overlying mucosa is intact (Figs. 21 and 22). These foci are usually <1.0 cm and appear as discrete, sessile nodules or plaques. This pattern is rarely associated with radiographic or clinical abnormalities. It is almost always an incidental finding at endoscopy, autopsy, or abdominal surgery, and there is little chance that the pathologist would confuse it with a neoplastic process.

The second form of pancreatic heterotopia presents as a localized submucosal nodule or umbilicated mass measuring up to 3 cm in diameter, usually in the periampullary region of the duodenum or in the gastric antrum. Although this vari-

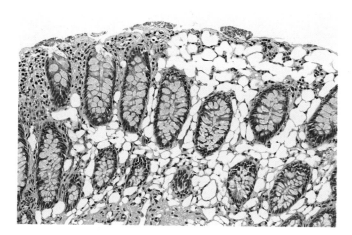

**FIG. 19.** Mucosal pseudolipomatosis. There is an intramucosal cluster of uniform, empty spaces that simulate fat cells.

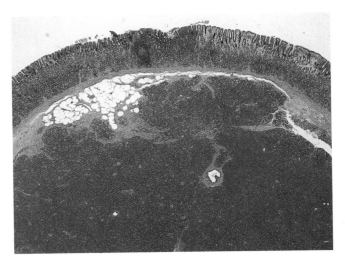

**FIG. 21.** Pancreatic heterotopia. A circumscribed nodule of pancreatic tissue is present in the submucosa of the gastric fundus.

ant of pancreatic ectopy may be an incidental finding in asymptomatic patients, it is sometimes discovered because of epigastric pain, bleeding, or biliary obstruction. In the latter scenarios, one observes a mixture of epithelial elements—including acinar and ductular structures—with a proliferation of smooth muscle that is derived from the muscularis (Fig. 23). This pattern has been described using the terms *myoepithelial hamartoma* and *adenoleiomyomatous hamartoma* (76,77). The relative proportion of acinar and ductular structures varies, and some cases appear to consist entirely of ducts that are surrounded by smooth muscle. This pattern is sometimes dubbed that of an adenomyoma, in likeness to a microscopically similar lesion in the gallbladder (78,79).

Recently, another pattern in ectopic pancreatic tissue was reported that was designated *pancreatic (acinar) metaplasia of the gastric mucosa* (80). In contrast to pancreatic hetero-

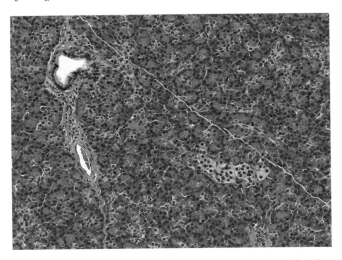

**FIG. 22.** Pancreatic heterotopia. A higher magnification showing well-formed acini, ducts, and small islets.

topia, this lesion did not present as a localized mass of acinar and ductular elements but was an incidental microscopic finding in grossly normal gastric mucosa. Nests of cells were found amid the gastric epithelium that had the morphologic and ultrastructural features of pancreatic acinar cells but that may have been misinterpreted as a microadenomatosis. The constituent cells were reactive for lipase and trypsinogen by immunohistochemical analysis. Pancreatic metaplasia was correlated with chronic gastritis and the concurrent presence of intestinal metaplasia. Subsequent to the appearance of this report, we also identified this lesion in a gastric biopsy from a patient with reflux esophagitis (Figs. 24 and 25). This finding has also been reported in the metaplastic epithelium of Barrett's esophagus.

### Infections of the Gut Presenting as Pseudotumors

#### *Syphilis (Lues)*

*Syphilis* is a rare but well-recognized cause of gastrointestinal pseudotumor formation. Until recently, infection by *Treponema pallidum* was considered a disease that was primarily of historic interest only, but its incidence has risen markedly in the past decade (81). This appears to be a reflection of the increased incidence of sexually transmitted infections in general; although some patients are coinfected with the human immunodeficiency virus (HIV), the recent surge in luetic disease is not necessarily related to the acquired immunodeficiency syndrome (AIDS) epidemic (82). Gastric involvement by syphilis is well documented, but the early studies of gastrointestinal syphilis were based largely on autopsy material, and involvement of the gut was considered a complication of tertiary lues only. Recent reports of the endoscopic findings in patients with syphilis, however, have shown significant pathologic changes at earlier stages as well.

In tertiary syphilis, there is marked fibrotic thickening of the gastric wall with pyloric outlet obstruction and an "hourglass" radiographic appearance that closely simulates that of adenocarcinoma of the linitis plastica type (83–85). Discrete syphilitic gummas are rare in the stomach. In secondary lues, a small percentage of patients has diffuse, nonspecific gastritis with erythema, nodular thickening of gastric folds, and occasional small ulcers (86). These patients most commonly present with symptoms of several weeks to several months duration, including vomiting, weight loss, and abdominal pain (87).

Histologic examination of gastric biopsies in syphilis reveals intense acute and chronic inflammation with dense plasma cell infiltrates that may simulate those seen in plasmacytic neoplasia. These two disorders are separable diagnostically using immunostains for light chain immunoglobulins; lues exhibits polytypic expression of the latter proteins, whereas plasma cell neoplasms are monoclonal. In some cases of syphilis, numerous spirochetes can be identi-

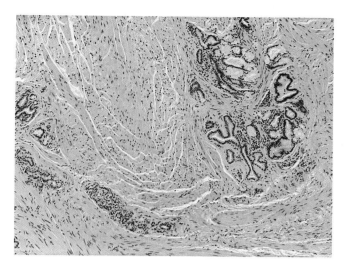

**FIG. 23.** Adenomyoma of the duodenum (pancreatic heterotopia). There is a collection of ductular and glandular structures surrounded by large bundles of smooth muscle.

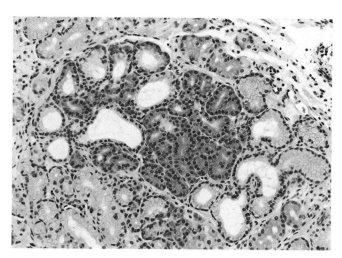

**FIG. 25.** Pancreatic (acinar) metaplasia of the gastric mucosa. Higher magnification showing apical cytoplasmic granules.

fied in the tissue with silver impregnation stains and immunofluorescence-based antibody-mediated methods (88). It should be remembered that diverse spirilliform organisms (including *Helicobacter*) can be demonstrated in gastric biopsies from patients who do *not* have syphilis, and this finding must therefore be correlated with other serologic and

histologic information. Anorectal syphilis is also well recognized as a lesion that may present as a mass with the potential to simulate a plasmacytic malignancy (89–91).

## PSEUDOTUMORS OF THE ESOPHAGUS

### Fibrovascular Polyp

*Fibrovascular polyp* of the esophagus (Table 3) is a very rare lesion, but one that has a characteristic clinical, radiographic, and gross appearance. Although polyps are reported to be the second most common benign "tumors" of the esophagus after leiomyomas, fewer than 100 cases have been reported. A variety of names have been applied to the former lesion, including *fibrous polyp, fibrolipomatous polyp, fibromyxoma,* and *pedunculated lipoma.* Fibrovascular polyp presents as an intraluminal mass that almost always arises from the upper third of the esophagus, most often near the cricoid cartilage. Some reported lesions have been surprisingly large, and thus many authors have used the term *giant fibrovascular polyp* in reference to them (92–94).

Fibrovascular polyps are usually solitary, soft, exophytic growths that range in size from 3 to 20 cm (average 5.0 cm). These masses can fill and distend the lumen, but even very large polyps remain attached to the esophageal wall by a narrow pedicle. It appears that the stalk of this slowly growing submucosal lesion is progressively elongated by continuous peristaltic action (19), and, in some cases, the polyp extends downward into the stomach. Regurgitation into the upper aerodigestive tract can also occur, however, with dramatic clinical consequences (95,96).

Microscopic examination of the esophageal fibrovascular polyp reveals an unencapsulated mass of fibrovascular tissue that is covered by an intact layer of benign squamous mucosa. The surface epithelium is unremarkable, and ulceration

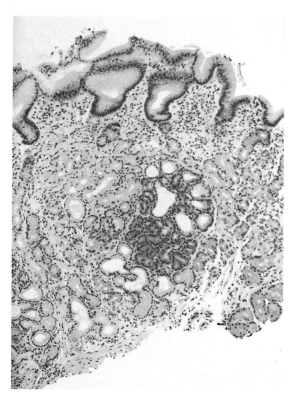

**FIG. 24.** Pancreatic (acinar) metaplasia of the gastric mucosa. A nest of cells within the gastric mucosa that resembles pancreatic acinar cells.

**TABLE 3.** *Pseudotumors of the esophagus*

Mucosal plaques and "bumps"
   Gastric heterotopia ("inlet patch")
   Glycogenic acanthosis
Polyps
   Fibrovascular polyp
   Inflammatory esophagogastric polyp (117)
Submucosal and intramural lesions
   Duplication cysts
   Esophageal intramural pseudodiverticulosis (118,119)

is unusual. The stroma may be myxoid or densely fibrous, and it typically contains scattered, stellate-shaped fibroblasts and many blood vessels. Inflammatory cells are usually sparse, but when present such elements are located near foci of mucosal ulceration. A characteristic feature of fibrovascular polyp is the presence of variable quantities of adipose tissue in the stroma (Fig. 26). In some instances, matrical fat is abundant and accounts for most of the volume of the mass, leading to potential confusion with an adipocytic neoplasm on microscopic grounds.

Fibrovascular polyp should be distinguished from inflammatory fibroid polyp. As reviewed above, IFP also presents as a pedunculated, submucosal, fibrovascular mass, but it usually occurs in the stomach and small intestine and only rarely involves the esophagus (4,97). The surface of inflammatory fibroid polyps is frequently ulcerated, and there are many inflammatory cells distributed throughout the lesion. In contrast, fibrovascular polyps do not show extensive surface erosion or inflammatory infiltrates, and are almost exclusively confined to the upper third of the esophagus. In addition, adipose tissue is not prominent in IFP, as it is in fibrovascular polyps.

The etiology of fibrovascular polyp is uncertain, but an interesting theory suggests these lesions are the end result of prolonged peristaltic action on loose, submucosal redundancies of the esophagus (98). Although they are uniformly benign lesions that do not recur after excision, deaths have been reported due to regurgitation of the polyp, with subsequent airway restriction and asphyxiation (99,100). Therefore treatment should consist of complete excision of the mass and its stalk (101).

## PSEUDONEOPLASTIC LESIONS OF THE STOMACH

A list of pseudotumors of the stomach is given in Table 4.

### Focal Lymphoid Hyperplasia of the Stomach (Gastric Pseudolymphoma)

Lymphoid hyperplasia of the gastrointestinal tract is actually a heterogeneous group of conditions that includes focal lymphoid hyperplasia of the stomach (gastric pseudolymphoma), focal lymphoid hyperplasia of the small intestine, focal lymphoid hyperplasia of the rectum (benign lymphoid polyp), and nodular lymphoid hyperplasia (102). The most

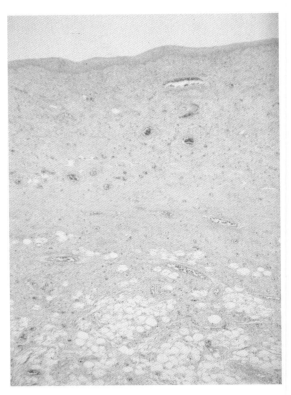

**FIG. 26.** Fibrovascular polyp of the esophagus. The stroma is composed of hyalinized fibrous tissue and fat.

common of these proliferations, and the one that most closely simulates neoplasia, is gastric pseudolymphoma. Prominent mucosal lymphocytic infiltrates can also be associated with such inflammatory disorders as *Helicobacter pylori*-associated gastritis, idiopathic inflammatory bowel disease, diverticulitis, and infections, but these conditions do not commonly simulate malignant lymphoma.

For many years it has been known that extensive, apparently reactive mucosal lymphoid infiltrates presenting as mass lesions can be found in the stomach in patients who have peptic ulcer disease (102–106) (Figs. 27–30). Recent studies have shown that many of these individuals are infected with *H. pylori* (107). Lymphoid infiltrates may appear as incidental microscopic findings adjacent to an otherwise unremarkable gastric ulcer, or they may present as large, ul-

**TABLE 4.** *Pseudotumors of the stomach*

Mucosal plaques and "bumps"
   Fundic gland polyp
   Pancreatic heterotopia
   Xanthoma (xanthelasma)
Polyps
   Inflammatory fibroid polyp
   Gastritis cystica profunda
Ulcers
   Gastric "pseudolymphoma"
Diffuse lesions
   Eosinophilic gastroenteritis
   Gastric syphilis
   Pseudotumoral enterocolitis

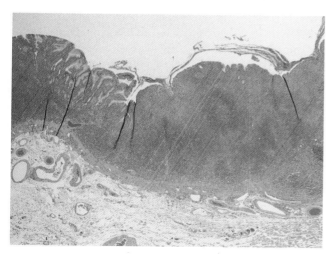

**FIG. 27.** MALToma ("pseudolymphoma") of the stomach. There is an extensive lymphoid infiltrate that is almost exclusively confined to the mucosa.

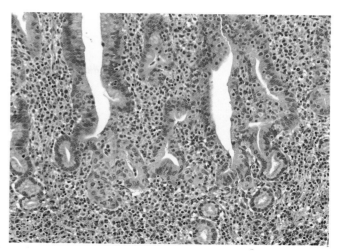

**FIG. 29.** MALToma ("pseudolymphoma") of the stomach. Lymphoid cells focally extend into the gastric glands, and small lymphoepithelial lesions are present.

cerated masses that closely simulate gastric cancer radiographically and endoscopically. Similar lesions have been described in other parts of the gut (108–110) (Fig. 31).

Histologic examination shows a mixed lymphocytic infiltrate consisting of small, round to slightly irregular lymphocytes, as well as numerous reactive-appearing lymphoid follicles with germinal centers. The latter structures are distributed throughout the lesion, as are diverse inflammatory cells. There may also be considerable fibrosis, especially at the margins of ulcers. Morphologic differences that have been used to distinguish gastric lymphoma from pseudolymphoma are summarized in Table 5.

The "benign" cytologic attributes of the lymphocytic infiltrate, the close association with gastric ulcers, the absence of involvement of regional lymph nodes, and the indolent clinical course have all contributed to the conclusion that

these lesions are exuberant but benign lymphoid reactions to mucosal injury. When reports of overt lymphoma in patients with gastric pseudolymphoma began to appear, it was postulated that the preceding condition was either a premalignant lesion or merely an associated but unrelated process (111–114). In recent years, however, a number of immunologic and molecular studies of gastric pseudolymphoma have revealed the presence of monoclonal populations of B lymphocytes in most cases, suggesting that they actually represent B-cell lymphomas (115–121). Histologic review of such cases occasionally discloses obvious features of intestinal lymphoma such as lymphoepithelial lesions and foci of large atypical lymphoid cells. However, even in cases that do not show these features, highly sensitive techniques such as the polymerase chain reaction can identify immunoglobulin gene rearrangements that define clonal B-cell populations (122). It now appears that most gastric pseudolymphomas

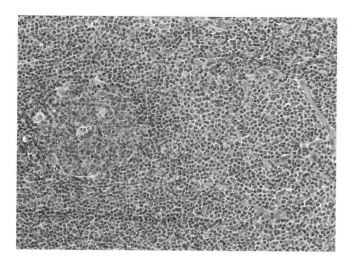

**FIG. 28.** MALToma ("pseudolymphoma") of the stomach. The infiltrate contains small lymphocytes and numerous reactive-appearing follicles.

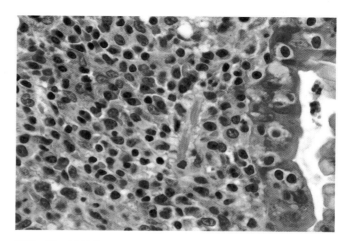

**FIG. 30.** MALToma ("pseudolymphoma") of the stomach. Note the mixture of cells including small and large lymphocytes and plasma cells.

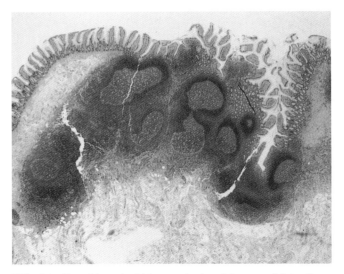

**FIG. 31.** Focal lymphoid hyperplasia of the small intestine. This lesion was present immediately proximal to an intestinal stricture caused by endometriosis in a 33-year-old woman.

represent a particular pattern of malignant lymphoma that has been designated *low-grade B-cell lymphoma of mucosa-associated lymphoid tissue (MALT)*. Moreover, the association of overt gastric lymphoma with preexisting pseudolymphoma probably represents a transformation of low-grade lymphoma into a more aggressive neoplasm. In light of these findings, many authors have suggested that pseudolymphoma is no longer an appropriate diagnostic classification and they have advocated that this term be abandoned (123–125).

Low-grade lymphoma of mucosa-associated lymphoid tissue, which is sometimes referred to as "MALToma," has characteristic clinical, morphologic, and immunophenotypic features (126). It should be remembered that this designation refers to a specific lesion and does not include all types of gastrointestinal lymphomas (Table 6). MALT lymphomas (or closely related tumors) occur in many extranodal sites including the thyroid gland, salivary glands, and orbits, but they are most common in the stomach. There is compelling evidence that in the stomach these lymphoid proliferations are caused by chronic antigenic stimulation due to infection with *H. pylori* (127). They have an indolent clinical course with rare dissemination beyond the gastrointestinal tract and a prolonged disease-free survival after treatment (128). Morphologic features in this disease group include prominent, reactive-appearing lymphoid follicles that are distributed throughout the masses, widened mantle zones that contain a mixture of small mature and atypical lymphocytes, and infiltration of the adjacent epithelium by lymphoid cells (130). MALT lymphomas feature monotypic expression of immunoglobulin light chains and have characteristic immunophenotypes. Because this pattern of low-grade lymphoma cannot be reliably diagnosed by morphologic features alone, immunophenotypic and cell surface marker studies should be performed on all florid gastrointestinal lymphoproliferative lesions to distinguish MALT lymphoma from reactive lymphoid hyperplasia.

## PSEUDONEOPLASTIC VASCULAR LESIONS

Vascular abnormalities are rarely manifest as gastrointestinal pseudotumors, but several malformations in that group can present as localized lesions. These are mentioned in Table 7 for completeness. The principal neoplasm with which such lesions may be confused is that of mucosal or mural hemangioma. However, attention to strict morphologic criteria is typically sufficient to distinguish between them diagnostically.

## PSEUDONEOPLASTIC LESIONS OF THE INTESTINES (TABLE 8)

### Pseudotumors Associated with Mucosal Prolapse

The *mucosal prolapse syndrome* (or solitary rectal ulcer syndrome) refers to a constellation of signs and symptoms thought to be related to prolapse of the rectal mucosa (130–131). The disorder is most commonly found in young or middle-aged women who have a history of chronic constipation with rectal pain and bleeding. In its classic form, there is a failure of relaxation of the puborectalis muscle dur-

**TABLE 5.** *Histologic features distinguishing gastric pseudolymphoma from lymphoma*

| Feature | Pseudolymphoma | Lymphoma |
|---|---|---|
| Cellular infiltrate | Polymorphous cellular infiltrate with lymphocytes, granulocytes, and histiocytes | Monomorphous lymphocytic infiltrate with atypia |
| Lymphoid follicles | Many follicles throughout the lesion | Follicles present only at periphery of lesion |
| Mucosa | Ulcer in 90% | Variable, usually superficial ulcers |
| | Glands not involved | Infiltration of glands by atypical lymphocytes |
| Lymphoepithelial lesions | Absent | Present |

Modified from Lewin (141).

**TABLE 6.** *Gastrointestinal lymphoproliferative disorders*

Solitary
  MALT lymphoma ("pseudolymphoma")
  Focal lymphoid hyperplasia (Fig. 33)
Multifocal
  Nodular lymphoid hyperplasia
  Multiple lymphomatous polyposis
  Immunoproliferative small intestinal disease
  Enteropathy-associated T-cell lymphoma
  Secondary non-Hodgkin's lymphoma

**TABLE 8.** *"Pseudotumors" of the intestines and rectum*

Mucosal plaques of "bumps"
  Gastric metaplasia
  Mucosal pseudolipomatosis
  Malakoplakia
Polyps
  Inflammatory fibroid polyp
  Inflammatory cloacogenic polyp
  Mucosal prolapse
  Hypertrophic anal papilla
  Lipomatous hypertrophy of the ileocecal valve
  Lymphoid polyp of the rectum
  Polypoid prolapsing mucosal folds of diverticular disease
Submucosal and intramural masses
  Inflammatory myofibroblastic tumor
  Pancreatic and gastric heterotopia
  Endometriosis
  Colitis cystica profunda
  Solitary (cecal) diverticulum
  Anorectal syphilis
  Angiostrongyliasis
Extrinsic lesions
  Retrorectal cysts
  Oil granuloma
  Giant colonic diverticulum

ing defecation, causing a functional obstruction at the anorectal junction. This leads to chronic straining at stool with increased intraabdominal pressure and eventual prolapse and ulceration of the mid-rectal mucosa, particularly anteriorly. The mucosa is raised, nodular, and reddened, and, despite the name of the syndrome, patients may have no ulcerations or more than one.

Mucosal prolapse is associated with a variety of characteristic histologic changes. These include varying combinations of crypt hyperplasia (sometimes with a villiform configuration), inflammation with epithelial ulceration, fibromuscular replacement of the lamina propria, and hypertrophy of the muscularis mucosae (Figs. 32–34). Mucosal crypts are elongated and distorted, and they often have a serrated luminal configuration. The lamina propria exhibits a mixture of inflammation and fibrosis, and smooth muscle cells extend upward into the lamina propria from the underlying muscularis mucosae. These changes may be confused with the features of hyperplastic polyps, villoglandular adenomas, and hamartomatous polyps.

In addition to the classic mucosal prolapse syndrome, there are several other closely associated clinicopathologic entities that share the above-cited histologic attributes. These include colitis cystica profunda and inflammatory cloacogenic polyps.

### Colitis Cystica Profunda

*Colitis cystica profunda* is characterized by the presence of benign colonic mucosa in the wall of the colon or rectum, deep to the muscularis mucosae (Figs. 35 and 36). The lesion is thought to be a reparative phenomenon that results from damage to the muscularis mucosae, with subsequent reepithelialization extending into submucosal defects. It occurs

**TABLE 7.** *Nonneoplastic vasoformative lesions of the gastrointestinal tract*

Angiodysplasia
Arteriovenous malformations
Caliber persistent artery of the stomach (Dieulafoy's aneurysm)
Gastric antral vascular ectasia
Varices

as two major subtypes (133,134). The more common form is a localized lesion that occurs in the rectum in association with mucosal prolapse, and has been referred to as localized colitis cystica profunda or *hamartomatous inverted polyp of the rectum* (135). The second, much less frequently encountered form is a diffuse or multifocal process in the colon or small intestine in patients who have acute or chronic inflammatory diseases such as ulcerative colitis or Crohn's disease (137,138). When the multifocal variant form involves the small intestine, it is sometimes referred to as *enteritis cystica profunda*. A similar lesion may be observed in the stomach proximal to gastroenterostomal anastomoses and is desig-

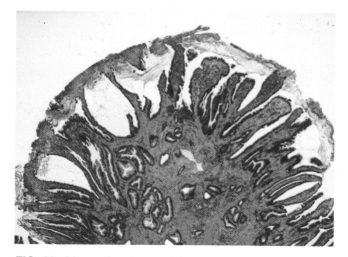

**FIG. 32.** Mucosal prolapse of the rectum. Note the polypoid configuration of the mucosa with dilated crypts and a surface exudate.

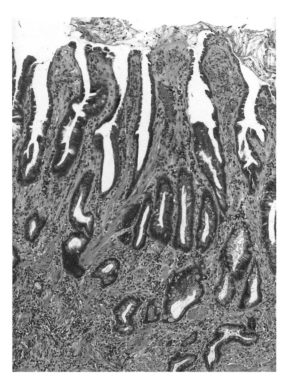

**FIG. 33.** Mucosal prolapse of the rectum. Higher magnification showing crypt hyperplasia with a villiform architecture, superficial mucosal erosion, and patchy fibromuscular replacement of the lamina propria.

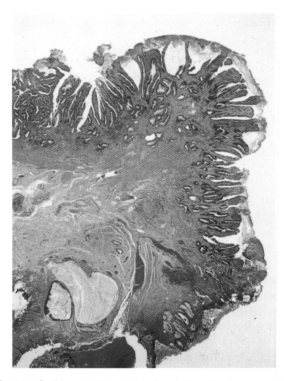

**FIG. 35.** Colitis cystica profunda. A localized mucosal excrescence in the rectum in a patient with mucosal prolapse. Note the mucus-filled cyst in the submucosa.

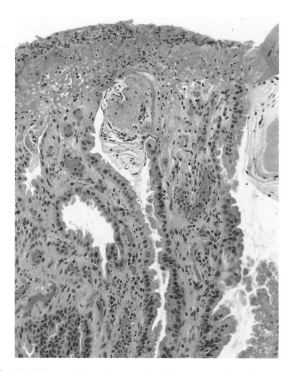

**FIG. 34.** Mucosal prolapse. Another example of mucosal prolapse showing more severe acute inflammation and mucosal necrosis with a thickened surface exudate. The crypts are lined by a serrated epithelium that simulates hyperplastic polyps.

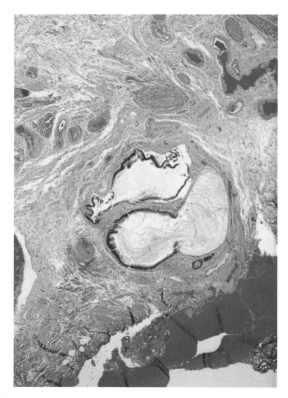

**FIG. 36.** Colitis cystica profunda. The mucus-filled cysts are lined by a single layer of epithelial cells without significant atypia or desmoplasia.

nated *gastritis cystica profunda* (138) (Fig. 37). Although colitis cystica profunda is usually small and clinically inapparent, examples of this lesion have been reported that presented as large, cystic masses that were mistaken for carcinoma on both macroscopic and histologic levels (139).

Microscopically, colitis cystica profunda is characterized by epithelial microcysts that penetrate the muscularis mucosae and extend into the submucosa or muscularis externa. The overall lesion varies in maximal size from a few millimeters to several centimeters, and, when grossly identifiable, appears as a raised, fluctuant submucosal mass. The stroma surrounding the cysts shows little fibrosis and variable degrees of inflammation. The locules of the lesion are lined by benign colonic epithelium, which often shows hyperplastic changes with villiform architecture and serrated glands. This tissue appears to be regenerative in nature and may show slight to moderate cytologic atypia. The presence of aberrant colonic epithelium and abundant mucus within the wall of the colon may strongly suggest mucinous adenocarcinoma, an erroneous suspicion that may be further supported by the presence of a localized mass.

Indeed, the most important differential diagnostic consideration in cases of colitis cystica profunda is that of well-differentiated adenocarcinoma. Histologic features that favor a benign interpretation include the presence of normal- or hyperplastic-appearing epithelium without adenomatous change or dysplasia, and coexistent acute and chronic inflammation. In addition, colitis cystica profunda would not be expected to incite the desmoplastic stromal response that is characteristic of invasive adenocarcinoma. Another lesion that shares some characteristics of colitis cystica profunda is the *giant inflammatory polyp* of inflammatory bowel disease (140). The latter is a large, nearly circumferential polypoid mass that most commonly arises in patients with Crohn's disease. Although it is thought merely to represent an exaggerated variant of common inflammatory pseudopolyps, giant inflammatory polyp is classified separately because of its gross similarity to intestinal neoplasia and the frequency of severe signs and symptoms (such as anemia and pain) with which it is associated.

## Inflammatory Cloacogenic Polyp

*Inflammatory cloacogenic polyp (ICP)* arises in the anal transition zone, most often at or very near the anorectal junction. It appears to be a localized expression of the mucosal prolapse syndrome (141–144) (Fig. 38). Histologic examination of the lesion reveals the same features described above in reference to mucosal prolapse. In addition, the base of the colonic crypts in ICP may be cystically dilated, and cysts may be observed in the submucosa as well, in likeness to colitis cystica profunda (145). Nonulcerated portions of the polyp may be composed of squamous epithelium, glandular elements, or both, and the lamina propria contains a mixture of smooth muscle, fibrous tissue, and inflammatory cells. Differential diagnostic considerations again include villoglandular polyps as well as well-differentiated adenocarcinoma. In examples of ICP that contain squamous epithelial elements, one may also be tempted to make an erroneous interpretation of anal transition zone carcinoma.

There have been several reports of nearly identical polypoid lesions outside the anal canal in patients who have clinical symptoms suggestive of acute inflammatory bowel disease (146,147). These individuals have numerous polyps in the rectum or sigmoid colon, all of which show the histologic features of mucosal prolapse. These include serrated tubules, fibromuscular replacement of the lamina propria, and surface ulceration with an inflammatory pseudomembrane. This constellation of findings has been used to define *eroded polypoid hyperplasia of the rectosigmoid* and *inflammatory "cap" polyps.*

## Malakoplakia

*Malakoplakia* is an unusual but well-defined inflammatory disease that is most commonly observed in the genitourinary tract (148,149). It has been reported in many other locations as well, including the adrenal gland, lung, lymph nodes, and gut (150–154), and the condition may clearly

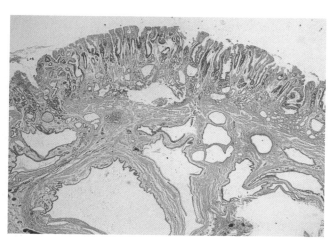

**FIG. 37.** Gastritis cystica profunda. Multiple epithelial-lined cysts of varying size are present throughout the submucosa.

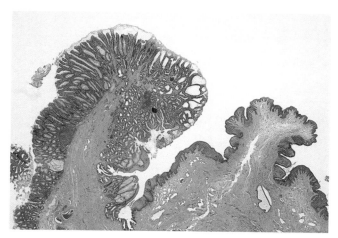

**FIG. 38.** Inflammatory cloacogenic polyp. A pedunculated polyp at the squamocolumnar junction shows the histologic features that are associated with mucosal prolapse.

simulate carcinoma on gross and microscopic levels (155). Gastrointestinal involvement usually affects the colon and rectum, and is most often found in association with another, preexisting intestinal disease such as idiopathic inflammatory bowel disease or adenocarcinoma (149,156–158). Malakoplakia only rarely presents in the gut as an isolated finding (159). In contrast to patients with renal lesions of this type, who show a striking female predominance, there is no apparent sex predilection in gastrointestinal malakoplakia.

In the alimentary tract, this condition is usually represented by soft, tan or yellow, plaque-like nodules on the surface of the mucosa. However, there may be more extensive involvement, with large discrete masses. The histologic features of enteric malakoplakia are similar to those of this condition in the urinary tract or elsewhere. Biopsy specimens typically show masses of histiocytes with abundant, granular, pale-staining cytoplasm and large numbers of neutrophils (Figs. 39–41). The macrophages, which are known as "von Hansemann cells," contain small, round, basophilic, PAS-positive, intracytoplasmic inclusions that measure 1–3 $\mu$m in diameter. Electron micrographic studies have shown that these structures represent giant phagolysosomes that contain a heterogeneous mixture of intact and partially degraded structures including bacteria, cell membranes, and myelin-like figures (160). In addition to these small inclusions, some histiocytes contain larger spherules that have a concentric lamellar appearance and measure 3–10 $\mu$m. These larger inclusions, referred to as Michaelis–Gutmann bodies, are phagolysosomes that have become encrusted with calcium and iron salts; they are considered diagnostic of malakoplakia. Michaelis–Gutmann bodies stain with methods such as the von Kossa and alizarin red techniques, and occasionally with Perl's procedure as well. Because the fully developed inclusions of malakoplakia may not be found in early stages of the disease, their presence is not required di-

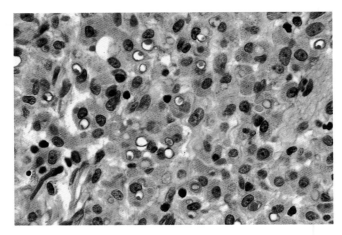

FIG. 40. Malakoplakia of the colon. Many of the polygonal histiocytes (von Hansemann cells) contain pale-staining, intracytoplasmic inclusions.

agnostically. The differential diagnosis of malakoplakia includes other histiocytic infiltrative disorders that involve the gastrointestinal tract; these are summarized in Table 2.

Malakoplakia, which is often identified in patients with immune suppression (161,162), appears to involve deranged bactericidal activity by monocytes and macrophages. The disease is thought to be caused by an acquired defect in lysosomal function, possibly due to abnormally low levels of cyclic guanosine monophosphate (GMP) (163). This defect is associated with decreased resistance to infection, particularly with enteric organisms such as *Escherichia coli,* and it results in the formation of large histiocytic aggregates. Although experimental evidence suggests that the disorder is correctable by administration of cholinergic agonists (to restore cyclic GMP to normal levels), the standard treatment for malakoplakia is long-term antibiotic therapy.

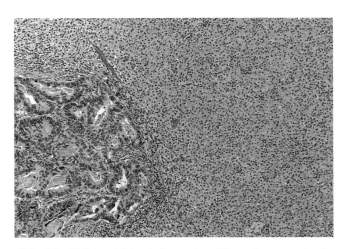

FIG. 39. Malakoplakia of the colon. There is a poorly circumscribed nest of large, eosinophilic cells adjacent to an invasive colonic adenocarcinoma.

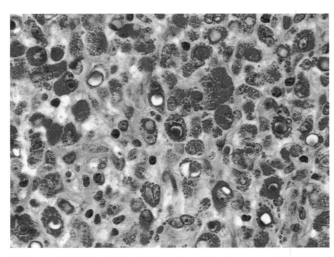

FIG. 41. Malakoplakia of the colon. The intracytoplasmic inclusions are PAS-positive and have a distinct target-like appearance.

## Tumefactive Endometriosis

*Endometriosis* is defined as the presence of endometrial glands and stroma in extrauterine sites. As such, this condition involves the gastrointestinal tract in roughly 10% of women who have endometriosis elsewhere (164–169). It is usually an incidental finding in the gut, but some examples present themselves as an obstructing tumefactive mass that closely simulates an intestinal neoplasm. The most common sites of gastrointestinal involvement are the rectum and sigmoid colon, distal ileum, and appendix, where the disease is usually limited to the serosal surfaces. As is true of those with more "typical" endometriosis, most affected patients are premenopausal, and the average age is 40 years. Most women with intestinal endometriosis have pelvic involvement as well, and the clinical signs and symptoms are therefore rarely localized or specific to the alimentary tract. Those that are referable to the gut include recurrent abdominal cramps; rectal bleeding, diarrhea, and constipation are much more uncommon.

Gastrointestinal endometriosis typically takes the form of small serosal or subserosal implants that measure <1 cm in greatest dimension. There may be scattered contiguous serosal fibrous adhesions, but these are usually not associated with strictures. Larger foci of endometriosis may extend through the muscularis externa and elicit an extensive sclerotic reaction, with marked concomitant hypertrophy of smooth muscle (Figs. 42 and 43). Such cases may present with bowel obstruction because of narrowing of the intestinal lumen, and, since preoperative diagnosis of enteric endometriosis by mucosal biopsy is uncommon, a segmental resection of bowel is usually performed (170).

Gross examination in such cases reveals a poorly circumscribed, constricting mass that is eccentrically located in the intestinal wall. Although the mucosa is rarely involved, this feature may be difficult to evaluate due to luminal distortion, secondary inflammatory changes, and ulceration.

Once endometrioid glands and stroma are identified in extrauterine tissues, the interpretation of endometriosis is easily made. The most difficult diagnostic scenario, however, arises when these elements are obliterated or otherwise masked by fibrosis, hemorrhage, smooth muscle proliferation, and other changes. Cases with these characteristics may be misinterpreted as a stromal or smooth muscle tumor, a metastatic adenocarcinoma, or a stricture caused by Crohn's disease, irradiation, or ischemia. In doubtful circumstances, additional sampling and examination of several microscopic sections of blocked tissues should be undertaken, either in the frozen section laboratory or in "routine" sign-out of the case. Often, simple thoroughness will enable one to identify the characteristic glands and stroma of endometriosis, as well as associated findings such as xanthomatized foci of chronic inflammation, hemorrhage, and hemosiderin deposition.

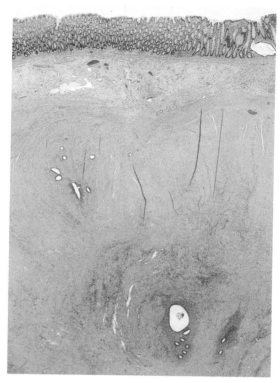

**FIG. 42.** Endometriosis of the colon. There are scattered glandular structures throughout the thickened muscularis externa.

## Pseudotumors Associated with Diverticular Disease

Diverticular disease of the colon—which includes both diverticulosis and diverticulitis—is a frequent cause of abdominal pain, intestinal hemorrhage, and obstruction of the gut in Western countries. Although all parts of the large intestine can be affected, the disorder most commonly affects

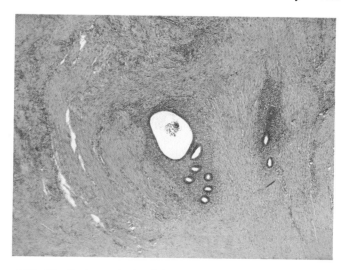

**FIG. 43.** Endometriosis of the colon. Endometrial glands and stroma are surrounded by hyperplastic bundles of smooth muscle.

the sigmoid colon. An important attribute of colonic diverticular disease is the particular pattern of hypertrophy seen in the muscularis externa. This change is probably essential to the very formation of diverticula and to clinical expression of the disease, and it is largely responsible for the typical morphologic findings of the disorder.

In patients with diverticular disease, the muscularis externa of the involved colon (particularly the longitudinal layer) becomes markedly thickened as a result of increased intraluminal pressure and increased peristaltic action. This compartmental hypertrophy is associated with tonic muscular contracture of the colon, which then leads to shortening of the affected bowel segment and thickening of the bowel wall. The circular layer of the muscularis externa may also be thickened, yielding a corrugated gross appearance. In typical cases, two rows of pulsion diverticula are found along the margins of the teniae between the mesenteric and antimesenteric borders of the bowel.

There are several complications of colonic diverticular disease that are properly considered in a discussion of pseudotumors at a clinical level. Perhaps the most common is acute diverticulitis with the formation of a peridiverticular abscess. This often results in a large, pericolonic inflammatory mass with secondary bowel obstruction. Acute diverticulitis with organizing abscesses can also be associated with a prominent fibrosing reaction. The latter process produces a firm, intramural colonic mass that is easily mistaken by the surgeon for adenocarcinoma (171). This pattern has been called "stenosing localized diverticulitis," a term that has little pathologic significance. It is unlikely to be confused with a neoplasm by pathologists on microscopic examination, although errors may indeed be made in this context by macroscopic analysis alone.

### Polypoid Prolapsing Mucosal Folds of Diverticular Disease

In addition to causing shortening and thickening of the bowel wall, tonic muscular contraction appears capable of producing polypoid, exophytic projections of the colonic mucosa (172–174). These excrescences are commonly located adjacent to diverticular ostia and have been designated as *polypoid prolapsing mucosal folds of diverticular disease* (Figs. 44 and 45). These folds represent mucosal redundancies that are thought to result from a combination of muscular contraction and prolonged traction by the fecal stream. As might be expected, such folds display the same histologic appearances as those associated with mucosal prolapse. These include mucosal hyperplasia with elongation of the epithelial crypts, serration of surface epithelium, "muscularization" of the lamina propria mucosa, and variable mucin depletion of the glandular epithelium. Confusion with adenomatous neoplasms or hamartomas is a possibility.

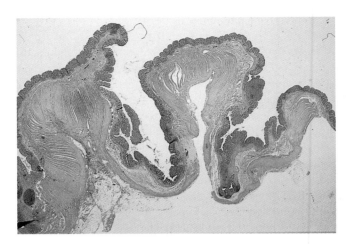

**FIG. 44.** Polypoid prolapsing mucosal folds of diverticular disease. A polypoid mucosal excrescence protrudes adjacent to a colonic diverticulum.

### Solitary Cecal Diverticulitis

*Cecal diverticulitis* is a very rare condition, but it appears to show distinct clinical and pathologic differences from diverticulitis of the left colon (175). Diverticula of the cecum occur at a younger mean age than those in sigmoid diverticulitis and are usually solitary. Patients with cecal diverticular disease most often present with right lower quadrant abdominal pain and are clinically thought to have acute appendicitis. At surgery, one third to one half of patients are found to have a cecal mass that is initially thought to represent adenocarcinoma on gross inspection. This is particularly true when the diverticulum is confined in the right iliac fossa, a finding called "hidden diverticulum." Peridiverticular inflammation and fibrosis may distort the local mucosa

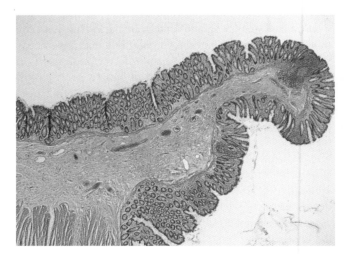

**FIG. 45.** Polypoid prolapsing mucosal folds of diverticular disease. The epithelium of the excrescence shows only mild histologic abnormalities.

and incite the presence of striking epithelial regeneration, passingly simulating invasive carcinoma histologically. However, close scrutiny fails to disclose the usual microscopic companions of the latter condition.

## Hypertrophic Anal Papilla

Anal papillae are located along the anal columns, between the anal sinuses. In patients with hemorrhoids and anal fissures, chronic inflammation and mucosal edema lead to hypertrophy of the papillae. These then protrude as polypoid masses into the anal lumen. Hypertrophic anal papillae are also called *fibroepithelial papillomas, anal tags*, and *skin tags,* and they are pedunculated masses that arise from the pectinate line. Experienced clinicians typically have little difficulty in recognizing these lesions, but they should be distinguished from adenomatous polyps.

Microscopic examination reveals a central pedicle of variably cellular fibrous tissue that is covered by a hyperplastic layer of keratinizing squamous epithelium (Fig. 46). Most hypertrophic anal papillae have dense, almost hyalinized cores with little edema or inflammation. As in inflammatory mucosal polyps at other sites, benign but cytologically atypical stromal cells are not unusual in hypertrophic anal papillae, and the surface epithelium may also demonstrate regenerative atypicality (56). One may be tempted by these findings to render mistaken diagnoses of a stromal tumor or carcinoma *in situ.*

## Pseudoneoplastic Conditions in the Retrorectal Space

The retrorectal or presacral area is a virtual space that is bounded by the rectum anteriorly, the sacrum posteriorly, the peritoneal reflection superiorly, and the levator ani and coccygeal muscles inferiorly. A variety of lesions may be identified in this compartment, but in a large study of "primary" retrorectal masses, Jao et al. found that cysts were the most common (176). These include *cystic teratoma or dermoid cyst, enteric duplication or enterogenous cyst, retrorectal cystic hamartoma, cloacal cyst,* and *developmental tailgut cyst.* There are probably no meaningful differences between retrorectal cystic hamartomas and developmental tailgut cysts (177). In the largest single study of tailgut cysts (178), Hjermstad and Helwig found that they occurred predominantly in adult women, most of whom had rectal pain. These fluctuant masses are usually palpable by rectal examination.

Tailgut cysts are typically multiloculated, and they are lined by a mixture of squamous, columnar, and transitional epithelium (Fig. 47). They are thought to represent cystic malformations that arise from remnants of the embryonic tailgut; however, these lesions are rarely identified in children. Although tailgut cysts are benign, incomplete excision is often associated with recurrence. Rare cases have been reported in which carcinoma appeared to arise in a preexisting tailgut cyst (179). Differential diagnosis includes true ter-

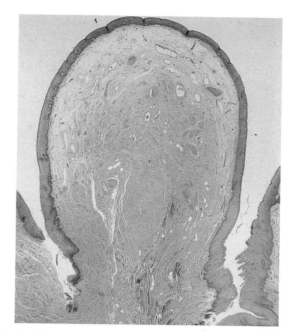

**FIG. 46.** Hypertrophic anal papilla. The papilla is composed of dense fibrovascular tissue covered by benign squamous epithelium.

atoma as well as invasive well-differentiated adenocarcinoma of the posterior rectal wall. These two entities are recognized by identification of tissues from at least two germ lines or destructive growth by overtly atypical epithelium, respectively.

## Elastofibromatous Lesions

There have been two reports of *elastofibromatous change* occurring in the gut. Although these did not present with

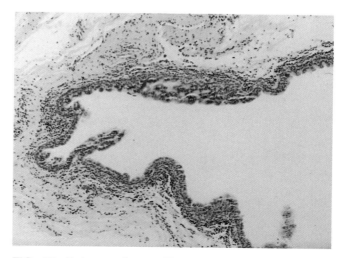

**FIG. 47.** Retrorectal cyst. The cyst is lined by a simple columnar epithelium and surrounded by loose fibrovascular tissue.

clinically apparent gastrointestinal masses, both cases showed histologic features that were identical to those of elastofibroma of soft tissue. One lesion occurred in the stomach adjacent to a benign gastric ulcer in a patient who also had elastofibroma dorsi (180). The second was an incidental finding in a random biopsy of the rectum in a patient thought to have amyloidosis (181). Although it is known that elastofibromas of any site may not, in fact, be true neoplasms, these lesions are nonetheless included here for the sake of completeness.

## Smooth Muscle Pseudotumors

*Smooth muscle pseudotumor* is a name given by Dankwa and Davies to a histologic finding that is occasionally observed in rectal biopsies (182). These authors demonstrated that "nodules" of smooth muscle seen in such specimens were actually avulsed, balled-up muscularis propria. Hence, they are an artifact of the biopsy procedure that may be misinterpreted as a gastrointestinal stromal neoplasm.

## REFERENCES

1. Vanek J. Gastric submucosal granuloma with eosinophilic infiltration. *Am J Pathol* 1949;25:397.
2. Helwig EB, Ranier A. Inflammatory fibroid polyps of the stomach. *Surg Gynecol Obstet* 1953;96:355–367.
3. Bullock WK, Moran ET. Inflammatory fibroid polyps of the stomach. *Cancer* 1953;6:488–493.
4. Leand PM, Murray GF, Zuidema GD, et al. Obstructing esophageal polyp with eosinophilic infiltration. *Am J Surg* 1968;116:93–96.
5. Assarian GS, Sundareson A. Inflammatory fibroid polyp of the ileum. *Hum Pathol* 1985;16:311–312.
6. Benjamin SP, Hawk WA, Turnbull RB. Fibrous inflammatory polyps of the ileum and cecum. Review of five cases with emphasis on differentiation from mesenchymal neoplasm. *Cancer* 1977;39:1300–1305.
7. Shimer GR, Helwig EB. Inflammatory fibroid polyps of the intestine. *Am J Clin Pathol* 1984;81:708–714.
8. Kim YI, Kim WH. Inflammatory fibroid polyps of gastrointestinal tract. Evolution of histologic patterns. *Am J Clin Pathol* 1988;89:721–727.
9. LiVolsi VA, Perzin KH. Inflammatory pseudotumors (inflammatory fibrous polyps) of the small intestine. *Dig Dis* 1975;20:325–336.
10. Blackshaw AJ, Levison DA. Eosinophilic infiltrates of the gastrointestinal tract. *J Clin Pathol* 1986;39:1–7.
11. Johnstone JM, Morson BC. Inflammatory fibroid polyp of the gastrointestinal tract. *Histopathology* 1978;2:349–361.
12. Navas-Palacios JJ, Colina-Ruizdelgado F, Sanchez-Larrea MD, Cortes-Cansino J. Inflammatory fibroid polyps of the gastrointestinal tract. An immunohistochemical and electron microscopic study. *Cancer* 1983;51:1682–1690.
13. Mori M, Tamura S, Enjoji M, Sugimachi K. Concomitant presence of inflammatory fibroid polyp and carcinoma or adenoma in the stomach. *Arch Pathol Lab Med* 1988;112:829–832.
14. Trillo AA, Rowden G. The histogenesis of inflammatory fibroid polyps of the gastrointestinal tract. *Histopathology* 1991;19:431–436.
15. Suster S, Robinson MJ. Inflammatory fibroid polyp of the small intestine: ultrastructural and immunohistochemical observations. *Ultrastruct Pathol* 1990;14:109–119.
16. van de Rijn M, Hendrickson MR, Rouse RV. An immunohistochemical study of inflammatory fibroid polyps of the gastrointestinal tract. *Appl Immunohistochem* 1994;2:54–59.
17. Kolodziejczyk P, Yao T, Tsuneyoshi M. Inflammatory fibroid polyp of the stomach. A special reference to an immunohistochemical profile of 42 cases. *Am J Surg Pathol* 1993;17:1159–1168.
18. Suen KC, Burton JD. The spectrum of eosinophilic infiltration of the gastrointestinal tract and its relationship to other disorders of angiitis and granulomatosis. *Hum Pathol* 1979;10:31–43.
19. Ming S-C. *Tumors of the esophagus and stomach*. 2nd series, fascicle 7. Washington DC: Armed Forces Institute of Pathology, 1973.
20. Caldwell JH, Mekhjian HS, Hurtubise PE, Berman FM. Eosinophilic gastroenteritis with obstruction: Immunologic studies of seven patients. *Gastroenterology* 1978;74:825–829.
21. Lewin KJ, Riddell RH, Weinstein WM. Small bowel mucosal disease. In: *Gastrointestinal pathology and its clinical implications.* New York: Igaku–Shoin, 1992;782–784.
22. Talley NJ, Shorter RG, Phillips SF, Zinsmeister AR. Eosinophilic gastroenteritis: a clinicopathological study of patients with disease of the mucosa, muscle layer, and subserosal tissues. *Gut* 1990;31:54–58.
23. Johnstone JM, Morson BC. Eosinophilic gastroenteritis. *Histopathology* 1978;2:335–348.
24. DeSchryver-Kecskemeti K, Clouse RE. A previously unrecognized subgroup of "eosinophilic gastroenteritis." Association with connective tissue diseases. *Am J Surg Pathol* 1984;8:171–180.
25. Male PJ, de Toledo F, Widgren S. Pseudotumoral enterocolitis and massive eosinophilia. *Gut* 1983;24:345–350.
26. Cohen MS, Jaques PF, Wall SD, Walker DH. A fatal eosinophilic process in a Laotian refugee. *Am J Clin Pathol* 1983;80:738–743.
27. Darby I, Skalli O, Gabbiani G. α-Smooth muscle actin is transiently expressed by myofibroblasts during experimental wound healing. *Lab Invest* 1990;63:21–29.
28. Schurch W, Seemayer TA, Gabbiani G. Myofibroblast. In: Sternberg SS, ed. *Histology for pathologists*. New York: Raven Press, 1992;109–144.
29. Skalli O, Schurch W, Seemayer TA, et al. Myofibroblasts from diverse pathologic settings are heterogeneous in their content of actin isoforms and intermediate filament proteins. *Lab Invest* 1989;60:275–285.
30. Mori K, Shinya H, Wolff WI. Polypoid reparative mucosal proliferation at the site of healed gastric ulcer: sequential gastroscopic, radiological, and histlogical observations. *Gastroenterology* 1971;61:523–529.
31. Dail DH. Plasma cell granuloma–histiocytoma complex. In: Dail DH, Hammar SP, eds. *Pulmonary pathology*. New York: Springer–Verlag, 1988;889–893.
32. Scully RE, Mark EJ, McNeely BU. Case records of the Massachusetts Hospital (Case 13–1984). *N Engl J Med* 1984;310:839–845.
33. Day DL, Sane S, Dehner LP. Inflammatory pseudotumor of the mesentery general and small intestine. *Pediatr Radiol* 1986;16:210–215.
34. Meis JM, Enzinger FM. Inflammatory fibrosarcoma of the mesentery and retroperitoneum. A tumor closely simulating inflammatory pseudotumor. *Am J Surg Pathol* 1991;15:1146–1156.
35. Pisciotto PT, Gray GF, Miller DR. Abdominal plasma cell pseudotumor. *J Pediatr* 1978;93:628–630.
36. Freud E, Bilik R, Yaniv I, et al. Inflammatory pseudotumor in childhood. *Arch Surg* 1991;126:653–655.
37. Gonzalez-Crussi F, deMello DE, Sotelo-Avila C. Omental-mesenteric myxoid hamartomas. Infantile lesions simulating malignant tumors. *Am J Surg Pathol* 1983;7:567–578.
38. Maves CK, Johnson JF, Bove K, Malott RL. Gastric inflammatory pseudotumor in children. *Radiology* 1989;173:381–383.
39. Tada T, Wakabayashi T, Kishimoto H. Plasma cell granuloma of the stomach. A report of a case associated with gastric cancer. *Cancer* 1984;54:541–544.
40. Isaacson P, Buchanan R, Mepham BL. Plasma cell granuloma of the stomach. *Hum Pathol* 1978;9:355–358.
41. Tang TT, Segura AD, Oechler HW, et al. Inflammatory myofibrohistiocytic proliferation simulating sarcoma in children. *Cancer* 1990;65:1626–1634.
42. Kojimahara K, Mukai M, Yamazaki K, et al. Inflammatory pseudotumor of the stomach: report of a highly infiltrative case with electron microscopic and immunohistochemical studies. *Acta Pathol Jpn* 1993;43:65–70.
43. Anand A, Vuitch F, Gould E, Albores-Saavedra J. Colonic pseudosarcomatous myofibroblastic proliferation. *Mod Pathol* 1991;4:33A.
44. Wolf BC, Khettry U, Leonardi HK, Neptune WB, Bhattacharyya AK, Legg MA. Benign lesions mimicking malignant tumors of the esophagus. *Hum Pathol* 1988;19:148–154.
45. Pettinato G, Manivel JC, DeRosa N, Dehner LP. Inflammatory myofibroblastic tumor (plasma cell granuloma). Clinicopathologic study

of 20 cases with immunohistochemical and ultrastructural observations. *Am J Clin Pathol* 1990;94:538–546.

46. Dehner LP. Extrapulmonary inflammatory myofibroblastic tumor: the inflammatory pseudotumor as another expression of the fibrohistiocytic complex. *Lab Invest* 1986;54:15A.

47. Coffin CM, Watterson J, Priest J, Dehner LP. Inflammatory myofibroblastic tumor: a clinicopathologic and immunohistochemical study of 73 cases. *Mod Pathol* 1994;7:5A.

48. Uzoaru I, Chou P, Reyes-Mugica M, Shen-Schwartz S, Gonzalez-Crussi F. Inflammatory myofibroblastic tumor of the pancreas. *Surg Pathol* 1993;5:181–188.

49. Souid AK, Ziemba MC, Dubansky AS, et al. Inflammatory myofibroblastic tumor in children. *Cancer* 1993;72:2042–2048.

50. Treissman SP, Gillis DA, Lee CLY, Giacomantonio M, Resch L. Omental-mesenteric inflammatory pseudotumor. *Cancer* 1994;73:1433–1437.

51. Jones EC, Clement PB, Young RH. Inflammatory pseudotumor of the urinary bladder. *Am J Surg Pathol* 1993;17:1193–1194.

52. Dirschmid K, Walser J, Hugel H. Pseudomalignant erosion in hyperplastic gastric polyps. *Cancer* 1984;54:2290–2293.

53. Nash S. Benign lesions of the gastrointestinal tract that may be misdiagnosed as malignant tumors. *Semin Diagn Pathol* 1990;7:102–114.

54. Jessurun J, Paplanus SH, Nagle R, Hamilton SR, Yardley JH, Tripp M. Pseudosarcomatous changes in inflammatory pseudopolyps of the colon. *Arch Pathol Lab Med* 1986;110:833–836.

55. Khekitka KM, Helwig EB. Deceptive bizarre stromal cells in polyps and ulcers of the gastrointestinal tract. *Cancer* 1991;67:2111–2117.

56. Schinella RA. Stromal atypia in anal papillae. *Dis Colon Rectum* 1976;19:611.

57. Bhatha PS, Chetty R, Clark SP, Wall AJ, Williams RA. Atypical mesenchymal (bizarre stromal) reaction in the gastrointestinal tract. *Int J Surg Pathol* 1993;1:145.

58. Coletta U, Sturgill BC. Isolated xanthomatosis of the small bowel. *Hum Pathol* 1985;16:422–424.

59. Ashfaq R, Timmons CF. Xanthomatous pseudotumor of the small intestine following treatment for Burkitt's lymphoma. *Arch Pathol Lab Med* 1992;16:299–301.

60. Beutler SM, Fretzin DF, Jao W, et al. Xanthomatosis resembling scleroderma in multiple myeloma. *Arch Pathol Lab Med* 1978;102:567.

61. Osborne BM, Hagemeister FB, Butler JJ. Extranodal gastrointestinal sinus histiocytosis with massive lymphadenopathy. Clinically presenting as a malignant tumor. *Am J Surg Pathol* 1981;5:603–611.

62. Foucar E, Rosai J, Dorfman R. Sinus histiocytosis with massive lymphadenopathy (Rosai–Dorfman disease): review of the entity. *Semin Diagn Pathol* 1990;7:19–73.

63. Mast A, Elewant A, Mortier G, et al. Gastric xanthoma. *Am J Gastroenterol* 1976;65:311–317.

64. Domellof L, Eriksson S, Helander HF, Janunger KG. Lipid islands in the gastric mucosa after resection for benign ulcer disease. *Gastroenterology* 1977;72:14–18.

65. Terruzzi V, Minoli G, Butti GC, Rossini A. Gastric lipid islands in the gastric stump and in non-operated stomach. *Endoscopy* 1980;12:58–62.

66. Kimura K, Hiramoto T, Buncher CR. Gastric xanthelasma. *Arch Pathol* 1969;87:110–117.

67. Weisberg T, Feldman M. Lipomas of the gastrointestinal tract. *Am J Clin Pathol* 1955;25:272–281.

68. Snover DC, Sandstad J, Hutton S. Mucosal pseudolipomatosis of the colon. *Am J Clin Pathol* 1985;84:575–580.

69. Segal GH, Petras RE. Small intestine. In: Sternberg SS, ed. *Histology for pathologists*. New York: Raven Press, 1992;547–571.

70. McGregor DH, Tawfik OW. Lipohyperplasia of the ileocecal valve. *Am J Clin Pathol* 1990;93:440.

71. Boquist L, Bergdahl L, Andersson A. Lipomatosis of the ileocecal valve. *Cancer* 1972;29:136–140.

72. Edwards M, Zangara H. Lipomatous hypertrophy of the ileocecal valve. *Am J Surg* 1951;82:533–537.

73. Dolan RV, ReMine WH, Dockerty MB. The fate of heterotopic pancreatic tissue. *Arch Surg* 1974;109:762–765.

74. Busard JM, Walters W. Heterotopic pancreatic tissue. *Arch Surg* 1950;60:674–682.

75. Lai EC, Tompkins RK. Heterotopic pancreas. Review of 26 year experience. *Am J Surg* 1986;151:697–700.

76. Clarke BE. Myoepithelial hamartoma of the gastrointestinal tract: a report of eight cases with comment concerning genesis and nomenclature. *Arch Pathol* 1940;30:143–152.

77. Attanoos R, Williams GT. Epithelial and neuroendocrine tumors of the duodenum. *Semin Diagn Pathol* 1991;8:149–162.

78. Lasser A, Koufman WB. Adenomyoma of the stomach. *Am J Dig Dis* 1977;22:965–969.

79. Gal R, Rath-Wolfson L, Ginzburg M, Kessler E. Adenomyomas of the small intestine. *Histopathology* 1991;18:369–371.

80. Doglioni C, Laurino L, Dei Tos AP, et al. Pancreactic (acinar) metaplasia of the gastric mucosa. Histology, ultrastructure, immunocytochemistry, and clinicopathologic correlations of 101 cases. *Am J Surg Pathol* 1993;17:1134–1143.

81. Rolfs RT, Nakashima AK. Epidemiology of primary and secondary syphilis in the United States, 1981 through 1989. *JAMA* 1990;264:1432–1437.

82. Winters HA, Notar-Francesco V, Bromberg K, et al. Gastric syphilis: five recent cases and a review of the literature. *Ann Intern Med* 1992;116:314–319.

83. Abdu RA, Carter K, Pomidor WJ. Gastric syphilis mimicking linitis plastica. *Arch Surg* 1993;128:103–104.

84. Jones BV, Lichtenstein JE. Gastric syphilis: radiologic findings. *AJR* 1993;160:59–61.

85. Anai H, Okada Y, Okubo K, et al. Gastric syphilis simulating linitis plastica type of gastric cancer. *Gastrointest Endoscop* 1990;36:624–626.

86. Butz WC, Watts JC, Rosales-Quintana S, Hicklin MD. Erosive gastritis as a manifestation of secondary syphilis. *Am J Clin Pathol* 1975;63:895–900.

87. Schlossberg D, Rudy FR, Jackson FW, Dumalag LB. Syphilitic enteritis. *Arch Intern Med* 1984;144:811–812.

88. Sachar DB, Klein RS, Swerdlow F. Erosive syphilitic gastritis: dark-field immunofluorescent diagnosis from biopsy specimens. *Ann Intern Med* 1974;80:512–514.

89. Bassi O, Cosa G, Colavolpe A, Argentieri R. Primary syphilis of the rectum—endoscopic and clinical features. Report of a case. *Dis Colon Rectum* 1994;34:1024–1026.

90. Faris MR, Perry JJ, Westermeier TG, Redmond J. Rectal syphilis mimicking histiocytic lymphoma. *Am J Clin Pathol* 1983;80:719–721.

91. Drusin LM, Singer C, Valenti AJ, et al. Infectious syphilis mimicking neoplastic disease. *Arch Intern Med* 1977;137:156–160.

92. Patel J, Kieffer RW, Martin M, Avant GR. Giant fibrovascular polyp of the esophagus. *Gastroenterology* 1984;87:953–956.

93. Vrabec DP, Colley AT. Giant intraluminal polyps of the esophagus. *Ann Otol Rhinol Laryngol* 1983;92:344–348.

94. Avezzano EA, Fleischer DE, Merida MA, Anderson DL. Giant fibrovascular polyps of the esophagus. *Am J Gastroenterol* 1990;85:299–302.

95. Jang GC, Clouse ME, Fleishner FG. Fibrovascular polyp—a benign intraluminal tumor of the esophagus. *Radiology* 1969;92:1196–1200.

96. Postlethwait RW, Lowe JE. Benign tumors and cysts of the esophagus. In: Orringer MB, ed. *Shackelford's surgery of the alimentary tract*. 3rd ed. Philadelphia: WB Saunders, 1991;335–352.

97. LiVolsi VA, Perzin KH. Inflammatory pseudotumors (inflammatory fibrous polyps) of the esophagus: a clincopathology study. *Dig Dis* 1975;20:475–481.

98. Appleman HD. Mesenchymal tumors of the gastrointestinal tract. In: Ming S-C, Goldman H, eds. *Pathology of the gastrointestinal tract*. Philadelphia: WB Saunders, 1992;339–342.

99. Petras R, Whitman G, Winkelman E, Falk G, Rice T. Fibrovascular polyp of the esophagus: a report of four cases and review of the literature. *Mod Pathol* 1990;3:79A.

100. Allen MS, Talbot WH. Sudden death due to regurgitation of a pedunculated esophageal lipoma. *J Thorac Cardiovasc Surg* 1967;54:756–758.

101. Timmons B, Sedwitz JL, Oller DW. Benign fibrovascular polyp of the esophagus. *South Med J* 1991;84:1370–1372.

102. Ranchod M, Lewin KJ, Dorfman RF. Lymphoid hyperplasia of the gastrointestinal tract. A study of 26 cases and review of the literature. *Am J Surg Pathol* 1978;2:383–400.

103. Wright CJE. Pseudolymphoma of the stomach. *Hum Pathol* 1973;4:305–318.

104. Rubin A, Isaacson PG. Florid reactive lymphoid hyperplasia of the terminal ileum in adults: a condition bearing a close resemblance to low grade malignant lymphoma. *Histopathology* 1990;17:19–26.

105. Hyjek E, Kelenyi G. Pseudolymphomas of the stomach: a lesion characterized by progressively transformed germinal centres. *Histopathology* 1982;6:61–68.

106. Brooks JJ, Enterline HT. Gastric pseudolymphoma: its three subtypes and relation to lymphoma. *Cancer* 1983;51:476–486.
107. Genta RM, Hamner HW, Graham DY. Gastric lymphoid follicles in *Helicobacter pylori* infection: frequency, distribution and response to triple therapy. *Hum Pathol* 1993;24:577–583.
108. Sheahan DG, West AB. Focal lymphoid hyperplasia (pseudolymphoma) of the esophagus. *Am J Surg Pathol* 1985;9:141–147.
109. Strodel WE, Cooper R, Eckhauser F, et al. Pseudolymphoma masquerading as colonic malignancy. *Dis Colon Rectum* 1983;26:68–72.
110. Lewin KJ. Disorders of the lymphoid system. In: Ming S-C, Goldman H, eds. *Pathology of the gastrointestinal tract*. Philadelphia: WB Saunders, 1992;281–290.
111. Wolf JA, Spjut HJ. Focal lymphoid hyperplasia of the stomach preceding gastric lymphoma: a case report and review of the literature. *Cancer* 1981;48:2518–2523.
112. Scoazed JY, Brousse N, Potet F, Jeulain JF. Focal malignant lymphoma in gastric pseudolymphoma: histologic and immunohistochemical study of a case. *Cancer* 1986;57:1330–1336.
113. Tokunaga O, Watanabe T, Morimatsu M. Pseudolymphoma of the stomach. A clinicopathologic study of 15 cases. *Cancer* 1987;59:1320–1327.
114. Schwartz MS, Sherman H, Smith T, Janis R. Gastric pseudolymphoma and its relationship to malignant gastric lymphoma. *Am J Gastroenterol* 1989;84;1555–1559.
115. Eimoto T, Futami K, Naito H, et al. Gastric pseudolymphoma with monotypic cytoplasmic immunoglobulin. *Cancer* 1985;55:788–793.
116. Burke JS, Sheibani K, Nathwani BN, et al. Monoclonal small (well differentiated) lymphocytic proliferations of the gastrointestinal tract resembling lymphoid hyperplasia. A neoplasm of uncertain malignant potential. *Hum Pathol* 1987;18:1238–1245.
117. Mori N, Oka K, Ishido T, Nakamura K. Primary gastric mantle zone lymphoma. A report of two cases. *Arch Pathol Lab Med* 1991;115:603–606.
118. Sigal SH, Saul SH, Auerbach HE, et al. Gastric small lymphocytic proliferation with immunoglobulin gene rearrangement in pseudolymphoma versus lymphoma. *Gastroenterology* 1989;97:195–201.
119. Sanchez L, Algara P, Villuendas R, et al. B-cell clonal detection in gastric low-grade lymphomas and regional lymph nodes: an immunohistologic and molecular study. *Am J Gastroenterol* 1993;88:413–419.
120. Sweeney JF, Muus C, McKeown PP, Rosemurgy AS. Gastric pseudolymphoma. Not necessarily a benign lesion. *Dig Dis Sci* 1992;37:939–945.
121. Schulman H, Sickel J, Kleinman MS, Adams JT. Gastric "pseudolymphoma" with restricted light chain expression in a patient with obscure gastrointestinal blood loss. *Dig Dis Sci* 1991;36:1495–1499.
122. Takano Y, Kato Y, Sato Y, Okudaira M. Clonal Ig-gene rearrangement in some cases of gastric RLH detected by PCR method. *Pathol Res Pract* 1992;188:973–980.
123. Harris NL. Extranodal lymphoid infiltrates and mucosa-associated lymphoid tissue (MALT). A unifying concept. *Am J Surg Pathol* 1991;15:879–884.
124. Hall PA, Levison DA. Malignant lymphoma in the gastrointestinal tract. *Semin Diagn Pathol* 1991;8:163–177.
125. van der Valk P, Lindeman J, Meijer CJLM. Non-Hodgkin's lymphomas of the gastrointestinal tract: a review with special reference to the gut-associated lymphoid tissue. In: Watanabe S, Wolff M, Sommers SC, eds. *Digestive Diseases and Pathology*. vol 1. Philadelphia: Field and Wood, 1988;105–119.
126. Zukerberg LR, Medeiros JL, Ferry JA, Harris NL. Diffuse low-grade B-cell lymphomas. Four critically distinct subtypes defined by a combination of morphologic and immunophenotypic features. *Am J Clin Pathol* 1993;100:373–385.
127. Wotherspoon AC, Doglioni C, Diss TC, et al. Regression of primary low-grade B-cell lymphoma of mucosa-associated lymphoid tissue type after eradication of Helicobacter pylori. *Lancet* 1993;342:575–577.
128. Blazquez M, Haioun C, Chaumette MT, et al. Low grade B cell mucosa associated lymphoid tissue lymphoma of the stomach: clinical and endoscopic features, treatment, and outcome. *Gut* 1992;33:1621–1625.
129. Isaacson P, Spencer J. Malignant lymphoma of mucosa-associated lymphoid tissue. *Histopathology* 1987;11:445–462.
130. Saul SH, Sollenberger LC. Solitary rectal ulcer syndrome. Its clinical and pathological underdiagnosis. *Am J Surg Pathol* 1985;9:411–421.
131. Ford MJ, Anderson JR, Gilmour HM, et al. Clinical spectrum of "solitary ulcer" of the rectum. *Gastroenterology* 1983;84;1533–1540.
132. Womack NR, Williams NS, Holmfield JHM, Morrison JFB. Pressure and prolapse—the cause of solitary rectal ulceration. *Gut* 1987;28:1228–1233.
133. Martin JK, Culp CE, Werland LH. Colitis cystica profunda. *Dis Colon Rectum* 1980;23:488.
134. Wayte DM, Helwig EB. Colitis cystica profunda. *Am J Clin Pathol* 1967;48:159–169.
135. Allen MS. Hamartomatous inverted polyps of the rectum. *Cancer* 1966;19:257–265.
136. Saul SH, Wong LK, Zinsser KR. Enteritis cystica profunda: association with Crohn's disease. *Hum Pathol* 1986;17:600–603.
137. Kyriakos M, Condon SC. Enteritis cystica profunda. *Am J Clin Pathol* 1978;69:77–85.
138. Franzin G, Novelli P. Gastritis cystica profunda. *Histopathology* 1981;5:535–547.
139. Bentley E, Chandrasoma P, Cohen H, et al. Colitis cystica profunda: presenting with complete intestinal obstruction and recurrence. *Gastroenterology* 1985;89:1157–1161.
140. Kelly JK, Langevin JM, Price LM, Hershfield NB, Share S, Blustein P. Giant and symptomatic inflammatory polyps of the colon in idiopathic inflammatory bowel disease. *Am J Surg Pathol* 1986;10:420–428.
141. Lobert PF, Appelman HD. Inflammatory cloacogenic polyp. A unique inflammatory lesion of the anal transition zone. *Am J Surg Pathol* 1981;5:761–766.
142. Saul SH. Inflammatory cloacogenic polyp: relationship to solitary rectal ulcer syndrome/mucosal prolapse and other bowel disorders. *Hum Pathol* 1987;18:1120–1125.
143. DuBoulay CEH, Fairbrother J, Isaacson PG. Mucosal prolapse syndrome—a unifying concept for solitary rectal ulcer syndrome and related disorders. *J Clin Pathol* 1983;36:1264–1268.
144. Allen-Mersh TG, Henry MM, Nicholls RJ. Natural history of anterior mucosal prolapse. *Br J Surg* 1987;74:679–682.
145. Levine DS. Solitary rectal ulcer syndrome. Are "solitary" rectal ulcer syndrome and "localized" colitis cystica profunda analogous syndromes caused by rectal prolapse? *Gastroenterology* 1987;92:243–253.
146. Burke AP, Sobin LH. Eroded polypoid hyperplasia of the rectosigmoid. *Am J Gastroenterol* 1990;85:975–980.
147. Bhatal PS, Macrae F, Slavin J. Rectosigmoid inflammatory "cap" polyps. *Int J Surg Pathol* 1993;1:149.
148. Stanton MJ, Maxted WC. Malakoplakia: a study of the literature and current concepts of pathogenesis, diagnosis and treatment. *J Urol* 1981;125:139–141.
149. McClure J. Malakoplakia. *J Pathol* 1983;140:275–330.
150. Nakabayashi H, Ito T, Izutsu K, et al. Malakoplakia of the stomach. Report of a case and review of the literature. *Arch Pathol Lab Med* 1978;102:136–139.
151. Gonzalez-Angulo A, Corral E, Garcia-Torres R, Quijano M. Malakoplakia of the colon. *Gastroenterology* 1965;48:383–387.
152. Finlay-Jones LR, Blackwell JB, Papadimitriou JM. Malakoplakia of the colon. *Am J Clin Pathol* 1968:50:320–329.
153. Ranchod M, Kahn LB. Malakoplakia of the gastrointestinal tract. *Arch Pathol* 1972;94:90–97.
154. Terner MY, Lattes R. Malakoplakia of colon and retroperitoneum. *Am J Clin Pathol* 1965;44:22–31.
155. Ghosh S, Pattnaik S, Jalan R, Maitra TK. Malakoplakia simulating rectal carcinoma. *Am J Gastroenterol* 1990;85:910–911.
156. Moran CA, West B, Schwartz IS. Malakoplakia of the colon in association with colonic adenocarcinoma. *Am J Gastroenterol* 1989;84:1580–1582.
157. Radin DR, Chandrasoma P, Halls JM. Colonic malakoplakia. *Gastrointest Radiol* 1984;9:359–361.
158. Ng IO, Ng M. Colonic malakoplakia: unusual association with ulcerative colitis. *J Gastroenterol Hepatol* 1993;8:110–115.
159. Lewin KJ, Riddell RH, Weinstein WM. Miscellaneous diseases. In: *Gastrointestinal pathology and its clinical implications*. New York: Igaku-Shoin, 1992;1134–1139.
160. Lewin KJ, Harrell GS, Lee AS, Crowley LG. Malakoplakia. An electron microscopic study: demonstration of bacilliform organisms in malacoplakic macrophages. *Gastroenterology* 1974;66:28–45.
161. Mir-Madjlessi HS, Towassolil H, Kamalian N. Malakoplakia of the colon and recurrent colonic strictures in a patient with primary hypogammaglobulinemia. *Dis Colon Rectum* 1982;25:723–727.
162. Yang CC, Huang T, Tsung SH, Dan DC. Rectal malakoplakia in a patient with Hodgkin's disease. *Dis Colon Rectum* 1983;26:129–132.
163. Abdou MI, NaPombejara C, Sagawa A, et al. Malakoplakia: evidence for monocyte lysosomal abnormality correctable by cholinergic agonist in vitro and in vivo. *N Engl J Med* 1977;297:1413–1419.

164. Earnest DL, Schneiderman DJ. Other diseases of the colon and rectum. In: Sleisenger MH, Fordtran JS, eds. *Gastrointestinal disease.* 4th ed. Philadelphia: WB Saunders, 1989;1592–1595.

165. Weed JC, Ray JE. Endometriosis of the bowel. *Obstet Gynecol* 1987;69:727–730.

166. Boles RS, Hodes PJ. Endometriosis of the small and large intestine. *Gastroenterology* 1958;34:367–380.

167. Parr NJ, Murphy C, Holt S, et al. Endometriosis and the gut. *Gut* 1988;29:1112–1115.

168. Aronchuck CA, Brooks FP, Dyson WL, et al. Ileocecal endometriosis presenting with abdominal pain and gastrointestinal bleeding. *Dig Dis Sci* 1983;28:566–572.

169. Clement PB. Pathology of endometriosis. *Pathol Annu* 1990;1:245–295.

170. Sievert W, Sellin JH, Stringer CA. Pelvic endometriosis simulating colonic malignant neoplasm. *Arch Intern Med* 1989;149:935–938.

171. Wood DA. *Tumors of the intestines.* Series 1. Fascicle 22. Washington, DC: Armed Forces Institute of Pathology, 1967.

172. Kelly JK. Polypoid prolapsing mucosal folds in diverticular disease. *Am J Surg Pathol* 1991;15:871–878.

173. Franzin G, Fratton A, Manfrini C. Polypoid lesions associated with diverticular disease of the sigmoid colon. *Gastrointest Endosc* 1985;31:196–199.

174. Mathus-Vliegen EMH, Tytgat GNJ. Polyp simulating mucosal prolapse syndrome in (Pre)-diverticular disease. *Endoscopy* 1986;18:84–86.

175. Asch MJ, Markowitz AM. Cecal diverticulitis: report of 16 cases and review of the literature. *Surgery* 1969;65:906–910.

176. Jao S-W, Beart RW, Spencer RJ, Reiman HM, Ilstrup DM. Retrorectal tumors. Mayo Clinic experience, 1960–1979. *Dis Colon Rectum* 1985;28:644–652.

177. Mills SE, Walker AN, Stallings RG, Allen S. Retrorectal cystic hamartoma. Report of three cases, including one with a perirenal component. *Arch Pathol Lab Med* 1984;108:737–740.

178. Hjermstad BM, Helwig EB. Tailgut cysts. Report of 53 cases. *Am J Clin Pathol* 1988;89:139–147.

179. Marco V, Autonell J, Farre J, Fernandez-Layos M, Doncel F. Retrorectal cyst-hamartomas. Report of two cases with adenocarcinoma developing in one. *Am J Surg Pathol* 1982;6:707–714.

180. Enjoji M, Sumiyoshi K, Sueyoshi K. Elastofibromatous lesion of the stomach in a patient with elastofibroma dorsi. *Am J Surg Pathol* 1985;9:233–237.

181. Goldblum JR, Beals T, Weiss SW. Elastofibromatous change of the rectum. A lesion mimicking amyloidosis. *Am J Surg Pathol* 1992;16:793–795.

182. Dankwa EK, Davies JD. Smooth muscle pseudotumors: a potentially confusing artifact of rectal biopsy. *J Clin Pathol* 1988;41:737–741.

## ADDENDUM REFERENCES

### *Inflammatory Fibroid Polyps*

Bradley B, Molloy PJ, Glick K, Kania RJ. Ileal intussusception and obstruction as presentation of inflammatory fibroid polyp. *Dig Dis Sci* 1995;40:812–813.

Dewailly A, Vandermolen P, Klein O, Andre JM, Lecomte-Houcke M, Colombel JF. Obstructive inflammatory fibroid polyp of the cardia. *Gastroenterol Clin Biol* 1995;19:646–647.

Gooszen AW, Tjon A, Tham RT, Veselic M, Bolk JH, Lamers CB. Inflammatory fibroid polyp simulating malignant tumor of the colon in a patient with multiple hamartoma syndrome (Cowden's disease). *Am J Roentgenol* 1995;165:1012–1013.

### *Inflammatory Myofibroblastic Tumor (Inflammatory Pseudotumor)*

Sfairi A, Farah A, Patel JC. Inflammatory pseudotumor of the small intestine: an unusual cause of intestinal intussusception in adults. *Presse Med* 1995;24:1909.

### *Syphilic Pseudotumors*

Long BW, Johnston JH, Wetzel W, Flowers RH III, Haick A. Gastric syphilis: endoscopic and histological features mimicking lymphoma. *Am J Gastroenterol* 1995;90:1504–1507.

### *Esophageal Fibrovascular Polyp*

Behar PM, Arena S, Marrangoni AG. Recurrent fibrovascular polyp of the esophagus. *Am J Otolaryngol* 1995;16:209–212.

Halfhide BC, Ginai AZ, Spoelstra HA, Dees J, Vuzevski VD. A hamartoma presenting as a giant esophageal polyp. *Br J Radiol* 1995;68:85–88.

### *Tumefactive Lymphoid Hyperplasia*

Spodaryk M, Mrukowicz J, Stopyrowa J, Czupryna A, Kowalska-Duplaga K, Fyderek K, Miezynski W. Severe intestinal nodular lymphoid hyperplasia in an infant. *J Pediatr Gastroenterol Nutr* 1995;21:468–473.

### *Vascular Malformations of the Gastrointestinal System*

Jaspersen D, Korner T, Schorr W, Brennenstuhl M, Hammar CH. Extragastric Dieulafoy's disease an an unusual source of intestinal bleeding: esophageal visible vessels. *Dig Dis Sci* 1994;39:2558–2560.

### *Colitis Cystica Profunda*

Ng WK, Chan KW. Postirradiation colitis cystica profunda: case report and literature review. *Arch Pathol Lab Med* 1995;119:1170–1173.

### *Inflammatory Cloacogenic Polyps*

Bass J, Soucy P, Walton M, Nizalik E. Inflammatory cloacogenic polyps in children. *J Pediatr Surg* 1995;30:585–588.

Carr NJ, Monihan JM, Nzeako UC, Murakata LA, Sobin LH. Expression of proliferating cell nuclear antigen in hyperplastic polyps, adenomas, and inflammatory cloacogenic polyps of the large intestine. *J Clin Pathol* 1995;48:46–52.

### *Tumefactive Endometriosis*

Daya D, O'Connell G, DeNardi F. Rectal endometriosis mimicking solitary rectal ulcer syndrome. *Mod Pathol* 1995;8:599–602.

Leutloff UC, Roeren T, Feldmann K, Sillem M, Rabe T, Kauffmann G. Symptomatic endometriosis of the large intestine: a case report. *Rontgenpraxis* 1996;49:115–117.

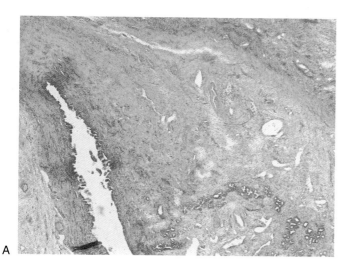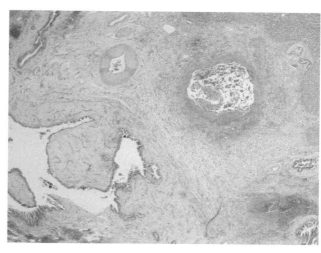

A                                                                                                                          B

**FIG. 2.** Recurrent pyogenic cholangiohepatitis. **A:** A left lobe resection from an Oriental woman with recurrent fever and chills shows many large bile ducts surrounded by fibrosis and lymphocytes. Many of the fibrous areas contain numerous small bile duct structures typical of collapse of liver (with hepatocytes disappearing) secondary to secondary thrombosis and infarction of large areas. **B:** Another left lobe resection specimen with abscess formation (central cavity is filled with neutrophils). The remaining viable hepatocellular component is the geographic margin at the periphery of the illustration.

primary or metastatic sarcomas, benign mesenchymal neoplasms including schwannoma and leiomyoma, fibrogenic variants of Rosai–Dorfman disease, epithelioid hemangioendothelioma, angiomyolipoma, and lobar or localized hepatic atrophy.

Hepatic abscesses are usually multiple and, unlike HIPs, they demonstrate central zones of necrosis. The former lesions are commonly associated with an underlying disease such as appendicitis or diverticulitis, and roughly 50% yield positive culture results for bacterial organisms, which are often mixed in nature (e.g., gram-negative enteric bacilli and gram-positive anaerobic cocci). The portion of abscesses that most closely imitates the microscopic appearance of IMT is their peripheral wall of granulation tissue and fibrosis, but the presence of confluent areas of acute inflammation should sway diagnostic opinion away from the latter lesion. Pyogenic cholangiohepatitis is an important cause of hepatic abscess formation that is associated with biliary obstruction (usually by intraductal calculi) (Fig. 2) (20). The inflammatory reaction around affected bile ducts in this condition is virtually identical microscopically to that of IMT (21). Again, however, the presence of confluent zones of suppurative inflammation and prominent periductal fibrosis is inconsistent with that interpretation (20,22). Amoebic abscesses likewise may contain foci that superficially resemble IMT, but the former lesions may be recognized by their content of amoebic trophozoites and cysts as well as acute inflammatory cells. After successful treatment, organizing amoebic abscesses may more closely simulate idiopathic HIPs, and historical data may become more crucial to their proper pathologic diagnosis.

Granulomatous hepatic disorders may also yield mass lesions with general pathologic characteristics that are capable of simulating those of IMT. In particular, infection with *Mycobacterium tuberculosis* is capable of doing so, as is sarcoidosis. Both conditions have been associated with fibrogenic nodular tumefactions that measured between 2 and 6.5 cm in maximum dimension (23,24).

Hepatic involvement by Rosai–Dorfman disease also has the potential to closely imitate the morphologic features of HIP (Fig. 3) (25,26). In the former of these disorders, variable numbers of large histiocytes are admixed with lymphoid

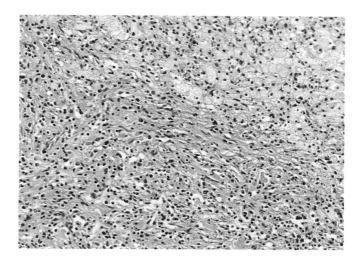

**FIG. 3.** Rosai–Dorfman (RD) lesion involving the liver. The usual RD hepatic lesion exhibits only small portal area changes but this reported case included a grossly visible nodule (8 mm). The histologic features of the hepatic lesion are identical to those of inflammatory pseudotumor with a mixture of fibroblastic cells, lymphocytes, and histiocytes in a myxoid stroma. The usual diagnostic trabecular pattern of sinusoidal histiocytes is not present anywhere in this large section. (Courtesy of Juan Rosai, M.D., New York. From ref. 26.)

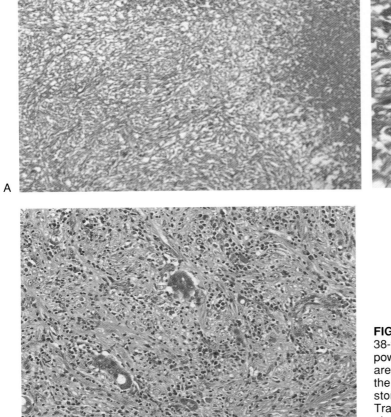

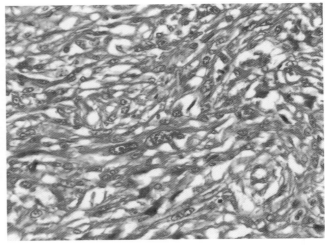

**FIG. 4.** Malignant fibrous histiocytoma primary in liver. This 38-year-old man had a 7-cm hard mass resected. **A:** Low power shows small areas of necrosis intermingled with solid areas of spindle cell proliferation. **B:** Spindle cells showing the large nuclei with prominent nucleoli. There are areas of storiform growth and a minor lymphocytic component. **C:** Trapped bile ducts within the stroma. The hepatocytes are absent with only a few ductal structures remaining from the former portal areas. (Courtesy of M. Fukayama.)

cells and myxofibrous stromal tissue. It is notable, however, that sinus histiocytosis with massive lymphadenopathy in the liver is virtually always accompanied by extrahepatic lesions as well, making clinical information critical to this differential diagnosis (27).

Metastases of the liver from such sarcomas as fibrosarcoma or malignant fibrous histiocytoma (MFH) usually occur in the context of previously documented tumor in the soft tissues and demonstrate obvious nuclear atypia in the proliferating spindle cells (Fig. 4). However, occasional cases of primary hepatic MFH may exhibit a relatively bland cytologic image (28) and they may require extensive sampling to document obviously malignant areas. Likewise, we have seen cases of primary epithelioid hemangioendothelioma of the liver (Fig. 16) that were "masked" by reactive proliferations of banal spindle cells.

Hepatic lymphomas are usually secondary in nature and therefore access to clinical data is the best means of avoiding their confusion with IMT of the liver. However, sclerosing malignant lymphomas are capable of bearing a strong resemblance to HIPs, and special studies (see above) may be required to distinguish between these disorders.

Benign mesenchymal neoplasms of the liver are extraordinarily rare, and they characteristically lack inflammatory cells as expected in IMTs. Moreover, immunostains for S-100 protein are capable of identifying schwannomas and excluding HIPs (29); a similar statement pertains to desmin immunoreactivity and hepatic leiomyomas.

*Biological Evolution of Hepatic Inflammatory Pseudotumors*

The great majority of patients with HIPs pursue an uncomplicated course after surgical intervention, culminating in complete recovery. However, occasional cases have proven fatal because of complicating postoperative disorders (14). In light of the latter information, it is noteworthy that the spontaneous regression of hepatic IMTs has been documented (30,31), as has partial resolution of such masses after administration of exogenous corticosteroids (32). Thus, conservative nonoperative management may be chosen in circumstances where surgery is relatively contraindicated.

A previously reported case of IMT had dramatic recurrence 30 months after initial resection by hemihepatectomy. Two new large (10 cm) lesions were resected and numerous special studies were completed which led to a diagnosis of "follicular dendritic cell tumor." The basic histologic features included a syncytia of large pleomorphic cells admixed with small lymphocytes and histiocytes (one lesion) and another lesion had a storiform fascicular pattern. Mitosis were uncommon. Reactivity with antibodies CD21, CD35, R4/23, and Ki-M4 are helpful. Frozen tissue may be necessary for reliable results (96). These results suggested that IMT may progress to follicular dendritic cell tumor (FDCT). A second case report of FDCT indicated a clonal Epstein Barr virus proliferation as well (97).

## Angiomyolipoma of the Liver

Angiomyolipoma (AML) of the liver is included in this discussion because of the authors' opinion that it represents a hamartomatous growth rather than a true neoplasm. This tumefaction is analogous to lesions seen in the kidney and soft tissues in tuberous sclerosis. It should also be distinguished from other adipocytic masses of the liver, including myelolipoma, tumefactive focal fatty metamorphosis, lipoma, and pseudolipoma.

### Clinical Features

The ages of patients with hepatic AMLs has ranged from 30 to 72 years, with no preference for either gender. The lesions have typically been found incidentally during radiographic evaluations done for unrelated conditions. There is a more tenuous association between AMLs of the liver and tuberous sclerosis than that which applies to renal lesions of that type, but AMLs of both sites were seen in up to 10% of patients in some series (33,34). The CT appearance of hepatic angiomyolipoma is said to be distinctive (35), and it may obviate the need for surgical therapy.

### Pathologic Findings

In a study from the Armed Forces Institute of Pathology (AFIP) (33), the size of AMLs of the liver varied between 1 and 20 cm; one half showed a maximal dimension of <3 cm. All of the lesions were solitary, except for the concurrent presence of three separate masses in one case. The vast majority of hepatic AMLs are located deep in the parenchyma and are therefore most accessible to needle biopsy. However, a pedunculated and superficial gross configuration has indeed been documented. The cut surfaces of resected AMLs are yellow–white and relatively homogeneous, and the lesions demonstrate sharp demarcation from the surrounding hepatic parenchyma.

The mixture of adipocytic, vascular, and smooth muscle components of AML is highly variable from case to case, and even between different areas of the same mass. Either the fatty or leiomyoma-like constituents may be predominant; the former elements may assume a hibernoma-like appearance if brown fat is observed in the lesion, and the smooth muscle components are capable of an alarming degree of cellularity and atypia that bring a diagnosis of leiomyosarcoma to the forefront of consideration. However, mitotic figures are sparse, nucleoli are absent, and a characteristic blending of the myogenous spindle cells with the walls of aberrantly shaped intralesional blood vessels provides another clue to the identity of hepatic AML (Fig. 5). Secondary fibrosis, epithelioid change in the smooth muscle elements, and extramedullary hemopoiesis represent additional potential findings in this pathologic entity.

### Results of Special Studies

As just cited above, epithelioid features in the myogenic component of AML may cause diagnostic confusion with carcinomas. Application of the periodic acid–Schiff (PAS) method may be beneficial in this setting inasmuch as both the fusiform and polygonal cells of angiomyolipoma often contain PAS-positive, rod-shaped crystalloids (36); these are not expected in HCC or metastatic carcinomas. In accord with immunohistochemical attributes of AML in other organs, hepatic lesions of this type show reactivity with HMB45 (a monoclonal antibody usually regarded as a melanocyte marker), as well as antibodies to desmin, $\alpha$-actin, and vimentin. S-100 protein may also be seen in adipocytic elements, but keratin, epithelial membrane antigen (EMA), neuroendocrine determinants, carcinoembryonic antigen, and AFP are uniformly absent (36,37). Electron microscopy shows the presence of cytoplasmic dense bodies and skeins of myogenous thin filaments in the spindle cells of hepatic AML, and, interestingly, premelanosome-like organelles have been demonstrated in epithelioid cells in some of these lesions (36). Whether they do in fact pursue melanocytic differentiation is a controversial and unsettled issue at present.

### Differential Diagnostic Considerations

In our experience and that of others (33), those examples of hepatic AML that contain a sizable number of epithelioid cells most often lead to mistakes in diagnosis. In most instances, the erroneous interpretation is that of HCC. Consideration also may be given to primary embryonal sarcoma of the liver, primary or secondary MFH, metastatic melanoma, or metastatic leiomyosarcoma, in cases where cellular pleomorphism is extreme. However, the lack of spontaneous necrosis and mitotic activity militates against the latter lesions, as does the characteristic admixture of adipocytic components—with or without hematopoietic elements—that is seen in AMLs. Nevertheless, it is worth emphasizing that several tissue blocks may need to be examined before these features are well visualized.

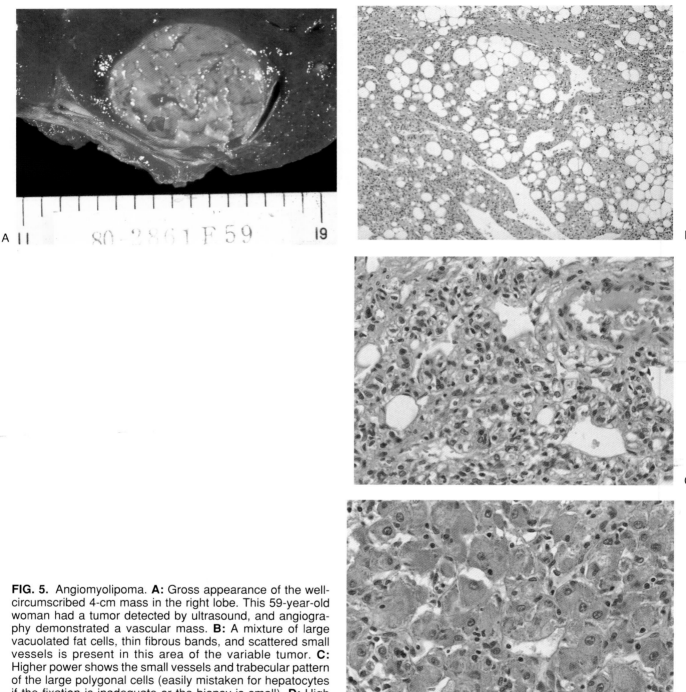

**FIG. 5. Angiomyolipoma. A:** Gross appearance of the well-circumscribed 4-cm mass in the right lobe. This 59-year-old woman had a tumor detected by ultrasound, and angiography demonstrated a vascular mass. **B:** A mixture of large vacuolated fat cells, thin fibrous bands, and scattered small vessels is present in this area of the variable tumor. **C:** Higher power shows the small vessels and trabecular pattern of the large polygonal cells (easily mistaken for hepatocytes if the fixation is inadequate or the biopsy is small). **D:** High power shows that the large epithelioid smooth muscle cells with abundant cytoplasm have small nuclei with no nucleoli and the trabecular growth pattern lacks lining cells.

Another possibility in lipocyte-rich variants of AML is the lesion known as hepatic "pseudolipoma." The latter entity simply represents entrapped epiploic appendages within the capsule of the liver and lacks spindle cell constituents (38).

*Biological Evolution*

The long-term behavior of hepatic AML has not been detailed extensively in the available literature on approximately 30 such lesions. However, malignant transformation is apparently unknown, and most masses of this type appear to remain relatively stable in size or enlarge slowly over time. Rupture has not been described, even with large AMLs. Conversely, spontaneous regression and shrinkage has occasionally been observed. In any event, resection of the lesion should not be considered mandatory once the diagnosis is secure.

**Tumefactive Focal Fatty Metamorphosis**

Tumefactive focal fatty metamorphosis (TFFM) refers to a localized collection of hepatocytes that have undergone marked fatty change and that are distinctly different from the adjacent nonfatty hepatic parenchyma. Because of this peculiarity, the condition may be mistaken for a neoplasm by both radiologists and pathologists.

*Clinical Features*

TFFM is a relatively common disorder that is usually detected by abdominal CT or MRI that is done for other reasons (39). The lesions may either be solitary or multifocal, and are seen in adult patients of all ages. There is no predilection for either gender. TFFM is seen mainly in individuals who have an underlying condition that predisposes to dyslipidemia, such as diabetes mellitus, morbid obesity, alcoholism, exogenous steroid use, and hyperalimentation. Confusion of this disorder with metastases is well known in the radiologic literature (40), and this problem may even pertain to surgeons and pathologists as well (see below). The CT appearance of TFFM is that of irregular low-attenuation nodules that blend at their peripheral aspects with the surrounding liver. Radionuclide scans (particularly with labeled xenon) show no hepatic defects, and this is a helpful observation in excluding clinical concerns over metastatic disease (41,42). It is currently unknown as to why some patients store hepatic lipid in this peculiar fashion and others exhibit more diffuse fatty change.

*Pathologic Findings*

The liver is normal in size and texture in cases of TFFM, but one or several lesions are apparent on cut surface. These are pale, yellow–white, and soft, measuring up to 4 cm in greatest dimension. They may be visible on peritoneoscopy or gross inspection of Glisson's capsule, against the dark red–brown background of the normal hepatic parenchyma. Microscopically, one simply observes marked fatty change in hepatocytes that is regional in distribution. Large cytoplasmic vacuoles of fat fill the affected parenchymal cells and displace their nuclei peripherally. Degenerative foci may also demonstrate a foreign body–type granulomatous response to spilled extracellular lipid. Portal triads are spared and show no particular abnormalities; the adjacent liver is likewise histologically unremarkable, and there is no fibrous capsular interface between it and the foci of TFFM.

*Biological Evolution*

The course of tumefactive fatty metamorphosis is dependent on the evolution of the underlying metabolic diseases. If systemic disturbances in lipid processing are corrected, the hepatic lesions may regress (40,45). However, one more commonly observes maintenance of a relatively stable size or gradual enlargement of the fatty deposits on follow-up CT of the abdomen.

**Mesenchymal Hamartoma of the Liver**

Many terms have been used to describe a distinctive mesenchymal lesion of the liver that can be confused with a true neoplasm. "Mesenchymal hamartoma" is the preferred designation for this proliferation, but it has also been called "bile duct fibroadenoma," "giant lymphangioma," and "cystic hamartoma."

*Clinical Features*

Mesenchymal hamartoma of the liver (MHL) is typically seen in childhood, but we have also observed rare examples of this lesion in young adults. It commonly attains a large size before coming to clinical attention. In a series by Ishak and Stocker on MHL (43), 69% arose in boys at an average age of 15 months (range: 1 day to 10 years). Most of these lesions present as a palpable mass, which is readily seen on CT or MRI of the abdomen as a tumefaction with low attenuation and some internal variability in density. In some cases, the serum level of AFP may be elevated, causing concern over possible diagnoses of juvenile HCC or hepatoblastoma. There is no association between MHL and congenital malformations in other organ systems.

*Pathologic Findings*

For unknown reasons, the majority of MHLs arise in the right hepatic lobe, and they are roughly symmetric spherical

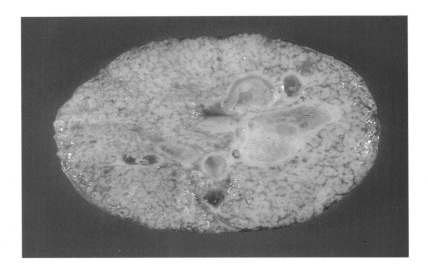

**FIG. 6.** Gross photograph of mesenchymal hamartoma of the liver. Note the relatively uniform tan color, with a glistening character reflecting the mucoid nature of the stroma. (Courtesy of Dr. Louis P. Dehner, Washington University, St. Louis, Missouri.)

masses. However, pedunculated forms that protrude from the surface of the liver have also been described. The weights of these lesions are variable, with a spectrum between 230 and 6800 g. The cut surfaces of MHL are gray–tan to brown or amber, with a multifocally mucomyxoid nature (Fig. 6) and cysts measuring from 3 mm to 14 cm in diameter.

Histologically, one observes edematous loose connective tissue that has an embryonic myxoid character, admixed with unremarkable interlobular bile ducts, clusters and cords of immature or mature hepatocytes, and fibrous bands (1) (Figs. 7 and 8). Dilated blood vessels may also be prominent in some examples, helping to explain the former classification of some MHLs as "lymphangiomas." Intralesional cysts are typically lined with nondescript cuboidal epithelium and mantled by condensed myxoid mesenchyme. Extramedullary hemopoiesis is common in the interstices of these masses, and areas showing chronic inflammatory cell infiltrates may also be evident. Mitotic activity is distinctly unusual, and pathologic division figures are essentially never found in MHL. Similarly, the nuclei of constituent spindle cells and epithelium are banal in nature. Heterologous mesenchymal differentiation (e.g., into cartilage, osteoid, or myogenous tissues) is uniformly absent.

### Differential Diagnosis

Examples of torsed-hepatic lobes in infants have assumed some of the characteristics of MHL in selected reports (44); these features have included a fibromyxoid stroma, cholangiolar proliferation, and isolation of hepatocytic nests in a myxedematous background. Nonetheless, they also demonstrated central foci of necrobiosis, hemorrhage, and fibrosis, none of which would be expected in mesenchymal hamartomas. Histologic mimicry of hepatoblastoma or hepatocellular carcinoma may be a problem if MHLs are subjected to needle biopsies, depending on the specific microscopic patterns that are sampled. However, neither of the former two

entities commonly contains much myxoid stroma, and that component should therefore sway the observer toward an interpretation of MHL. Embryonal sarcoma of the liver is capable of imitating many of the generic histologic attributes of mesenchymal hamartomas, but the first of these two lesions shows a much higher degree of nuclear anaplasia and pleomorphism in proliferating spindle cells. The PAS stain (with diastase) may also be used to demonstrate cytoplasmic hyaline globules in embryonal sarcoma, but these structures are lacking in MHL.

### Biological Evolution

Hepatic mesenchymal hamartomas pursue an innocuous clinical course, even if they are only subtotally removed surgically (1). Indeed, partial excision is not an uncommon

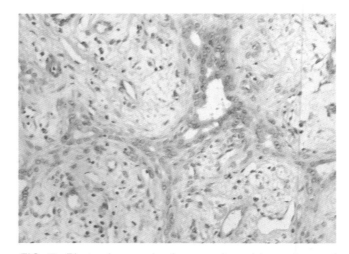

**FIG. 7.** Photomicrograph of mesenchymal hamartoma of the liver, demonstrating delicate fibrovascular stroma and mucomyxoid stroma, among which bland fusiform and stellate cells are distributed. (Courtesy of Dr. Louis P. Dehner, Washington University, St. Louis, Missouri.)

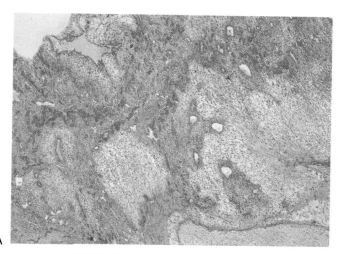 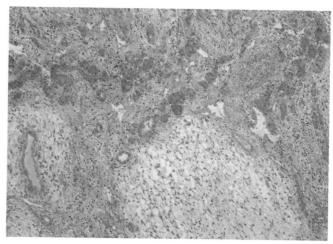

A                                                          B

**FIG. 8.** Mesenchymal hamartoma. **A:** The loose edematous stroma has many cystic spaces surrounded by myxoid tissue. **B:** Small islands of hepatocytes appear trapped near the periphery of the tumor.

eventuality inasmuch as the lesions are extremely vascular and may bleed profusely (81, 82). There are no documented examples of malignant transformation of MHLs.

## EPITHELIAL PROLIFERATIONS

Distinction of focal nodular hyperplasia (FNH) from hepatocellular adenoma (HCA) can be challenging in a few selected cases but more often limited sampling of a lesion causes difficulty in classification. A needle biopsy with characteristic ductular proliferation is an important clue to FNH, but broad fields of hepatocytes without ductules is nondiagnostic of a specific lesion. Therefore, complete review of the radiographic changes, gross appearance at surgery or by video (if laparoscopic surgery performed) and palpation may assist in the correct diagnosis.

### Focal Nodular Hyperplasia of the Liver

In the past, synonymous terms for FNH have included "focal cirrhosis," "benign hepatoma," and "hamartoma." Of these, only the first is of practical interest because FNH is recognizable only against a background of normal hepatic architecture. Because of the similarity of this hyperplastic proliferation to cirrhosis, its presence in the latter condition is unprovable!

### Clinical Findings

FNH shows a striking predilection for female patients, most of whom are between 20 and 50 years of age (range 20–57 years; mean 35 years). For every man with this lesion, approximately 20 women will be similarly affected. This fact may be related to the relatively common use of oral con-traceptives and other exogenous steroids by adult women in the United States. In roughly half of all cases, a mass is discovered incidentally during abdominal imaging or surgical procedures; even retrospectively, only 25% of patients are in any way symptomatic (7). Radiographic studies are capable of producing a definitive diagnosis in 50% of cases, based on an uptake of sulfur colloid in radionuclide scans and a characteristic central zone of fibrosis as seen with CT or MRI (83). However, these attributes may not be well seen in lesions that are <3 cm in dimension, and the latter are therefore those that are most commonly resected. Focal calcifications have been reported in a small number of FNH (5 cases in a series of 357 lesions) and thus are not a definite clue for fibrolamellar carcinoma (91).

### Pathologic Features

Although FNH may certainly assume the form of a solitary hepatic parenchymal nodule, multiple concomitant lesions (up to 4) are observed in 10–15% of cases; this observation underscores their probable hyperplastic nature. The masses range in size from 1 to 14 cm (Fig. 9). The cut surfaces of FNH resemble those of normal liver or MRNs, except that there is a grossly visible zone of roughly stellate white–gray fibrosis in approximately two thirds of cases (47).

Needle biopsies of FNH that are interpreted in the absence of adequate clinical information are inconclusive or misleadingly suggest a diagnosis of cirrhosis. Also, both nodular hyperplasia and hepatocellular "adenoma" show clusters and sheets of banal hepatocytes—sometimes with clear-cell change—separated by sinusoidal blood vessels. Nuclei are oval to round with small nucleoli and dispersed chromatin, and mitotic activity is sparse or absent.

As mentioned earlier, the diagnostic feature of FNH is the presence of a central zone of fibrous "scarring," in which cholangiolar and vascular proliferation is also apparent (Fig.

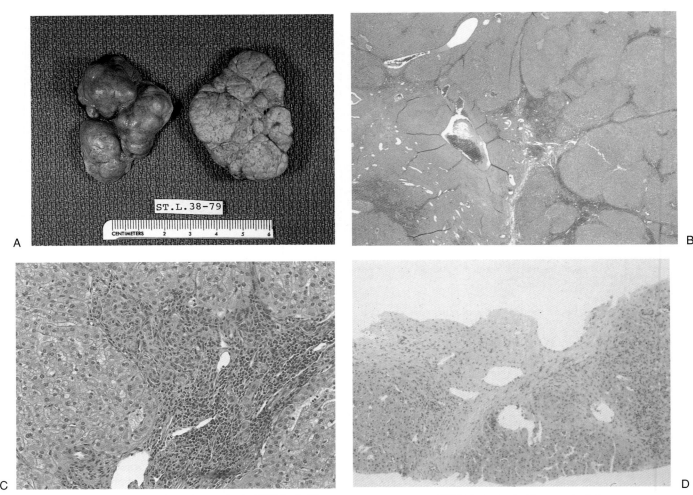

**FIG. 9.** Focal nodular hyperplasia (FNH). **A:** The gross appearance of FNH is typical with a central dimpling on the surface with the cut surface showing the radial scar. **B, C, D:** The central scar and major vessels. The fibrosis contains numerous cholangiolar structures (not true bile ducts) and lymphocytes. In C, a needle biopsy of FNH has sampling problems, and this needle biopsy shows the prominent fibrosis with scattered large vessels and a few areas of cholangiolar proliferation. Additional clinical information was required to establish a confident diagnosis. A diagnosis of cirrhosis is also possible but the large vessels (without major bile ducts) are typical of FNH.

9). The cholangioles are histologically bland and, in all likelihood, metaplastic because they are sometimes spatially dissociated from the lesional blood vessels and are not connected to the biliary drainage system (49). Prominent lymphoid infiltrates may be associated with them, simulating the appearance of inflamed portal tracts. The central proliferative vascular component of FNH may be complex, and it has been postulated that it reflects a vaso-occlusive-ischemic pathogenesis for this lesion (50). The peripheral aspects of FNH feature a "bulging" growth pattern of the hepatocytic cords without fibrous encapsulation, as is also seen in many hepatocellular "adenomas."

Because of the particular details of its microanatomy, FNH cannot be accurately recognized by the pathologist without access to suitable radiographic data and clinical information. We have previously cited the utility of viewing videotapes of selected surgical procedures on the liver, and this undertaking is particularly appropriate in the diagnosis of open or peritoneoscopically directed biopsies of FNH.

*Results of Special Procedures*

In general, adjunctive procedures are not necessary in the interpretation of focal nodular hepatic hyperplasia. However, one may on occasion wish to perform immunostains for low molecular weight keratin to highlight foci of ductular proliferation in the central aspects of this lesion.

*Biological Evolution*

Malignant change has not been described in connection with FNH. Uncommonly, pedunculated variants of this lesion—as well as (rarely) some deeply seated examples—

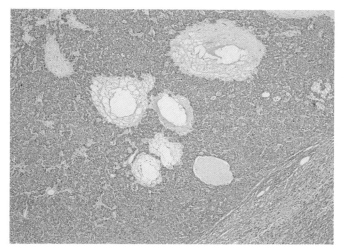 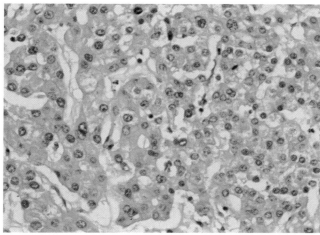

**FIG. 10.** Hepatocellular adenoma. **A:** The large sheets of hepatocytes are interrupted by dilated sinusoidal areas (pelioid change). Higher power (**B**) shows the thin cords (two cells thick). Hepatocytes have normal nuclear/cytoplasmic ratio, and there is no acinar formation.

may undergo painful infarction and intralesional hemorrhage, prompting emergent surgical excision. In general, however, FNH may be managed by "benign neglect," without concern over potential complications. Exceptionally, the surgeon may wish to excise very large lesions that are located immediately beneath the hepatic capsule because of the possibility of rupture after minor trauma. Otherwise, FNH may be expected to remain stable in size or even regress spontaneously with the passage of time. An unusual case has been labeled "progressive type," in which a large resected FNH occurred in a woman with recurrent multiple FNH lesions, some of which had spontaneous infarction and consequent abdominal pain (92). A uniform pattern of X chromosome inactivation indicated many FNH lesions are monoclonal. Thus these lesions may be due to a vascular anomaly; clonal epithelial proliferation apparently occurs (93).

### Clinical Findings

There are some well-recognized etiologic factors that have been associated with the development of HCA. These include exogenous estrogen or anabolic steroid usage, as well as inborn errors of metabolism affecting the liver. Estrogen-related lesions of this type were most commonly seen during the 1970s but are less often encountered nowadays, perhaps because of changes in the formulation of steroid-based medications or in their schedules of administration. For example, it has been stated that 5 years of continuous usage of exogenous steroids places patients at significant risk for HCA (51).

In accord with the foregoing statements, it should be no surprise that HCA is by far a disease of female patients, and it is seen during the childbearing years (15 to 45 years). Up to half of these masses are discovered because of abdominal

pain or rupture into the peritoneal cavity with attendant hemorrhage. Another 30% produce a palpable but asymptomatic abdominal mass, 10–20% are discovered incidentally during radiographic procedures done for unrelated diseases, and the scant remainder of cases are diagnosed in association with concomitant hepatocellular carcinomas in patients who have glycogen storage diseases. Whether or not the malignant hepatocellular neoplasms eventuate from HCA is an unresolved point of contention.

### Pathologic Features

Most HCAs are solitary lesions—with the exceptions having been noted above—and they are easily seen through Glisson's capsule as discrete spherical masses. The sizes of these lesions range from 2–3 cm to >10 cm (52) and in our experience they may weigh in excess of 2 kg. Cut surfaces of HCAs show a variegated appearance; large nodules often contain central foci of hemorrhage or spontaneous gelatinous degeneration with cyst formation, whereas smaller lesions may have a relatively uniform, tan, granular fabric.

Microscopically, one observes sheets and clusters of mature, unremarkable hepatocytes without any interspersed portal tracts or fibrous septa. There may a thin connective tissue capsule around a portion of the lesion, and some trabeculae of constituent cells may contain numerous small blood vessels. The central scars that are associated with FNH are lacking. Large and centrally degenerate lesions demonstrate extracellular accumulations of proteinaceous material and amorphous fibromyxoid stroma (Fig. 10). Some HCAs may contain dilated sinusoidal vascular channels, mimicking peliosis hepatis. In regard to the constituent cells themselves, nuclear to cytoplasmic ratios are normal but focal nucleolar prominence and nuclear hyperchromasia may accompany degenerative changes. Mitotic figures are notably absent, and one does not observe the "nodules in a nodule" pattern of growth that may be associated with HCC. Other more unusual findings include prominent fatty metamorphosis in the lesional cells; clear-cell change with cellular glycogenesis; abundant cytoplasmic Mallory-type hyaline, acinar formations in HCAs that are seen in the context of anabolic steroid usage; and perilesional foreign body–type granulomatous reactions.

### Results of Special Procedures

There is usually no need to implement adjunctive studies in the diagnosis of HCA. It might be expected that flow cytometric or image analytic measurement of DNA content might assist in the distinction between the latter lesion and well-differentiated HCC, but in our experience this task can be accomplished by conventional histologic evaluation.

### Differential Diagnosis

If sufficient tissue is available, the distinction of FNH from HCA is usually reliable. A crucial problem is the segregation of well-differentiated HCC from HCA. The procurement of several biopsy samples may be valuable in this context because our experience has shown that small foci of obvious carcinoma are often admixed with very low-grade (HCA-like) HCC. In addition, cytoplasmic basophilia, nuclear crowding, and mitotic activity all favor an interpretation of HCC over one of HCA.

### Biological Evolution

In keeping with the premise that HCAs are in fact nonneoplastic, discontinuation of exogenous steroid use has been associated with regression of many of these lesions (53). In cases where the mass is large and in danger of rupture, surgical excision or debulking should be undertaken. This also allows for thorough tissue sampling, with the aim of excluding well-differentiated HCC (54).

### Macroregenerative Hepatocellular Nodules

Many of the salient features of MRNs have been cited in the introductory section of this chapter. However, other details merit further discussion at this point.

As currently defined, MRN refers to a circumscribed nodular proliferation of hepatocytes that is larger than 8 mm, with banal cytologic features and "entrapped" portal triads at the peripheral aspects of the lesion. Other terms used for such nodules in the past have included "adenomatous hyperplasia" and "atypical regenerative nodule." MRNs arise in the context of cirrhosis in most instances, but a few cases are encountered in the setting of recovery from acute liver diseases featuring submassive hepatocellular necrosis (1).

The difficulty with which some examples of MRN are dis-tinguished from small HCCs is reflected in the fact that a review panel was convened to address that topic alone. Its consensus statement recommended use of the term "borderline hepatocellular nodule" for lesions that show clinicopathologic features that are intermediate to those of MRN and HCC (55).

In the authors' opinion, popularization of MRN as a distinct pathologic entity may be credited to Edmondson (56), who drew on his own considerable personal experience and pertinent radiologic data (57) in characterizing the lesion. In recent years, a great deal of additional information on MRN has been contributed by investigators in Japan, including results of biopsy studies, clinical surveillance, and postmortem examinations (58).

### Clinical Findings

Patients at highest risk for the development of MRNs are those who have cirrhosis, particularly in the setting of chronic infection with hepatitis B or C viruses. These individuals are often monitored for the appearance of HCC with sequential CT, radionuclide studies of the liver, ultrasonography, or MRI. Unfortunately, while these studies are effective in detecting the emergence of focal architectural aberrations in the hepatic parenchyma, they are incapable of distinguishing between MRNs, FNH, small HCCs, fibrous scars, and metastatic tumors in many instances (59).

The advent of laparoscopic surgery has increased the frequency with which pathologists receive biopsies of MRNs, and they are also frequent findings in explanted livers from patients who have received orthotopic hepatic allografts. Approximately 20–25% of those specimens will demonstrate large regenerative hepatocellular nodules if careful gross examinations are done at 5- to 10-mm intervals (60,61). Another 25% of cases show multiple nodules that are not obvious macroscopically but that have microscopic features that are generally similar to those of MRN. A proportion of the grossly visible lesions actually are better classified as "borderline hepatocellular nodules" or small HCCs that were clinically inapparent.

### Pathologic Features

On gross inspection of resected liver tissue, MRNs can be separated from the surrounding parenchyma because of dissimilarities in color and texture. Some of these lesions may be bile-stained; others are surrounded by a prominent fibrous pseudocapsule; and selected examples show a more uneven consistency and a tan–gray color. All such nodules require extensive sampling, including submission en toto for histologic study in some cases.

Microscopically, one group of MRNs shows clearly benign cytomorphologic features, with orderly cords and nests of mature hepatocytes that lack nuclear atypia, abnormal nu-

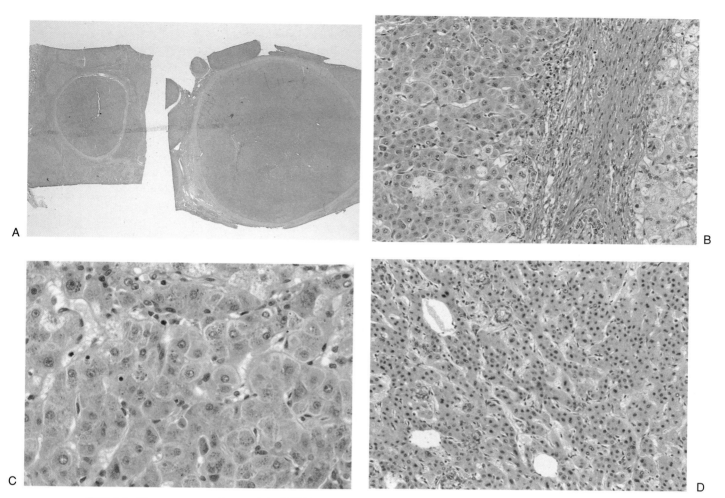

**FIG. 11.** Macroregenerative nodule (MRN) and look-alikes. **A:** A large distinctive nodule is surrounded by small cirrhotic nodules. Trapped portal areas are present within the larger central nodule. **B:** The capsule is thin and the cord pattern is regular (1–2 cells thick). The hepatocytes are not arranged in an acinar growth pattern. **C:** A higher power of the thin cords shows hepatocytes without atypia. **D:** An atypical MRN has thin cords but a few scattered acini composed of hepatocytes surrounding a central cavity. The atypia is a matter of degree. If the acini were numerous and the hepatocytes demonstrated increased nuclear/cytoplasmic ratios, carcinoma would be the favored diagnosis. (Courtesy of Linda Ferrell, M.D., San Francisco.)

clear-to-cytoplasmic ratios, and mitotic activity (Fig. 11). Often, however, step sectioning of tissue blocks will reveal areas that fit the description just given, whereas other foci—in the same nodule—demonstrate acinar formations; bile production; cytoplasmic Mallory's hyaline, "nodule-in-nodule" growth patterns; and anisonucleosis; all of this raises the specter of HCC. Still other examples of MRN show histologic features that are indeterminate for malignancy throughout the entirety of the lesion. The latter are most properly categorized as "borderline" or "dysplastic" MRNs.

### Results of Special Studies

In the analysis of MRNs whose morphologic properties are indeterminate, flow cytometric determination of DNA content may offer some assistance in ascertaining biological potential. DNA aneuploidy may be tentatively used to support an interpretation of malignancy in this context, although some dysplastic nodules are also aneuploid and well-differentiated HCCs may be diploid. Image analysis of various morphologic features such as nuclear roundness and size variation, width of cellular trabeculae, nuclear-to-cytoplasmic ratios, cellular density, and others also demonstrates considerable overlap between MRN and HCC. Multivariate logistic analysis may yet reveal consistent differences that could be helpful diagnostically (62), but this possibility remains to be seen. Cytophotometric DNA measurement of MRNs, borderline nodules, and small HCCs has indicated a gradation of nuclear density in this group of lesions and offers the most telling indirect evidence that MRN may be a precursor to hepatic carcinoma (63). Monoclonality of any given hepatocellular nodule may be discerned by assessing the cellular integration of episomal DNA from hepatitis B or C viruses, but because this phenomenon is seen in cirrhosis as well as some HCCs it does not equate with the presence of neoplastic transformation (64). Finally, there is preliminary evidence to suggest that immunohistochemical evaluation of proliferation markers (e.g., with Ki-67 or antiproliferating cell nuclear antigen) may assist the pathologist in separating MRN from more aggressive hepatic lesions (65).

### Biological Evolution

Follow-up of recipients of hepatic allografts has shown no evidence of hepatocellular proliferations, even though their explanted native livers contained MRNs, borderline hepatocellular nodules, or small HCCs (68). However, we are indeed aware of examples of MRN that, by serial fine needle aspiration biopsies, were demonstrated to have evolved into HCC. This information makes one consider surgical resection of any lesion that is felt to be in this spectrum. However, it should also be remembered that many cirrhosis-associated MRNs show regression over time, and others remain stable for prolonged periods (66). Hence, the recommended approach to such lesions is that of regular clinical, radiographic, and biochemical evaluation. Even though MRN is probably a precursor to HCC, the former of these lesions does not produce steadily increasing values of AFP as seen in primary carcinomas of the liver. It should also be remembered that MRN and HCC may coexist (67).

## PROLIFERATIVE AND PSEUDOPROLIFERATIVE LESIONS OF THE INTRAHEPATIC BILE DUCTS

### Congenital Hepatic Fibrosis

Congenital hepatic fibrosis (CHF) is a term that was introduced by Kerr in 1961, as a synonym for biliary fibroadenomatosis, cholangiodysplastic pseudocirrhosis, and hepatobiliary fibropolycystic disease (69). This disorder actually represents a proliferation of biliary epithelium as much as it does an excess in intrahepatic tissue. It is principally detected in young patients, but is increasingly being recognized in adults as well in biopsy specimens.

### Clinical Findings

Portal hypertension is a principal clinical manifestation of CHF, often with associated esophageal varices and splenomegaly. Another common mode of presentation is with recurrent cholangitis—caused by Caroli's disease (dilatation of the intrahepatic bile ducts) (70)—and occasional cases demonstrate all of these problems. Still other patients are asymptomatic (71). Biochemical tests of hepatic function

are paradoxically normal in this condition, regardless of its biological phenotype.

Renal disease, usually represented by autosomal dominant (adult) polycystic disease, is present in 60–90% of cases of CHF. Some individuals have symptoms and signs relating principally to the urinary tract, with relatively few if any complaints that are referable to the liver. Because of the above-cited associations and variable presentation of CHF, some authors have suggested that it does not represent a single clinicopathologic entity. Instead, they prefer the view that CHF is actually a spectrum of anomalies involving the biliary and renal tubular epithelia (72,73).

### Pathologic Features

The liver is typically enlarged in CHF, with several depressions on its surface. These are usually only a few millimeters in maximal size, with irregular margins. After fixation in formalin, the lesions assume a gray color and are distinct from the surrounding liver tissue. If wedge biopsies of the liver are received from patients with CHF, or one is dealing with an autopsy specimen, it is advisable to section through the tissue at close intervals to evaluate the possible presence of biliary cysts (74). These often are well seen on CT of the abdomen and are typical of Caroli's disease. The degree of hepatic abnormality in CHF is highly variable from case to case, and even in different areas of the liver in the same patient (75,76).

On microscopic examination, the portal tracts are widened by abundant fibrous tissue, and they also contain proliferating bile ducts and ductules that assume a convoluted profile (Fig. 12). Many of the ducts contain concretions of bile. The ductular structures are evenly spaced and do not have a back-to-back configuration, as expected in cholangiocarcinoma. Similarly, there is no cytologic atypia, a desmoplastic stromal reaction is lacking, and mitotic activity is nil. Results of a serial-section study performed by Nakanuma et al. (75) suggests that the biliary radicals in CHF connect to the major bile ducts, potentially accounting for the diffuse cholangitis that may be a part of the syndrome. Associated inflammation is, however, highly variable, as stated previously.

### Differential Diagnosis

Wedge or needle biopsies of CHF may be misdiagnosed as showing cirrhosis because of the interportal fibrosis that characterizes this condition. However, one does not see the formation of regenerative hepatocellular nodules in CHF, as expected in cirrhosis; portal triads contain abnormal (usually sclerotic) portal veins; and the bile ductular proliferation described above is histologically distinctive. Another pitfall in the diagnosis of CHF is potential confusion with metastatic carcinoma because of the gross features of the disease and possible errors in interpreting the biliary epithelial profiles as adenocarcinoma. Attention to the gland-to-gland relation-

Monga G, Ramponi A, Falzoni PU, Boldorini R. Renal and hepatic angiomyolipomas in a child without evidence of tuberous sclerosis. *Pathol Res Pract* 1994;190:1208–1213.

Nonomura A, Mizukami Y, Kadoya M. Angiomyolipoma of the liver: a collective review. *J Gastroenterol* 1994;29:95–105.

Nonomura A, Mizukami Y, Kadoya M, Takayanagi N, Hirono T. Multiple angiomyolipoma of the liver. *J Clin Gastroenterol* 1995;20:248–251.

Terris B, Flejou JF, Picot R, Belghiti J, Henin D. Hepatic angiomyolipoma: a report of four cases with immunohistochemical and DNA-flow cytometric studies. *Arch Pathol Lab Med* 1996;120:68–72.

### *Focal Pseudotumorous Fatty Change in the Liver*

Imaoka S, Sasaki Y, Nakano H, Iwanaga T. Lipomatous tumors (lipoma, angiomyolipoma, myelolipoma, focal fatty change) in the liver. *Ryoikibetsu Shokogun Shirizu* 1995;7:288–291.

Kawamori Y, Matsui O, Takahashi S, Kadoya M, Takashima T, Miyayama S. Focal hepatic fatty infiltration in the posterior edge of the medial segment associated with aberrant gastric venous drainage: CT, US, and MR findings. *J Comput Asst Tomogr* 1996;20:356–359.

Kreft B, Stark D, Schild H. Atypical focal fatty liver. *Aktuelle Radiol* 1995; 5:372–373.

Layfield LJ. Focal fatty change of the liver: cytologic findings in a radiographic mimic of metastases. *Diagn Cytopathol* 1994;11:385–389.

Lee PJ, Leonard JV, Dicks-Mireaux C. Focal fatty liver change in glycogenosis type 1A. *Eur J Pediatr* 1995;154:332.

Lilenbaum RC, Lilenbaum AM, Hryniuk WM. Interleukin 2-induced focal fatty infiltrate of the liver that mimics metastases. *J Natl Cancer Inst USA* 1995;87:609–610.

Nakanuma Y. Non-neoplastic nodular lesions in the liver. *Pathol Int* 1995; 45:703–714.

Verhille R, Marchal G, Baert AL, Fevery J. Focal fatty infiltration of the liver associated with important mass effect. *J Belge Radiol* 1994;77: 10–12.

### *Hepatic Mesenchymal Hamartoma*

Chau KY, Ho JW, Wu PC, Yuen WK. Mesenchymal hamartoma of liver in a man: comparison with cases in infants. *J Clin Pathol* 1994;47:864–866.

de Chadarevian JP, Pawel BR, Faerber EN, Weintraub WH. Undifferentiated (embryonal) sarcoma arising in conjunction with mesenchymal hamartoma of the liver. *Mod Pathol* 1994;7:490–493.

Helal A, Nolan M, Bower R, Mair B, Debich-Spicer D. Mesenchymal hamartoma of the liver. *Arch Pediatr Adolesc Med* 1995;149:315–316.

Mascarello JT, Krous HF. Second report of a translocation involving 19q13.4 in a mesenchymal hamartoma of the liver. *Cancer Genet Cytogenet* 1992;58:141–142.

Nakanuma Y. Non-neoplastic nodular lesions in the liver. *Pathol Int* 1995; 45:703–714.

Otal TM, Hendricks JB, Pharis P, Donnelly WH. Mesenchymal hamartoma of the liver: DNA flow cytometric analysis of eight cases. *Cancer* 1994; 74:1237–1242.

Sarihan H, Yildiz K, Ozoran Y. An unusual case of ectopic mesenchymal hamartoma of the liver. *South Afr J Surg* 1994;32:152–153.

Tepetes K, Selby R, Webb M, Madariaga JR, Iwatsuki S, Starzl TE. Orthotopic liver transplantation for benign hepatic neoplasms. *Arch Surg* 1995; 130:153–156.

### *Focal Nodular Hyperplasia of the Liver*

Altmann HW. Hepatocellular nodular hyperplasias, adenomas, and carcinomas. *Verhandl Deutsch Gesellsch Pathol* 1995;79:84–108.

Caseiro-Alves F, Zins M, Mahfouz AE, Rahmouni A, Vilgrain V, Menu Y, Mathieu D. Calcification in focal nodular hyperplasia: a new problem for differentiation from fibrolamellar hepatocellular carcinoma. *Radiology* 1996;198:889–892.

Gaffey MJ, Iezzoni JC, Weiss LM. Clonal analysis of focal nodular hyperplasia of the liver. *Am J Pathol* 1996;148:1089–1096.

Nakanuma Y. Non-neoplastic nodular lesions in the liver. *Pathol Int* 1995; 45:703–714.

Reymond D, Plaschkes J, Luthy AR, Leibundgut K, Hirt A, Wagner HP. Focal nodular hyperplasia of the liver in children: review of followup and outcome. *J Pediatr Surg* 1995;30:1590–1593.

Sakatoku H, Hirokawa Y, Inoue M, Kojima M, Yabana T, Sakurai M. Focal nodular hyperplasia in an adolescent with glycogen storage disease type I with mesocaval shunt operation in childhood: a case report and review of the literature. *Acta Paediatr Jpn* 1996;38:172–175.

### *Macroregenerative Hepatocellular Nodules*

Altmann HW. Hepatocellular nodular hyperplasias, adenomas, and carcinomas. *Verhandl Deutsch Gesellsch Pathol* 1995;79:84–108.

Faccioli S, Chieco P, Gramantieri L, Stecca BA, Bolondi L. Cytometric measurement of cell proliferation in echo-guided biopsies from focal lesions of the liver. *Mod Pathol* 1996;9:120–125.

Hytiroglou P, Theise ND, Schwartz M, Mor E, Miller C, Thung SN. Macroregenerative nodules in a series of adult cirrhotic liver explants: issues of classification and nomenclature. *Hepatology* 1995;21:703–708.

Patriarca C, Roncalli M, Viale G, Alfano RM, Braidotti P, Guddo F, Coggi G. Extracellular matrix proteins, integrin receptors (VLA-beta 1, VLA-alpha 2, and VLA-alpha 5) and growth fraction in atypical macroregenerative nodules of the liver: an immunocytochemical case study. *Histochemistry* 1994;102:29–36.

Riegler JL. Preneoplastic conditions of the liver. *Semin Gastrointest Dis* 1996;7:74-87.

Terada T, Nakanuma Y. Multiple occurrence of borderline hepatocellular nodules in human cirrhotic livers: possible multicentric origin of hepatocellular carcinoma. *Virchows Arch A* 1995;427:379–383.

Theise ND. Macroregenerative (dysplastic) nodules and hepatocarcinogenesis: theoretical and clinical considerations. *Semin Liver Dis* 1995;15: 360–371.

### *Congenital Hepatic Fibrosis*

Bauman ME, Pound DC, Ulbright TM. Hepatocellular carcinoma arising in congenital hepatic fibrosis. *Am J Gastroenterol* 1994;89:450–451.

Bertheau P, Degott C, Belghiti J, Vilgrain V, Renard P, Benhamou JP, Henin D. Adenomatous hyperplasia of the liver in a patient with congenital hepatic fibrosis. *J Hepatol* 1994;20:213–217.

Besnard M, Pariente D, Hadchouel M, Bernard O, Chaumont P. Portal cavernoma in congenital hepatic fibrosis: angiographic reports of 10 pediatric cases. *Pediatr Radiol* 1994;24:61–65.

Lewis SM, Roberts EA, Marcon MA, Harvey E, Phillips MJ, Chuang SA, Buncic JR, Clarke JT. Joubert syndrome with congenital hepatic fibrosis: an entity in the spectrum of oculo-encephalo-hepato-renal disorders. *Am J Med Genet* 1994;52:419–426.

Lipschitz B, Berdon WE, Defelice AR, Levy J. Association of congenital hepatic fibrosis with autosomal dominant polycystic kidney disease: report of a family with review of the literature. *Pediatr Radiol* 1993;23: 131–133.

Marmorale A, Mainguene C, Gavelli A, Huguet C. Pure angiocholitic form of congenital hepatic fibrosis. *Gastroenterol Clin Biol* 1996;20:211–212.

Perisic VN. Long-term studies on congenital hepatic fibrosis in children. *Acta Paediatr* 1995;84:695–696.

Ramirez-Mayans JA, Mata-Rivera N, Mora-Tiscareno MA, Cervantes-Bustamante R, Vargas-Gomez MA, Aguinaga V, Rocio G. Congenital hepatic fibrosis: study of 26 cases. *Acta Gastroenterol Latinoam* 1994; 25:297–303.

### *Bile Duct Hamartoma and Bile Duct Adenoma*

Bhathal PS, Hughes NR, Goodman ZD. The so-called bile duct adenoma is a peribiliary gland hamartoma. *Am J Surg Pathol* 1996;20:858–864.

Hasebe T, Sakamoto M, Mukai K, Kawano N, Konishi M, Ryu M, Fukamachi S, Hirohashi S. Cholangiocarcinoma arising in bile duct adenoma with focal area of bile duct hamartoma. *Virchows Arch A* 1995;426: 209–213.

Nakanuma Y. Non-neoplastic nodular lesions in the liver. *Pathol Int* 1995; 45:703–714.

### *Pseudoneoplastic Hepatic Atrophy*

Lory J, Schweizer W, Blumgart LH, Zimmermann A. The pathology of the atrophy/hypertrophy complex (AHC) of the liver: a light microscopic and immunohistochemical study. *Histol Histopathol* 1994;9:541–554.

### *Bacillary Peliosis of the Liver*

Koehler JE, Cederberg L. Intraabdominal mass associated with gastrointestinal hemorrhage: a new manifestation of bacillary peliosis. *Gastroenterology* 1995;109:2011–2014.

Thonnard J, Carreer F, Delmee M. Rochalimaea henselae, Afipia felis, and cat-scratch disease. *Acta Clin Belg* 1994;49:158–167.

## Sclerotic Cavernous Hemangioma of the Liver

Jager HJ, Cataneda F, Hasse F, Gotz F. Incidental finding in ultrasound: uncertain epigastric tumor. Giant cavernous hemangioma of the left liver lobe. *Radiologe* 1995;35:481–484.

Mitsudo K, Watanable Y, Saga T, Dohke M, Sato N, Minami K, Shigeyasu M. Nonenhanced hepatic cavernous hemangioma with multiple calcifications: CT an pathologic correlation. *Abdom Imag* 1995;20:459–461.

Saegusa T, Ito K, Oba N, Matsuda M, Kojima K, Tohyama K, Matsumoto M, Miura K, Suzuki H. Enlargement of multiple cavernous hemangiomas of the liver in association with pregnancy. *Intern Med* 1995;34:207–211.

## Sclerosing (Cirrhosiform) Hepatocellular Carcinoma

Kita K, Saito S, Tsuchida T, Shimizu Y, Nambu S, Higuchi K, Takahara T, Watanabe A, Koizumi F. Hepatic metastases of pancreatic gastrinoma associated with sclerosing hepatocellular carcinoma. *Jpn J Gastroenterol* 1996;93:377–381.

Yamashita Y, Fan ZM, Yamamoto H, Matsukawa T, Arakawa A, Miyazaki T, Harada M, Takahashi M. Sclerosing hepatocellular carcinoma: radiologic findings. *Abdom Imag* 1993;18:347–351.

Yamashita Y, Iwao T, Torimura T, Tanaka M, Hirai K, Abe M, Toyonaga A, Sugihara S, Kojiro M, Tanikawa K. Sclerosing hepatocellular carcinoma with hypercalcemia: a case report. *Kurume Med J* 1992;39:113–116.

Yoshida J, Takayama T, Yamamoto J, Shimada K, Kosuge T, Yamasaki S, Hasegawa H, Moriyama N, Takayasu K, Muramatsu Y, et al. Computed tomography of sclerosing hepatocellular carcinoma. *Comput Med Imag Graphics* 1992;16:125–130.

## Sclerosing Epithelioid Hemangioendothelioma of the Liver

Botella MT, Cabrera T, Sebastian JJ, Navarro MJ, Alvarez R, Uribarrena R. Epithelioid hemangioendothelioma: a rare hepatic tumor. *Rev Espan Enferm Dig* 1995;87:749–751.

Hidaka H, Nakamura K, Tsuneyoshi M. Hepatic epithelioid hemangioendothelioma. *Rad Med* 1995;13:43–45.

Madariaga JR, Marino IR, Karavias DD, Nalesnik MA, Doyle HR, Iwatsuki S, Fung JJ, Starl TE. Long-term results after liver transplantation for primary hepatic epithelioid hemangioendothelioma. *Ann Surg Oncol* 1995;2:483–487.

*Pathology of Pseudoneoplastic Lesions,*
edited by M. R. Wick, P. A. Humphrey, and J. H. Ritter.
Lippincott-Raven Publishers, Philadelphia © 1997.

# CHAPTER 7

# Pseudoneoplastic Lesions of the Kidneys and Ureters

John N. Eble

**Renal Angiomyolipoma**
   Clinical Features
   Pathologic Features
   Differential Diagnosis
**Juxtaglomerular Cell Tumor**
   Clinical Features
   Pathologic Features
   Differential Diagnosis
**Renomedullary Interstitial Cell Tumor**
   Clinical Features
   Pathologic Features
   Differential Diagnosis
**Cystic Nephroma**
   Clinical Features

   Pathologic Features
   Differential Diagnosis
**Xanthogranulomatous Pyelonephritis**
   Clinical Features
   Pathologic Features
   Differential Diagnosis
**Renal Malakoplakia**
   Clinical Features
   Pathologic Features
**Other Inflammatory Pseudotumors**
**Renal Pelvis and Ureter**
**Conclusions**
**References**

The kidneys are the site of several peculiar mass lesions, the neoplastic natures of which remain unsettled. Most prominent among such proliferations are renal angiomyolipoma, juxtaglomerular cell tumor, renomedullary interstitial cell tumor, and cystic nephroma. Renal angiomyolipoma is clearly benign and has long been regarded as a hamartomatous combination of blood vessels, smooth muscle, and fat. However, it occasionally extends into the renal vein and vena cava or appears in lymph nodes draining the kidney, mimicking an aggressive cancer with the capacity for metastasis. For this reason, it is included in this chapter on pseudotumors of the kidney. Juxtaglomerular cell tumors form mass lesions and often cause dramatic hypertension. Whether or not they are neoplastic is called into question by the observation that none has been multiple or recurred and that there is no evidence for a malignant counterpart to them. For this reason, they are discussed here under the umbrella of "pseudotumors." Renomedullary interstitial cell tumors

are common in the kidneys of adults but it remains unclear as to whether they are neoplasms, hyperplastic nodules, or hamartomas. As small mass lesions they simulate renal neoplasia and merit discussion below. Conversely, cystic nephroma is usually regarded as a neoplasm, albeit on scant evidence. Because it is benign and can be confused with cystic nephroblastoma or cystic renal cell carcinoma, it is also included. The first part of this chapter is devoted to discussion of these lesions. The diagnostic problems posed by pseudoneoplastic spindle cell proliferations elsewhere in the urinary tract very seldom arise in the kidneys. However, the inflammatory conditions of xanthogranulomatous pyelonephritis and malakoplakia sometimes mimic renal neoplasms radiologically, clinically, and pathologically. These processes and the diagnostic problems they present are considered in the second part of the discussion.

   J. N. Eble: Department of Pathology and Laboratory Medicine, Indiana University School of Medicine, and Richard L. Roudebush Veterans Affairs Medical Center, Indianapolis, Indiana 46202-2884.

## RENAL ANGIOMYOLIPOMA

Renal angiomyolipomas are rare lesions that are composed (as their name conveys) of a variable mixture of blood vessels, smooth muscle, and fat. Reported series (1–8) rarely exceed 40 cases (Table 1). Their mixed nature has prompted most authorities to consider them hamartomas rather than true neoplasms. However, as presented below, they do have many of the properties of neoplasms, including a potential for attainment of a great size and growth that may be invasive and may destroy adjoining structures. When accompanied by angiomyolipomas in regional lymph nodes, they may closely mimic metastatic sarcoma.

## Clinical Features

Renal angiomyolipoma has long been known to occur in two disparate settings: in association with tuberous sclerosis and as a sporadic proliferation. Tuberous sclerosis is a complex genetic disorder, the classic symptoms of which include severe mental retardation and grand mal seizures, sometimes resulting in death in childhood. It was among such patients that an association with renal angiomyolipoma was discovered early in this century. However, subsequent study has revealed a spectrum of lesions and severity in this syndrome and it is now clear that the disease has many forms. Gomez (9) has proposed that the diagnosis may be made definitively on the basis of any one of the findings listed in Table 2, or provisionally if any two of the features in Table 3 are present. This construct has muddied the dichotomy between tuberous sclerosis–associated and sporadic angiomyolipomas because most reports dismiss the question of whether or not the patient had tuberous sclerosis with a statement to the effect that the patient had "no stigmata of tuberous sclero-

**TABLE 2.** *Findings pathognomonic of tuberous sclerosis*

Cortical tuber
Multiple subependymal glial nodules
Retinal hamartoma
Cutaneous angiofibromas (adenoma sebaceum) on the face
Ungual fibroma
Fibrous plaques in the skin of the forehead or scalp
Multiple renal angiomyolipomas

sis," without specifying the details of the evaluation. This topic is discussed in more detail below in the section on differential diagnosis.

In cases that are treated surgically, patients with angiomyolipomas are much more likely to be women than men (see Table 1); the ratio of females to males is approximately 3:1. This ratio holds among the 19 patients with tuberous sclerosis in the series summarized in Table 1. The great majority of angiomyolipomas have been found in adults. The mean age among those patients who have tuberous sclerosis is approximately 25 years, about two decades younger than the patients without tuberous sclerosis (Table 1). Renal angiomyolipoma has often been reported in children with tuberous sclerosis, including a congenital case in a premature infant (10). However, it is rare in children without tuberous sclerosis (see Table 1). Two children, both aged 12 years, are cited as the youngest known examples of sporadic angiomyolipoma (1,11). However, this claim is questionable in light of the short follow-up and the frequent late development of signs of tuberous sclerosis. It is fair to say that renal an-

**TABLE 1.** *Age and gender in 228 cases of renal angiomyolipoma*

| Citation | Cases | Female/male | Age |
|---|---|---|---|
| Price & Mostofi (1) | | | |
|   With tuberous sclerosis | | Excluded | |
|   Without tuberous sclerosis | 30 | 21:9 | 12–69 mean 41 |
| Hajdu & Foote (2) | | | |
|   With tuberous sclerosis | 0 | | |
|   Without tuberous sclerosis | 27 | 25:2 | 41–80 |
| Farrow et al. (3) | 32 | 23:9 | |
|   With tuberous sclerosis | 10 | | 6–80 |
|   Without tuberous sclerosis | 22 | | 26–72 |
| Jardin et al. (4) | 15 | 9:6 | |
|   With tuberous sclerosis | 5 | 3:2 | 20–36 mean 29 |
|   Without tuberous sclerosis | 10 | 6:4 | 34–71 mean 48 |
| Blute et al. (5) | 44 | 39:5 | |
|   With tuberous sclerosis | 4 | 4:0 | 4–46 mean 24 |
|   Without tuberous sclerosis | 40 | 35:5 | 17–80 mean 55 |
| Tong et al. (6) | 24 | 17:7 | |
|   With tuberous sclerosis | 4 | 4:0 | 10–28 mean 22 |
|   Without tuberous sclerosis | 20 | 13:7 | mean 45 |
| Cozar Olmo et al. (7) | 39 | 30:9 | |
|   With tuberous sclerosis | 5 | 4:1 | 17–30 mean 26 |
|   Without tuberous sclerosis | 34 | 26:8 | 28–71 mean 47 |
| Mukai et al. (8) | 17 | 11:6 | |
|   With tuberous sclerosis | 3 | 3:0 | 22–31 mean 27 |
|   Without tuberous sclerosis | 14 | 8:6 | 29–67 mean 51 |

**TABLE 3.** *Features supporting a presumptive diagnosis of tuberous sclerosis*

Central Nervous System
  Infantile spasms
  Myoclonic, tonic, or atonic seizures
  Wedge-shaped cortical-subcortical calcification
  Multiple subcortical hypomyelinated lesions
  Peripapillary retinal hamartoma not distinguishable
    from drusen
Skin and Oral Cavity
  Hypomelanotic macules
  Shagreen patches
  Gingival fibromas
  Enamel pits
Viscera
  Multiple renal tumors
  Renal cysts
  Cardiac rhabdomyoma
  Pulmonary lymphangiomyomatosis
  Radiographic "honeycomb" lungs
History
  First-degree relative with tuberous sclerosis

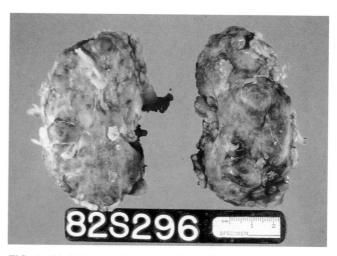

**FIG. 1.** Multiple small renal angiomyolipomas in the kidneys of a patient with tuberous sclerosis.

giomyolipoma is essentially unknown in children who lack the signs of tuberous sclerosis, and the diagnosis of that syndrome should be vigorously and persistently sought when a child is found to have renal angiomyolipoma.

Many angiomyolipomas are asymptomatic and are discovered incidentally through radiologic examinations that are done for unrelated problems. When present, symptoms are usually related to mass effects. Angiomyolipomas are benign and incapable of metastasis. This is so generally agreed on that many such lesions that are detected by imaging are merely followed (12). Moreover, kidneys from which angiomyolipomas have been resected have been used as donor organs for transplantation (13). Although they are incapable of metastasis, angiomyolipomas are not entirely innocuous. The abundant and abnormal elastin-poor vascularity of angiomyolipomas makes them prone to hemorrhage into the retroperitoneum (14,15), sometimes with fatal results (16). In some cases there is a history of trivial trauma, but in most the hemorrhage appears to be spontaneous (17). Pregnancy, with attendantly increased intraabdominal pressure and increased blood volume, has also been associated with rupture and hemorrhage of renal angiomyolipomas (18).

Although most angiomyolipomas are confined to the kidney or Gerota's space, some do infiltrate into surrounding structures. Farrow et al. (3) mentioned two patients in whom such lesions could not be resected completely because of extensive extrarenal invasion. One of these patients later developed a recurrence in the flank. Kragel and Toker (19) similarly described a 52-year-old woman with unresectable bilateral renal angiomyolipomas, in whom the lesions extended from the pelvic brim to the diaphragm with infiltration of the colon, diaphragm, and aortic adventitia, ultimately causing her death.

**Pathologic Features**

Angiomyolipomas range in size from small lesions that are found incidentally in autopsy or nephrectomy specimens (Fig. 1) to massive lesions that replace much of the kidney and extend into the retroperitoneum (Fig. 2). Grossly, their color depends on the proportions of the constituent tissue elements. Those composed mostly of fat are predominantly yellow and may therefore resemble renal cell carcinoma. Others in which smooth muscle is a prominent component are more pink or tan, with the ability to simulate mesenchymal neoplasms. Angiomyolipomas may occur as solitary or multiple tumors, and likewise can be unilateral or bilateral. Whereas radiographic examination will often discover multiplicity, very small lesions may not be detectable preoperatively or before autopsy examination. Inasmuch as the difference between two or more angiomyolipomas and a solitary lesion currently represents the difference between a confirmed diagnosis of tuberous sclerosis (9) (see Table 2)

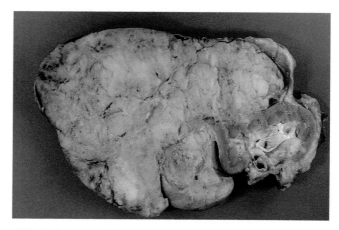

**FIG. 2.** Large angiomyolipoma arising in the kidney and filling the retroperitoneum.

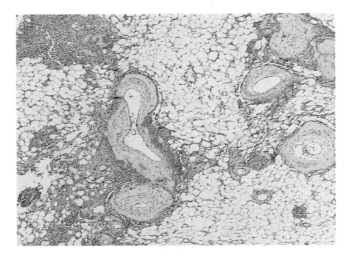

**FIG. 3.** Angiomyolipoma with fat, smooth muscle, and clusters of thick-walled blood vessels.

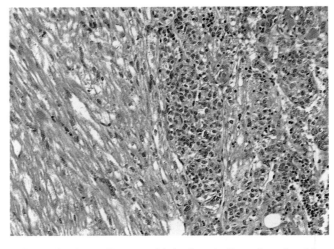

**FIG. 5.** Angiomyolipoma with both spindle cell and epithelioid smooth muscle.

and a sporadic benign proliferation with no long-term consequences, it is of great importance for the pathologist examining a kidney bearing an angiomyolipoma to make every effort to find additional lesions, even if they are very small.

Histologically, angiomyolipomas have varied appearances, depending on the relative proportions of the three constitutive elements. Fat or smooth muscle usually predominates, and in some lesions one of these tissues may be so dominant as to raise the possibility of renal lipoma or leiomyoma. The vascular component usually includes thick-walled tortuous vessels, which are often clustered in groups (Fig. 3). Although these vessels resemble arteries microscopically, their walls are poor in elastic fibers. The fat in angiomyolipomas is usually ordinary mature adipose tissue, although areas resembling fetal fat have been de-

scribed in a few lesions. The appearance of the smooth muscle component varies from fascicles of spindle cells to epithelioid cells that are arranged in sheets interspersed with vessels and fat cells (Figs. 4 and 5). In areas where smooth muscle is not the predominant element, it may form cuffs about the intralesional blood vessels. Epithelioid cells in angiomyolipomas contain cytoplasm that is either finely granular and eosinophilic or relatively clear (Fig. 6). Nuclear pleomorphism is sometimes prominent (Fig. 7) and mitotic figures may be present. Observation of these features has occasionally resulted in an erroneous diagnosis of sarcoma or sarcomatoid carcinoma. The borders of angiomyolipomas are usually well circumscribed, and either abut directly on the adjacent kidney or are limited by a thin fibrous pseudocapsule. A few renal tubules may be entrapped in the

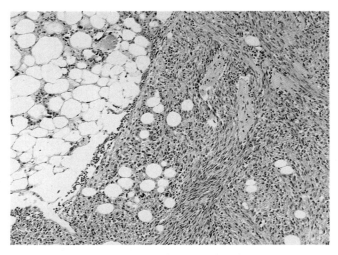

**FIG. 4.** Angiomyolipoma with highly cellular sheets of smooth muscle.

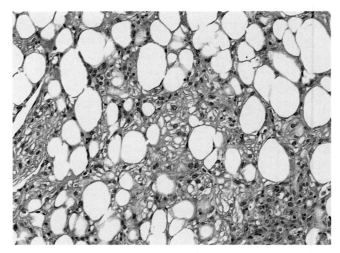

**FIG. 6.** Angiomyolipoma showing smooth muscle cells with clear cytoplasm.

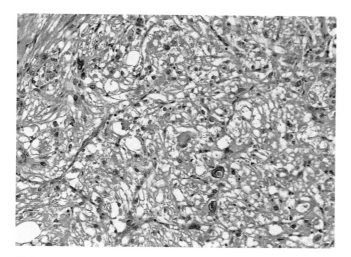

**FIG. 7.** Angiomyolipoma showing smooth muscle cells with nuclear atypia.

these observations, finding granules and crystalloids in the cytoplasm of large epithelioid smooth muscle cells in 11 of 17 cases. Ultrastructurally, the cytoplasm of some such cells contains aggregates of pleomorphic granules, some of which resemble melanosomes (21) and others that more closely resemble renin granules (21,22).

Immunohistochemically, the most distinctive finding in angiomyolipomas is their reactivity with HMB45 (21,23–25), which is generally considered a marker of melanocytes. This observation is most prominent in epithelioid smooth muscle cells (23), but under optimal conditions diffuse immunolabeling is demonstrable (21). Reactivity for HMB45 is unusual in other mesenchymal proliferations but has been found in other lesions that are part of the tuberous sclerosis complex, including lymphangiomyomatosis of the lung and lymph nodes (24) and cardiac rhabdomyoma (21). Additionally, reactivity for actins can usually be demonstrated in the smooth muscle cells of angiomyolipomas (25), including those that also react with HMB45 (26). Vimentin, desmin, and neuron-specific enolase are also demonstrable in 50% or more of cases (25). The lesions fail to stain with antibodies to cytokeratins and epithelial membrane antigen (25); reactivity for renin similarly has not been demonstrated (8).

most peripheral aspects of the lesions. An infiltrative growth pattern may be mimicked by marked multiplicity of angiomyolipomas of variable sizes that make contact with one another at some points but maintain islands of renal tissue between them in other areas. Recognition of this pattern as one of multifocality rather than infiltration by a single angiomyolipoma is important for the diagnosis of tuberous sclerosis (see Table 2).

Tweeddale et al. (20) discovered diastase-sensitive periodic acid–Schiff (PAS)–reactive granules in most smooth muscle cells of angiomyolipomas. Mukai et al. (8) extended

### Differential Diagnosis

The most important differential diagnostic consideration in cases of angiomyolipoma is that of malignancy, including renal cell carcinoma, a true renal or retroperitoneal sarcoma,

**TABLE 4.** *Renal angiomyolipoma associated with angiomyolipoma in regional lymph nodes*

| Citation | Age/sex | Elements | Extent | Tuberous sclerosis | Follow-up (months) |
|---|---|---|---|---|---|
| Campbell (27) | 28/F | M + V + F | 1 node | No | NA |
| Scott (28) | 12/M | M + V + F | 1 node | Yes | NA |
| Busch (29) | 21/M | M + V + F | Several | No | NA |
| | 49/F | M + F | 1/16 | No | NA |
| Bloom (30) | 19/F | M | 6/14 | Yes | 36 A&W |
| | 11/M | M + V + F | Several | Yes | 36 A&W |
| Dao (31) | 24/M | M + V + F | 7/12 | Yes | 12 A&W |
| Hulbert (32) | 24/M | M + V + F | NA | No | NA |
| Sant (33) | 6.5/F | V + F | 1/11 | Yes | 108 A&W |
| | 49/F | M + V + F | 2/22 | No | 36 A&W |
| Brecher (34) | 63/F | M + F | 1/2 | No | 180 A&W |
| Manabe (35) | 27/F | M + V + F | Several | No | 24 A&W |
| Taylor (36) | 9/F | NA | All nodes | Yes | 20 A&W |
| | 15/M | NA | Several | Yes | 24 A&W |
| | 25/F | NA | 9/10 | Yes | 96 A&W |
| Ro (37) | 53/F | M + V + F | 2 nodes | No | 12 A&W |
| | 49/M | M + V + F | 1 node | No | 216 A&W |
| | 58/F | M + V + F | 2 nodes | No | 24 A&W |
| Ansari (38) | 46/F | M + V + F | 9/9 | No | 2 A&W |
| Tallarigo (26) | 14/M | M + V + F | 5/5 | Yes | 24 A&W |
| | 29/F | M + V + F | 1 node | No | 20 A&W |
| | 56/F | M + V + F | 3/6 | No | NA |

and a sarcoma arising in angiomyolipoma. In most angiomyolipomas, the lack of nuclear atypia and circumscription of the mass leaves no question as to its nature. However, when the smooth muscle component exhibits epithelial features, a renal cell carcinoma may be considered as a possible diagnosis. Moreover, some renal angiomyolipomas are associated with angiomyolipomas in regional lymph nodes and, especially when the renal angiomyolipoma shows nuclear pleomorphism or mitotic activity, it can be mistaken for sarcoma or sarcomatoid renal cell carcinoma. This association was recognized in early references on the tumor (20), but lymph nodal angiomyolipomas associated with renal tumors of the same type were not described again until 1974 (27). Eighteen examples have subsequently been described (26,28–38) (Table 4). The deposits in the nodes are histologically identical to the renal lesions, and no patient with this constellation has developed remote or visceral lesions that would indicate the presence of metastasis. Based on these facts, this phenomenon is presently viewed as multifocal angiomyolipoma rather than a single angiomyolipoma spread from the lesion in the kidney to the lymph nodes. Invasion of the renal vein and vena cava by angiomyolipoma have been reported (39–48) in 10 cases; however, none of these patients developed distant disease. Thus, in the absence of remote metastases, the diagnoses of mixed sarcoma of kidney or sarcoma arising in angiomyolipoma should be regarded with great circumspection. Only two credible cases of sarcoma arising from angiomyolipoma are known (49,50) and in both cases the neoplasm was a leiomyosarcoma.

Another consideration in the differential diagnosis is that of lymphangiomyomatosis, a rare disease characterized by proliferation of smooth muscle in the lungs, lymphatic ducts, and lymph nodes. In similarity to angiomyolipoma, it predominantly affects women of childbearing age. Rarely, this lesion may occur in the kidneys (51) and paraaortic lymph nodes (Figs. 8 and 9). It differs histologically from an-

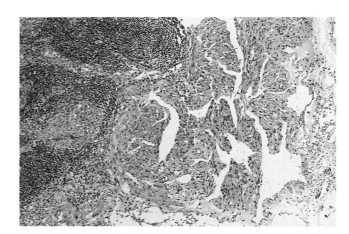

**FIG. 9.** Lymphangiomyoma in paraaortic lymph node. (Courtesy of M. Saegusa, Hiroshima.)

giomyolipoma, being composed of smooth muscle cells surrounding irregular and anastomosing slit-like vascular spaces. Additionally, there is a strong association between lymphangiomyomatosis and renal angiomyolipoma. Among 27 patients with pulmonary lymphangioleiomyomatosis seen at the Mayo Clinic from 1976 to 1989, Kerr et al. (52) found 7 with angiomyolipoma of the kidney. None of these individuals had any of the other findings that are characteristic of tuberous sclerosis. Other cases of lymphangioleiomyomatosis in association with renal angiomyolipoma have been described (53–55). Ansari et al. (38) found deposits resembling lymphangioleiomyomatosis in the regional lymph nodes of a 46-year-old woman with renal and lymph nodal angiomyolipoma.

## JUXTAGLOMERULAR CELL TUMOR

In 1967, Robertson et al. (56) reported the case of a hypertensive youth whose hypertension was cured by resection of an unusual renal lesion. A similar case was described nearly simultaneously by Kihara et al. (57,58), who proposed the term "juxtaglomerular cell tumor" (JCT). A synonym that has been used for this mass is "reninoma," a name similar to those given to a number of other endocrinologically active tumors. Since those initial descriptions were given, 59 more cases have been reported (some more than once) (59–118) as compiled in Table 5. Corvol et al. (98) demonstrated the rarity of these lesions, finding only 7 in a population of 30,000 new hypertensive patients.

### Clinical Features

Clinically, JCTs occur mainly in young adults and adolescents; the average age at resection is 27 years. The youngest patient was 7 years old (114) and the oldest 69 (95). Only 10

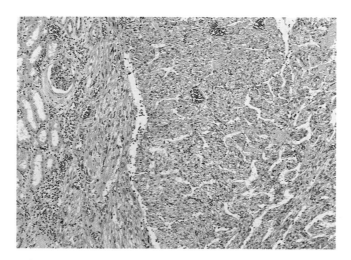

**FIG. 8.** Renal lymphangiomyoma showing smooth muscle with slit-like vascular spaces. (Courtesy of M. Saegusa, M.D., Hiroshima.)

**TABLE 5.** *Sixty-one juxtaglomerular cell tumors*

| Age at onset of hypertension | Age at resection | Sex/side | Size (cm) | Ref. |
|---|---|---|---|---|
| 15 | 16 | M/L | 3 | Robertson (56) |
| 23 | 23 | F/L | 2 | Kihara (57,58) |
| 13 | 13 | M/R | — | Lee (59) |
| 37 | 43 | F/R | 4 × 4 | Eddy (60) |
| 13 | 14 | M/R | 3.5 × 2.5 × 2 | Bonnin (61), Phillips (62) |
| 13 | 18 | M/R | 1.5 | Conn (63), MacCallum (64) |
| 24 | 29 | M/R | 2.0 | Schambelan (65) |
| 8 | 8 | F/L | 0.8 | More (66), Davidson (67), Lindop (68), Brown (69) |
| 23 | 38 | F/L | 2 | Gherardi (70) |
| 10 | 10 | M/R | 0.2 × 0.15 | Hirose (71) |
| 25 | 23 | M/L | 0.9 × 1.1 | Ørjavik (72) |
| 15 | 15 | F/R | 0.9 | Connor (73), Barajas (74) |
| 17 | 17 | F/L | 4.2 × 3.4 × 3.2 | Takahashi (75), Kida (76) |
| 22 | 26 | F/R | 2.5 | Baldet (77,78), Mimran (79) |
| 18 | 18 | F/L | 0.7 | Bonnin (80) |
| 15 | 16 | F/L | 1.2 | Warshaw (81) |
| 47 | 47 | M/R | — | Hanna (82) |
| 16 | 18 | F/R | 1.5 | Valdés (83) |
| 22 | 30 | F/L | 1.5 | El Matri (84,85) |
| 17 | 20 | F/L | 3.5 | Lam (86) |
| 18 | 40 | F/R | 4 × 4 | Moss (87), Jordan (88) |
| 29 | 29 | F/R | 2 × 1.5 | Sanfilippo (89), Jordan (88) |
| 33 | 33 | F/L | 6 × 4 | Furusato (90) |
| 13 | 14 | F/R | 3.0 | Dunnick (91) |
| 15 | 15 | F/R | 4.0 | Dunnick (91) |
| 19 | 21 | F/L | 3.5 | Dunnick (91) |
| 20 | 28 | F/R | 4.5 | Dunnick (91) |
| — | 29 | M/R | 4.0 | Dunnick (91) |
| 29 | 29 | F/R | 2.0 | Dunnick (91) |
| 18 | 41 | F/R | 4.0 | Dunnick (91) |
| 38 | 47 | F/L | 3.5 | Dunnick (91) |
| — | 57 | M/R | 6.5 | Dunnick (91) |
| 19 | 19 | F/L | 0.4 × 0.5 | Baldet (78) |
| 50 | 57 | M/R | 4.5 | Squires (92) |
| 16 | 21 | F/L | 2.5 | Hradec (93) |
| 25 | 27 | M/R | 1.5 | Galen (94) |
| 22 | 27 | F/L | 5 × 3 | Camilleri (95), Baruch (96,97) Corvol (98) |
| 17 | 21 | M/R | 3 | Camilleri (95), Baruch (96,97) Corvol (98), Raynaud (99) |
| 53 | 69 | F/L | 3 | Camilleri (95), Baruch (96,97) Corvol (98), Raynaud (99) |
| 31 | 36 | M/L | 2.5 × 2 × 2 | Têtu (100,101) |
| 11 | 11 | F/L | 5 × 4 × 2.2 | Dennis (102) |
| 26 | 30 | M/— | — | Jordan (88) |
| 30 | 33 | F/R | 2 | Hermus (103), van den Berg (104) |
| 27 | 27 | F/L | 2.9 × 3.0 | Handa (105) |
| — | 36 | F/L | 2.5 × 2.2 × 2 | Guo (106) |
| 22 | 22 | F/L | 4.5 | Martinéz Amenós (107) |
| 21 | 23 | M/R | 1.0 | Pedrinelli (108) |
| 21 | 26 | F/R | 2.5 | Tierney (109) |
| 19 | 20 | M/— | 1.5 | Corvol (98) |
| 19 | 24 | M/— | 1.3 | Corvol (98) |
| 17 | 35 | F/— | 1.0 | Corvol (98) |
| 13 | 22 | F/— | 3.0 | Corvol (98) |
| 20 | 20 | F/L | 8 × 6 × 6 | Remynse (110) |
| 32 | 44 | M/L | 2.3 | Schonfeld (111) |
| 22 | 24 | M/L | 6 × 4 × 3 | Lopéz G-Asenjo (112) |
| 15 | 21 | M/L | 2 | Rossi (113) |
| 7 | 7 | M/L | 0.5 | Garel (114) |
| 31 | 36 | M/L | 6.5 × 5 | Kreutz (115) |
| 25 | 25 | F/R | 2.8 | Uno (116,117) |
| 38 | 44 | M/R | 3.5 | Têtu (101) |
| 23 | 23 | M/R | 3 | Armato (118) |

have been 40 years old or more, whereas 26 have been in their third decade of life and 19 have been 20 or younger at diagnosis. A review of the patients' histories reveals that in many cases hypertension had been present for years before the renal lesion was identified and resected. For example, a 41-year-old woman reported by Dunnick et al. (91) had been hypertensive for 23 years. The average age of first symptoms is 22, 5 years younger than the mean age at the time of resection. Thirty-six patients with JCT have been female and 25 were male, yielding a ratio of approximately 3:2. The left and right kidneys are affected equally frequently by this lesion.

All reported individuals with JCT have been hypertensive, and resection of their tumors has almost invariably produced a marked reduction in blood pressure. No instance of metastasis or local invasion has occurred. Two patients whose tumors were found at autopsy died of uncontrollable hypertension (70,88). Whereas nephrectomy was chosen in early cases or when the tumor could not be localized precisely, a number of patients with JCT have been treated successfully with partial nephrectomy or enucleation of the lesion (78,83,84,89,96,105,108).

**Pathologic Features**

Grossly, JCTs are usually small. In some instances, surgery has been done based only on measurements of renal vein renin (71,72,81,83,96). In the case reported by Hirose et al. (71), no lesion was found on initial examination of the specimen but a small proliferation of juxtaglomerular cells was subsequently detected. The largest tumor was 8 cm in diameter (91) and a few others have had diameters of 4.5 cm or more (90–92,95,102,107,110,112,115). Generally, the lesions have been <3 cm and some have even been invisible when examining the surface of the renal cortex after stripping the capsule. With this in mind, when a juxtaglomerular cell tumor is suspected, the kidney must be sectioned at close intervals and any grossly abnormal area submitted for histologic study. In all reported cases, the tumor has been unilateral and solitary. Larger tumors are usually circumscribed by zones of dense fibrous tissue. The cut surfaces range from pale gray–white to light yellow. The tissue is firm and rubbery and sometimes contains small cyst-like cavities (82,92) (Fig. 10).

Microscopically, JCTs have variable appearances. Some consist of irregular trabeculae of eosinophilic cells set in a background of loose edematous or myxoid connective tissue (Fig. 11); others show round epithelioid cells with clear or eosinophilic cytoplasm arranged in nodules or sheets (Fig. 12), or tubular structures lined with low cuboidal cells. Spindle cell elements have also been reported (95). Furosato et al. (90) found that approximately 50% of juxtaglomerular cell tumors contained tubules and that these tended to occur in younger patients. Lymphocytic infiltrates are frequently present diffusely or as aggregates (Fig. 13). Often, mast cells

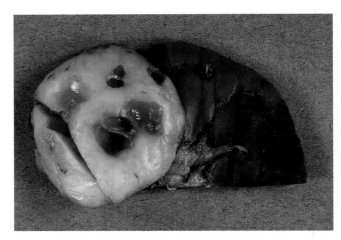

**FIG. 10.** Juxtaglomerular cell tumor composed of firm tan tissue with scattered cavities.

are numerous in JCTs (62,64). The cyst-like cavities seen grossly appear to be degenerative and are usually not lined by epithelium (Fig. 14). Uncommonly, areas with papillary architecture may be present (101). Mild nuclear pleomorphism (92) and rare mitotic figures have been reported. The tumors are quite vascular and the blood vessels are variable in size and mural thickness, ranging from thick-walled (66) to sinusoidal (64).

Use of Bowie's stain (modified for juxtaglomerular cell granules) reveals intracytoplasmic granules in many of the cells in JCT, as does immunofluorescent staining using thioflavin T (56,57,60). The granules are also positive with the periodic acid–Schiff (PAS) method. Immunohistochemical methods have shown that the lesional cells contain renin (68,86,95,100,102). Chemical analyses have been done on tissue from some lesions; these have revealed renin levels ranging from 200 to 2000 times those of normal renal tissue, and large quantities of inactive renin as well (66,79).

**FIG. 11.** Juxtaglomerular cell tumor with lacy pattern of compact cells in edematous background.

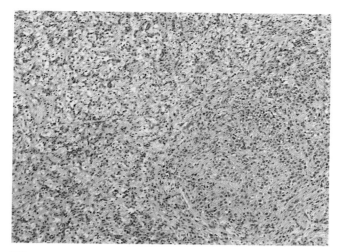

**FIG. 12.** Juxtaglomerular cell tumor showing focus of epithelioid round cells with clear cytoplasm.

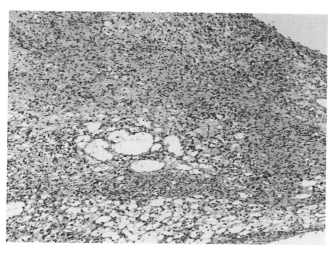

**FIG. 14.** Juxtaglomerular cell tumor with small and large cavities.

The cytoplasmic granules that are characteristic of juxtaglomerular cells (119) are visible ultrastructurally (64). Developing into round or ovoid inclusions (Fig. 15) by a process of aggregation (62), these structures begin as rhomboidal granules (see Fig. 15) that have an internal crystalline structure with a periodicity of approximately 60 Å (62,77). Furosato et al. (90) studied the ultrastructure of the cells lining the tubular elements in one lesion and found that they resembled the immature epithelium found in nephroblastomas. Barajas et al. (74) observed unmyelinated neural elements with terminals in contact with juxtaglomerular tumor cells. The combination of these diverse types of tissue has led some investigators (65,71,100) to conclude that these tumors are hamartomas or "pseudotumors," but this viewpoint is controversial.

**Differential Diagnosis**

Renin-containing cells have been found in nephroblastoma (120,121), clear cell renal cell carcinoma (122), and congenital mesoblastic nephroma (123,124). In angiomyolipoma (21,22), granules similar to those of JCT have been found by electron microscopy. Lindop et al. (125) used a panel of polyclonal and monoclonal antibodies to evaluate the presence of immunoreactive renin in a wide range of human tumors and normal tissues, and found renin-containing cells only in the kidney, renal cell carcinoma, and nephroblastoma. Renin secretion by Wilms' tumor, renal cell carcinoma, and congenital mesoblastic nephroma has similarly produced clinical hypertension that was cured by resection of the tumors (121–123).

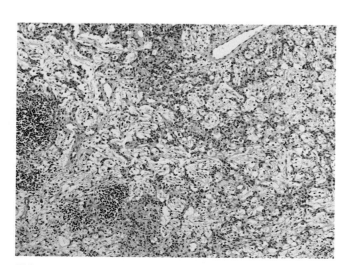

**FIG. 13.** Juxtaglomerular cell tumor showing clusters of lymphocytes.

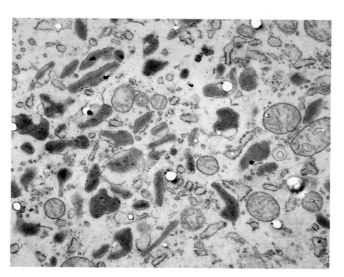

**FIG. 15.** Juxtaglomerular cell tumor. Ultrastructural appearance of rhomboid and pleomorphic granules.

## RENOMEDULLARY INTERSTITIAL CELL TUMOR

Small pale tumors of the renal medulla have long been recognized at the time of autopsy and often have been called "fibromas." More recently, ultrastructural studies have shown that these lesions are composed of renomedullary interstitial cells (126,127) and this concept of their nature is now generally accepted (128). Renomedullary interstitial cells contain vasodepressor substances that are believed to have important antihypertensive functions (129), but the relationship, if any, of renomedullary interstitial cell tumors to hypertension has remained controversial. It has been suggested that these nodules are hyperplastic (pseudoneoplastic), arising in reaction to the stimulus of chronic hypertension (126,127). However, Stuart et al. (130) found no significant difference in heart weight or blood pressure in two groups of 160 autopsied patients with and without renomedullary interstitial cell tumors, and a similarly negative result was found by Martin and Tiltman in another study (131). Carrying this line of investigation further, Zimmermann et al. (132) found that patients with hypocellular amyloid-containing renomedullary interstitial cell tumors had increased heart weights relative to others with amyloid-free lesions and to control patients without lesions. Zimmermann et al. hypothesized that the secretory activity of cellular renomedullary interstitial cell tumors may be sufficient to counteract rises in blood pressure but that the deposition of amyloid within the lesions resulted in reduced endocrine function and the development of hypertension.

### Clinical Features

Renomedullary interstitial cell tumors are common autopsy findings. In a study of 800 kidneys from 400 autopsies in which the kidneys were cut in 1.5-mm slices, Warfel and Eble (133) found 447 renomedullary interstitial cell tumors in 218 kidneys from 152 patients. The incidence of the lesions in individuals who were 20 years or older was 46% for males and 44% for females. None was found in a patient younger than 18 years. Multiplicity was common among patients with renomedullary interstitial cell tumors, and 57% had more than one lesion. Reis et al. (134) observed 108 lesions among 89 patients in a series of 500 autopsies, in which the kidneys were sectioned at 2-mm intervals. Allowing for differences in examination techniques, these results agree with those of other necropsy studies (135–137).

### Pathologic Features

As elucidated by autopsy series, most renomedullary interstitial cell tumors are small white nodules in the renal medullary pyramids (Fig. 16). In one large autopsy analysis (133), <15% were larger than 3 mm and the largest was 6 mm. For this reason, it is rare that they cause symptoms or are discovered by imaging techniques. In kidneys that are re-

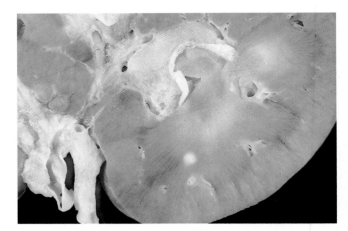

**FIG. 16.** Renomedullary interstitial cell tumor. Typical appearance of small pale nodule within a medullary pyramid.

sected for other reasons, renomedullary interstitial cell tumors are sometimes found incidentally; large lesions of this type may occasionally cause concern until their identity is recognized pathologically (Fig. 17).

Histologically, renomedullary interstitial cell tumors are well-circumscribed nodules (Fig. 18) that are composed of small stellate or polygonal renomedullary interstitial cells. These are set in a background of loose faintly basophilic stroma that is reminiscent of renal medullary matrix (Fig. 19). At the periphery, renal medullary tubules are often entrapped in the lesions (Fig. 20). Interlacing bundles of delicate fibers are usually also present. In amyloid-containing renomedullary interstitial cell tumors, the delicacy of the stroma is lost, and irregular deposits of amyloid are apparent. Although these lesions have been called "fibromas," most contain little collagen (Fig. 21).

A few cases have been documented that may represent symptomatic renomedullary interstitial cell tumors

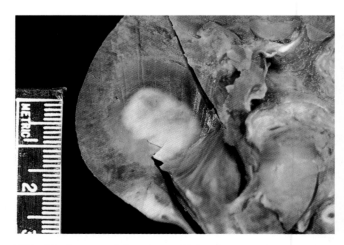

**FIG. 17.** Renomedullary interstitial cell tumor. An exceptionally large lesion discovered in a transplanted kidney was resected for rejection.

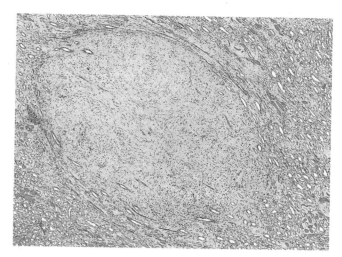

**FIG. 18.** Renomedullary interstitial cell tumor showing sharp circumscription from surrounding renal medulla.

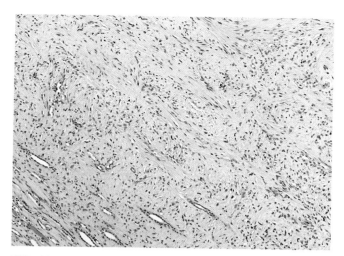

**FIG. 20.** Renomedullary interstitial cell tumor composed of interlacing bundles of spindle cells with a few entrapped medullary tubules.

(138–146). These are summarized in Table 6. Most presented as pedunculated masses extending into the renal pelvic cavity (138,140–144,146). Although early cases were called renal pelvic "fibromas"(138–143), the three most recent reports (144–146) on such lesions have recognized the medullary origin of the tumors. Histologically, they are submucosal lesions consisting of stroma with variable cellularity, containing loosely interwoven collagen bundles. In some cases, the matrix has been myxoid or edematous. The cellular component consists of spindle cells that resemble fibroblasts. In a number of examples, tubules resembling those of the renal medulla have been present deep within the tumors or in their peripheral portions (139,145,146). While some of the lesions in Table 6 may be fibroepithelial polyps of the type more commonly found in the ureters, the predominance of females (70% of patients with fibroepithelial polyps are male) and the gross appearance of caliceal origin of some of the lesions support the notion that these are probably renomedullary interstitial cell tumors.

### Differential Diagnosis

Other than renomedullary interstitial cell tumors, few mass lesions arise in the renal medullary pyramids (133). Most of the latter are either carcinomas of the collecting ducts (147) or hemangiomas (148), with which renomedullary interstitial cell tumors are unlikely to be confused.

Drut and De Cusminsky (149) described a widely metastatic and fatal renal sarcoma in a 70-year-old man that was composed of pleomorphic spindle cells containing Sudan IV–positive droplets and toluidine blue–reactive granules. Chemical analyses showed that the tumor contained prostaglandins. They proposed the name "renomedullary interstitial cell sarcoma" for this previously unknown neoplasm, but its relationship, if any, to benign interstitial cell nodules is unproven at present.

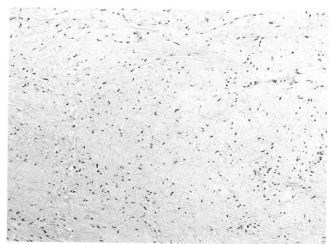

**FIG. 19.** Renomedullary interstitial cell tumor showing sparse cellularity with delicate spindle and stellate cells.

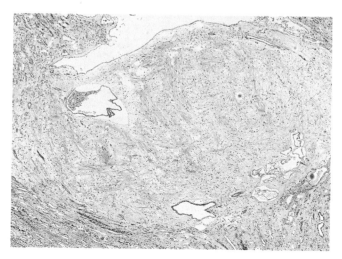

**FIG. 21.** Renomedullary interstitial cell tumor. This Trichrome-stained section shows a paucity of collagen.

**TABLE 6.** *Symptomatic renomedullary interstitial cell tumors*

| Age | Sex | Comment | Ref. |
|-----|-----|---------|------|
| 29 | F | 2 cm, pedunculated | Boross and Puhr (138) |
| 20 | F | 22-lb tumor, 13 × 11 × 5 in. | Gordon-Taylor (139) |
| 32 | F | 7 × 1.5 cm, pedunculated | Immergut and Cottler (140) |
| 60 | M | 3.5 × 2 × 2 cm, pedunculated | Shucksmith (141) |
| 42 | F | 4 × 4 × 2 cm, pedunculated | Bernier et al. (142) |
| 29 | F | 2.5 cm, pedunculated | Cassimally (143) |
| 31 | F | 1.3 cm, pedunculated | Lennox and Clark (144) |
| 70 | F | 8 × 13 × 14 cm | Polga (145) |
| 54 | F | 2.9 × 2.8 × 2 cm, pedunculated | Glover and Buck (146) |

## CYSTIC NEPHROMA

Cystic nephroma, also called "multilocular cyst" and "multilocular cystic nephroma," is a rare and controversial renal lesion found both in children and in adults. It was first described and illustrated in 1892 by Edmunds (150), but it remained for Powell et al. (151) and Boggs and Kimmelstiel (152) to propose criteria by which these lesions can be distinguished from other cystic lesions of the kidneys (Table 7). With the recognition of cystic renal cell carcinoma and cystic, partially differentiated nephroblastoma as distinct variants of renal cell carcinoma and Wilms' tumor, the guide-lines for the diagnosis of cystic nephroma have been further complicated. This point is discussed further in the section on differential diagnosis.

### Clinical Features

Cystic nephromas are benign and effectively treated by conservative surgery. Castillo et al. (153) reviewed 187 cases, including 29 from their own institution; these authors found a male predominance of almost 2:1 in patients younger than 2 years of age and a female predominance of more than 3:1 among adults. Although the original definition (151) of this entity required that it be unilateral, bilateral lesions do occur rarely.

### Pathologic Features

The original illustration published by Edmunds (150) in 1892 shows beautifully the gross features most characteristic of cystic nephroma (Fig. 22). The lesions are well circumscribed by a fibrous capsule and are composed of multiple discrete locules that do not communicate with one another. These have smooth inner surfaces and contain clear yellowish fluid (Fig. 23). Solid areas are absent or scanty and the septa range from paper thin to a few millimeters in thickness.

Microscopically, the stromal partitions in cystic nephroma are composed of fibrous tissue that may include foci of calcification (Fig. 24). The septa may also contain differentiated tubules (as opposed to primitive tubules with the morphology characteristic of Wilms' tumor), inflammatory cells, and reactive fibroblasts. The cysts are usually lined with flattened or low cuboidal epithelium with small amounts of cytoplasm (Fig. 25); occasionally, the lining cells have a hobnail configuration.

**TABLE 7.** *Diagnostic features of cystic nephroma*

*1951 Criteria of Powell, Shackman, and Johnson (151)*
1. The lesion should be unilateral.
2. The lesion should be solitary.
3. The lesion should be multilocular.
4. The cavities should not communicate with the renal pelvis.
5. The loculi should not communicate with one another.
6. The loculi should have a definite epithelial lining.
7. There should be no renal elements within the lesion.
8. Residual kidney, if present, should be normal.

*1956 Criteria of Boggs and Kimmelstiel (152)*
1. The lesion must be multilocular.
2. The cysts must, for the most part, be lined by epithelium.
3. The cysts must not communicate with the renal pelvis.
4. The residual renal tissue should be essentially normal, except for pressure atrophy.
5. Fully developed, mature nephrons or portions of such should not be present within the septa of the lesion.

*1989 Criteria of Joshi and Beckwith (154)*
1. The lesion is composed entirely of cysts and their septa.
2. It forms a discrete mass, well-demarcated from the remainder of the kidney.
3. The septa are the sole solid component of the lesion and conform to the contours of the cysts, without solid, expansive nodules.
4. The cysts are lined by flattened, cuboidal, or hobnail epithelium.
5. The septa are composed of fibrous tissue in which well-differentiated tubules may be present.

*1993 Criteria of Kajani, Rosenberg, and Bernstein (155)*
1. Well-circumscribed tumor containing multiple cysts lined with epithelium.
2. Septa containing no normal tissue.
3. Surrounding tissue normal except for compression.

### Differential Diagnosis

The morphologic definition of cystic nephroma that was offered by Powell et al. (151) (see Table 7) was based on a small number of cases and was designed to exclude malfor-

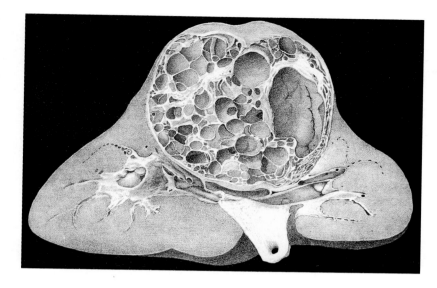

**FIG. 22.** Cystic nephroma. Gross appearance as illustrated by Edmunds (150).

mations and infectious cystic lesions. A modification by Boggs and Kimmelstiel (152) (see Table 7) removed the arbitrary criteria of unilaterality and solitude, and permitted the intraseptal immature renal elements found in one of their two cases (in a 5-month-old boy). The latter provision blurred the distinction from cystic nephroblastoma, which on clinical, radiographic, and pathologic grounds is the most important differential diagnostic consideration in children. Joshi and Beckwith (154), using the case material of the National Wilms' Tumor Study Pathology Center, addressed this point (see Table 7) and classified lesions with immature elements in the stromal septa as "cystic, partially differentiated nephroblastomas" (Fig. 26). When nodular solid areas of immature tissue were present, they considered the tumors nephroblastomas with multifocal cystic change. They believed that cystic nephroma and cystic partially differentiated nephroblastoma are closely related but distinct entities, differing in the degree of differentiation of their component

tissues. Kajani et al. (155) conversely regarded the distinction between the two lesions as artificial in light of their similarly benign behaviors. The latter investigators proposed a more simplified and unitarian set of diagnostic criteria (see Table 7). They believed that cystic partially differentiated nephroblastoma and cystic nephroma merely represent the poles of a spectrum of cellularity between lesions in children and adults.

Although the problem of the relationship of cystic nephroma to nephroblastoma is a thorny one, the relationship of the former of these lesions to cystic renal cell carcinoma is also problematic. Multilocular cystic renal cell carcinomas constitute a recently recognized (156–162) group of tumors that grossly resemble cystic nephromas. However, they differ by containing clear cells that are identical to those of clear cell renal cell carcinoma (Fig. 27). These epithelia typically line some of the intralesional locules, and they may form small collections in the septa as well. Multi-

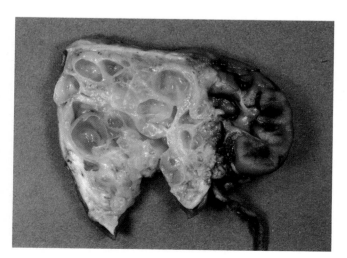

**FIG. 23.** Cystic nephroma composed of many locules with smooth linings and thin septa.

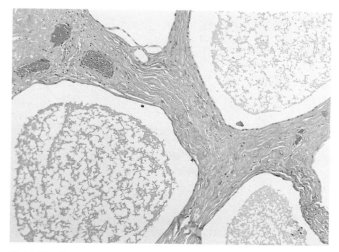

**FIG. 24.** Cystic nephroma. Septa is composed of fibrous tissue, and the locules contain eosinophilic fluid.

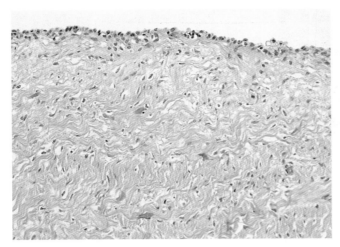

**FIG. 25.** Cystic nephroma. The lining epithelium is simple, cuboidal, and atrophic.

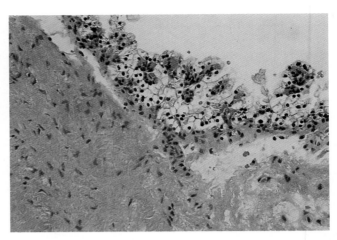

**FIG. 27.** Multilocular cystic renal cell carcinoma with fibrous septa focally covered by cells with clear cytoplasm identical to those of low-grade clear cell renal cell carcinoma.

locular renal adenocarcinomas appear to have a very favorable prognosis.

The relationship of Wilms' tumor, cystic partially differentiated nephroblastoma, cystic nephroma, and multilocular cystic renal cell carcinoma is incompletely understood and controversial. One unifying concept (154,155,163) links nephroblastoma, cystic partially differentiated nephroblastoma, and cystic nephroma in a spectrum of differentiation within a family of tumors, in a manner that is somewhat analogous to the grouping of neuroblastoma, ganglioneuroblastoma, and ganglioneuroma. Although this idea is attractive, the truth may not be so simple. Beckwith and Joshi (154) found that mature heterologous elements (particularly skeletal muscle) are common in cystic partially differentiated nephroblastoma but not in cystic nephroma. This observa-

tion is difficult to reconcile with the concept that cystic nephroma is a more differentiated form of cystic partially differentiated nephroblastoma. The dramatic difference in the gender distribution between childhood and adulthood is also a troublesome flaw in the unitarian hypothesis. In the end, it may prove to be the case that several tumors of different origins have very similar gross and microscopic appearances but show essential histologic differences. A simplifying factor is derived from knowing that renal cell carcinoma arises in a variety of longstanding cystic diseases of the kidney (164–169). By analogy, it is possible that that neoplasm may in the same way occasionally take origin in the cysts of cystic nephroma, accounting for some multilocular cystic renal cell carcinomas.

## XANTHOGRANULOMATOUS PYELONEPHRITIS

Xanthogranulomatous pyelonephritis (XP) is an uncommon inflammatory condition that can be mistaken clinically or pathologically for renal cell carcinoma or nephroblastoma (170–172). Kobayashi et al. (173) observed that its similarities to renal cell carcinoma may pose particular diagnostic difficulties in aspiration biopsy specimens. More than 600 cases of XP have been reported (174) individually or in series since the disease was first described by Schlagenhaufer in 1916 (175) and named by Österlind in 1944 (176). In Table 8, 378 cases from 11 large series (177–187) are represented.

Experimentally, ligation of the ureter and intravenous injection of a suspension of *Escherichia coli* have produced xanthogranulomatous pyelonephritis in rats (188). Although some aspects of the pathogenesis of XP in humans remain controversial, it is generally accepted that obstruction and infection are important etiologic factors.

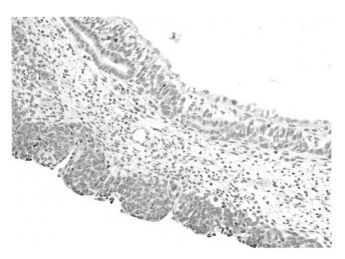

**FIG. 26.** Cystic partially differentiated nephroblastoma with blastema in the septa. (Courtesy of B. Beckwith, M.D., National Wilms' Tumor Study Pathology Center, Loma Linda, CA.)

**TABLE 8.** *Large series of xanthogranulomatous pyelonephritis*

| Ref. | Number of cases | Sex M/F | Age Range | Age Mean |
|------|----------------|---------|-----------|----------|
| Goodman et al. (184) | 23 | 7:16 | 16–70 | 44 |
| Malek et al. (179) | 18 | 9:9 | 15–70 | 48 |
| Flynn et al. (186) | 28 | 10:18 | 18–71 | 43 |
| Tolia et al. (182) | 29 | 8:21 | 9–87 | 57 |
| Roggia et al. (183) | 22 | — | 33–72 | 47 |
| McDonald (180) | 40 | 9:31 | 21–94 | 48 |
| Parsons et al. (178) | 87 | 14:73 | 13–85 | 54 |
| Rosi et al. (177) | 62 | 23:39 | 14–75 | 47 |
| Kural et al. (185) | 16 | 6:10 | 6–58 | 23 |
| Antonakopoulos et al. (181) | 17 | 7:10 | 23–85 | 62 |
| Chuang et al. (187) | 36 | 10:26 | 19–75 | 50 |
| *Aggregates* | 378 | 103:253 | 6–94 | 49 |

## Clinical Features

In approximately two thirds of XP cases, the patient is female (see Table 8). Although a number of small series of pediatric cases (189–194) have been reported, and children are included in the majority of the series reported in Table 8, most affected individuals are adults, and the mean age is approximately 49. Typically, the patient presents with multiple symptoms, commonly including flank pain, recurring fever, malaise, anorexia, weight loss, and, occasionally, hematuria (179,184). This constellation of complaints has much in common with those seen in many renal cell carcinomas. In a majority of XP cases, physical examination demonstrates a mass in the flank (178,179,182,195) or abdomen (184). Imaging usually shows a nonfunctioning kidney containing calculi (178). Pyuria and bacteriuria are common, but 25% of patients have sterile urine (184). *Proteus mirabilis* and *E. coli* are the most common bacterial organisms observed. Thus, the preoperative diagnosis of XP is difficult. Rarely, this condition may be associated with systemic amyloidosis (196).

## Pathologic Features

The resected kidney in XP is usually enlarged and an obstruction to urinary outflow is almost always present (178) (Fig. 28). Most often, this is caused by calculi; the second most frequent cause of obstruction is congenital obstruction of the ureteropelvic junction (178). Because these are the most common etiologies, most cases of XP are unilateral. The kidney is hydronephrotic and the lesions of XP consist of yellow or orange tissue surrounding the renal pelvis and calyces. Its consistency, color, infiltrative appearance, and distortion and destruction of the surrounding parenchyma can closely mimic the appearance of renal cell carcinoma (Fig. 29). Abscesses are also common and the renal pelvis is often filled with pus and necrotic debris.

Based on the extent of renal involvement, Malek et al. (179) proposed that XP could be divided into three stages:

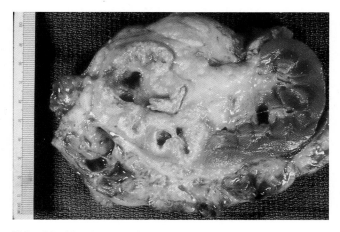

**FIG. 28.** Xanthogranulomatous pyelonephritis replacing much of the kidney and extending into perirenal fat. Note calculus in renal pelvis.

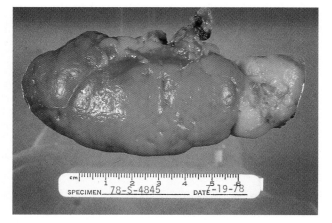

**FIG. 29.** Xanthogranulomatous pyelonephritis forming a mass at one renal pole, grossly mimicking renal cell carcinoma.

*Stage I—Nephric.* In this stage, the disease is confined to the kidney.

*Stage II—Nephric and Perinephric.* In this stage of XP, the inflammation extends into the fat of Gerota's fascia.

*Stage III—Nephric, Perinephric, and Paranephric.* The inflammation in this phase of XP extends massively into the retroperitoneal fat, with considerable distortion of neighboring structures.

Only roughly 25% of lesions are stage I at diagnosis. In fact, in the series of Parsons et al. (178,197), two thirds of the cases were stage III. Most often, the entire kidney was affected in that study; XP was found to be focal within the parenchyma in only 2 of 87 cases.

Microscopically, the abnormalities seen in XP range from submucosal plaques to coalescing nodules involving most of the kidney. The inflammatory infiltrate consists predominantly of macrophages (Fig. 30), with most having foamy cytoplasm, but some contain eosinophilic granular cytoplasm. Both cell types stain with oil red O (181). Cholesterol clefts and foreign body giant cells may also be present. Where the process extends beyond the renal capsule, fat necrosis is common and there are frequently extracellular aggregates of lipid globules (178). Later in the process, fibrotic organization takes place. Variant forms occur in which the xanthoma cells are spindle-shaped or in which there are large numbers of multinucleated giant cells (178). Rarely, granulomatous pyelonephritis associated with renal calculi may closely simulate the histologic appearance of tuberculosis (198).

**Differential Diagnosis**

The most important consideration in the differential diagnosis of XP is confusion with clear cell renal cell carcinoma.

**FIG. 30.** Xanthogranulomatous pyelonephritis composed of sheets of polygonal histiocytes with clear cytoplasm. Note that blood vessels are not prominent.

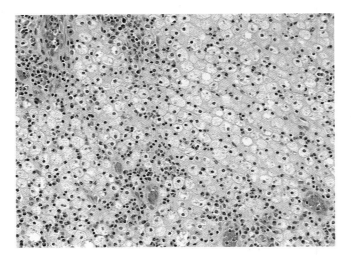

**FIG. 31.** Xanthogranulomatous pyelonephritis. At high magnification the clear cytoplasm is seen to be foamy.

The sheets of foamy histiocytes of XP may resemble the latter tumor, particularly on low-magnification microscopy or in frozen sections. Closer examination shows that the lesions of XP lack the delicate vessels and pattern of vascularity that are typical of renal cell carcinoma. Moreover, the cytoplasm of the foamy histiocytes is filled with many small vesicles (Fig. 31), whereas that of the tumor cells in renal cell carcinoma has an empty appearance.

Although some renal cell carcinomas also exhibit pleomorphic nuclei that would be inconsistent with those of histiocytes, this observation is of inconsistent help because many carcinomas do show small regular nuclei resembling those of histiocytes. Iskandar et al. (199) have noted that the converse problem of mistaking renal cell carcinoma for XP may also be encountered. These problems are further exacerbated by the occasional concurrence (in 3–10% of cases) of XP with renal cell carcinoma and other urologic neoplasms (174). Under these circumstances, immunostains for keratin or epithelial membrane antigen might be necessary to identify renal epithelial tumors with certainty.

**RENAL MALAKOPLAKIA**

Malakoplakia is an uncommon inflammatory lesion that can cause tumefactive masses in the kidney, simulating a primary renal neoplasm (200–202). First described in 1902 and 1903 by Michaelis and Gutmann (203) and by von Hansemann (204), malakoplakia occurs most frequently in the urinary bladder, where it is visible as yellow–white, soft, raised plaques on the mucosal surface. It was this appearance, combined with a reluctance to speculate on the pathogenesis of the disorder, that prompted von Hansemann to combine the

Greek roots for plaque ("plakos") and soft ("malakos") to coin the word "malakoplakia" for the condition (205).

## Clinical Features

More than 50 cases of renal parenchymal malakoplakia have been reported (202,205). Approximately 80% of these have occurred in women (205). McClure (205) reviewed 49 cases, concerning patients whose ages ranged from 3 to 81 years with a mean of 44 years. Malakoplakia has been present bilaterally in more than 25% of cases (205–208) and many patients have died either of the disease directly or of the uremia it can produce (206). In patients with malakoplakia of the kidney, concurrent extrarenal malakoplakia is also common. It most frequently involves the urinary bladder, ureter, or retroperitoneum (205). A number of these individuals have had iatrogenic immunosuppression in conjunction with organ transplantation (209) or have been immunosuppressed for other reasons. Deridder et al. (206) noted that anemia was common in patients with renal malakoplakia, but the cause of this association is unclear.

## Pathologic Features

The appearance of the resected kidney in malakoplakia cases varies from that of diffuse multinodular cortical enlargement (202,206) to a cancer-like configuration consisting of a large yellowish mass with apparent perinephric infiltration (201). Abscesses and cyst-like spaces are also occasionally evident within such lesions (205).

Histologically, malakoplakia in the kidney resembles that seen in the urinary bladder and other organ sites (Fig. 32). Smith (210) identified three phases in the development of malakoplakia and Esparza et al. (202) have confirmed their presence in the kidney.

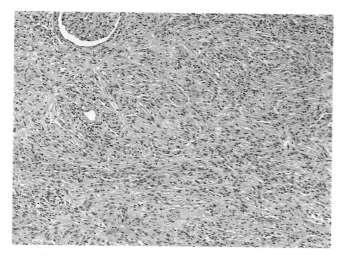

**FIG. 32.** Malakoplakia diffusely infiltrating and expanding the renal interstitium. (Courtesy of A. R. Esparza, M.D., Providence, RI.)

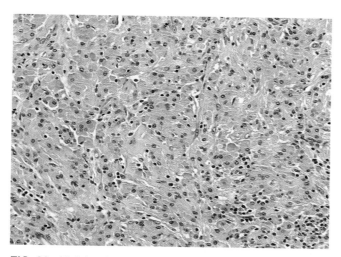

**FIG. 33.** Malakoplakia with sheets of epithelioid Hansemann histiocytes. (Courtesy of A. R. Esparza, M.D., Providence, RI.)

### Early Phase

This form of the disease is characterized by a spectrum of inflammation ranging from a predominance of plasma cells to large numbers of vacuolated macrophages to the presence of plump macrophages with granular cytoplasm (Fig. 33). Calcospherites (Michaelis–Gutmann bodies) are absent in this phase.

### Classic Phase

In this stage, lesions of malakoplakia are packed with large, plump histiocytes (von Hansemann histiocytes), and Michaelis–Gutmann bodies are present within such cells and are also seen lying free in the extracellular spaces (Fig. 34).

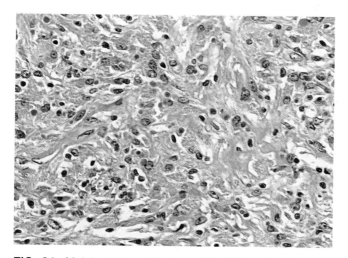

**FIG. 34.** Malakoplakia with basophilic Michaelis–Gutmann bodies. (Courtesy of A. R. Esparza, M.D., Providence, RI.)

Plasma cells, lymphocytes, and multinucleated giant cells may be present in variable numbers.

### Fibrosing Phase

Fibroblasts and collagen are present in aggregates, between which histiocytes, lymphocytes, and occasional Michaelis–Gutmann bodies are distributed in this phase of the disorder.

Lacking Michaelis–Gutmann bodies, the early phase is diagnosed on the basis of finding diffuse infiltrates of von Hansemann histiocytes with destruction of the renal tubular architecture. The cytoplasm of these cells is distinctly granular and eosinophilic, and the cells may contain round colorless intracytoplasmic inclusions, thought to correspond to the glycolipid aggregates that are the precursors of Michaelis–Gutmann bodies (202). "Megalocytic interstitial nephritis" is a term that was proposed in 1945 for a few cases that resembled malakoplakia but lacked Michaelis–Gutmann bodies and in which there was no association with vesical malakoplakia (211). Presently, it appears that megalocytic interstitial nephritis is the same condition as early phase malakoplakia (202,211), and some reviews have dropped it from use as a distinct diagnostic entity (212,213).

It is in the classic phase that Michaelis–Gutmann bodies, the specific hallmark of malakoplakia, are most readily found. These inclusions are calcospherites that are caused by the crystallization of hydroxyapatite on anionic constituents, within phagolysosomes in the cytoplasm of the von Hansemann histiocytes (214). Experimentally, lesions that are indistinguishable from malakoplakia have been induced by injection of a lipopolysaccharide extract of *E. coli* into the kidneys of rats (215). This biochemical substrate appears to provide the anionic sites for mineralization. In sections stained with hematoxylin and eosin, Michaelis–Gutmann bodies consist of a basophilic matrix that often appears to be surrounded by a halo, giving a characteristic "bird's-eye" or targetoid appearance (see Fig. 34).

Histochemical stains can be helpful when Michaelis–Gutmann bodies are scarce or difficult to appreciate in routine sections. The von Kossa stain is effective, and highlights the inclusions as dark brown–black bodies against a pale background (Fig. 35). Von Hansemann histiocytes are diffusely PAS-positive, and the intensity of this reaction may obscure the Michaelis–Gutmann bodies within them.

Ultrastructurally, the phagolysosomes of the von Hansemann histiocytes contain a matrix consisting of whorled fragments of membranous and myelin figures (216). A form that is intermediate between the phagolysosome and the Michaelis–Gutmann body consists of an outer ring of mineralization surrounding a central kernel of lipid-rich cellular debris (202). Michaelis–Gutmann bodies range from 5 to 10 $\mu$m in diameter and consist of a crystalline core surrounded by a less dense zone. Usually, this portion of the inclusion is

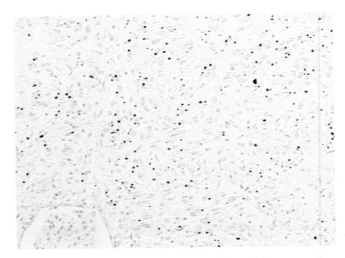

**FIG. 35.** Malakoplakia. Section stained for calcium revealing many Michaelis-Gutmann bodies. (Courtesy of A. R. Esparza, M.D., Providence, RI.)

granular or homogeneous, but sometimes it consists of myelin figures (216). The X-ray diffraction pattern of the crystalline core is consistent with that of hydroxyapatite, and electron probe microanalysis has shown that it contains calcium, phosphorus, and iron (216).

Esparza et al. (202) have noted that the fibrosing phase of malakoplakia may resemble a pleomorphic sarcoma. However, recognition of Michaelis–Gutmann bodies in sections stained with the hematoxylin and eosin or von Kossa techniques resolves this differential diagnosis.

## OTHER INFLAMMATORY PSEUDOTUMORS

Inflammatory lesions that are more circumscribed than xanthogranulomatous pyelonephritis and malakoplakia rarely produce tumefactions in the kidney (217–219). De-

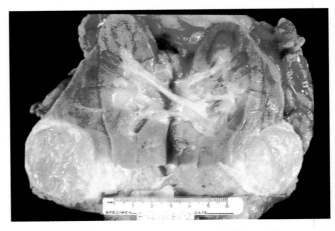

**FIG. 36.** Fibrous pseudotumor of the kidney (plasma cell granluoma). (Photograph courtesy of Dr. Mark A. Weiss, Cincinnati, OH.)

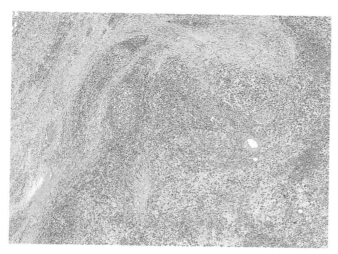

**FIG. 37.** Fibrous pseudotumor of the kidney. The lesion is circumscribed and consists of fibrous tissue with a dense population of lymphocytes and plasma cells. (Courtesy of Dr. Mark A. Weiss, Cincinnati, OH.)

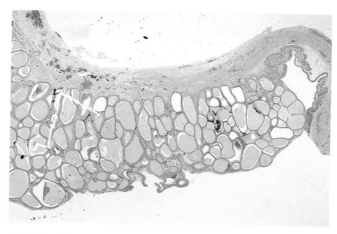

**FIG. 39.** Florid von Brunn's nests and early ureteritis cystica forming a tumor-like nodule on the ureteral mucosa. (Courtesy of Dr. Robert H. Young, Boston, MA.)

pending on their composition and resemblance to various inflammatory processes that are more common in other organs, these proliferations have been designated "plasma cell granuloma," "inflammatory pseudotumor," and "myxoid inflammatory pseudotumor." Related symptoms include flank pain and painless hematuria, and adults and children have been equally affected.

Grossly, such lesions are well-circumscribed masses (Fig. 36) that range in color from yellow-brown to off-white. Some have a gelatinous character, whereas at least one example was extensively calcified. Histologically, their composition ranges from partially hyalinized fibrous tissue—in which there are dense populations of plasma cells and lymphocytes (Fig. 37), with or without metaplastic bone—to a myxoid stroma containing many arborizing small blood vessels and a diffuse infiltrate of histiocytes, plasma cells, lymphocytes, and eosinophils. Old and new intralesional hemor-

rhage may be prominent as well. Although the nature of renal "pseudotumors" as inflammatory processes is relatively obvious in that part of the spectrum that features numerous plasma cells, myxoid lesions of this type may be seen in cellular areas, raising the possibility of a sarcoma, such as inflammatory malignant fibrous histiocytoma or myxoid liposarcoma. The bland nuclear features of myxoid inflammatory pseudotumors are helpful in making this distinction despite the fact that mitotic activity may be notable.

## RENAL PELVIS AND URETER

Many pseudoneoplastic lesions of the mucosa of the urinary bladder also occur in the renal pelvis and ureter. These include the ureteral counterpart of cystitis cystica (ureteritis cystica) (Fig. 38); von Brunn's nests (Fig. 39); nephrogenic

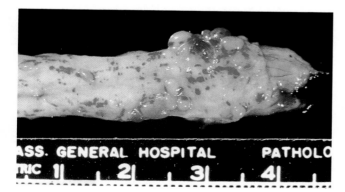

**FIG. 38.** Ureteritis cystica forming domed nodules protruding into the ureteral lumen. (Courtesy of Dr. Robert H. Young, Boston, MA.)

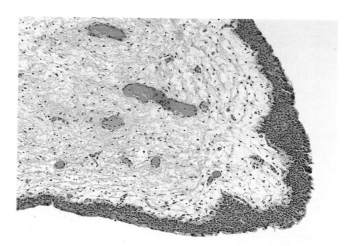

**FIG. 40.** Fibroepithelial polyp of the ureter is covered by essentially normal urothelium.

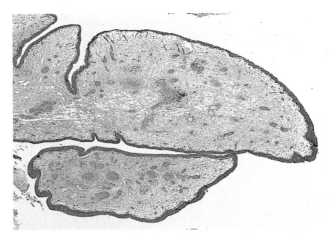

**FIG. 41.** Fibroepithelial polyp of the ureter. The core is composed of loose edematous connective tissue with prominent blood vessels.

adenoma (220,221); endometriosis (222); and other inflammatory conditions that are discussed in detail in Chapter 8.

Fibroepithelial polyps are more common in the ureters and renal pelvis than they are in the bladder. These lesions occur at all ages (223–227) (mean = approximately 40 years), with a male preponderance of 2:1 (228). Colicky pain and hematuria are the most common symptoms (226,228). Grossly, fibroepithelial polyps take the form of single or multiple, slender, smooth-surfaced vermiform polyps, which usually arise from a common base. The ureteropelvic junction is a common site of origin, and the lesions may cause obstruction at that anatomic point (226). Rarely, they may be bilateral (229). Microscopically, fibroepithelial polyps are surfaced by bland urothelium (Fig. 40) that may be focally eroded. The cores of the polyps are composed of loose edematous and vascular stroma with a scant population of inflammatory cells (Fig. 41).

## CONCLUSIONS

The foregoing discussion should make it apparent that hamartomatous, hyperplastic, and inflammatory reactive lesions are all represented among the pseudoneoplastic proliferations of the kidney. Whereas these are usually readily recognizable on the basis of conventional morphologic analysis, some examples will require the application of special adjunctive studies to secure a definitive diagnosis. Because the overwhelming majority of renal tumors are malignant, the clinical importance of accurately identifying pseudoneoplastic lesions of the kidney cannot be overemphasized.

## REFERENCES

1. Price EB Jr, Mostofi FK. Symptomatic angiomyolipoma of the kidney. *Cancer* 1965;18:761–774.
2. Hajdu SI, Foote FW Jr. Angiomyolipoma of the kidney. Report of 27 cases and review of the literature. *J Urol* 1969;102:396–401.
3. Farrow GM, Harrison EG Jr, Utz DC, Jones DR. Renal angiomyolipoma. A clinicopathologic study of 32 cases. *Cancer* 1968;22:564–570.
4. Jardin A, Richard F, Le Duc A, Chatelain C, Le Guillou M, Fourcade R, Camey M, Küss R. Diagnosis and treatment of renal angiomyolipoma (based on 15 cases). Arguments in favor of conservative surgery (based on 8 cases). *Eur Urol* 1980;6:69–82.
5. Blute ML, Malek RS, Segura JW. Angiomyolipoma. Clinical metamorphosis and concepts for management. *J Urol* 1988;139:20–24.
6. Tong YC, Chieng PU, Tsai TC, Lin SN. Renal angiomyolipoma. Report of 24 cases. *Br J Urol* 1990;66:585–589.
7. Cozar Olmo JM, Martínez-Piñeiro JA, Navarro J, Moreno JA, Martínez-Piñeiro L, Cisneros J, Avellana JA, de la Peña J. Angiomiolipoma renal. Estudio de 39 pacientes y revisión de conjunto. *Actas Urol Esp* 1992;16:749–758.
8. Mukai M, Torikata C, Iri H, Tamai S, Sugiura H, Tanaka Y, Sakamoto M, Hirohashi S. Crystalloids in angiomyolipoma. 1. A previously unnoticed phenomenon of renal angiomyolipoma occurring at a high frequency. *Am J Surg Pathol* 1992;16:1–10.
9. Gomez MR. Criteria for diagnosis. In: Gomez MR, ed. *Tuberous sclerosis*. 2nd ed. New York: Raven Press, 1988;9–19.
10. Pratt-Thomas HR. Tuberous sclerosis with congenital tumors of heart and kidney. Report of a case in a premature infant. *Am J Pathol* 1947;23:189–199.
11. Weaver RG, Carlquist JH. Two rare tumors of the renal parenchyma. *J Urol* 1957;77:351–357.
12. Oesterling JE, Fishman EK, Goldman SM, Marshall FF. The management of renal angiomyolipoma. *J Urol* 1986;135:1121–1124.
13. Bissada NK, Bissada SA, Fitts CT, Rajagopalan PR, Nelson R. Renal transplantation from living related donor after excision of angiomyolipoma of the donor kidney. *J Urol* 1993;150:174–175.
14. Vasko JS, Brockman SK, Bomar RL. Renal angiomyolipoma. A rare cause of spontaneous massive retroperitoneal hemorrhage. *Ann Surg* 1965;161:577–581.
15. Daghfous MH, Messeddi H, Guermassi M, Hached M, Ben Achour D, Robbana A, Horchani A, Ben Jaafar M. Complications hémorragiques révélatrices d'angiomyolipome rénal, à propos de deux cas. *J Urol (Paris)* 1992;98:175–177.
16. Burkitt R. Fatal haemorrhage into a perirenal liposarcoma. *Br J Surg* 1949;36:439.
17. Parry GW, McWilliam J, Ragoonan C, Harvey JS. Renal angiomyolipoma. Diagnosis and management. *Br J Clin Pract* 1991;45:290–293.
18. Valvo JR, Feinstein MJ, Wallinga H, Cockett AT. Spontaneous intrapartum rupture of renal hamartoma. *Urology* 1983;22:286–289,
19. Kragel PJ, Toker C. Infiltrating recurrent renal angiomyolipoma with fatal outcome. *J Urol* 1985;133:90–91.
20. Tweeddale DN, Dawe CJ, McDonald JR, Culp OS. Angiolipoleiomyoma of kidney. Report of a case with observations on histogenesis. *Cancer* 1995; 764–770.
21. Weeks DA, Chase DR, Malott RL, Chase RL, Zuppan CW, Beckwith JB, Mierau GW. HMB-45 staining in angiomyolipoma, cardiac rhabdomyoma, other mesenchymal processes, and tuberous sclerosis–associated brain lesions. *Int J Surg Pathol.* 1994; 1:191–198.
22. Yum M, Ganguly A, Donohue JP. Juxtaglomerular cells in renal angiomyolipoma. *Urology* 1984;24:283–286.
23. Pea M, Bonetti F, Zamboni G, Martignoni G, Riva M, Colombari R, Mombello A, Bonzanini M, Scarpa A, Ghimenton C, Donati LF. Melanocyte-marker-HMB-45 is regularly expressed in angiomyolipoma of the kidney. *Pathology* 1991;23:185–188.
24. Chan JKC, Tsang WYW, Pau MY, Tang MC, Pang SW, Fletcher CDM. Lymphangiomyomatosis and angiomyolipoma. Closely related entities characterized by hamartomatous proliferation of HMB-45 positive smooth muscle. *Histopathology* 1993;22:445–455.
25. Ashfaq R, Weinberg AG, Albores-Saavedra J. Renal angiomyolipoma and HMB-45 reactivity. *Cancer* 1993;71:3091–3097.
26. Tallarigo C, Baldassarre R, Bianchi G, Comunale L, Olivo G, Pea M, Bonetti F, Martignoni G, Zamboni G, Mobilio G. Diagnostic and therapeutic problems in multicentric renal angiomyolipoma. *J Urol* 1992;148:1880–1884.
27. Campbell EW, Brantley R, Harrold M, Simson LR. Angiomyolipoma presenting as fever of unknown origin. *Am J Med* 1974;57:843–846.
28. Scott MB, Halpern M, Cosgrove MD. Renal angiomyolipoma. Two varieties. *Urology* 1975;6:768–773.

29. Busch FM, Bark CJ, Clyde HR. Benign renal angiomyolipoma with regional lymph node involvement. *J Urol* 1976;116:715–717.

30. Bloom DA, Scardino PT, Ehrlich RM, Waisman J. The significance of lymph nodal involvement in renal angiomyolipoma. *J Urol* 1982;128:1292–1295.

31. Dao AH, Pinto AC, Kirchner FK, Halter SA. Massive nodal involvement in a case of renal angiomyolipoma. *Arch Pathol Lab Med* 1984;108:612–613.

32. Hulbert JC, Graf R. Involvement of the spleen by renal angiomyolipoma. Metastasis or multicentricity. *J Urol* 1983;130:328–329.

33. Sant GR, Ucci AA Jr, Meares EM Jr. Multicentric angiomyolipoma. Renal and lymph node involvement. *Urology* 1986;28:111–113.

34. Brecher ME, Gill WB, Straus FH II. Angiomyolipoma with regional lymph node involvement and long-term follow-up study. *Hum Pathol* 1986;17:962–963.

35. Manabe T, Moriya T, Kimoto M. Benign renal angiomyolipoma with regional lymph node involvement, report of a case showing enlargement five years after nephrectomy. *Acta Pathol Jpn* 1987;37:1853–1858.

36. Taylor RS, Joseph DB, Kohaut EC, Wilson ER, Bueschen AJ. Renal angiomyolipoma associated with lymph node involvement and renal cell carcinoma in patients with tuberous sclerosis. *J Urol* 1989;141:930–932.

37. Ro JY, Ayala AG, El-Naggar A, Grignon DJ, Hogan SF, Howard DR. Angiomyolipoma of kidney with lymph node involvement, DNA flow cytometric analysis. *Arch Pathol Lab Med* 1990;114:65–67.

38. Ansari SJ, Stephenson RA, Mackay B. Angiomyolipoma of the kidney with lymph node involvement. *Ultrastruct Pathol* 1991;15:531–538.

39. Kutcher R, Rosenblatt R, Mitsudo S, Goldman M, Kogan S. Renal angiomyolipoma with sonographic demonstration of extension into the inferior vena cava. *Radiology* 1982;143:755–756.

40. Brantley RE, Mashni JW, Bethards RE, Chernys AE, Chung WM. Computerized tomographic demonstration of inferior vena caval tumor thrombus from renal angiomyolipoma. *J Urol* 1985;133:836–837.

41. Rothenberg DM, Brandt TD, D'Cruz I. Computed tomography of renal angiomyolipoma presenting as right atrial mass. *J Comput Assist Tomogr* 1986; 10:1054–1056.

42. Camúñez F, Lafuente J, Robledo R, Echenagusia A, Pérez M, Simo G, Gálvez F. CT demonstration of extension of renal angiomyolipoma into the inferior vena cava in a patient with tuberous sclerosis. *Urol Radiol* 1987;9:152–154.

43. Arenson AM, Graham RT, Shaw P, Srigley J, Herschorn S. Angiomyolipoma of the kidney extending into the inferior vena cava. Sonographic and CT findings. *AJR* 1988;151:1159–1161.

44. Byrne DJ, Hamilton Stewart PA, Lowe JW. Malignant angiomyolipoma of the kidney associated with hypercalcemia. *Br J Urol* 1988; 62:89–90.

45. Back W, Heine M, Potempa D. Intravaskuläre Form eines Angiomyolipoms der Niere, Fallbericht und Literaturübersicht. *Pathologe* 1992;13:212–214.

46. Umeyama T, Saitoh Y, Tomaru Y, Kitaura K. Bilateral renal angiomyolipoma associated with bilateral renal vein and inferior vena caval thrombi. *J Urol* 1992;148:1885–1887.

47. Honda N, Matsuoka K, Fujimoto K, Nishimura H, Abe T, Noda S, Hayabuchi N. Renal angiomyolipoma extending into inferior vena cava. MR demonstration. *J Comput Assist Tomogr* 1993;17:161–162.

48. Weiss H, Alken P, Wehner H, Schilp M. Gibt es metastasierende Angiomyolipome? *Ultraschall Med* 1993;14:112–116.

49. Ferry JA, Malt RA, Young RH. Renal angiomyolipoma with sarcomatous transformation and pulmonary metastases. *Am J Surg Pathol* 1991;15:1083–1088.

50. Lowe BA, Brewer J, Houghton DC, Jacobson E, Pitre T. Malignant transformation of angiomyolipoma. *J Urol* 1992;147:1356–1358.

51. Saegusa M, Sakuramoto K, Hashimoto H, Uno S, Aramaki K, Johsen T. Lymphangiomyomatosis involving the kidney. A case report. *Acta Urol Jpn* 1993;39:249–252.

52. Kerr LA, Blute ML, Ryu JH, Swensen SJ, Malek RS. Renal angiomyolipoma in association with pulmonary lymphangioleiomyomatosis. Forme fruste of tuberous sclerosis? *Urology* 1993;41:440–444.

53. Monteforte WJ Jr, Kohnen PW. Angiomyolipomas in a case of lymphangiomyomatosis syndrome. Relationships to tuberous sclerosis. *Cancer* 1974;34:317–321.

54. Lack EE, Dolan MF, Finisio J, Grover G, Singh M, Triche TJ. Pulmonary and extrapulmonary lymphangioleiomyomatosis. Report of a case with bilateral renal angiomyolipomas, multifocal lymphangioleiomyomatosis and a glial polyp of the endocervix. *Am J Surg Pathol* 1986;10:650–657.

55. McIntosh GS, Hamilton Dutoit S, Chronos NV, Kaisary AV. Multiple unilateral renal angiomyolipomas with regional lymphangioleiomyomatosis. *J Urol* 1989;142:1305–1307.

56. Robertson PW, Klidjian A, Harding LK, Walters G, Lee MR, Robb-Smith AHT. Hypertension due to a renin-secreting renal tumor. *Am J Med* 1967;43:963–976.

57. Kihara I, Kitamura S, Hoshino T, Seida H, Watanabe T. A hitherto unreported vascular tumor of the kidney. A proposal of "juxtaglomerular cell tumor." *Acta Pathol Jpn* 1968;18:197–206.

58. Kihara I. Juxtaglomerular and androsterone secreting renal tumor. *Nippon Rinsho* 1971;29:952–959.

59. Lee MR. Renin-secreting kidney tumours, a rare but remediable cause of serious hypertension. *Lancet* 1971;2:254–255.

60. Eddy RL, Sanchez SA. Renin-secreting renal neoplasm and hypertension with hypokalemia. *Ann Intern Med* 1971;75:725–729.

61. Bonnin JM, Hodge RL, Lumbers ER. A renin-secreting renal tumour associated with hypertension. *Aust N Z J Med* 1972;2:178–181.

62. Phillips G, Mukherjee TM. A juxtaglomerular cell tumor. Light and electron microscopic studies of a renin-secreting kidney tumor containing both juxtaglomerular cells and mast cells. *Pathology* 1972;4:193–204.

63. Conn JW, Cohen EL, McDonald WJ, Blough WM Jr, Lucas CP, Mayor GH, Eveland WC, Bookstein JJ, Lapides J. The syndrome of hypertension, hyperreninemia and secondary aldosteronism associated with renal juxtaglomerular cell tumor (primary reninism). *J Urol* 1973;109:349–355.

64. MacCallum DK, Conn JW, Baker BL. Ultrastructure of a renin-secreting juxtaglomerular cell tumor of the kidney. *Invest Urol* 1973; 11:65–74.

65. Schambelan M, Howes EL Jr, Stockigt JR, Noakes CA, Biglieri EG. Role of renin and aldosterone in hypertension due to a renin-secreting tumor. *Am J Med* 1973;55:86–92.

66. More IAR. Renin-secreting tumor associated with hypertension. *Cancer* 1974;34:2093–2102.

67. Davidson JK, Clark DC. Renin-secreting juxtaglomerular-cell tumour. *Br J Radiol* 1974;47:594–597.

68. Lindop GBM, Stewart JA, Downie TT. The immunocytochemical demonstration of renin in a juxtaglomerular cell tumor by light and electron microscopy. *Histopathology* 1983;7:421–431.

69. Brown JJ, Lever AF, Robertson JIS, Fraser R, Morton JJ, Tree M, Bell PRF, Davidson JK, Ruthven IS. Hypertension and secondary hyperaldosteronism associated with a renin-secreting renal juxtaglomerular cell tumour. *Lancet* 1973;2:1228–1232.

70. Gherardi GH, Arya S, Hickler RB. Juxtaglomerular body tumor. A rare occult but curable cause of lethal hypertension. *Hum Pathol* 1974; 5:236–240.

71. Hirose M, Arakawa K, Kikuchi M, Kawasaki T, Omoto T, Kato H, Nagayama T. Primary reninism with renal hamartomatous alteration. *JAMA* 1974;230:1288–1292.

72. Ørjavik OS, Aas M, Fauchald P, Hovig T, ystese B, Brodwall EK, Flatmark A. Renin-secreting renal tumour with severe hypertension. Case report with tumour renin analysis. Histopathological and ultrastructural studies. *Acta Med Scand* 1975;197:329–335.

73. Connor G, Bennett CM, Lindstrom R, Paul J, Brosman S, Barajas L. Benign hypertension and juxtaglomerular cell tumor. *Kidney Int* 1975; 8:437.

74. Barajas L, Bennett CM, Connor G, Lindstrom RR. Structure of a juxtaglomerular cell tumor. The presence of a neural component. A light and electron microscopic study. *Lab Invest* 1977;37:357–368.

75. Takahashi T, Miura T, Sue A, Saito K, Sakaue M, Yamagata Y, Fukuchi S, Sato Z, Hirai T, Terashima K, Oka K, Imai Y. A case of juxtaglomerular cell tumor diagnosed preoperatively. *Nephron* 1976; 17:483–495.

76. Kida T, Takahashi T. Preoperative scintigraphic evaluation of the location of juxtaglomerular cell tumor. *Eur J Nucl Med* 1985;10:382–385.

77. Baldet P, Mimran A. Tumeur bénigne du rein à sécrétion de rénine dite "de l'appareil juxtaglomérulaire" étude optique et ultrastructurale. *Ann Anat Pathol* 1977;22:21–40.

78. Baldet P, Mimran A, Granier M, Dupont M. Formes histologiques et

ultrastructurales des tumeurs bénignes du rein avec sécrétion de rénine. *Ann Pathol* 1983;3:225–234.

79. Mimran A, Leckie BJ, Fourcade JC, Baldet P, Navratil H, Barjon P. Blood pressure, renin-angiotensin system and urinary kallikrein in a case of juxtaglomerular cell tumor. *Am J Med* 1978;65:527–536.

80. Bonnin JM, Cain MD, Jose JS, Mukherjee TM, Perrett LV, Scroop GC, Seymour AE. Hypertension due to a renin-secreting tumour localised by segmental renal vein sampling. *Aust N Z J Med* 1977; 7:630–635.

81. Warshaw BL, Anand SK, Olson DL, Grushkin CM, Heuser ET, Lieberman E. Hypertension secondary to a renin-producing juxtaglomerular cell tumor. *J Pediatr* 1979;94:247–250.

82. Hanna W, Tepperman B, Logan AG, Robinette MA, Colapinto R, Phillips MJ. Juxtaglomerular cell tumour (reninoma) with paroxysmal hypertension. *Can Med Assoc J* 1979;120:957–959.

83. Valdés G, Lopez JM, Martinez P, Rosenberg H, Barriga P, Rodriguez JA, Otipka N. Renin-secreting tumor. Case report. *Hypertension* 1980;2:714–718.

84. El Matri A, Slim R, Hamida Ch, Chadli A, Ben Maiz H, Haddad S, Milliez P, Camilleri JP, Zmerli S, Ben Ayed H. Hypertension artérielle secondaire à une "tumeur à rénine." Une observation. *Nouv Presse Med* 1980;9:157–159.

85. Slim R, El Materi A, Ben Maiz H, Ben Ayed H, Fourati A. Aspects radiologiques de la tumeur à rénine. *J Radiol Electrol Med Nucl* 1979; 60:287–289.

86. Lam ASC, Bédard YC, Buckspan MB, Logan AG, Steinhardt MI. Surgically curable hypertension associated with reninoma. *J Urol* 1982; 128:572–575.

87. Moss AH, Peterson LJ, Scott CW, Winter K, Olin DB, Garber RL. Delayed diagnosis of juxtaglomerular cell tumor hypertension. *N C Med J* 1982;43:705–707.

88. Jordan JM, Gunnells JC. Juxtaglomerular apparatus tumor. A rare but curable cause of secondary hypertension. *South Med J* 1985;78: 1353–1356.

89. Sanfilippo F, Pizzo SV, Croker BP. Immunohistochemical studies of cell differentiation in a juxtaglomerular tumor. *Arch Pathol Lab Med* 1982;106:604–607.

90. Furosato M, Hayashi H, Kawaguchi N, Yokota K, Saito K, Aizawa S, Ishikawa E. Juxtaglomerular cell tumor, with special reference to the tubular component in regards to its histogenesis. *Acta Pathol Jpn* 1983;33:609–618.

91. Dunnick NR, Hartman DS, Ford KK, Davis CJ Jr, Amis ES Jr. The radiology of juxtaglomerular cell tumors. *Radiology* 1983;147: 321–326.

92. Squires JP, Ulbright TM, DeSchryver-Kecskemeti K, Engleman W. Juxtaglomerular cell tumor of the kidney. *Cancer* 1984;53:516–523.

93. Hradec E, Hork K. Nádor juxtaglomerulárního aparátu ledviny. *Rozhl Chir* 1984;63:262–268.

94. Galen FX, Devaux C, Houot AM, Menard J, Corvol P, Corvol MT, Gubler MC, Mounier F, Camilleri JP. Renin biosynthesis by human tumoral juxtaglomerular cells. Evidence for a renin precursor. *J Clin Invest* 1984;73:1144–1155.

95. Camilleri JP, Hinglais N, Bruneval P, Bariety J, Tricottet V, Rouchon M, Mancilla-Jimenez R, Corvol P, Menard J. Renin storage and cell differentiation in juxtaglomerular cell tumors. An immunohistochemical and ultrastructural study of three cases. *Hum Pathol* 1984;15: 1069–1079.

96. Baruch D, Corvol P, Alhenc-Gelas F, Dufloux M-A, Guyenne TT, Gaux J-C, Raynaud A, Brisset J-M, Duclos J-M, Menard J. Diagnosis and treatment of renin-secreting tumors. Report of three cases. *Hypertension* 1984;6:760–766.

97. Baruch D, Dufloux M, Guyenne TT, Gaux JC, Raynaud A, Brisset JM, Duclos JM, Corvol P, Ménard J. Trois cas de tumeur à rénine d'origine rénale. Méthodes diagnostiques et traitement. *Arch Mal Coeur* 1983;76:81–86.

98. Corvol P, Pinet F, Galen FX, Plouin PF, Chatellier G, Pagny JY, Corvol MT, Ménard J. Seven lessons from seven renin secreting tumors. *Kidney Int* 1988;Suppl 34, Suppl. 25:S-38–S-44.

99. Raynaud A, Chatellier G, Baruch D, Angel C, Menard J, Gaux JC. Radiologic features of renin-producing tumors. A report of two cases. *Ann Radiol* 1985;28:439–446.

100. Tetu B, Totovic V, Bechtelsheimer H, Smend J. Tumeur rénale à sécrétion de rénine, à propos d'un cas avec étude ultrastructurale et immunohistochimique. *Ann Pathol* 1984;4:55–59.

101. Têtu B, Vaillancourt L, Camilleri JP, Bruneval P, Bernier L, Tourigny R. Juxtaglomerular cell tumor of the kidney. Report of two cases with a papillary pattern. *Hum Pathol* 1993;24:1168–1174.

102. Dennis RL, McDougal WS, Glick AD, MacDonnell RC Jr. Juxtaglomerular cell tumor of the kidney. *J Urol* 1985;134:334–338.

103. Hermus ARMM, Pieters GFFM, Lamers APM, Smals AGH, Hanselaar AGJM, Van Haelst UJG, Kloppenborg PWC. Hypertension and hypokalemia due to a renin-secreting kidney tumour. *Neth J Med* 1986;29:84–91.

104. van den Berg JC, Hermus ARMM, Rosenbusch GR. Juxtaglomerular cell tumour of the kidney as cause of hypertension. A case report. *Br J Radiol* 1992;65:542–545.

105. Handa N, Fukunaga R, Yoneda S, Kimura K, Kamada T, Ichikawa Y, Takaha M, Sonoda T, Tokunaga K, Kuroda C, Onishi S. State of systemic hemodynamics in a case of juxtaglomerular cell tumor. *Clin Exp Hypertens [A]* 1986;8:1–19.

106. Guo JZ, Gong LS, Qiu XC. A case of juxtaglomerular cell tumor (reninism). Diagnostic methods and treatment. *Chung Hua Nei Ko Tsa Chih* 1986;25:25–27.

107. Martínez Amenós A, Carreras L, Rama H, Romero M, Sarrias X, Alsina J; Tumor de células del aparato yuxtaglomerular secretor de renina. *Med Clin (Barc)* 1987;88:157–159.

108. Pedrinelli R, Graziadei L, Taddei S, Lenzi M, Magagna A, Bevilacqua G, Salvetti A. A renin-secreting tumor. *Nephron* 1987;46:380–385.

109. Tierney JP, McClellan WT, Cuadra WD. Surgically curable hypertension associated with juxtaglomerular cell tumor. *W V Med J* 1988;84: 233–234.

110. Remynse LC, Begun FP, Jacobs SC, Lawson RK. Juxtaglomerular cell tumor with elevation of serum erythropoietin. *J Urol* 1989;142: 1560–1562.

111. Schonfeld AD, Jackson JA, Somerville SP, Johnson CF, Anderson PW. Renin-secreting juxtaglomerular cell tumor causing severe hypertension. Diagnosis by computerized tomography-directed needle biopsy. *J Urol* 1991;146:1607–1609.

112. López G-Asenjo JA, Blanco González J, Ortega Medina L, Sanz Esponera J. Juxtaglomerular cell tumor of the kidney. Morphological, immunohistochemical and ultrastructural studies of a new case. *Pathol Res Pract* 1991;187:354–359.

113. Rossi GP, Zanin L, Dessí-Fulgheri P, Savastano S, Cavazzana A, Prayer-Galetti T, Rappeli A, Pessina AC. A renin-secreting tumour with severe hypertension and cardiovascular disease. A diagnostic and therapeutic challenge. *Clin Exp Hypertens [A]* 1993;15:325–338.

114. Garel L, Robitaille P, Dubois J, Russo P. Pediatric case of the day. *Radiographics* 1993;13:477–479.

115. Kreutz R, Zhou H, Pfeifer U, Gasc JM, Ganten D, Kessler FJ. Primärer hyperreninismus. Eine seltene usache der sekundären arteriellen hypertonie. *Dtsch Med Wochenschr* 1993;118:1110–1114.

116. Uno M, Yamada S, Ozeki S, Okano M, Deguchi T, Kuriyama M, Ban Y, Kawada Y, Okumura N, Tanaka T, Hoshiyama N, Nojiri M. Renin-secreting renal tumor. A case report. *Nippon Hinyokika Gakkai Zasshi* 1993;84:1130–1133.

117. Tanaka T, Okumura A, Mori H. Juxtaglomerular cell tumor. *Arch Pathol Lab Med* 1993;117:1161–1164.

118. Armato U, D'Agostino D, Romano F, Salvetti A, Mantero F. Long-term preservation of renin-secreting ability by human adult juxtaglomerular tumor cells in explant culture. *Jpn J Cancer Res* 1993;84: 734–741.

119. Barajas L. The development and ultrastructure of the juxtaglomerular cell granule. *J Ultrastruct Res* 1966;15:400–413.

120. Lindop GBM, Fleming S, Gibson AAM. Immunocytochemical localisation of renin in nephroblastoma. *J Clin Pathol* 1984;37:738–742.

121. Ganguly A, Gribble J, Tune B, Kempson RL, Luetscher JA. Renin-secreting Wilms' tumor with severe hypertension. Report of a case and brief review of renin-secreting tumors. *Ann Intern Med* 1973;79: 835–837.

122. Hollifield JW, Page DL, Smith C, Michelakis AM, Staab E, Rhamy R. Renin-secreting clear cell carcinoma of the kidney. *Arch Intern Med* 1975;135:859–864.

123. Cook HT, Taylor GM, Malone P, Risdon RA. Renin in mesoblastic nephroma. An immunohistochemical study. *Hum Pathol* 1988;19: 1347–1351.

124. Tsuchida Y, Shimizu K, Hata J, Honna T, Nishiura M. Renin production in congenital mesoblastic nephroma in comparison with that in Wilms' tumor. *Pediatr Pathol* 1993;13:155–164.

*Pathology of Pseudoneoplastic Lesions,*
edited by M. R. Wick, P. A. Humphrey, and J. H. Ritter.
Lippincott-Raven Publishers, Philadelphia © 1997.

CHAPTER **8**

# Pseudoneoplastic Lesions of the Urinary Bladder, Prostate Gland, and Urethra

Robert H. Young

## THE URINARY BLADDER

A listing of pseudoneoplastic lesions of the urinary bladder is presented in Table 1. These include some, but not all, of the nonneoplastic lesions of the urinary bladder listed by the World Health Organization as epithelial abnormalities and tumor-like lesions (1). Those not responsible for pathologic misdiagnosis as a neoplasm are omitted, and several recently described entities are added. The lesions discussed may simulate a neoplasm clinically and/or pathologically, and emphasis here is placed on the diagnostic problems that they may pose for the surgical pathologist.

### Von Brunn's Nests

Von Brunn's nests are typically rounded, well-circumscribed, superficial nests of transitional cells devoid of significant atypia and in such cases pose no diagnostic difficulty. Diagnostic problems may arise when von Brunn's nests lie relatively deep in the lamina propria (Fig. 1), this

R. H. Young: Department of Pathology, Harvard Medical School and Massachusetts General Hospital, Boston, Massachussetts 02114.

**TABLE 1.** *Pseudoneoplastic lesions of the urinary bladder*

Von Brunn's nests
Cystitis glandularis (including mucinous metaplasia)
Nephrogenic adenoma
Papillary-polypoid cystitis
Fallopian tube prolapse
Giant cell cystitis
Radiation cystitis
Malakoplakia
Polyps
Hamartomas
Endocervicosis and Müllerianosis
Postoperative spindle cell nodule
Inflammatory pseudotumor
Paraganglia

displacement from the overlying epithelium occasionally resulting in a misdiagnosis of carcinoma. Although the bland histology of the cells in von Brunn's nests contrasts with the significant atypia seen in most invasive bladder cancers, it should be remembered that the epithelium in von Brunn's nests, like the surface epithelium, may exhibit hyperplasia and reactive atypia, including mitotic activity. It is helpful that invasive carcinoma of the bladder usually exhibits irregular infiltration of the stroma by nests of cells and single cells with moderate to marked atypia, often with an associated stromal response. Occasionally, however, invasive carcinoma has a pushing margin, or is composed of well-circumscribed nests of cells with slight atypia and has an appearance that may be difficult to distinguish from von Brunn's nests (2,3). Even when invasive carcinoma has relatively bland cytologic features, the cell nests generally have a more disorderly arrangement and more variation in size and shape than von Brunn's nests.

## Cystitis Glandularis (Including Mucinous Metaplasia)

Although usually a microscopic finding, cystitis glandularis is occasionally visible grossly. Worrisome-appearing, fleshy polypoid lesions may rarely be present, particularly in cases of the intestinal type of cystitis glandularis, and occasionally the radiologic and/or cystoscopic appearance of cystitis glandularis suggests a malignant tumor (4–10). On microscopic examination the lesion usually occurs in a nonpolypoid mucosa (Fig. 2) but occasionally an exuberant proliferation produces a papillary or polypoid lesion (4,6,10), helping to explain the occasional case that simulates a neoplasm at cystoscopy.

On microscopic examination problems usually arise in cases of the intestinal, rather than the typical, form of cystitis glandularis. Even with a very florid proliferation, the glands retain an essentially orderly arrangement (Fig. 3) and lack the irregular stromal infiltration that generally facilitates the diagnosis of adenocarcinoma. Additionally, the atypicality in most adenocarcinomas exceeds that seen in cystitis glandularis. However, cases are encountered in which distinction from adenocarcinoma has been very difficult. In one case (11), two distinguished pathologists disagreed over the benign or malignant nature of a glandular proliferation; in another case misinterpretation of cystitis glandularis led to an unnecessary cystectomy (12). Rarely, mucin extravasation into the stroma is seen in cases of cystitis glandularis (12A) (Fig. 3). Cases in which there is an irregular disposition of the glands in the stroma, glands deep in the lamina propria, and cytologic atypia, even if minor, increase the likelihood of glands being neoplastic (2). Finally, it should be noted that as cystitis glandularis of the intestinal type may progress to adenocarcinoma (13), cases meriting the designation "cystitis glandularis with atypia" are seen. Occasionally mucinous epithelium, including that showing intestinal metaplasia, may replace the lining urothelium (see Fig. 2). This is usually associated with underlying cystitis

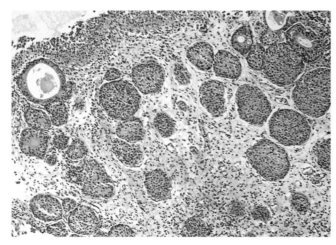

**FIG. 1.** Von Brunn's nests. Well-circumscribed round to oval nests of transitional cells are conspicuous, and extend deeply, within the lamina propria.

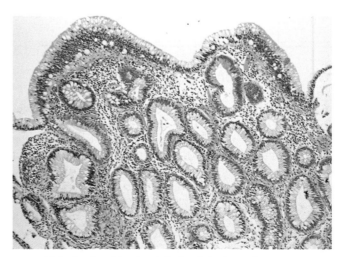

**FIG. 2.** Cystitis glandularis of the intestinal type.

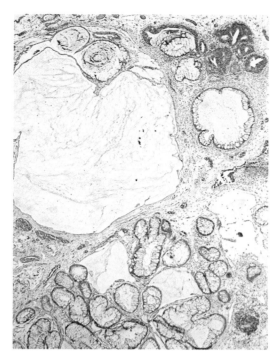

**FIG. 3.** Cystitis glandularis of the intestinal type. There is focal extravasation of mucin into the stroma.

glandularis of the typical or intestinal type but may be seen on its own. In the latter situation, the lesion should be referred to as mucinous metaplasia if the epithelium is nonintestinal in type, or intestinal metaplasia.

### Nephrogenic Adenoma (Nephrogenic Metaplasia, Adenomatous Metaplasia)

At cystoscopy nephrogenic adenoma may simulate a papillary, sessile, or in-situ carcinoma (14–23). Approximately 55% of the lesions are papillary, 10% polypoid, and 35% sessile. The lesions vary from incidentally discovered microscopic lesions to masses up to 7 cm in size. Approximately 60% are 1 cm or less, 30% between 1 and 4 cm, and 10% larger than 4 cm. They are typically single but almost 20% are multiple; rarely there is diffuse bladder involvement.

On microscopic examination tubular (Fig. 4), cystic (Fig. 5), polypoid (Fig. 6), papillary (Fig. 7), and rarely diffuse (solid) (Fig. 8) patterns are encountered. Occasionally the cells grow in cords (Fig. 9) or singly (Fig. 10). The tubules are usually small, round, and hollow but are occasionally larger, elongated, and solid. Occasionally the tubules have a complex branching pattern (Fig. 11). The tubules may grow in a striking band-like fashion (Fig. 12). They are sometimes surrounded by a prominent basement membrane (Fig. 13). The tubules frequently undergo varying degrees of cystic dilatation, and cysts, which are present in most cases, sometimes predominate (see Fig. 5). The tubules and cysts may contain an eosinophilic or basophilic secretion that is usually

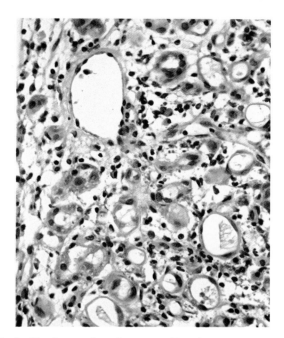

**FIG. 4.** Nephrogenic adenoma. Classic pattern of small tubules lined with cuboidal cells.

mucicarminophilic. Papillae are less common than tubules and cysts but are not rare. In some cases a striking pattern of numerous small papillae budding from larger papillae is seen (23) (Fig. 14). Occasionally larger, broader, polypoid structures are present (Fig. 15). Foci with a diffuse growth (see Fig. 8) are always limited in extent in my experience.

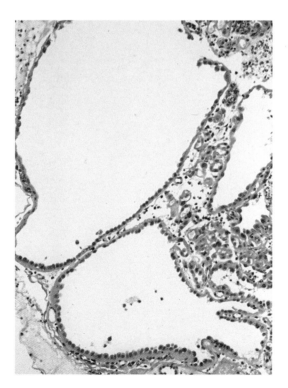

**FIG. 5.** Nephrogenic adenoma. Cystic pattern.

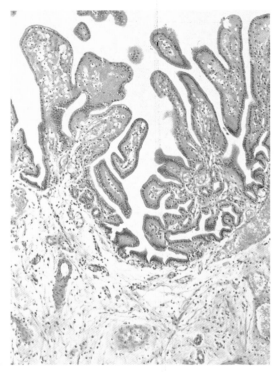

**FIG. 6.** Nephrogenic adenoma. Polypoid pattern. Note the minimal associated tubular component.

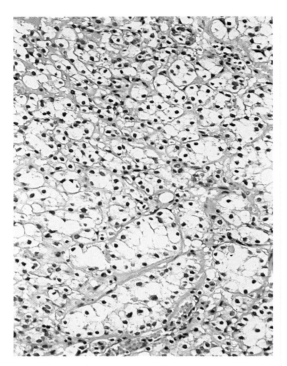

**FIG. 8.** Nephrogenic adenoma. Diffuse pattern *(top left)* and solid tubular pattern *(bottom* and *right)*. The cells have abundant clear cytoplasm.

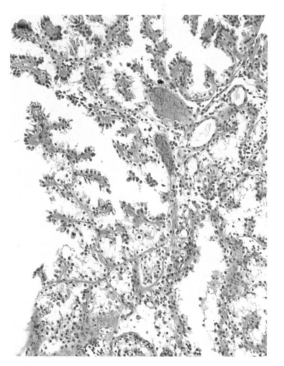

**FIG. 7.** Nephrogenic adenoma. Delicate thin papillae are present.

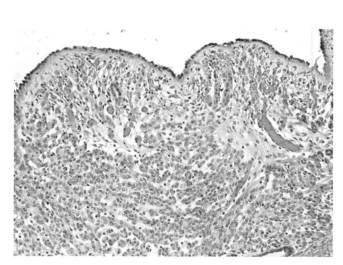

**FIG. 9.** Nephrogenic adenoma. There is a prominent pattern of thin cords.

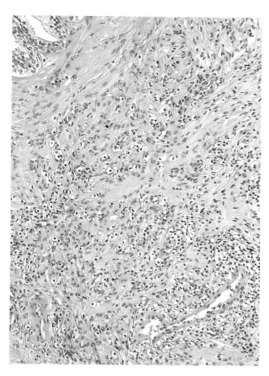

**FIG. 10.** Nephrogenic adenoma. The lesional cells are arranged in small clusters and singly.

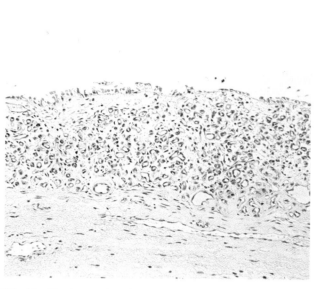

**FIG. 12.** Nephrogenic adenoma. The tubules are growing in a band-like fashion beneath the mucosa.

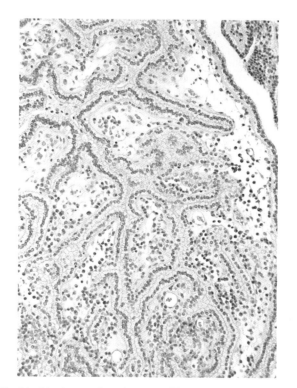

**FIG. 11.** Nephrogenic adenoma. The tubules have a complex branching pattern.

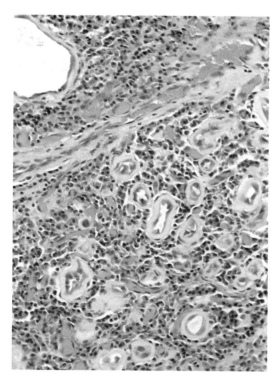

**FIG. 13.** Nephrogenic adenoma. The tubules have prominent basement membranes.

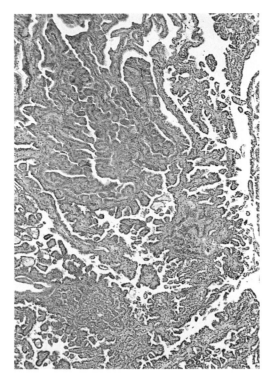

FIG. 14. Nephrogenic adenoma. There is a prominent papillary pattern with numerous small papillae budding off of larger papillae.

The majority of the cells lining the tubules, cysts, and papillae are cuboidal to low columnar with scant cytoplasm, but occasionally the lining cells or those in the solid areas have abundant clear cytoplasm. Hobnail cells line some tubules and cysts in up to 70% of the cases (Fig. 16) (23), and large cysts may be lined with flattened cells. Small amounts of mucin may be present in the cells of nephrogenic adenoma but glycogen is absent or scanty in our experience. Nuclear

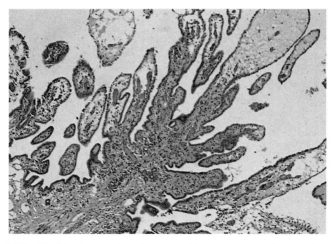

FIG. 15. Nephrogenic adenoma. There are prominent edematous polyps. A few small tubules are present at the base of the polyps and provide a clue to the diagnosis. (Courtesy of Dr. John Eble.)

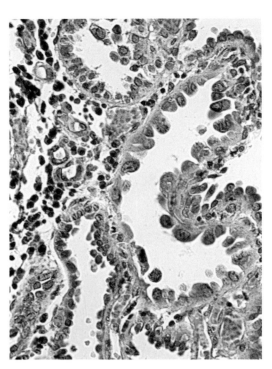

FIG. 16. Nephrogenic adenoma. Tubules and cysts are predominantly lined with hobnail cells.

atypia is uncommon, and when present appears degenerative. Mitoses are absent or rare.

Several features of nephrogenic adenoma may cause particular diagnostic difficulty. Tiny tubules containing mucin and apparently lined with a single layer of cells with compressed nuclei may simulate signet ring cells (Fig. 17); at least one nephrogenic adenoma was initially misdiagnosed as a signet ring cell adenocarcinoma (24). The haphazard distribution of the tubules or single cell growth (see Fig. 10) may also simulate the appearance of an invasive adenocarcinoma, a resemblance that is enhanced when the tubules are admixed with the muscle fibers that may be found in the lamina propria. Hobnail cells (see Fig. 16) may suggest the diagnosis of the rare clear cell carcinoma of the bladder, particularly because the latter, like nephrogenic adenoma, has tubular, cystic, and papillary patterns (25). A solid growth of cells with clear cytoplasm may also raise the possibility of clear cell carcinoma. A variety of clinical and pathologic differences as outlined in Table 2 should enable the distinction of these two lesions, although this is occasionally difficult. Clear cell carcinoma is less common in the bladder than in the urethra and in our experience distinction between nephrogenic adenoma and clear cell carcinoma is more troublesome in the urethra, particularly within a urethral diverticulum (see section on urethra). Although they persist or recur in about one third of the cases, nephrogenic adenomas are benign. Evidence suggesting that nephrogenic adenoma is a precursor of clear cell carcinoma of the bladder is not convincing. That clear cell carcinoma is much more common in the urethra and in women whereas nephrogenic ade-

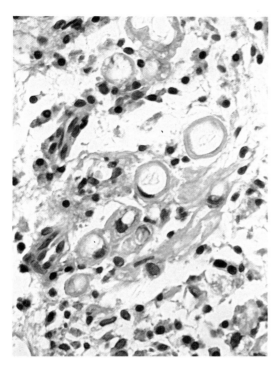

**FIG. 17.** Nephrogenic adenoma. Small tubules, some of which appear to be lined with a single cell, contain intraluminal mucin, and simulate signet ring cells.

noma is more common in the bladder and in men argues against such a relationship.

There has recently been an upsurge of appreciation that some low-grade transitional cell carcinomas may mimic nephrogenic adenoma. This arises in cases of transitional cell carcinoma with relatively bland-appearing tubules with lumens, suggesting the hollow tubules of nephrogenic adenoma, or tumors with nests (nested transitional cell carcinoma), suggesting the solid tubules that may be seen in nephrogenic adenoma (2,3). For example, case 1 in a series of carcinomas of the bladder with deceptively benign-appearing foci reported by Talbert and Young (2) was initially

misdiagnosed as nephrogenic adenoma because of the small tubules illustrated in figure 1 of that paper. A feature helpful in distinguishing these neoplastic tubules from those of nephrogenic adenoma is that the former often show a peripheral layer of one or more transitional cells whereas in nephrogenic adenoma there is a single, usually cuboidal to columnar cell lining the tubules without peripheral transitional cells. Additionally, in some nephrogenic adenomas an appreciable basement membrane around the tubules supports that interpretation, whereas that finding is absent around the tubules of transitional cell carcinoma. Finally, the carcinomas usually show focal, admittedly somewhat subtle, cytologic atypicality and lack the other patterns that are so often present in nephrogenic adenoma.

**Papillary-Polypoid Cystitis**

At cystoscopy or on microscopic examination this lesion may be confused with transitional cell carcinoma (26–29). The designation papillary cystitis is used when thin, finger-like papillae are present (Fig. 18), and the term polypoid cystitis is used when the lesions are edematous and broad-based (Fig. 19). In both papillary and polypoid cystitis there is typically prominent chronic inflammation in the stroma, and blood vessels, some of them ectatic, may be conspicuous. As papillary and polypoid cystitis are usually associated with inflammation, there may be metaplastic changes in the lesional or adjacent urothelium.

The two particular clinical settings that should suggest that an exophytic bladder lesion may be inflammatory are an indwelling catheter and a vesical fistula. Polypoid cystitis was found in 80% of the patients with an indwelling catheter in one study (28); although usually of microscopic size, grossly visible polypoid lesions up to 0.5 cm in diameter that typically involved the dome or posterior wall were seen in

**TABLE 2.** Comparison of nephrogenic adenoma and clear cell carcinoma of bladder

| Feature | Nephrogenic adenoma | Clear cell carcinoma |
|---|---|---|
| Sex distribution | Male predominance | Female predominance |
| Age distribution | One third under 30 y | Rare under 45 y |
| Predisposing factors | Common | Absent |
| Large size | Rare | Common |
| Diffuse pattern | Rare | Common |
| Clear cells | Rare | Common |
| Cytoplasmic glycogen | Rare | Abundant |
| Atypia/mitoses | Rare | Common |

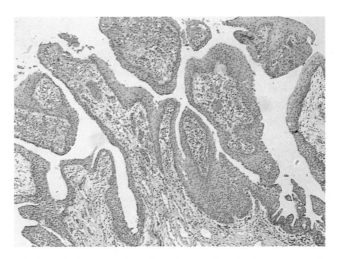

**FIG. 18.** Papillary cystitis. Papillae are lined with metaplastic squamous epithelium, and the cores of the papillae contain prominent blood vessels and inflammatory cells.

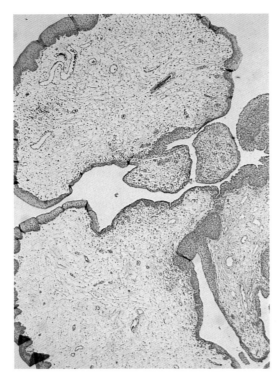

**FIG. 19.** Polypoid cystitis. Large, edematous polyps are covered by metaplastic squamous epithelium.

approximately one third of the cases. The entire bladder may be involved when a catheter has been present for a prolonged period, usually 6 months or more. Although a catheter is typically associated with polypoid cystitis, occasionally it is associated with papillary cystitis (29).

The mucosal changes associated with a vesical fistula may have the characteristics of polypoid cystitis (30–35) or, less commonly, papillary cystitis (32,36), or, occasionally, an inflammatory lesion may lack the specific features of papillary or polypoid cystitis but may mimic a neoplasm clinically (37,38). As extravesical symptoms are absent, at least initially, in approximately half of the cases, diagnostic difficulty may occur in these cases. For example, in one series of patients with bladder involvement secondary to Crohn's disease, 50% of the patients had symptoms of frequency, urgency, and dysuria before the diagnosis of inflammatory bowel disease was established (33). The cystoscopic appearance was considered suspicious for carcinoma in at least 4 of 30 cases of vesicointestinal fistula in one study (32), and on microscopic examination the appearances were characteristic of either papillary or polypoid cystitis. In another series 6 of 14 patients were referred with the diagnosis of a suspected bladder tumor (39) and lesions suspicious for carcinoma have been recorded by others (30).

The major differential diagnosis of papillary and polypoid cystitis is with papillary transitional cell carcinoma. Cases of papillary and polypoid cystitis without a history of catheterization are particularly likely to be considered carcinomas at

cystoscopy. On gross and microscopic examination, the fronds of polypoid cystitis are typically much broader than those of a papillary carcinoma, although the thin papillae of papillary cystitis are more difficult to distinguish from carcinoma. In both types of cystitis, the urothelium may be hyperplastic but usually is not as stratified as in a carcinoma; additionally, umbrella cells are more often present. The fibrovascular cores of the papillae of a transitional cell carcinoma typically lack the edema of polypoid cystitis and the prominent inflammation of both papillary and polypoid cystitis. Large papillae of a transitional cell carcinoma also often give rise to smaller papillae, a feature not associated with papillary or polypoid cystitis. Finally, significant cytologic atypia within a papillary lesion or the adjacent urothelium favors a diagnosis of carcinoma.

### Fallopian Tube Prolapse

In one remarkable case a patient with a vesicovaginal fistula that developed 3 months after a total abdominal hysterectomy was found to have a polypoid mass at the bladder base that was interpreted clinically as papillary carcinoma (40). However, microscopic examination showed fragments of fallopian tube (Fig. 20), the case representing a unique case of fallopian tube prolapse after hysterectomy.

### Giant Cell Cystitis

Atypical mononucleated or multinucleated mesenchymal cells are a relatively frequent finding in the lamina propria of the bladder (Fig. 21) (41). Wells (42) found them in one third

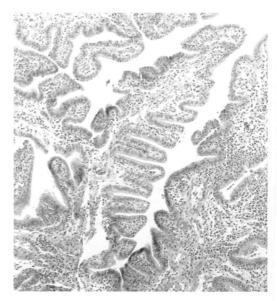

**FIG. 20.** Fallopian tube prolapse into bladder. (Courtesy of Dr. Bhagirath Majmudar.)

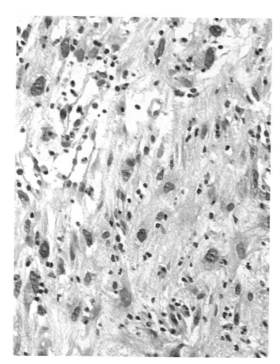

**FIG. 21.** Giant cell cystitis. Atypical mesenchymal cells are present in the superficial lamina propria.

of cases of cystitis at autopsy and applied the term "giant cell cystitis" to those cases. Cells of this type, which are relatively common in routine biopsies without significant cystitis, often have tapering eosinophilic cytoplasmic processes and may simulate both smooth or skeletal muscle cells. Their nuclei are typically hyperchromatic and often irregular in size and shape but mitotic figures are typically absent. The cells resemble those that may be seen in various benign mesenchymal tumors and in the stroma of the female genital tract. Similar cells may be seen in patients treated with chemotherapeutic agents (43) and radiation (44–46). These atypical stromal cells rarely cause serious diagnostic problems but may when found in the stroma of another lesion (see section on polyps).

## Radiation Cystitis

In cases of radiation cystitis the urothelium may show cytologic atypia (44,45). Cytoplasmic and nuclear vacuolation, karyorrhexis, and a normal nuclear/cytoplasmic ratio are features suggestive of radiation injury (46). Atypical mesenchymal cells similar to those seen in giant cell cystitis are also typically present in the lamina propria (Fig. 22). Other characteristic changes of radiation injury, including marked stromal edema or fibrosis (see Fig. 22), prominent telangiectatic vessels, hyalinization, and thrombosis of the vessels are also helpful.

## Malakoplakia

On gross examination the lesions in malakoplakia are often multiple (Fig. 23) and are typically soft yellow or yellow–brown plaques frequently with central umbilication and a hyperemic rim (47,48). They typically measure <2 cm; however, larger nodules are seen in approximately one quarter of the cases and occasionally striking papillary or polypoid tumor–like lesions are seen. On microscopic examination there is a characteristic infiltrate beneath a typically intact urothelium of mononuclear histiocytes with granular eosinophilic cytoplasm (Fig. 24) and the diagnostic intracytoplasmic Michaelis–Gutmann bodies (Fig. 25). In late stages of malakoplakia the picture may be complicated by extensive granulation tissue and fibrosis and in all stages a prominent inflammatory cell infiltrate may partially obscure the nature of the process. Carcinomas of the bladder containing cells with abundant eosinophilic cytoplasm are rare, and malakoplakia should be carefully excluded before such an uncommon tumor is diagnosed.

## Fibroepithelial Polyps

Atypical mesenchymal cells of the type sometimes seen in cases of cystitis have occurred in one fibroepithelial polyp (Fig. 26) (49) and suggested the possible diagnosis of sar-

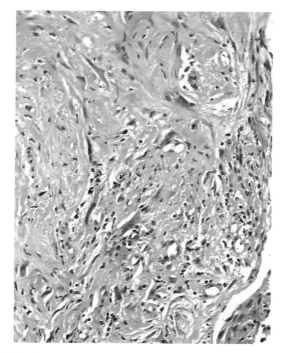

**FIG. 22.** Radiation cystitis. The lamina propria is fibrotic and hyalinized and contains scattered atypical mesenchymal cells.

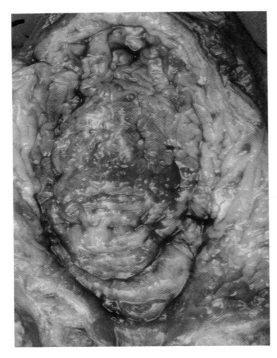

**FIG. 23.** Malakoplakia. Numerous small nodules are present in the bladder mucosa. (Courtesy of Dr. John Eble.)

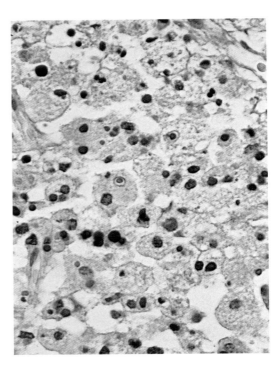

**FIG. 25.** Malakoplakia of the bladder. Several of the eosinophilic histiocytes (Von Hansemann cells) contain targetoid eosinophilic inclusions (Michaelis–Gutmann bodies).

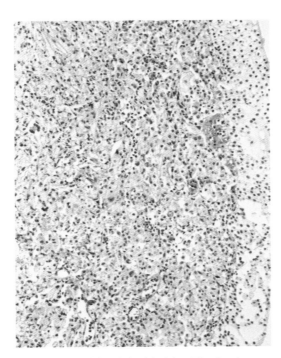

**FIG. 24.** Malakoplakia of the bladder. The lamina propria is effaced by a dense proliferation of histiocytes with abundant eosinophilic cytoplasm.

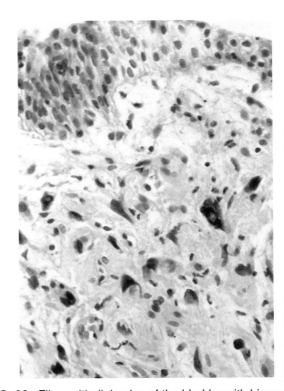

**FIG. 26.** Fibroepithelial polyp of the bladder with bizarre nuclei in stroma.

coma botryoides on microscopic examination. An absence of a cambium layer, rhabdomyoblasts and mitotic activity helped establish the diagnosis.

## Hamartomas

Hamartomas of the bladder have typically been polypoid and composed microscopically of foci resembling von Brunn's nests, cystitis glandularis, or cystitis cystica (Fig. 27) dispersed irregularly in a stroma that varies from muscular to fibrous or edematous. One case involved a markedly cellular stroma, particularly around the glandular component (50), suggesting the possible diagnosis of a low-grade neoplasm, but current evidence points to a nonneoplastic nature for these rare lesions.

## Endocervicosis and Müllerianosis

Recently six tumor-like glandular lesions characterized by a prominent component of endocervical-type epithelium that involved the wall of the urinary bladder in women of reproductive age were reported and one example of a similar lesion is present in the prior literature (51,52). Five patients presented with bladder symptoms. In each patient a mass that ranged from 2 to 5 cm was typically located in the posterior wall or posterior dome. Microscopic examination typically reveals extensive involvement of the involved bladder wall by irregularly disposed benign-appearing or mildly atypical endocervical-type glands, some of which are cystically dilated (Figs. 28 and 29). Occasionally one may find ciliated cells or a minor component of endometrioid glands and glands lined with nonspecific cuboidal or flattened cells with eosinophilic cytoplasm. In some cases the glands are associated with fibrosis, edema, or extravasated mucin in the adjacent stroma (Fig. 30). Although primarily intramural, mu-

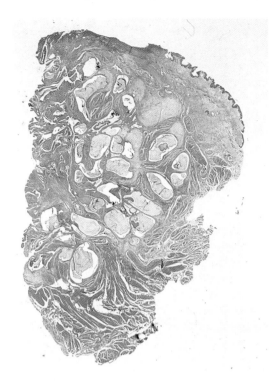

**FIG. 28.** Endocervicosis. Numerous mucinous glands and cysts permeate the bladder wall. (Courtesy of Dr. Philip B. Clement.)

cosal involvement may be seen (Fig. 31). Rarely there is a focal endometriotic stroma, indicating a relationship of this lesion to endometriosis. This and other features, such as an occasional association with a history of a cesarean section, indicate that this is a unique Müllerian lesion of the bladder and represents the mucinous analogue of endometriosis. Lack of awareness of this entity may lead to a misdiagnosis of adenocarcinoma.

Rarely, endosalpingiosis is seen in the bladder associated with endocervicosis or endometriosis leading to usage of the designation "Müllerianosis" (52).

## Postoperative Spindle Cell Nodule

This designation was given by Proppe et al. (53) in 1984 to a proliferative spindle cell lesion that developed in the lower urinary tract of five men and the lower genital tract of four women. All of the lesions developed within 3 months after a surgical procedure had been performed at the same site. Two of the lesions in men were in specimens obtained by transurethral resection of the bladder; both men had had a similar procedure performed two months previously. At cystoscopy a "heaped-up tumor" and a "friable vegetant mass" were noted, respectively.

Microscopic examination reveals intersecting fascicles of spindle cells (Fig. 32), which often show striking mitotic activity, resulting in a marked resemblance to a sarcoma, particularly leiomyosarcoma. The cells, however, do not exhibit

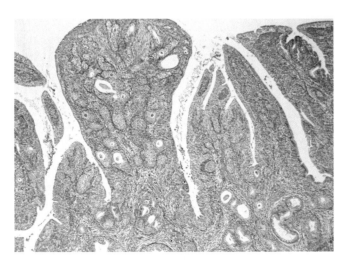

**FIG. 27.** Hamartoma of the bladder. Polyps are composed of nests of epithelium resembling von Brunn's nests, cystitis glandularis, and cystitis cystica. (Courtesy of Dr. Athanase Billis.)

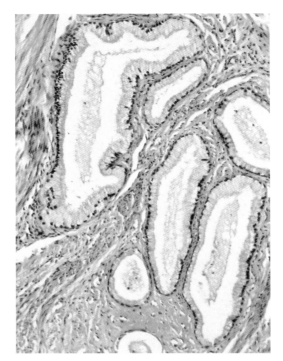

**FIG. 29.** Endocervicosis. Glands lined by benign columnar mucinous epithelium lie in the muscularis propria of the bladder.

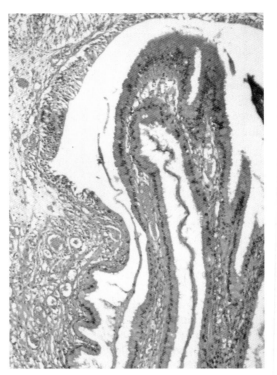

**FIG. 31.** Endocervicosis. Mucinous epithelium focally replaces the urothelium at the bottom left and a polypoid projection of the endocervicosis is present in the bladder lumen.

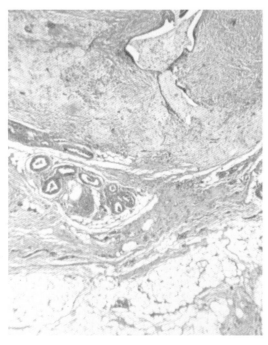

**FIG. 30.** Endocervicosis. The process has extended almost into the perivesical fat, which is seen at the bottom. Glands of endocervicosis are seen at the top. One of them has ruptured, and there is a reaction to extravasated mucin in the adjacent tissue.

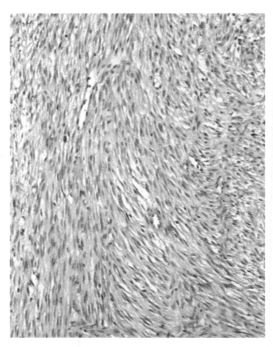

**FIG. 32.** Postoperative spindle cell nodule. Interlacing fascicles of spindle cells impart a resemblance to leiomyosarcoma.

significant cytologic atypia. Additional microscopic features that are often present include prominent blood vessels (Fig. 33), which are often small; scattered, acute and chronic inflammatory cells; small foci of hemorrhage; mild to moderate edema; and focal myxoid change in the stroma. The clinical association with a recent operation was the major initial clue that these lesions represented an exuberant reactive proliferation, an interpretation supported by the benign outcome after conservative management of the initially and subsequently reported cases (54,55).

Although other sarcomas, such as Kaposi's sarcoma, occasionally are suggested, leiomyosarcoma is usually the major consideration in differential diagnosis. Distinction from a moderate to poorly differentiated leiomyosarcoma is not difficult, as the atypia in these cases exceeds that seen in a postoperative spindle cell nodule (PSCN). However, some well-differentiated leiomyosarcomas do not appear much more atypical cytologically than a PSCN and may be less mitotically active than a PSCN. Although one might expect destructive growth to be helpful in this differential diagnosis, the PSCN may invade the muscular wall of the bladder. Although leiomyosarcomas may be vascular, the often prominent delicate network of small blood vessels that is seen in many PSCNs is, in our opinion, more in keeping with a diagnosis of PSCN than sarcoma. Myxoid change may be seen in both PSCN and leiomyosarcoma, and is not particularly helpful diagnostically, although extremely prominent myxoid change perhaps favors leiomyosarcoma. In our experience (56), PSCN has stained positively for cytokeratin in

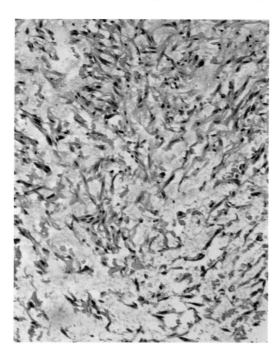

**FIG. 34.** Inflammatory pseudotumor. There is a loose, edematous appearance. Note occasionally enlarged nucleus.

some cases, whereas leiomyosarcomas of the bladder have been cytokeratin-negative. Ultimately, distinction between these two processes is very dependent on the clinical history of a recent operative procedure. In occasional cases in our experience it has been impossible to make a confident distinction between them, particularly when the interval between a prior operative procedure and the development of a spindle cell lesion is longer (more than 3 months) than in most cases of PSCN. In these cases careful clinical follow-up with repeat cystoscopy and further biopsies is indicated.

### Inflammatory Pseudotumor

Benign proliferative spindle cell lesions of the bladder that may microscopically suggest a sarcoma may also occur in patients without a recent history of an operation (57–62). A variety of designations have been used for the lesion in these cases. We prefer the term "inflammatory pseudotumor" (61) because it has been used for similar lesions occurring at other sites.

This lesion may occur at any age but typically occurs in young adults with an average age of 28 years. About twice as many women as men have been reported with this lesion. The size of the lesions may be quite variable, with some being striking polypoid intraluminal masses. On gross examination the majority have been exophytic but occasionally an endophytic gross appearance is observed. On microscopic examination the characteristic appearance is that of spindle cells, typically relatively widely separated in a vascular, myxoid, or sometimes basophilic stroma (Fig. 34). Less

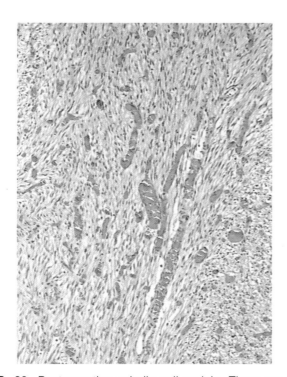

**FIG. 33.** Postoperative spindle cell nodule. There are numerous blood vessels.

commonly, a more compact cellular appearance is seen (Fig. 35) and when plasma cells are present the appearance is reminiscent of a plasma cell granuloma variant of inflammatory pseudotumor. Indeed it is probable that the occasional "plasma cell granuloma" of the bladder reported (63) is in this category of lesion. The cell type of inflammatory pseudotumor is similar to that seen in nodular fasciitis of the soft tissues (Fig. 36). Ultrastructural examination has typically shown the features of myofibroblasts, and flow cytometric DNA analysis gave diploid results in all six cases studied in one recent series (61). On microscopic examination, the differential diagnosis of this lesion is similar to that of the postoperative spindle cell nodule, including both myxoid sarcomas and myxoid areas in sarcomatoid carcinoma (64). With regard to the latter consideration, the age of the patient is also helpful as most sarcomatoid carcinomas occur in an older age group. It should be mentioned that occasional inflammatory pseudotumors, like the postoperative spindle cell nodule, have been immunoreactive for keratin (61). The diagnosis of a reactive mesenchymal lesion in the bladder should be made with great caution in these cases in which there is no history of a recent operation, which is so helpful in cases of postoperative spindle cell nodule.

### Paraganglia in the Bladder

Honma (65) was able to identify paraganglia in 51% of bladders at autopsy, finding them in all regions. Their presence in a bladder biopsy may cause confusion with a neo-

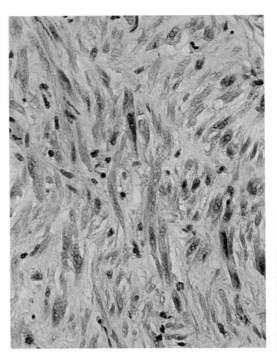

**FIG. 36.** Inflammatory pseudotumor. High-power examination shows spindle cells with abundant cytoplasm having a morphology consistent with that of myofibroblasts.

plasm (66), particularly if a small biopsy with artifact is obtained. The configuration of paraganglia, their sinusoidal vascular pattern, as well as the bland cytology of the cells and the absence of a surrounding stromal reaction (Fig. 37), are helpful in this differential diagnosis.

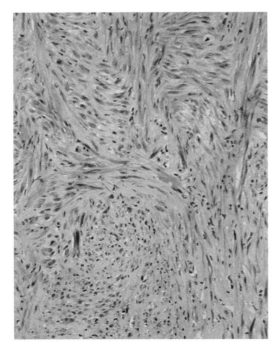

**FIG. 35.** Inflammatory pseudotumor. Compact cellular growth of spindle cells.

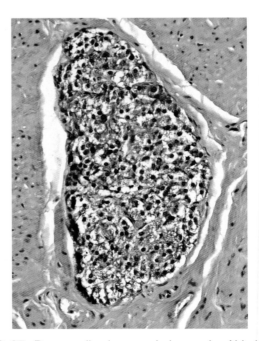

**FIG. 37.** Paraganglion in muscularis propria of bladder.

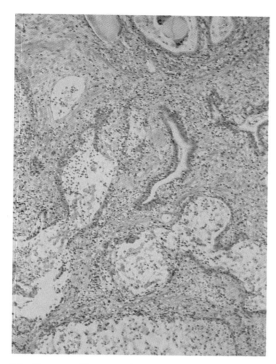

**FIG. 54.** Nonspecific granulomatous prostatitis. The ducts contain inspissated debris with inflammatory cells, have focally ruptured, and are associated with inflammation and reactive changes in the adjacent fibromuscular stroma.

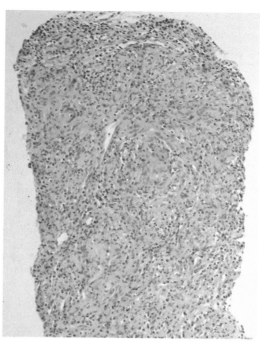

**FIG. 56.** Nonspecific granulomatous prostatitis. Low-power examination of a needle biopsy specimen shows a densely cellular infiltrate causing concern for malignancy.

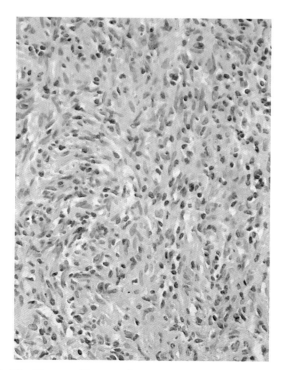

**FIG. 55.** Nonspecific granulomatous prostatitis. Many of the cells are spindle-shaped.

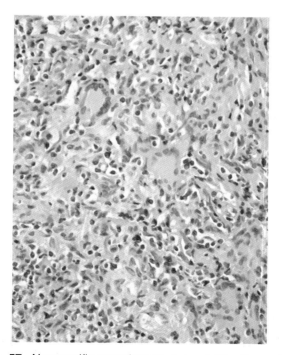

**FIG. 57.** Nonspecific granulomatous prostatitis. Several giant cells are present.

## Malakoplakia

Three quarters of patients with malakoplakia of the prostate have had prostatic enlargement and in several cases the process has initially been misdiagnosed as carcinoma by the pathologist (47,103–105). As with granulomatous prostatitis, the diffuse arrangement of the cells may lead to a misdiagnosis of high-grade carcinoma (Fig. 58). The microscopic appearance is somewhat similar to that of nonspecific granulomatous prostatitis but there is a more dominant population of histiocytes with eosinophilic cytoplasm and, in addition, Michaelis–Gutmann bodies (Fig. 59), which are required for the diagnosis.

## Xanthoma of the Prostate

Recently, Sebo and colleagues (106) described a series of cases and summarized previously reported cases (107,108) in which localized collections of cholesterol-laden histiocytes in the prostate caused some diagnostic difficulty. One of the seven cases of what they refer to as "prostatic xanthoma" occurred in a patient with mild hyperlipidemia. One of their cases was initially misinterpreted as adenocarcinoma but the histiocytic nature of the process was confirmed by immunohistochemical staining (106). The xanthomas consisted of demarcated cohesive nodular clusters of cells without evidence of gland formation and with small uniform nuclei and inconspicuous nucleoli (Fig. 60). These bland cytologic features and the foamy nature of the cytoplasm are important clues to the diagnosis.

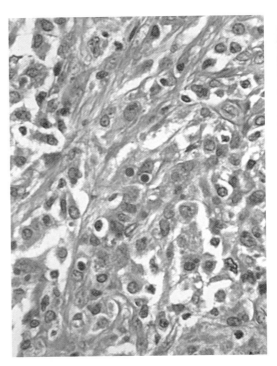

**FIG. 59.** Malakoplakia of the prostate. A PAS stain highlights two Michaelis–Gutmann bodies (center).

## Seminal Vesicle Tissue, Cowper's Glands, and Paraganglia in Prostate Specimens

The frequency with which seminal vesicle tissue is present in transurethral resections of the prostate has varied from 3% to 23% (109,110). It is also seen occasionally in needle biopsies. The acini of this organ are closely apposed (Fig. 61) and, as their cells typically exhibit striking nuclear hyperchromatism (Fig. 62) and pleomorphism (111,112), a neoplasm might be simulated. However, although atypical, the nuclei do not typically show mitotic activity and the changes appear degenerative. Appreciation of these features and the frequent presence of cytoplasmic golden brown lipofuscin pigment in the seminal vesicle epithelium (see Fig. 61) should help avoid a potentially serious diagnostic error. It should be emphasized that lipofuscin is not rare in prostatic epithelium, and this finding alone should not be considered diagnostic of seminal vesicle tissue (113).

Cowper's glands may also be present rarely within a prostatic specimen (Fig. 63) (114). The acini of Cowper's glands, however, have a lobular arrangement and are associated with excretory ducts and skeletal muscle. In addition, the cells lining the acini are not atypical and lack prominent nucleoli.

Another normal structure that may be present in prostate specimens and that may result in a misdiagnosis of cancer is paraganglia (66,115,116). As mentioned in the section on the bladder, however, their distinctive appearance should permit recognition; their typical presence in periprostatic soft tissue

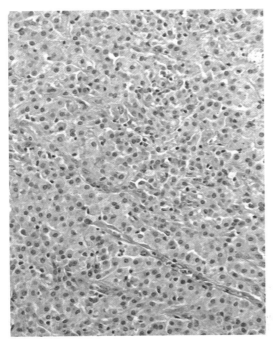

**FIG. 58.** Malakoplakia of the prostate. There is a diffuse growth of cells with appreciable eosinophilic cytoplasm.

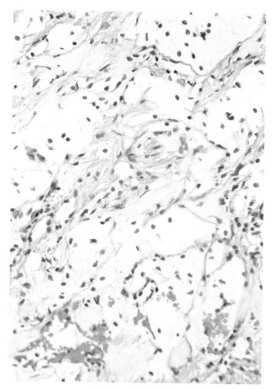

**FIG. 60.** Xanthoma of the prostate. Histiocytes with abundant foamy cytoplasm have small shrunken nuclei. (Courtesy of Dr. John Eble.)

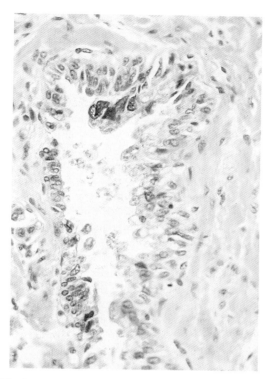

**FIG. 62.** Seminal vesicle tissue. Note atypical nuclei.

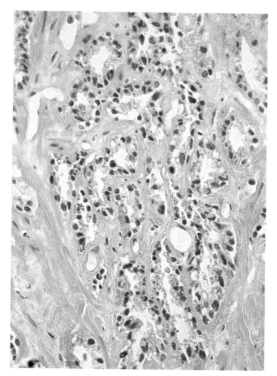

**FIG. 61.** Seminal vesicle tissue in prostatic transurethral resection material. The acini are closely apposed, focally have atypical nuclei, and contain abundant intracytoplasmic lipofuscin pigment.

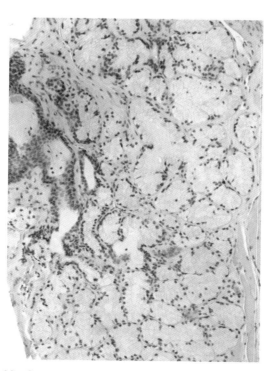

**FIG. 63.** Cowper's gland in prostatic needle biopsy specimen.

(Fig. 64) rather than in the prostate itself (116) decreases the likelihood of diagnostic errors.

## Benign Glands around Nerves and in Skeletal Muscle

Occasionally benign prostatic glands may be immediately adjacent to nerves, without appreciable intervening stroma, emphasizing the hazard of using perineural invasion as the sole criterion for malignancy in the prostate (117–119). Carstens (118) serially sectioned eight normal or hyperplastic prostates and found two or more foci of perineural invasion in seven of them. The glands never completely surrounded the nerve and were not seen in endothelium-lined spaces. In another study, benign glands were found in perineural spaces in 6 of 26 prostates (119). This phenomenon should be distinguished by cytologic criteria from the perineural invasion by malignant glands that often occurs in prostatic carcinoma. The presence of benign glands within the skeletal muscle that occurs normally in the prostate should also not lead to an erroneous diagnosis of malignancy (Fig. 65) (120–123).

## Radiation Effect

Bostwick et al. (124) found that the most common radiation-induced changes in the prostate were a decrease in the ratio of neoplastic glands to stroma as well as atrophy, squa-

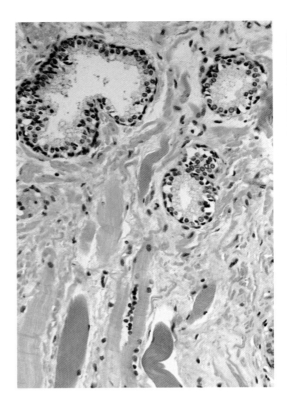

**FIG. 65.** Benign prostatic glands adjacent to skeletal muscle.

mous metaplasia, and atypia of nonneoplastic glands. Stromal fibrosis, atypical fibroblasts, and foreign body giant cells were also seen occasionally. Vascular changes included intimal proliferation of arteries and foam cells in vessel walls. Most problematic for the pathologist is the cytologic atypia of nonneoplastic glands that was present in 78% of the cases (151) (Fig. 66). The architectural arrangement of atypical nonneoplastic glands remains relatively normal—a helpful feature in excluding residual tumor. When other obvious changes of radiation injury are present, the presence of cytologic atypia should be conservatively interpreted. Additionally, although enlarged and hyperchromatic, the nuclei typically do not have prominent nucleoli. The transitional cells lining the prostatic urethra and prostatic ducts may also exhibit cytologic atypia following radiation, and such changes should also be evaluated cautiously.

## Squamous (and Transitional Cell) Metaplasia

The frequent association of prostatic infarcts with squamous metaplasia (Fig. 67) has in the past sometimes led to an erroneous diagnosis of squamous cell carcinoma of the prostate (125,126). Squamous metaplasia of the prostate (127,128) is also found with increased frequency in patients who have undergone a recent transurethral resection (126), and it is commonly found in the benign areas of the gland when the patient has received estrogens for prostatic carcinoma (129–131). Sometimes squamous metaplasia is found

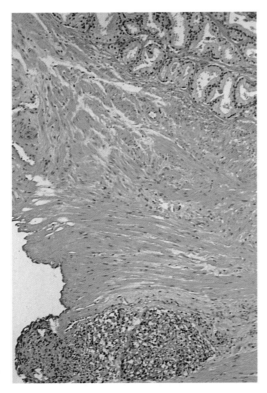

**FIG. 64.** Paraganglion (bottom) in periprostatic tissue.

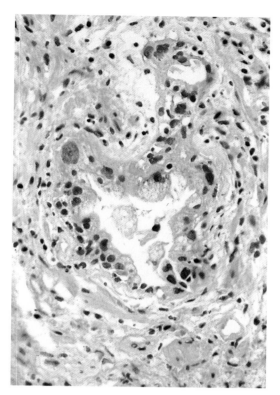

**FIG. 66.** Epithelial atypia in prostate of patient who received radiation for carcinoma of the bladder.

in the absence of any of these predisposing factors (Fig. 68) (126). Squamous cell carcinoma of the prostate is so rare that such a diagnosis should only be made after metaplasia has been carefully excluded.

Although transitional cells are usually only conspicuous in periurethral zones, occasionally they are seen in the central portion of the prostate. Their characteristic nuclear grooves and bland cytology should both enable their recognition and keep them from being misdiagnosed as prostatic intraepithelial uroplasia or carcinoma.

## Basaloid Lesions

### Typical Basal Cell Hyperplasia

Several papers in the last 14 years (132,133) have drawn attention to the occasional striking proliferation of the prostatic basal cells, producing an appearance that may be confused with carcinoma (Fig. 69). However, the cells usually appear bland cytologically (although there are exceptions, as discussed below), and as the pattern of this process differs significantly from those of typical prostatic adenocarcinoma, awareness of this entity should enable one to avoid its misinterpretation. Normal basal cells may have prominent nucleoli (Fig. 70). Sometimes the cells in basal cell hyperplasia have appreciable pale cytoplasm. Cases reported as embryonal hyperplasia of the prostate (134) appear similar to basal cell hyperplasia except for the presence of a loose, myxoid stroma. Basal cell hyperplasia has recently

been described as a frequent finding in patients treated for prostate cancer by luteinizing hormone–releasing hormone agonists and flutamide (135).

### Atypical Basal Cell Hyperplasia

Two papers have highlighted the fact that some cases of basal cell hyperplasia may show cytologic features such as prominent nucleoli and mitotic activity that cause concern (Figs. 71 and 72) but do not justify being called carcinoma (136–138). Nuclear prominence was present in 11 of 12 cases in one series; 2 cases exhibited hyperchromatism and nuclear pleomorphism and 6 had rare mitotic figures (136). In atypical basal cell hyperplasia a normal architecture is still retained (see Fig. 71), whereas architectural abnormalities indicative of stromal invasion are necessary to establish a diagnosis of basal cell carcinoma (137). Although some authors include a category of basal cell adenoma in their classification of basaloid lesions of the prostate, I favor the interpretation of these cases as basal cell hyperplasia occurring within adenomatous nodules rather than as benign neoplasms.

### Adenoid Cystic-like Lesions

Rarely a process that resembles adenoid cystic carcinoma of the salivary glands occurs within the prostate gland (139,140). A cribriform pattern of pseudocysts is most characteristic (Fig. 73) but glands, nests, and cords of basaloid cells are also encountered. In areas the appearance is indis-

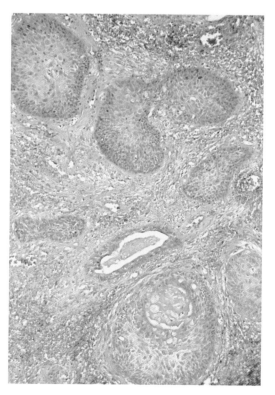

**FIG. 67.** Squamous metaplasia of the prostate. This is occurring in a zone of infarction.

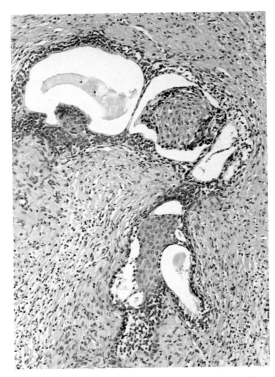

**FIG. 68.** Squamous metaplasia of the prostate. The metaplasia in this case was idiopathic.

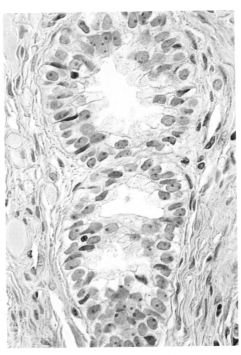

**FIG. 70.** Basal cell hyperplasia. A number of the basal cells have prominent nucleoli.

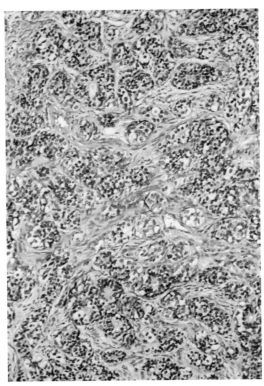

**FIG. 69.** Basal cell hyperplasia. Despite the florid basal cell proliferation the retention of an underlying orderly acinar architecture can be appreciated.

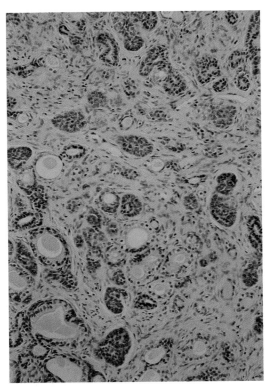

**FIG. 71.** Atypical basal cell hyperplasia. Note the retention of an orderly architecture.

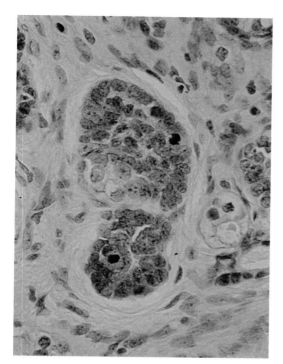

**FIG. 72.** Atypical basal cell hyperplasia. A nest of basal cells exhibits moderate cytologic atypia, and two mitotic figures are visible.

tinguishable from that of basal cell hyperplasia, due to the presence of nests of basaloid cells without prominent atypia or mitotic activity. The cribriform spaces surround basophilic secretion or hyalinized, eosinophilic material. Squamous metaplasia may be seen. Most of these cases have been interpreted as adenoid cystic carcinomas, but their malignant nature has been seriously questioned (139). The prognosis associated with this process is excellent on the basis of the limited experience to date.

## Postoperative Spindle Cell Nodule

This lesion (53) has been discussed in the section on the bladder and, as the features are similar in the prostate, it is not repeated here. One reported "sarcoma" of the prostate had features suggesting that it may have been this lesion (141).

## Atypical Stromal Cells

Bizarre nuclear changes of the type commonly seen in uterine smooth muscle tumors may be seen in the prostatic stromal cells (Fig. 74). These changes may be seen in the stroma of the unusual neoplasm that has been called cystosarcoma phyllodes of the prostate (142–143) or cystic epithelial-stromal tumor (144), and rarely within circumscribed stromal proliferations interpreted as leiomyomas (145). Cells with bizarre nuclei may also be distributed in the stroma of otherwise unremarkable cases of benign prostatic hyperplasia (146,147). The lack of a mass or mitoses and the benign course support the pseudoneoplastic nature of this change.

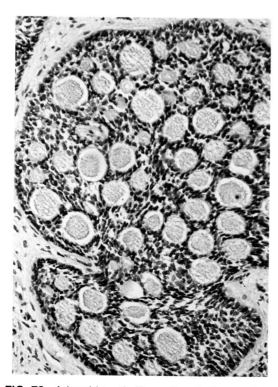

**FIG. 73.** Adenoid cystic-like pattern in the prostate.

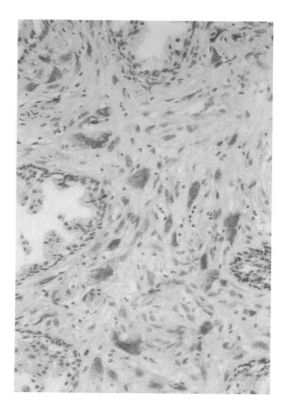

**FIG. 74.** Enlarged, bizarre nuclei in stroma of hyperplastic prostatic nodule.

# THE URETHRA

## Von Brunn's Nests and Urethritis Glandularis (Including Intestinal Metaplasia)

These common proliferations of urothelium most characteristically seen in the urinary bladder may be seen in the urethra. Von Brunn's nests, sometimes with glands reflecting urethritis glandularis, were found in as many as 74% of urethras from female patients with urethral symptoms in one study (148), and were similarly frequent in a series of men (149). They are rarely the source of diagnostic difficulty and when they are, features similar to those helpful in the bladder, as discussed earlier, facilitate the correct diagnosis.

Intestinal metaplasia is rarely seen in urethritis glandularis (149) and may also be seen as a surface phenomenon (150). Associated dysplasia (150), as in intestinal metaplasia of the bladder, has a significant association with adenocarcinoma (151,152).

## Caruncle

This common urethral lesion in women characteristically contains on microscopic examination varying components of hyperplastic epithelium, blood vessels, and inflammatory cells (Fig. 75) (153). This has led to their classification, particularly in the older literature, as papillomatous (or epithe-

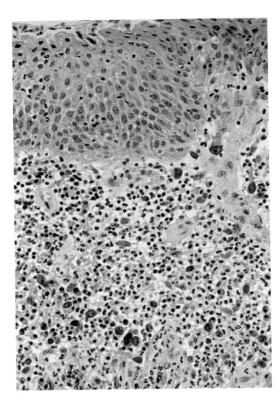

**FIG. 76.** Urethral caruncle. Note atypical stromal cells with associated inflammation.

lial), angiomatous, and granulomatous variants (154). However, there is such overlap that a specific subclassification is currently rarely applied. It is important, however, for pathologists to be aware that occasionally these proliferations can be exuberant microscopically (Fig. 75), and, as Herbut (154) noted many years ago, "to the unwary, nests of epithelial cells found within the core of a polypoid mass may offer some difficulty deciding whether the lesion is benign or malignant." However, as he noted, this worry should be "easily dispelled by the fact that the cells in a benign caruncle are always regular," i.e., cytologically benign. Olcott (155), in his series of caruncles, also noted that in almost 20% of cases conspicuous epithelial "infolding" raised the possibility of malignancy. Intestinal metaplasia may also rarely complicate the appearance of a caruncle (156), and intestinal epithelium interpreted as congenital has been described (157).

A rare pseudoneoplastic phenomenon that has recently been described within urethral caruncles is the presence of atypical stromal cells (Fig. 76), apparently of mesenchymal type, that may cause a striking, worrisome proliferation (Fig. 77) but that appear to be benign (146, 158). Numerous atypical cells, some of them elongated with moderate amounts of eosinophilic cytoplasm, were dispersed singly, in small groups and in sheets within the stroma of a urethral caruncle with a background of a mixed inflammatory cell infiltrate (146). Stains for lymphoid markers are negative. We favor

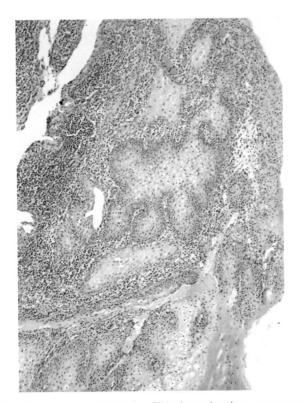

**FIG. 75.** Urethral caruncle. The invaginating squamous tongues may produce a superficially worrisome appearance.

Vieillefond A, Cakalir C, Paradis V, Bensadoun H, Benoit G. Ectopic prostatic polyp in the bladder: report of 2 cases. *Prog Urol* 1993;3:71–74.

## Hyperplasia of the Verumontanum

Gaudin PB, Wheeler TM, Epstein JI. Verumontanum mucosal gland hyperplasia in prostatic needle biopsy specimens: a mimic of low grade prostatic adenocarcinoma. *Am J Clin Pathol* 1995;104:620–626.

## Transitional Cell Hyperplasia of Prostatic Accessory Ducts

Akang EE, Aligbe JU, Olissa EG. Prostatic tumors in Benin City, Nigeria. *W Afr J Med* 1996;15:56–60.

Lepor H, Shapiro E, Wang B, Liang YC. Comparison of the cellular composition of benign prostatic hyperplasia in Chinese and Caucasian-American men. *Urology* 1996;47:38–42.

*Pathology of Pseudoneoplastic Lesions,*
edited by M. R. Wick, P. A. Humphrey, and J. H. Ritter.
Lippincott-Raven Publishers, Philadelphia © 1997.

CHAPTER 9

# Pseudoneoplastic Lesions of the Testis, Scrotum, and Penis

J. Carlos Manivel

The aim of this chapter is to review lesions of the male genitals that might be confused with neoplasms. These fall into two general categories: (a) reactive or inflammation-related pseudoneoplasias and (b) proliferations of vestigial but normally located structures. Some of these entities may confuse the clinician because they form palpable masses or are detected through radiologic studies, or because they become symptomatic by displacing or compressing adjacent structures.

A proportion of these lesions, principally reflected by those representing developmental abnormalities, are readily diagnosed and are treated only superficially herein. It is undeniably important to be familiar with entities in that category to avert unnecessarily aggressive treatment and to signal the possible presence of associated local or systemic abnormalities that may be life threatening. However, they are usually not confused with other processes morphologi-

  J. C. Manivel: Department of Laboratory Medicine and Pathology, University of Minnesota Hospitals and Clinics, Minneapolis, Minnesota 55455.

cally. Another category of lesions—and that which is most germane to the theme of this chapter—is reflected by those whose gross or microscopic appearance may mislead the pathologist into a diagnosis of neoplasia, with potentially catastrophic consequences.

## TESTIS

### Cysts of the Tunica Albuginea

Cysts of the tunica albuginea are most common between the fifth and eighth decades of life but can also occur in younger individuals (1). They are located in the anterolateral surface of the testis, measure from 0.5 to 4 cm in diameter, may be solitary or multiple, uni- or multiloculated, and contain serous or brown fluid (2). Microscopically, a dense fibrous wall is lined with single cuboidal or flattened epithelium. Most are probably derived from mesothelial inclusions, but an origin from efferent ductules and seminiferous tubules has also been suggested (3). These cysts should be distinguished from testicular germ cell tumors; the absence of teratomatous elements allows this distinction to be made, but thorough histological sampling is required to document this point. Occasionally, solid nests of cells with longitudinal nuclear grooves and a so-called coffee-bean appearance may undergo cystic change and produce pseudoneoplastic lesions of the tunic. These cellular aggregates have been designated "Walthard's rests" because of microscopic similarities to their counterparts in the fallopian tubes. Patients with cysts of the tunica albuginea have a high incidence of other genitourinary malformations, primarily exemplified by renal and testicular dysplasia.

### Infectious Orchitis

Most cases of bacterial orchitis are recognized as such clinically and they respond to antibiotic therapy. However, long-standing or diagnostically indeterminate examples of this disease may prompt an orchiectomy. Under such circumstances, histologic examination may demonstrate architectural distortion, fibrosis, and stromal inflammation with a pattern that occasionally may be confused with that of a neoplasm. Similarly, rare examples of viral diseases in which intense chronic orchitis is the sole or predominant manifestation, such as mumps, may sometimes be confused with a neoplasm on clinical, gross, and even microscopic grounds. Viral infection may particularly simulate a lymphoma or seminoma because of abundant lymphoid infiltrates and parenchymal distortion (4–7). Nevertheless, immunohistochemical and genotypic characterization of the lymphocytes in this setting demonstrate a polyclonal cellular population and exclude a hematopoietic malignancy. Similarly, the remaining germ cells in orchitis lack the placental-like alkaline phosphatase (PLAP) immunoreactivity and glycogen content that typify true neoplasms that comprise such elements.

### Nonimmune Granulomatous Orchitis

Granulomatous orchitis may produce firm, painless enlargement of the testis and thereby simulate a neoplasm on physical examination. Cases of granulomatous orchitis may be divided into idiopathic conditions, and those in which the etiology is known. Examples of the latter include tuberculosis, "atypical" mycobacterioses, brucellosis, leprosy, tertiary syphilis, fungal infections, schistosomiasis, and foreign body reactions (8–11). Sarcoidosis (12) (still regarded as a possibly infectious granulomatous disease) may also present in the testis. Procurement of appropriate serologic tests and microbiological cultures is essential to resolve the cited differential diagnosis. In addition, because prominent obscuring granulomatous inflammation may be observed in occasional germ cell tumors, the pathologist is well advised to sample such testes thoroughly for microscopic examination. Moreover, performance of immunostains for PLAP and the histochemical periodic acid–Schiff (PAS) method is advisable in identifying those neoplasms.

### Autoimmune Granulomatous Orchitis

The pathogenesis of autoimmune granulomatous orchitis (AGO) is probably related to exposure of sperm to the immune system through trauma to the testis or ischemic insults. Acid-fast lipid in sperm may be responsible for the granulomatous response. Scrotal swelling, with or without pain, is the usual mode of presentation; an indurated, enlarged testis may simulate a neoplasm clinically. Patients with AGO may have oligospermia or azoospermia. Most are in the fifth to sixth decades of life, but the condition under discussion may also occur outside of that age range. A recent history of gram-negative bacterial urinary tract infection or trauma is common (13–20). Macroscopically, the testis in AGO is enlarged and firm, and the tunica albuginea is frequently thickened. The cut surfaces show variable distortion of normal parenchymal architecture by yellow–tan to white–gray indurated areas that may superficially resemble the gross images of testicular lymphoma or seminoma. Involvement is usually diffuse, but AGO may sometimes present as a well-circumscribed, localized nodule. In approximately 50% of cases, the epididymis and spermatic cord are also affected and may contain sperm granulomas. The microscopic appearance depends on the stage of the disease; early in its evolution the seminiferous tubules are preserved, and germ cells and Sertoli cells are variably destroyed by epithelioid histiocytes that form noncaseating granulomas (Fig. 1A). In contrast to infectious granulomatous orchitis and sarcoidosis, the granulomas in AGO are predominantly intratubular rather than interstitial. Other inflammatory elements that are potentially present in this disorder include Langhans-type giant cells, lymphocytes, and eosinophils. In late stage disease, virtually all tubular elements are destroyed and the normal testicular architecture is replaced by histiocytes and scattered lymphocytes and plasma cells (Fig. 1B). Silver stains may, however, outline the remnants of seminiferous tubular

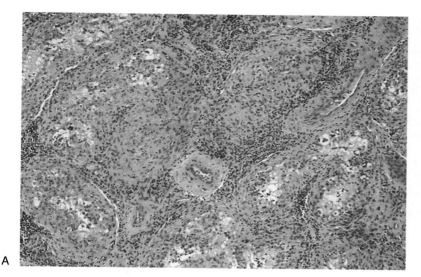

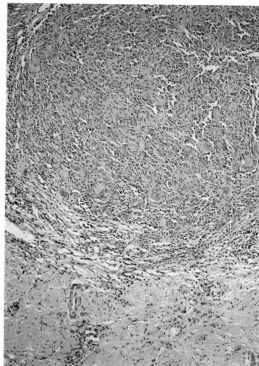

**FIG. 1.** Granulomatous orchitis. **A:** Early involvement. **B:** Late stage disease.

basement membranes. The testicular blood vessels may show thrombosis and arteritis.

The overall histologic appearance may superficially resemble that of a Sertoli cell tumor, a malignant lymphoma, or a germ cell neoplasm. In that context, performance of the techniques discussed above, namely, PAS stains and immunostains for PLAP, is once again advisable as a means of resolving differential diagnostic uncertainties.

### Tumefactive Malakoplakia (Greek: "Soft plaque")

Most cases of testicular malakoplakia occur between the ages of 30 and 70 years, but younger and older patients with this condition have also been observed. The clinical presentation of testicular malakoplakia (TM) may simulate that of acute or chronic epididymo-orchitis, but asymptomatic testicular enlargement in other cases may simulate a neoplasm on clinical grounds (21–27). Urine cultures frequently grow *Escherichia coli*. For unknown reasons, the right testis is affected twice as often as the left; moreover, all examples of TM are unilateral, and epididymal involvement frequently coexists. The disease is thought to be due to abnormal intracellular processing of phagocytized bacteria by the constituent histiocytes, probably because of an inherent lysosomal defect.

Grossly, the gonad in malakoplakia is enlarged and its cut surfaces show replacement of the testicular parenchyma by yellow–white to tan–brown nodules of variable consistency. Overt abscesses are frequently present. The microscopic ap-

pearance of TM is similar to that in other locations and is characterized by confluent aggregates of histiocytes with abundant granular eosinophilic cytoplasm (von Hansemann cells), and intra- and extracellular Michaelis–Gutmann bodies. The latter inclusions may be absent in early stages of the disease. Michaelis–Gutmann bodies are represented by round, solid or concentric, lamellated, basophilic inclusions of variable size (generally measuring 10–30 $\mu$m) (Fig. 2). They can be highlighted by use of the PAS technique or by stains for calcium (von Kossa; alizarin red) (Fig. 3) or iron (Perl's method). Polymorphonuclear leukocytes, lymphocytes, granulation tissue, and variable degrees of fibrosis are also apparent in TM.

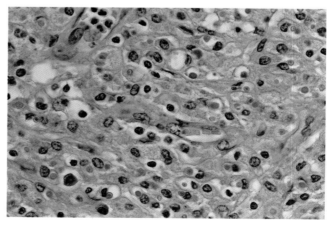

**FIG. 2.** Malakoplakia of the testis.

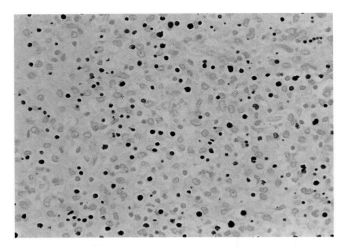

**FIG. 3.** Malakoplakia; von Kossa's stain.

The degree of parenchymal preservation in the affected testis depends on the age of the lesion; in well-developed malakoplakia, the seminiferous tubules may be largely effaced by the histiocytic infiltrate, and a striking resemblance to a Leydig cell tumor may be obtained. Nonetheless, the cytoplasmic Reinke's crystals that are often present in stromal tumors are lacking in TM; conversely, Leydig cell neoplasms do not exhibit formation of abscesses at a macroscopic level, or microscopic Michaelis–Gutmann bodies.

Ultrastructurally, the latter structures show a concentric appearance. An electron-dense core is surrounded by layers of variable density, as well as by radial spicules that are composed of hydroxyapatite. As stated above, the granules of the histiocytes in TM stain with PAS on conventional microscopy. Electron microscopy shows that they are phagolysosomes that contain ingested bacteria (frequently, *E. coli*). These organelles evolve into fully formed Michaelis–Gutmann bodies by becoming encrusted with calcium and iron salts.

## Testicular Cysts

Nonneoplastic cystic lesions of the testis include hydatid cyst (28), simple cyst, epidermoid cyst, cysts of the rete testis, and cystic dysplasia. Furthermore, ovotestes may exhibit the presence of cystic follicles in the ovarian tissue (29). These entities are discussed below.

### Simple Cysts

Simple testicular cysts affect patients over a wide age range. They produce painless testicular enlargement, and measure from 1 to several centimeters in maximal dimension. Grossly, these lesions are solitary and uniloculated, and contain clear serous fluid; their lining is glistening and smooth (30–33). Microscopically, they are lined with cuboidal or flattened epithelium, and the absence of other cell types distinguishes them from cystic teratomas. The adjacent testicular tissue shows compression atrophy, but it is devoid of intratubular germ cell neoplasia, as would be expected in many cases of true testicular teratoma.

### Epidermoid Cysts

The histogenesis of epidermoid cysts in the testis is controversial. Some observers regard these lesions as examples of "monodermal" (single-lineage) differentiation in teratomas. Other proposed histogenetic mechanisms center on squamous metaplasia of the rete testis or of epithelial inclusions in the tunica albuginea, or displacement of ectodermal tissue in a manner analogous to that causing epidermal inclusion cysts of the skin. Regardless of these considerations, "pure" epidermoid cyst of the testis is important to distinguish pathologically from true teratoma. The former of these two entities is innocuous, whereas testicular teratomas in adults behave as unequivocal malignancies (34–42).

Testicular epidermoid cysts affect males of various ages; however, most are encountered between the second and fourth decades of life, and produce painless testicular enlargement. These growths are responsible for approximately 1 in 100 cases of testicular enlargement.

Grossly, they typically show a diameter of 1–2 cm. The cut surface reveals an intraparenchymal location, usually in the periphery of the testis. The cyst has thin walls and contains yellow–white pasty material (Fig. 4A) . Microscopically, a thin fibrous wall is lined with mature squamous epithelium, and the cyst contents consist of keratin debris (Fig. 4B). The squamous lining may be focally ulcerated, resulting in foreign body reaction. Occasionally, the cyst wall shows calcification. Pathologic exclusion of a cystic teratoma is predicated on the absence of other somatic cell types, including dermal appendages, and relies on the fact that the capsule has been thoroughly sampled. The seminiferous tubules adjacent to a testicular epidermoid cyst may show compression atrophy, but they lack intratubular germ cell neoplasia (43).

When the diagnosis is suspected clinically and is supported by the results of ultrasonography, frozen section examination may be used to confirm the diagnosis, and a conservative local excision may be performed with gonadal preservation (44). Cysts that are adjacent to a macroscopic scar should *not* be handled in this manner, however, because those particular lesions may represent regressed germ cell tumors.

### Cysts of the Rete Testis

Only one example of a rete testis cyst has been reported; it presented as an asymptomatic testicular mass in an adult, and was lined with unremarkable rete epithelium (45). Again, the potential for confusion of such a lesion with true cystic teratoma exists, but notation of its specific anatomic location and the particulars of its microscopic features should allow

26. Baker WC, Bishai MB, de Vere White RW. Misleading testicular masses. *Urology* 1988;31:111–113.

27. Moriyama N, Kitamura T, Kuniyoshi N, et al. A case of malakoplakia of the testis and epididymis. *Jpn J Urol* 1989;80:740–743.

28. Kumar PVN, Jahanshahi SL. Hydatid cyst of testis. A case report. *J Urol* 1987;137:511–512.

29. Rutgers JL, Scully RE. Pathology of the testis in intersex syndromes. *Semin Diagn Pathol* 1987;4:275–291.

30. Schmidt SS. Congenital simple cyst of the testis: a hitherto undescribed lesion. *J Urol* 1966;96:236–238.

31. Tosi SE, Richardson JR Jr. Simple cyst of the testis: case report and review of the literature. *J Urol* 1975;114:473–475.

32. Takihara H, Valvo JR, Tokuhara M, et al. Intratesticular cysts. *Urology* 1982;20:80–82.

33. Dmochowski RR, Rudy DC, Weitzner S, et al. Simple cyst of the testis. *J Urol* 1989;142:1078–1081.

34. Kumar PVN, Khezri AA. Epidermoid cysts of the testis. *Br J Urol* 1986;58:463.

35. Zaitoon MM. Epidermoid cyst of the testis. *Urology* 1986;28:434–435.

36. Malek RS, Rosen JS, Farrow GM. Epidermoid cyst of the testis: a critical analysis. *Br J Urol* 1986;58:55–59.

37. Haas GP, Shumaker BP, Cerny JC. The high incidence of benign testicular tumors. *J Urol* 1986;136:1219–1220.

38. Johnson JW, Hodge EE, Radwin HM. Epidermoid cyst of testis: a case for orchiectomy. *Urology* 1987;29:23–25.

39. Kaasinen E, Taavitsainen M, Lehtonen T. Epidermoid cyst of the testis: case report with a review of the literature. *Eur Urol* 1988;15:141–143.

40. Thomsen H. Epidermoid cyst of the testis: benign teratoma in an adult. *Scand J Urol Nephrol* 1988;122:339–341.

41. Aitchison M, Blair J, Hutchison AG. Epidermoid cyst of the testis. *Br J Urol* 1989;63:324.

42. Reinberg Y, Manivel JC, Llerena J, Niehans G, Fraley E. Epidermoid cyst (monodermal teratoma) of the testis. *Br J Urol* 1990;66:648–651.

43. Manivel JC, Reinberg Y, Niehans GA, Fraley E. Intratubular germ cell neoplasia in testicular teratomas and epidermoid cysts: correlation with prognosis and possible biological significance. *Cancer* 1989;64:715–720.

44. Badalament RA, Haas GP, Cerny JC, et al. Conservative management of epidermoid cyst of testis. *Urology* 1986;28:28–30.

45. Tejada E, Eble JN. Simple cyst of the rete testis. *J Urol* 1988;139:376–377.

46. Leissring JC, Oppenheimer ROF. Cystic dysplasia of the testis. A unique congenital anomaly studied by microdissection. *J Urol* 1973;110:362–363.

47. Fisher JE, Jewett TC Jr, Nelson SJ, et al. Ectasia of the rete testis with ipsilateral renal agenesis. *J Urol* 1982;128:1040–1043.

48. Nistal M, Regadera J, Paniagua R. Cystic dysplasia of the testis: light and electron microscopic study of three cases. *Arch Pathol Lab Med* 1984;108:579–583.

49. Tesluk H, Blankenburg TA. Cystic dysplasia of testis. *Urology* 1987;29:47–49.

50. Nistal M, Santamaria L, Paniugua R. Acquired cystic transformation of the rete testis secondary to renal failure. *Hum Pathol* 1989;20:1065–1070.

51. Sharp SC, Batt MA, Lennington WJ. Epididymal cribriform hyperplasia: a variant of normal epididymal histology. *Arch Pathol Lab Med* 1994;118:1020–1022.

51a. Hartwick RW, Ro JY, Srigley JR, et al. Adenomatous hyperplasia of the rete testis: a clinicopathologic study of nine cases. *Am J Surg Pathol* 1991;15:350–357.

52. Rutgers JL, Young RH, Scully RE. The testicular 'tumor' of the adrenogenital syndrome: a report of five cases and review of the literature on testicular masses in patients with disorders of the adrenal glands. *Am J Surg Pathol* 1988;12:503–513.

53. Johnson RE, Scheithauer B. Massive hyperplasia of testicular adrenal rests in a patient with Nelson's syndrome. *Am J Clin Pathol* 1982;77:501–507.

54. Skoglund RW, McRoberts JW, Ragde H. Torsion of the spermatic cord: a review of the literature and an analysis of 70 new cases. *J Urol* 1970;104:604–607.

55. Guiney EJ, McGlinchey J. Torsion of the testes and the spermatic cord in the newborn. *Surg Gynecol Obstet* 1981;152:273–274.

56. Brewer ME, Glasgow BJ. Adult testicular torsion. *Urology* 1986;27:356–357.

57. Williamson RCN. Torsion of the testis and allied conditions. *Br J Surg* 1976;63:465–476.

58. Shurbaji MS, Epstein JI. Testicular vasculitis: implications for systemic disease. *Hum Pathol* 1988;19:186–189.

59. Huisman TK, Collins WJ Jr, Voulgarakis GR. Polyarteritis nodosa masquerading as a primary testicular neoplasm: a case report and review of the literature. *J Urol* 1990;144:1236–1238.

60. Nistal M, Paniagua R, Albaurrea MA, Santamaria L. Hyperplasia and the immature appearance of Sertoli cells in primary testicular disorders. *Hum Pathol* 1982;13:3–12.

61. Nistal M, Paniaguia R, Diez-Pardo JA. Histologic classification of undescended testes. *Hum Pathol* 1980;11:666–674.

62. Hadziselimovic F, Herzog B, Huff DS, Menardi G. The morphometric histopathology of undescended testes and testes associated with incarcerated inguinal hernia: a comparative study. *J Urol* 1991;146:627–629.

63. Melekos MD, Asbach HW. Epididymitis: aspects concerning etiology and treatment. *J Urol* 1987;138:83–86.

64. Kundert PR. Cholesteatoma of the epididymis. *J Urol* 1946;56:454–457.

65. Pingree LJ, Brown DE. Cholesteatoma of the epididymis. *J Urol* 1951;65:126–135.

66. McClure J. A case of malacoplakia of the epididymis associated with trauma. *J Urol* 1980;124:934–935.

67. Dubey NK, Tavadia HB, Hehir M. Malacoplakia: a case involving epididymis and a case involving a bladder complicated by calculi. *J Urol* 1988;139:359–361.

68. Wakeley CPG. Cysts of the epididymis, the so-called spermatocele. *Br J Surg* 1943;31:165–171.

69. Kuo T, Gomez LG. Monstrous epithelial cells in human epididymis and seminal vesicles. *Am J Surg Pathol* 1981;5:483–490.

70. Dahl EV, Bahn RC. Aberrant adrenal cortical tissue near the testis in human infants. *Am J Pathol* 1962;40:587–598.

71. Mares AJ, Shkolnik A, Sacks M, Feuchtwanger MM. Aberrant (ectoptic) adrenocortical tissue along the spermatic cord. *J Pediatr Surg* 1980;15:289–292.

71a. Wick MR, Cherwitz DL, McGlennen RC, Dehner LP. Adrenocortical carcinoma: an immunohistochemical comparison with renal cell carcinoma. *Am J Pathol* 1986;122:343–352.

72. Walker AN, Mills SE. Glandular inclusions in inguinal hernial sacs and spermatic cords: Müllerian-like remnants confused with functional reproductive structures. *Am J Clin Pathol* 1984;82:85–89.

73. Young RH, Scully RE. Testicular and paratesticular tumors and tumor-like lesions of ovarian common epithelial and Müllerian types: a report of four cases and review of the literature. *Am J Clin Pathol* 1986;86:146–152.

74. Civantos F, Lubin J, Rywlin AM. Vasitis nodosa. *Arch Pathol* 1972;4:355–361.

75. Kiser GC, Fuchs EF, Kessler S. The significance of vasitis nodosa. *Urology* 1986;136:42–44.

76. Balogh K, Travis WD. The frequency of perineural ductules in vasitis nodosa. *Am J Clin Pathol* 1984;82:710–713.

77. Goldman RL, Azzopardi JG. Benign neural invasion in vasitis nodosa. *Histopathology* 1982;6:309–315.

78. Balogh K, Travis WD. Benign vascular invasion in vasitis nodosa. *Am J Clin Pathol* 1985;83:426–430.

79. Balogh K, Argenyi ZB. Vasitis nodosa and spermatic granuloma of the skin: a histologic study of a rare complication of vasectomy. *J Cutan Pathol* 1985;12:528–533.

80. Arias-Stella J, Takano Moron J. Atypical epithelial changes in the seminal vesicles. *Arch Pathol* 1958;66:761–766.

81. Norris HJ, Yunis E. Age changes of seminal vesicles and deferentia in diabetics. *Arch Pathol* 1964;77:126–131.

82. Garret M, Hamm FC. Atypical cells of origin from the seminal vesicles complicating cytologic evaluations of prostatic secretions. *Am J Clin Pathol* 1963;39:265–272.

83. Koivuniemi A, Tyrkkö J. Seminal vesicle epithelium in fine needle as-

piration biopsies of the prostate as a pitfall in the cytologic diagnosis of carcinoma. *Acta Cytol* 1976;20:116–119.

83a. Manivel JC. Unpublished observations.

84. Dehner LP, Scott D, Stocker JT. Meconium periorchitis: a clinicopathologic study of four cases with a review of the literature. *Hum Pathol* 1986;17:807–812.

85. Oertel YC, Johnson FB. Sclerosing lipogranuloma of male genitalia: review of 23 cases. *Arch Pathol Lab Med* 1977;101:321–326.

86. Engelman ER, Herr HW, Ravera J. Lipogranulomatosis of external genitalia. *Urology* 1974;3:358–361.

87. Smetana HF, Bernhard W. Sclerosing lipogranuloma. *Arch Pathol* 1950;50:296–325.

88. Matsuda T, Shichiri Y, Hida S, et al. Eosinophilic sclerosing lipogranuloma of the male genitalia not caused by exogenous lipids. *J Urol* 1988;140:1021–1024.

89. Matsushima M, Tajima M, Maki A, et al. Primary lipogranuloma of male genitalia. *Urology* 1988;31:75–77.

90. Hollander JB, Begun FP, Lee RD. Scrotal fat necrosis. *J Urol* 1985;134:150–151.

91. Honoré LH. Nonspecific peritesticular fibrosis manifested as testicular enlargement: clinicopathological study of nine cases. *Arch Surg* 1978;113:814–816.

92. Goulding FJ, Traylor RA. Juvenile xanthogranuloma of the scrotum. *J Urol* 1983;129:841–842.

93. Sarlis I, Yakoymakis S, Rebelakos AG. Fibrous pseudotumor of the scrotum. *J Urol* 1980;124:742–743.

94. Nistal M, Paniagua R, Fuentes E, Regadera J. Histogenesis of adenomatoid tumor associated with pseudofibromatous periorchitis in an infant with hydrocele. *J Pathol* 1984;144:275–280.

95. Thompson JE, Van Der Walt JD. Nodular fibrous proliferation (fibrous pseudotumour) of the tunica vaginalis testis: a light, electron microscopic and immunocytochemical study of a case and review of the literature. *Histopathology* 1986;10:741–748.

96. Rosai J, Dehner LP. Nodular mesothelial hyperplasia in hernia sacs: a benign reactive condition simulating a neoplastic process. *Cancer* 1975;35:165–175.

96a. Walker AN, Mills SE. Surgical pathology of the tunica vaginalis testis and embryologically-related mesothelium. *Pathol Annu* 1988;23(2):125–152.

97. Harris CJ, Das S, Vogt PJ. Fibrous hamartoma of infancy in the scrotum. *J Urol* 1982;127:781–782.

98. Sharma TC, Kagan HN, Sheils JP. Malacoplakia of the male urethra. *J Urol* 1981;125:885–886.

99. Sloane BB, Figueroa TE, Ferguson D, et al. Malacoplakia of the urethra. *J Urol* 1988;129:1300–1301.

100. Zoon JJ. Balanoposthite chronique circonscrite benigne a plasmocytes. *Dermatologica* 1952;105:1–7.

101. Brodin M. Balanitis circumscripta plasmacellularis. *J Am Acad Dermatol* 1980;2:33–35.

## ADDENDUM REFERENCES

### Genital Epidermoid Cysts

Heidenreich A, Engelmann UH, Vietsch HV, Derschum W. Organ preserving surgery in testicular epidermoid cysts. *J Urol* 1995;153:1147–1150.

Koenigsberg RA, Kelsey D, Friedman AC. Case report: ultrasound and MRI findings in a scrotal epidermoid cyst. *Clin Radiol* 1995;50:576–578.

Malvica RP. Epidermoid cyst of the testicle: an unusual sonographic finding. *Am J Roentgenol* 1993;160:1047–1048.

Minakami H, Ito H, Miura N, Masui M, Kotake T, Sugano I. Cyst of the tunica albuginea testis: a case report. *Acta Urol Jpn* 1994;40:431–433.

Shapeero LG, Vordemark JS. Epidermoid cysts of testes and role of sonography. *Urology* 1993;41:75–79.

### Tumefactive Orchitis

Gillot JM, Brouillard M, Hatron PY, Devulder B. Testicular localization of systemic diseases. *Presse Medicale* 1995;24:691–694.

Huong DL, Papo T, Piette JC, Wechsler B, Bietry O, Richard F, Valcke JC, Godeau P. Urogenital manifestations of Wegener's granulomatosis. *Medicine* 1995;74:152–161.

Osca-Garcia JM, Alfaro-Ferreres L, Ruiz-Cerda JL, Moreno-Pardo B, Martinez-Jabaloyas J, Jimenez-Cruz JF. Idiopathic granulomatous orchitis. *Acta Urol Espan* 1993;17:53–56.

Stein A. Granulomatous orchitis associated with retrograde ejaculation. *Am J Clin Pathol* 1995;104:232.

Terao T, Kura N, Ohashi H, Mizuo T, Kameda N. Syphilitic orchitis: report of a case. *Acta Urol Jpn* 1993;39:973–976.

Wegner HE, Loy V, Dieckmann KP. Granulomatous orchitis: an analysis of clinical presentations, pathological anatomic features, and possible etiologic factors. *Eur Urol* 1994;26:56–60.

### Testicular Malakoplakia

Kajbafzadeh AM. Malakoplakia of the testis. *Br J Urol* 1995;76:276.

Masuda M, Yamanaka N. Testicular malakoplakia: case report. *Jpn J Urol* 1993;84:906–909.

Stevens SA. Malakoplakia of the testis. *Br J Urol* 1995;75:111–112.

### Tumefactive Hyperplasia of the Rete Testis

Bale PM, Watson G, Collins F. Pathology of osseous and genitourinary lesions of Proteus syndrome. *Pediatr Pathol* 1993;13:797–809.

Butterworth DM, Bisset DL. Cribriform intratubular epididymal change and adenomatous hyperplasia of the rete testis: a consequence of testicular atrophy? *Histopathology* 1992;21:435–438.

Cooper K, Govender D. Adenomatous hyperplasia of rete testis. *Histopathology* 1994;24:101–102.

### Genital Masses in the Adrenogenital Syndromes

Davis JM, Woodroof J, Sadasivan R, Stephens R. Case report: congenital adrenal hyperplasia and malignant Leydig cell tumor. *Am J Med Sci* 1995;309:63–65.

Roos G, Oehler U, Bodeker J, Helpap B. Unilateral testicular tumor in adrenogenital syndrome. *Pathologe* 1994;15:119–123.

### Genital Masses in the Testicular Feminization (Androgen Insensitivity) Syndrome

Jockenhovel-Rutgers JK, Mason JS, Griffin JE, Swerdloff RS. Leydig cell neoplasia in a patient with Reifenstein syndrome. *Exp Clin Endocrinol* 1993;101:365–370.

Sultan C, Lobaccaro JM, Belon C, Terraza A, Lumbroso S. Molecular biology of disorders of sex differentiation. *Hormone Res* 1992;38:105–113.

### Pseudoneoplastic Lesions in Cryptorchidism

Allen FJ, Van Vollenhoven F. Leydig cell tumor of intraabdominal testis. *Urology* 1993;42:729–731.

Bosland MC. Hormonal factors in carcinogenesis of the prostate and testis in human and in animal models. *Prog Clin Biol Res* 1996;394:309–352.

Huff DS, Hadziselimovic F, Snyder HM III, Blythe B, Ducket JW. Histologic maldevelopment of unilaterally cryptorchid testes and their descended partners. *Eur J Pediatr* 1993;152 (Suppl):S11–S14.

Kirsch AJ, Bastian W, Cohen HL, Glassberg KI. Precocious puberty in a child with unilateral Leydig cell tumor of the testis following orchiopexy. *J Urol* 1993;150:1483–1485.

Safak M, Adsan O, Baltaci S, Beduk Y. Bilateral Leydig cell tumors with unilateral cryptorchidism: case report. *Scand J Urol Nephrol* 1994;28:433–434.

### Tumefactive Epididymitis

Butterworth DM, Bisset DL. Cribriform intratubular epididymal change and adenomatous hyperplasia of the rete testis: a consequence of testicular atrophy? *Histopathology* 1992;21:435–438.

Hori S, Tsutsumi Y. Histological differentiation between chlamydial and bacterial epididymitis: nondestructive and proliferative versus destructive and abscess-forming: immunohistochemical and clinicopathological findings. *Hum Pathol* 1995;26:402–407.

### Adrenal Heterotopia of the Spermatic Cord

Roca-Suarez A, Alvarez-Ossorio JL, Del Toro-Bacerra JA, Maximiano-Vaszuez R, Gordon-Laporte R. Adrenal ectopia in the spermatic cord. *Acta Urol Espan* 1993;17:584–587.

### Pseudotumors of the Spermatic Cord

Tsukikawa M, Miki T, Takayama H, Gotou T, Tsujimura A, Sugao H, Takaha M, Takeda M, Kurata A. Intrascrotal fibrous pseudotumor accompanied by pelvic kidney with ectopic ureteral opening: a case report. *Acta Urol Jpn* 1995;41:489–492.

## Mullerian Rests in the Male Genitalia

Lamesch AJ. Monorchidism or unilateral anorchidism. *Langenbecks Arch Fur Chir* 1993;379:105–108.

Minh HN, Belaisch J, Smadja A. Female pseudohermaphroditism. *Presse Med* 1993;22:1735–1740.

## Tumefactive Vasitis

Onishi N, Honjoh M, Takeyama M, Sakaguchi H. Vasitis nodosa suspected as a spermatic cord tumor: a case report. *Acta Urol Jpn* 1992;38:595–597.

Ralph DJ, Lynch MJ, Pryor JP. Vasitis nodosa due to torture. *Br J Urol* 1993;72:515–516.

Schmidt SS, Minckler TM. The vas after vasectomy: comparison of cauterization methods. *Urology* 1992;40:468–470.

## Scrotal Pseudotumors

Fetsch JF, Montgomery EA, Meis JM. Calcifying fibrous pseudotumor. *Am J Surg Pathol* 1993;17:502–508.

Golomb J, Kopolovic J, Siegel Y. Sclerosing lipogranuloma of the external male genitalia. *Br J Urol* 1992;70:575.

Gosselin P, Delaporte E, Catteau B, Cotten H, Lecombe-Houcke M, Piette F, Bergoend H. Sclerosing lipogranuloma in a male. *Ann Dermatol Venereol* 1995;122:682–685.

Grebenc ML, Gorman JD, Sumida FK. Fibrous pseudotumor of the tunica vaginalis testis: imaging appearance. *Abdom Imag* 1995;20:379–380.

Imazu T, Takayama H, Tsukikawa M, Tsujimura A, Sugao H, Takaha M, Takeda M, Kurata A. Cysts in the cavum tunica vaginalis testis: a case report. *Acta Urol Jpn* 1994;40:725–728.

Irisawa C, Hamasaki T, Kantou S, Yamada Y, Kondou Y, Mouri J, Chiga R, Yamaguchi O, Shiraiwa Y. Two cases of primary sclerosing lipogranuloma in the scrotum: review of 63 cases reported in Japan. *Acta Urol Jpn* 1994;40:169–173.

Kizer JR, Bellah RD, Schnaufer L, Canning DA. Meconium hydrocele in a female newborn: an unusual case of a labial mass. *J Urol* 1995;153:188–190.

Radner M, Vergesslich KA, Weninger M, Eilenberger M, Ponhold W, Pollak A. Meconium peritonitis: a new finding in rubella syndrome. *J Clin Ultrasound* 1993;21:346–349.

Saginoya T, Yamaguchi K, Toda T, Kiyuna M. Fibrous pseudotumor of the scrotum: MR imaging findings. *Am J Roentgenol* 1996;167:285–286.

Salle JL, De Fraga JC, Wojciechowski M, Antunes CR. Congenital rupture of scrotum: an unusual complication of meconium peritonitis. *J Urol* 1992;148:1242–1243.

Takahara H, Takahashi M, Ueno T, Ishihara T, Naito K. Sclerosing lipogranuloma of the male genitalia: analysis of the lipid constituents and histological study. *Br J Urol* 1993;71:58–62.

Takahashi M, Kawano H, Ishihara T, Uchino F, Takihara H, Baba Y. Membranocystic lesion in sclerosing lipogranuloma of the scrotum: an ultrastructural study. *Ultrastruct Pathol* 1992;16:641–649.

## Scrotal Angiokeratoma

Gioglio L, Porta C, Moroni M, Nastasi G, Gangarossa I. Scrotal angiokeratoma (Fordyce): histopathological and ultrastructural findings. *Histol Histopathol* 1992;7:47–55.

Hisa T, Taniguchi S, Goto Y, Teramae H, Osato K, Kakudo K, Takigawa M. Scrotal angiokeratoma in a young man. *Acta Dermatovenereol* 1996;76:75.

Taniguchi S, Inoue A, Hamada T. Angiokeratoma of Fordyce: a cause of scrotal bleeding. *Br J Urol* 1994;73:589–590.

## Scrotal Cutaneous Hamartomas

Hsiao GH, Chen JS. Acquired genital smooth muscle hamartoma: a case report. *Am J Dermatopathol* 1995;17:67–70.

Popek EJ, Montgomery EA, Fourcroy JL. Fibrous hamartoma of infancy in the genital region: findings in 15 cases. *J Urol* 1994;152:990–993.

Sotelo-Avila C, Bale PM. Subdermal fibrous hamartoma of infancy: pathology of 40 cases and differential diagnosis. *Pediatr Pathol* 1994;14:39–52.

Stock JA, Niku SD, Packer MG, Krous H, Kaplan GW. Fibrous hamartoma of infancy: a report of two cases in the genital region. *Urology* 1995;45:130–131.

## Plasma Cell Infiltrates of the Penile Skin

Haedersdal M, Wulf HC. Plasma cell balanitis treated with a copper vapour laser. *Scand J Plast Reconstr Surg Hand Surg* 1995;29:357–358.

Jolly BB, Krishnamurty S, Vaidyanathan S. Zoon's balanitis. *Urol Int* 1993;50:182–184.

Vohra S, Badlani G. Balanitis and balanoposthitis. *Urol Clin N Amer* 1992;19:143–147.

Yoganathan S, Bohl TG, Mason G. Plasma cell balanitis and vulvitis (of Zoon): a study of 10 cases. *J Reproduc Med* 1994;39:939–944.

*Pathology of Pseudoneoplastic Lesions,*
edited by M. R. Wick, P. A. Humphrey, and J. H. Ritter.
Lippincott-Raven Publishers, Philadelphia © 1997.

# CHAPTER 10

# Pseudoneoplastic Lesions of the Female Genital Tract and Peritoneum

## Philip B. Clement and Robert H. Young

P. B. Clement: Department of Pathology, Vancouver Hospital and Health Sciences Centre and the University of British Columbia, Vancouver, British Columbia, Canada V5Z 1M9.

R. H. Young: Department of Pathology, Massachusetts General Hospital, Harvard Medical School, Boston, Massachusetts 02114.

In this chapter, we have endeavored to cover all lesions that could be misinterpreted as a neoplasm on gross or microscopic examination. What lesions are considered pseudoneoplastic is somewhat subjective, but we believe that the disorders we include meet one or both of these criteria based on our own experience and that in the literature. Organizing the material caused difficulty, as some entities (such as pregnancy luteoma) are unique to one organ, whereas others (such as endometriosis) may be seen at any of the sites considered here. In order to minimize repetition, some topics, such as cervical epithelial lesions, are considered by anatomic site, whereas other disorders are grouped together regardless of their anatomic location. The cervical epithelial lesions with which we begin (HPV-related and preneoplastic lesions are not included) probably account for more problems of the type under discussion than any other group of lesions in the female genital tract.

## EPITHELIAL LESIONS OF THE UTERINE CERVIX

Most of the pseudoneoplastic lesions covered in this section (Table 1) are glandular. As mentioned above, for organizational reasons some of them are considered elsewhere in this chapter: Arias-Stella reaction, endometriosis, and endocervicosis.

### Florid Squamous Metaplasia

Conventional squamous metaplasia should rarely cause diagnostic difficulty, but florid examples with involvement of many endocervical glands and clefts may pose a considerable challenge. Indeed, in an old text an eminent pathologist illustrates a case of "early epidermoid carcinoma" arising in a cervical polyp that is, we believe, probably florid squamous metaplasia (1). Reassuring features in these cases are the occurrence of the process in foci consistent with replaced endocervical glands, the smooth contours of the squa-

**TABLE 1.** *Pseudoneoplastic epithelial lesions of the uterine cervix*

Florid squamous metaplasia
Postbiopsy pseudoinvasion of squamous epithelium
Transitional cell metaplasia
Papillary endocervicitis
Tunnel clusters
Deep glands and cysts
Microglandular hyperplasia
Mesonephric hyperplasia
Diffuse laminar endocervical glandular hyperplasia
Glandular hyperplasia, not otherwise specified
Metaplasias (tubal, endometrioid, intestinal)
Changes secondary to extravasation of mucin
Arias–Stella reaction
Endometriosis
Endocervicosis
Reactive atypias

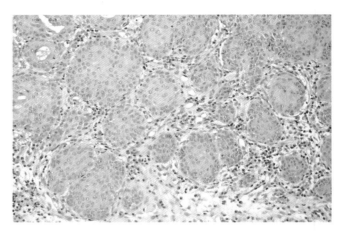

**FIG. 1.** Florid squamous metaplasia.

mous nests in contrast to the irregular shapes seen in invasive carcinoma, the bland cytology, and an absence of a stromal response (Fig. 1). Sometimes the focal identification of mucinous epithelial cells or mucin in the midst of squamous cells reinforces the diagnosis of squamous metaplasia.

### Postbiopsy "Pseudoinvasion" of Squamous Epithelium

In these cases, nests of squamous epithelium are present in the stroma, having been implanted there at the time of a prior biopsy (Fig. 2). Their occasional presence deep in the wall and the lack of an association with endocervical glands may suggest squamous carcinoma, particularly as the biopsy has often been performed for a preneoplastic squamous abnormality. Additionally, the squamous nests may be somewhat irregular in shape and may be associated with a fibrotic stroma secondary to postbiopsy scarring. The correct diagnosis is usually suggested by the small number of nests (often solitary), an absence of abnormal epithelium between the

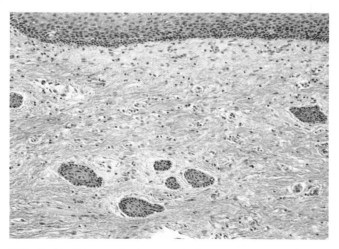

**FIG. 2.** Postbiopsy displacement of squamous nests in cervical stroma. Note the lack of continuity with the overlying epithelium, which is not dysplastic.

deep nests and the overlying mucosa, the presence of bland nuclear features, and an absence of any abnormalities of the overlying epithelium (Fig. 2). A potentially more difficult diagnostic problem can arise when noninvasive but dysplastic squamous epithelium is artifactually displaced into vascular spaces. This pseudoinvasion of vascular spaces was attributed to cervical lidocaine injection prior to loop diathermy in one recently described case (2).

## Transitional Cell Metaplasia

Transitional (urothelial) cell metaplasia of the cervix is quite common, particularly in postmenopausal females. On low-power examination the lack of maturation may impart an appearance that initially suggests dysplasia (Fig. 3). This change is usually seen in the surface mucosa, but involvement of endocervical glands may result in an appearance resembling that of Walthard's nests, and indeed cases have been reported as such (3). On microscopic examination transitional cell metaplasia is distinguished from dysplasia by the uniformity of the cells, lack of significant mitotic activity, and characteristic nuclear grooves within many of the nuclei (3A, 3B) (Fig. 4). Changes similar to those of transitional cell metaplasia were found in a series of female-to-male transsexuals who had been treated with large doses of androgens (4). It should be noted that transitional cells in the cervix may become dysplastic and may rarely even be the presumed origin of both benign and malignant transitional cell tumors (5).

## Papillary Endocervicitis

A florid papillary pattern is occasionally encountered in chronic endocervicitis (6). Stromal papillae that are usually relatively regular and that contain chronic inflammatory cells are covered by a single layer of benign endocervical

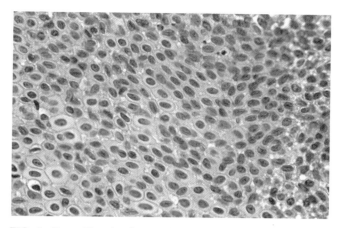

**FIG. 4.** Transitional cell metaplasia. Note the bland cytologic features and the regular nuclei, some of which have longitudinal nuclear grooves.

columnar epithelium (Fig. 5). This pattern is similar to that of endocervical villoglandular adenocarcinomas (7), but those tumors usually exhibit focal cellular stratification and always show more cytologic atypia than seen in papillary endocervicitis.

## Tunnel Clusters

Tunnel clusters occur in the cervix of approximately 10% of adult multigravida women (8–11). Fluhmann (8,9) de-

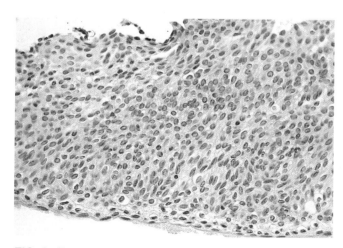

**FIG. 3.** Transitional cell metaplasia. The stratification that is apparent on low power may suggest the erroneous diagnosis of dysplasia.

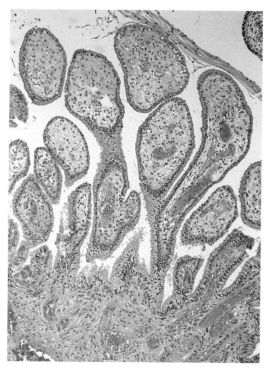

**FIG. 5.** Papillary endocervicitis. The papillae are lined with a single layer of bland columnar cells.

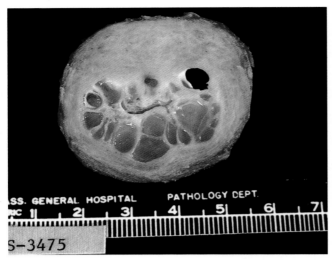

**FIG. 6.** Tunnel clusters. Many cysts containing inspissated mucin involve most of the cervical wall in the lower half of the illustration.

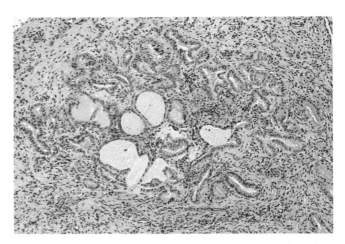

**FIG. 8.** Tunnel cluster. Note admixture of cystic and noncystic glands.

scribed two types of tunnel clusters, one noncystic and lined with columnar epithelium (type A), and the other cystic and lined with cuboidal or flattened epithelium (type B). In one recent study of tunnel clusters (11) that was restricted to cystic lesions they were observed grossly in approximately 40% of cases (Fig. 6).

Tunnel clusters are typically discrete, <5 mm in diameter (but occasionally up to 20 mm), rounded foci composed of 20–50 closely packed tubules that may be oval, round, or irregular, and of varying size (Figs. 7 and 8). Multiple foci are present in about 80% of cases (11), and occasionally the tunnel clusters are confluent. The tubules, which typically contain mucin, are separated by scanty connective tissue, and the tunnel cluster is surrounded by normal endocervical stroma. In occasional cases (6,11), mild nuclear atypia and occasional mitotic figures have led to the misdiagnosis of adenoma malignum ("minimal deviation adenocarcinoma") (12,12A). The lobulated appearance of tunnel clusters is a

helpful diagnostic feature not observed in adenoma malignum. Tunnel clusters also lack the infiltrative pattern and frequent desmoplasia of adenoma malignum (12). Like other benign disorders of the endocervical glands, tunnel clusters may occasionally extend deeply into the cervical wall, and the distinction of deep cystic tunnel clusters from deep Nabothian cysts (see below) is sometimes arbitrary. Type A tunnel clusters, in particular, may show some cytologic atypia that is occasionally problematic (12A).

**Deep Glands and Cysts**

Endocervical glands occasionally lie deep in the cervical stroma (13–16). Such deep glands are usually few in number and resemble normal endocervical glands, but rarely they are numerous, exhibit slight variability in size and shape, and extend into the outer third of the cervical wall (Fig. 9) (16). Similarly, Nabothian cysts may extend through most of the cervical wall (Fig. 10) (17). In the latter cases, gross exami-

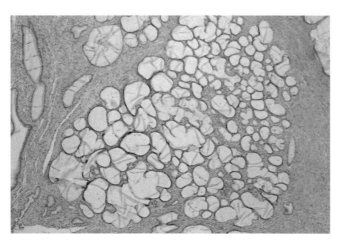

**FIG. 7.** Tunnel clusters.

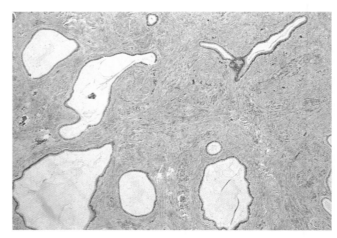

**FIG. 9.** Deep glands and cysts. The glands and cysts are unassociated with a stromal reaction and have bland cytologic features.

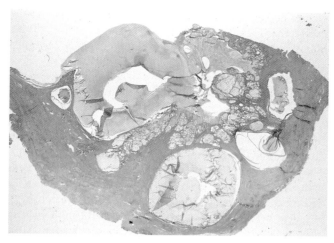

**FIG. 10.** Deep Nabothian cysts. The cysts extend into the outer aspect of the cervical wall.

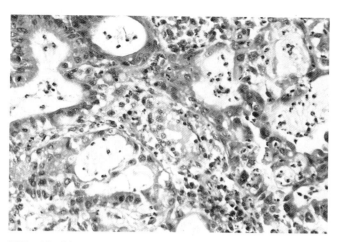

**FIG. 12.** Microglandular hyperplasia. The glands contain mucin with inflammatory cells, and the lining epithelium exhibits reactive atypia.

nation of the cervix shows numerous mucin-filled cysts measuring up to 1 cm in diameter replacing the endocervical wall. Histologic examination shows cysts lined with benign columnar or cuboidal to flattened endocervical epithelium devoid of mitotic activity.

Deep glands and cysts may be confused with adenoma malignum. Adenoma malignum, however, is usually associated with a suspicious mass, and its neoplastic glands typically exhibit a wide range of sizes and shapes, a periglandular stromal response, and focal cytologic atypia—features absent in deep glands and cysts. Additional features that support or are diagnostic of adenoma malignum include perineural invasion, vascular invasion, and cytoplasmic immunoreactivity for carcinoembryonic antigen (CEA) (12).

## Microglandular Hyperplasia

Microglandular hyperplasia (MGH) is usually related to progesterone stimulation, most commonly oral contracep-

tives and, less frequently, pregnancy (18–25). It may also be seen in a patient receiving only estrogen, or in a nonpregnant patient not on hormonal therapy, and Greeley et al. have recently questioned the hormonal basis of MGH (26). The lesion typically occurs in young women (mean age 33.5 years), but approximately 5% of the cases have occurred in postmenopausal women (18–25). The patients are usually asymptomatic but may complain of abnormal vaginal bleeding or vaginal discharge. MGH is typically an incidental microscopic finding, but occasionally it has the clinical appearance of an erosion, an ordinary cervical polyp, or a polypoid mass that is sometimes friable and suspicious for carcinoma (23).

On microscopic examination (Figs. 11–19) MGH may be nonpolypoid or polypoid (Fig. 11), either as a pure lesion or as part of an endocervical polyp. The lesion characteristically consists of closely packed glands that vary from small and round to large, irregular, and cystically dilated (Figs. 11

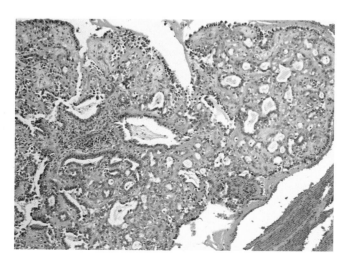

**FIG. 11.** Microglandular hyperplasia. A polyp contains numerous glands of varying sizes in its stroma.

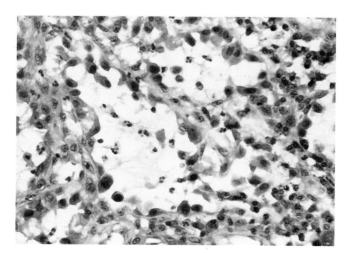

**FIG. 13.** Microglandular hyperplasia. There is a loose "reticular" pattern scattered inflammatory cells. Note occasional hobnail cells.

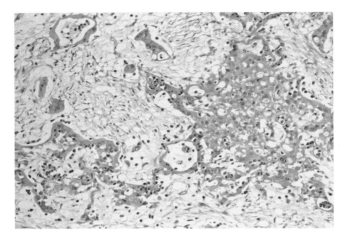

**FIG. 14.** Microglandular hyperplasia. There is a pseudoinfiltrative pattern within an edematous stroma.

and 12). They usually contain a basophilic or eosinophilic mucinous secretion. There may be an extensive infiltrate of acute and chronic inflammatory cells in the mucin and intervening stroma (Figs. 12 and 13); the latter is occasionally extensively hyalinized (Fig. 19). In some cases, small nests and large aggregates of epithelial cells are irregularly distributed in a myxoid stroma, imparting a pseudoinfiltrative pattern (Fig. 14). MGH may also manifest a reticular pattern, in which the cells, some of which may be spindle-shaped, are loosely dispersed in an edematous stroma (Fig. 13), or grow as solid sheets of cells (Figs. 15 and 16), often with eosinophilic cytoplasm (27). Exceptionally the cells are arranged in trabeculae or small cords. The cells lining the glands and cysts are usually low columnar, cuboidal, or flat, with faintly basophilic or granular cytoplasm. Occasionally the cells have abundant eosinophilic cytoplasm or resemble hobnail cells (Fig. 13). Subnuclear vacuoles, which stain positively for mucin but are negative for glycogen, are often present and may be conspicuous (Fig. 19). Rarely some cells within the solid foci have pale mucinous cytoplasm and ec-

centric nuclei, simulating the signet ring cells of an adenocarcinoma (Figs. 17 and 18) (27). The nuclei of the cells are almost always small and regular. Rarely they may be mildly or even moderately atypical, but this atypia generally has a degenerative appearance. In such cases, nucleoli may be visible but are only rarely conspicuous; mitotic figures are rare (25).

Clear cell adenocarcinoma is the neoplasm most likely to be confused with MGH because, like MGH, it may have tubular, cystic, and solid patterns, with a hyalinized stroma. The solid foci of clear cell carcinoma usually consist of cells with abundant, clear, glycogen-rich cytoplasm whereas the constituent cells in solid foci of MGH never have conspicuous clear cytoplasm. Additionally, clear cell carcinomas almost always have at least focal severe cytologic atypia, of a degree that is inconsistent with MGH. Rare adenocarcinomas, both cervical and endometrial, have focal microglandular patterns, extensive acute inflammation, and glands filled with mucin, creating a superficial resemblance to MGH (28,29). However, the degree of nuclear atypicality and mitotic activity in the microglandular areas, at least focally, exceeds that of MGH. CEA negativity favors a diagnosis of MGH in contrast to cervical adenocarcinomas, which are usually CEA-positive, but this is not a reliable distinguishing characteristic, as occasional cervical adenocarcinomas are negative or only focally positive for CEA (12,30–32).

### Mesonephric Hyperplasia

Hyperplastic mesonephric remnants are occasionally so florid that the diagnosis of adenocarcinoma is suggested, especially in those cases accompanied by cytologic atypia and mitotic activity (33,34). Ferry and Scully (33) have divided mesonephric hyperplasia into three categories: lobular mesonephric hyperplasia (75% of their cases), diffuse mesonephric hyperplasia (20%), and pure mesonephric ductal hyperplasia (5%) (Figs. 20–26).

In lobular hyperplasia, round to oval, occasionally dilated,

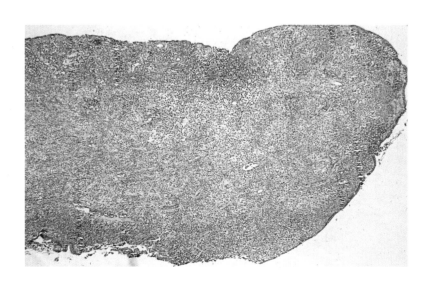

**FIG. 15.** Microglandular hyperplasia. A cervical polyp from a pregnant woman has been replaced by a solid proliferation of cells.

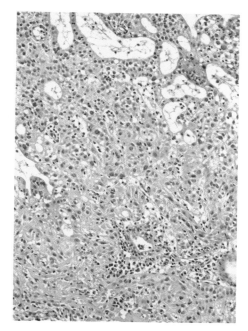

**FIG. 16.** Microglandular hyperplasia. A solid proliferation of cells with eosinophilic cytoplasm occupies most of the illustration, but more typical microglandular hyperplasia is present at the top.

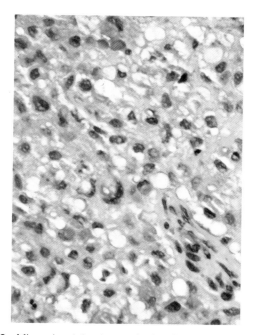

**FIG. 18.** Microglandular hyperplasia. Signet ring–like cells contain mucin (mucicarmine stain).

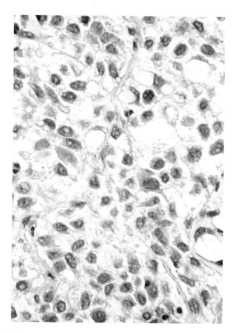

**FIG. 17.** Microglandular hyperplasia. Several signet ring–like cells are present.

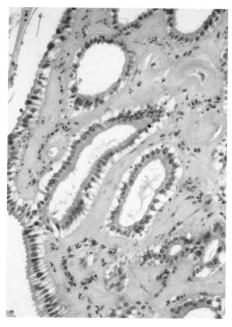

**FIG. 19.** Microglandular hyperplasia. Many of the cells lining glands have prominent subnuclear vacuoles, and there is conspicuous stromal hyalinization.

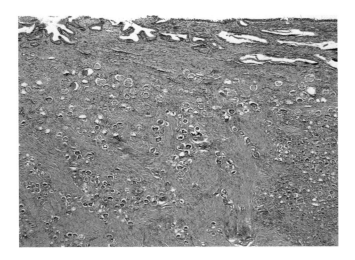

**FIG. 20.** Mesonephric hyperplasia. The cervical stroma contains numerous small tubules in a lobular pattern.

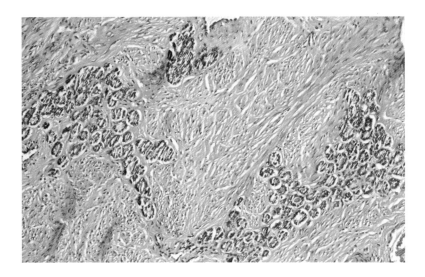

**FIG. 21.** Mesonephric hyperplasia. Two distinct lobular aggregates of small tubules unassociated with any alteration of the cervical stroma are present.

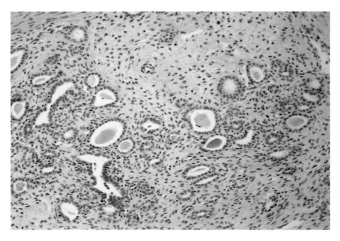

**FIG. 22.** Mesonephric hyperplasia. Cuboidal cells with bland nuclear features line the tubules, which contain a colloid-like eosinophilic secretion.

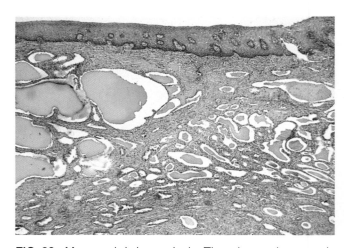

**FIG. 23.** Mesonephric hyperplasia. There is prominent cystic dilatation of the tubules.

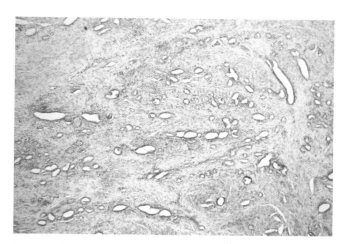

**FIG. 24.** Mesonephric hyperplasia. The tubules have a pseudoinfiltrative pattern and lack the typical eosinophilic intraluminal secretion.

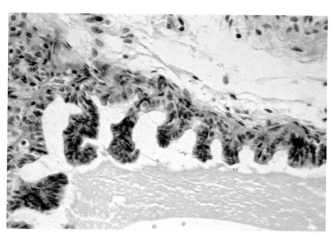

**FIG. 26.** Mesonephric ductal hyperplasia. High-power view of small papillae seen in Fig. 25.

tubules are arranged in at least vaguely lobular aggregates (Figs. 20–22). These tubules characteristically contain intraluminal bright pink, periodic acid–Schiff (PAS)–positive, hyaline material. In diffuse hyperplasia no lobular grouping is apparent, and the irregular distribution of the tubules and their presence deep in the cervical wall may create a very worrisome appearance, particularly if the characteristic intraluminal eosinophilic material is absent (Figs. 23 and 24). Approximately three quarters of cases of lobular and diffuse hyperplasia demonstrate an additional component of ductal hyperplasia, characterized by one or more large round or elongated ducts (depending on the plane of section) lined by pseudostratified epithelium, which often forms small regular papillae (Figs. 25 and 26). The tubular forms of mesonephric hyperplasia are most likely to be misinterpreted as invasive adenocarcinoma, but ductal hyperplasia, particularly when pure, is usually misdiagnosed as a premalignant glandular le-

sion. The elongated form of the ducts and the lack of an association with endocervical glands are initial clues to their nature, and high-power scrutiny reveals no significant cytologic atypia. Finally, the micropapillae seen in ductal hyperplasia are distinctive and with rare exceptions are not a feature of premalignant glandular lesions.

Mesonephric hyperplasia must be distinguished from mesonephric adenocarcinoma, a problem compounded by the usual origin of the latter on a background of mesonephric hyperplasia (35). In contrast to mesonephric hyperplasia, which is almost always an incidental microscopic finding, mesonephric carcinomas usually produce grossly visible lesions. On microscopic examination, the tubules of the carcinomas are at least focally confluent, may be associated with a stromal reaction, and are lined with cells with more atypia and mitotic activity than seen in mesonephric hyperplasia. Additionally, most mesonephric carcinomas have other pat-

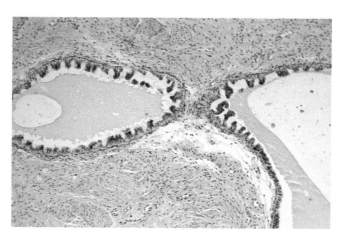

**FIG. 25.** Mesonephric ductal hyperplasia. Two ducts contain many small papillae.

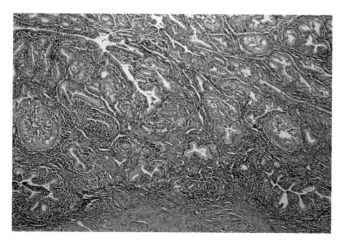

**FIG. 27.** Diffuse laminar endocervical glandular hyperplasia. There is a sharp demarcation of the lesion with the subjacent cervical stroma.

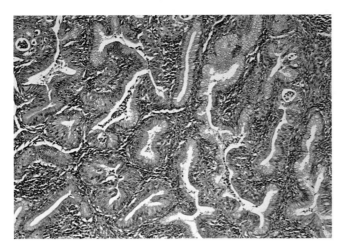

**FIG. 28.** Diffuse laminar endocervical gland hyperplasia. There are prominent lymphoid cells between the glands. Note the lack of cytologic atypia.

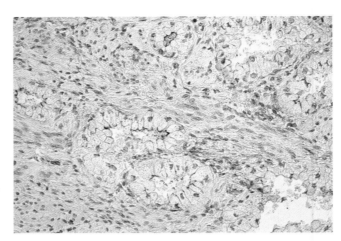

**FIG. 30.** Endocervical glandular hyperplasia, not otherwise specified. An immunohistochemical stain for carcinoembryonic antigen shows only glycocalyceal staining.

terns (retiform, papillary, solid, or trabecular), and in some cases a component of neoplastic spindle cells, features absent in mesonephric hyperplasia (35).

Mesonephric hyperplasia may be also confused with adenoma malignum, clear cell adenocarcinoma, and, rarely, metastatic adenocarcinoma. The glands in adenoma malignum (12) are much more irregular in size and shape than the tubules of mesonephric hyperplasia, are lined with mucinous cells, and are often surrounded by an edematous or desmoplastic stroma that is absent in mesonephric hyperplasia. The tubules in mesonephric hyperplasia may resemble the tubular glands of many clear cell adenocarcinomas, and the tubules in mesonephric hyperplasia may undergo cystic dilatation (Fig. 23), suggesting the tubulocystic pattern of clear cell carcinoma. In contrast to mesonephric hyperplasia, at least some of the cells lining the glands and cysts of clear

cell carcinoma have conspicuous clear, glycogen-rich cytoplasm or are hobnail cells. Other patterns of clear cell carcinoma contain similar cells, which also exclude mesonephric hyperplasia. Metastatic adenocarcinomas may occasionally be composed of small tubular glands reminiscent of those of mesonephric hyperplasia; in most cases the former will, at least focally, have architectural and cytologic features inconsistent with mesonephric hyperplasia.

### Diffuse Laminar Endocervical Glandular Hyperplasia

This form of endocervical glandular hyperplasia is characterized by a diffuse distribution of endocervical glands typically appearing as a discrete layer sharply demarcated from the underlying cervical stroma (Figs. 27 and 28) (36). The affected patients have been of reproductive age and, with only one exception, lacked a history of exogenous hormone exposure. Microscopic examination of the lesions,

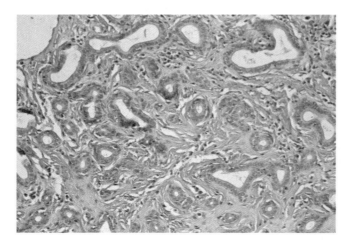

**FIG. 29.** Endocervical glandular hyperplasia, not otherwise specified. The glands have a somewhat orderly arrangement, and there is no stromal reaction.

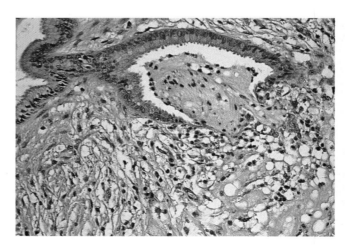

**FIG. 31.** Rupture of endocervical gland with stromal reaction to extravasated mucin.

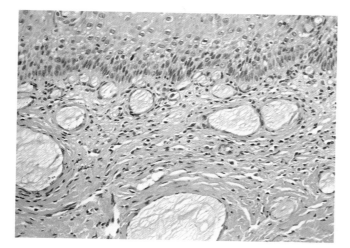

**FIG. 32.** Extravasated mucin in endocervical stroma.

which have all been incidental histologic findings, reveals a proliferation of moderately sized, closely packed endocervical glands in the inner third of the cervical wall. Mild reactive cytologic atypia has been present in some cases. A marked inflammatory response and focal stromal edema have been present in most of the cases, but a desmoplastic stroma has not. The last feature, as well as a lack of irregular or deep stromal infiltration, and an absence of at least focal malignant cytologic features, aids in the distinction of this process from adenoma malignum.

## Glandular Hyperplasia, Not Otherwise Specified

The endocervical epithelium may be hyperplastic, sometimes floridly so, without exhibiting any of the special histologic patterns already discussed (Figs. 29 and 30) (37,38). Changes may include glandular irregularity and, rarely, a cribriform pattern. Lack of deep invasion, an orderly, sometimes lobulated arrangement of the glands, a well-demarcated margin with the adjacent cervical stroma, a usual lack

of a stromal reaction, and bland nuclear features are all characteristics that indicate the nonneoplastic nature of this process.

## Changes Secondary to Extravasation of Mucin

Although the lack of a stromal response often supports the benign nature of an endocervical glandular lesion, the stroma adjacent to benign glands may exhibit reactive changes in response to mucin extravasated from a ruptured gland (Fig. 31). A foreign body giant cell reaction is sometimes seen in these cases, and in some of the cases foamy histiocytes are conspicuous. In one apparently unique case gland rupture was associated with dissection of mucin into the stroma and vascular lumens; the resulting appearance raised initial concern about a primary or metastatic adenocarcinoma (Fig. 32) (37). Michael and colleagues (38) described another case of a pseudoneoplastic glandular lesion with an unusual appearance interpreted by them as being due, at least in part, to the extravasation of mucin.

## Metaplasias

### Tubal and Tuboendometrioid Metaplasia

Tubal metaplasia was found in 31% of cone biopsy and hysterectomy specimens in a recent series (39). "Tuboendometrioid metaplasia" has been found in 25% of hysterectomy specimens when a prior cone biopsy had been performed, suggesting that it may be a reparative response in at least some cases (40). In tubal metaplasia, endocervical surface or glandular epithelium is replaced by a single layer of ciliated cells, nonciliated cells, and peg cells (Figs. 33–35). Tuboendometrioid metaplasia is similar but has rare ciliated cells (Fig. 36). Usually the glands involved by tubal and tuboendometrioid metaplasia otherwise resemble normal endocervical glands, but one or more unusual features, such as variability in size and shape, cystic dilatation, focal crowd-

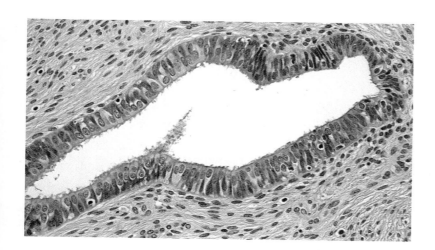

**FIG. 33.** Tubal metaplasia.

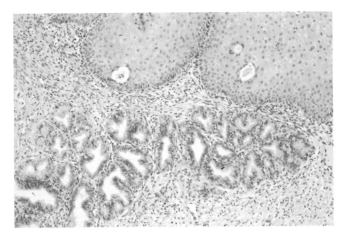

**FIG. 34.** Tubal metaplasia. Metaplasia in a tunnel cluster produces a picture on low power that causes concern for endocervical glandular dysplasia or *in situ* adenocarcinoma.

ing (Figs. 34 and 35), a deep location, and periglandular stromal hypercellularity (Fig. 36) or edema (41), may raise the possibility of a well-differentiated invasive adenocarcinoma. The admixture of cell types, including prominence of ciliated cells, as well as the lack of atypia, mitotic activity, and a desmoplastic stromal reaction, facilitate the correct diagnosis in these and more typical cases of tubal metaplasia.

### Endometrioid Metaplasia

Benign endometrioid glands, interpreted as ectopic endometrial glands, were found deep in the wall in 1% of cervices examined in one series (15). Endometrioid glands arising by a process of metaplasia of the mucinous endocervical epithelium may also be seen. In our experience, pure endometrioid metaplasia is rare (42), there usually being an additional component of tubal metaplasia such that the term

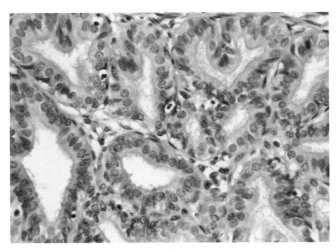

**FIG. 35.** Tubal metaplasia. Cilia are visible. High-power of Fig. 34.

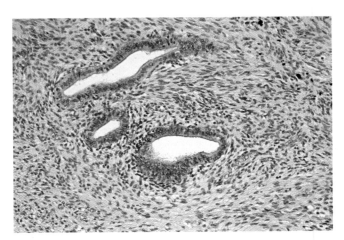

**FIG. 36.** Tuboendometrioid metaplasia. There is a cellular stroma around the glands.

"tuboendometrioid" metaplasia (see above) is more appropriate (40).

### Intestinal Metaplasia

Intestinal metaplasia is the rarest cervical glandular metaplasia and is characterized by the focal presence of goblet and argentaffin cells within the endocervical glands (43). Intestinal metaplasia in the cervix is seen much more commonly in adenocarcinoma *in situ* (44) and in invasive adenocarcinomas and can occasionally occur in benign neoplasms (45,46).

### Reactive Atypia

As elsewhere in the body, reactive atypia in association with marked inflammation is occasionally seen within endocervical glandular cells. This may occur in the epithelium of otherwise normal glands or within any of the specific lesions discussed above. In some cases the atypical nuclei are large and hyperchromatic. In contrast to *in situ* adenocarcinoma, the nuclei often have a smudgy appearance and are often present in cells with abundant eosinophilic cytoplasm (46A). In comparison to *in situ* adenocarcinoma, the cells of reactive atypia are more variable in size and shape, they tend to be separated by more normal-appearing cells, and mitotic figures are rare. Perhaps some of these changes have a viral etiology: Brown and Wells (47) described bizarre multinucleated giant cells within endocervical glands with evidence of HPV infection elsewhere in the cervix. The authors concluded that the changes were secondary to viral infection.

## ENDOMETRIAL EPITHELIAL METAPLASIAS

With the possible exception of the first entity considered here, the lesions discussed in this section are unquestionably metaplasias. In our experience the most common problem associated with them is the underdiagnosis of a significant associated lesion, usually hyperplasia or carcinoma. However, in some cases striking degrees of metaplasia may result in an overdiagnosis of hyperplasia or carcinoma, a problem that initially led Hendrickson and Kempson to highlight these lesions in their seminal contribution (48).

## Papillary Syncytial Change

Papillary syncytial change (PSC) involves the endometrial surface epithelium and less commonly the superficial endometrial glands (48–51). Cells with eosinophilic cytoplasm, indistinct cell borders, and bland nuclear features are arranged in syncytial aggregates, cellular buds, and papillae lacking stromal cores (Fig. 37). Normal mitotic figures were present in 20% of cases in one series (50). PSC is commonly associated with active endometrial bleeding with evidence of glandular and stromal breakdown, including cell necrosis, aggregates of closely packed small stromal cells, and neutrophils (50). PSC, therefore, probably represents a regenerative phenomenon following ovulatory or anovulatory menstrual bleeding (51,52), although others consider it a metaplasia (48) or a "retrogressive" change (50). Its microscopic size, usual confinement to the endometrial surface, and benign nuclear features facilitate distinction of PSC from papillary carcinomas. In this context, however, it is noteworthy that two studies have shown that endometrial adenocarcinomas are frequently associated with PSC or can exhibit a PSC-like change on their surface (29,53). In some but not all of these cases, the PSC or PSC-like change exhibited nuclear atypia greater than that usually encountered in PSC, although the atypia was typically less than that of the underlying carcinoma. For these reasons, a careful search for an associated carcinoma should be undertaken when PSC or a PSC-like change is prominent, especially in post-

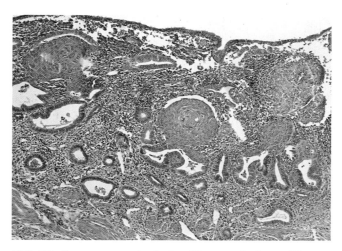

FIG. 38. Squamous metaplasia of the morular type of the endometrium.

menopausal women, and a repeat curettage may be indicated (29).

## Squamous Metaplasia

Squamous metaplasia of the morular type (acanthosis) may be related to unopposed estrogen stimulation, chronic endometritis, pyometra, or a foreign body (such as an intrauterine device), although most cases lack these associations. It usually takes the form of nests (morules) of immature squamous cells that typically have indistinct cell borders and bland nuclear features. The nests occupy, and often obliterate, glandular lumina (Fig. 38), sometimes forming confluent masses of squamous epithelium that occasionally is centrally necrotic (48,54–56). Adenocarcinoma with squamous metaplasia may be misdiagnosed when florid squamous metaplasia occurs within a complex atypical hyperplasia ("adenoacanthosis") if sufficient attention is not paid to the features of the associated glandular component.

Extensive replacement of the surface endometrium by mature keratinizing squamous epithelium without morule formation ("ichthyosis uteri") (54) is usually secondary to pyometra. This process has bland nuclear features, and no mitoses or invasion, excluding the usual primary endometrial squamous cell carcinoma. However, only the last feature is absolutely reliable, as some endometrial squamous cell carcinomas are exceptionally well differentiated. For example, we have encountered two cases in which curettings in a postmenopausal woman revealed fragments of normal-appearing, glycogenated squamous epithelium devoid of cellular atypia, but both lesions invaded the myometrium and one metastasized to several pelvic lymph nodes.

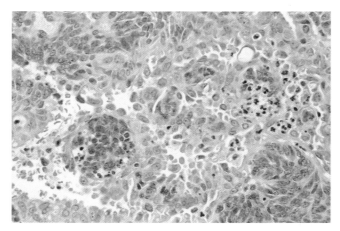

FIG. 37. Papillary syncytial change. Note the admixed nests of degenerating stromal cells.

## Mucinous Metaplasia

In mucinous metaplasia, endometrial glands are lined with columnar cells with mucin-rich cytoplasm (48,57). The cells typically mimic endocervical epithelium on routine sections, histochemical staining, and ultrastructural examination, but can rarely be constituted by goblet cells (58). Rare cases may be accompanied by mucometra (59) or mucinous lesions elsewhere in the female genital tract; in one case, the patient also had bilateral borderline mucinous ovarian tumors, mucinous epithelial inclusions within pelvic lymph nodes, and papillary mucinous proliferations within endocervical glands (60). When mucinous epithelium is atypical, extensive, or both, there should be a high index of suspicion for mucinous adenocarcinoma, as many of the latter are well differentiated.

## Ciliated Metaplasia

As small numbers of ciliated cells are found lining normal proliferative endometrial glands, the term "ciliated metaplasia" should be restricted to cases in which ciliated cells are the dominant or sole cell type. The ciliated cells have uniform round nuclei and often strikingly eosinophilic cytoplasm. They usually line the gland as a single layer but occasionally stratify. The absence of architectural complexity and atypical nuclear features separates ciliated metaplasia from rare examples of atypical hyperplasia with a prominent component of ciliated cells, or ciliated adenocarcinoma (61).

## Eosinophilic Metaplasia

In this type of metaplasia, glands are lined with nonciliated cells with abundant eosinophilic cytoplasm (Fig. 39) (48) that may be oncocytic (62). The uniformity of the round

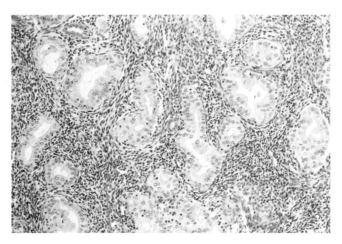

**FIG. 39.** Eosinophilic metaplasia of endometrium.

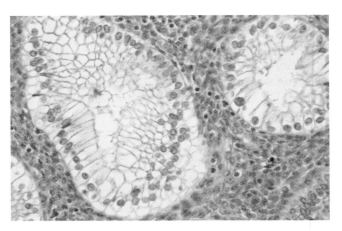

**FIG. 40.** Clear cell metaplasia of endometrium in nonpregnant patient.

central nuclei and paucity of mitotic figures distinguish this alteration from hyperplasia with atypia or occasional adenocarcinomas in which the cells have abundant eosinophilic cytoplasm (63).

## Hobnail Cell and Clear Cell Metaplasia

Rarely, endometrial glands exhibiting hobnail cell or clear cell metaplasia (Fig. 40) are an isolated finding with no apparent cause in a nonpregnant patient (48). The former cell type may also occur as a reactive change (see next section). The differential diagnosis of clear cell and hobnail cell metaplasia is with clear cell carcinoma, but the focal microscopic distribution of the metaplastic glands, the usual occurrence as a surface phenomenon unassociated with architectural complexity, and the absence of mitotic activity are criteria that distinguish this lesion from carcinoma. Similar metaplastic changes occurring in pregnancy (Arias-Stella reaction) are discussed below.

## ENDOMETRIAL TUMOR–LIKE CHANGES ASSOCIATED WITH MENSES, HYPERPLASIA, POLYPS, AND CURETTAGE

The marked fragmentation and crowding of endometrial glands and surface epithelium that occur at the time of menses, which may be accentuated by the curettage procedure, are changes that have been confused with complex hyperplasia or even adenocarcinoma (Fig. 41). The associated stromal findings (see below), the fragmented nature of the epithelium, the frequent presence of residual secretory changes in the epithelium, and the absence of nuclear atypicality argue against a diagnosis of carcinoma or a precancerous lesion. The stromal changes noted above that are characteristic of an anovulatory or postovulatory menstrual

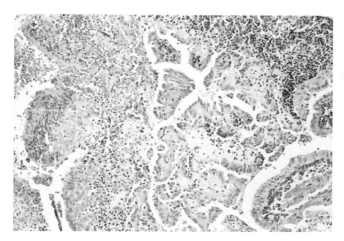

**FIG. 41.** Menstrual endometrium. There is marked fragmentation. This specimen was initially misdiagnosed as adenocarcinoma.

endometrium take the form of compact, densely cellular nests of endometrial stromal cells (64). The degenerating stromal cells have scanty cytoplasm and irregular, sometimes spindled, hyperchromatic nuclei, an appearance that can be mistaken for a small cell carcinoma or stromal sarcoma (Fig. 42). The nests are often surrounded by larger epithelial cells; both cell types lack features of malignancy and mitotic activity. Papillary syncytial change (see above) may also be present. Awareness of these menstrual changes and attention to the features noted above facilitate the correct diagnosis.

Menstrual endometrium may occasionally be found within uterine blood vessels (Fig. 43). In 1927, Sampson illustrated intravascular menstrual endometrium in two uteri from women who were menstruating at the time of hysterec-

tomy (65). More recently, Banks et al. described a case in which numerous foci of menstrual endometrium were found within parametrial blood vessels of a hysterectomy specimen, the appearance simulating vascular invasion by a poorly differentiated malignant tumor (66).

Rarely, the sinusoidal thrombosis and stromal breakdown that may accompany endometrial hyperplasia (usually cystic hyperplasia) are associated with reactive epithelium and stromal atypia (Figs. 44–46). The focality, background, and associated hemorrhage and fibrin are all clues to the nature of the process in these cases. Similar regenerative and reparative endometrial changes in uteri removed shortly after a D&C should not be confused with a cancerous or precancerous lesion. Such changes are characterized by epithelial atypia, which may be striking. The alterations are typically confined to the surface epithelium and superficial glands, and include focal nuclear enlargement, hyperchromasia, and prominent nucleoli; some of the cells may have a hobnail appearance (Fig. 46). Papillary syncytial change (see above) may also represent a postcurettage reparative response. Awareness of a recent curettage, the superficial location of the changes, an absence of significant architectural changes in the underlying glands, and, in some cases, inflammatory changes in the stroma will facilitate the diagnosis. A final example of reactive epithelial atypia that is worth noting is the epithelial atypia that may be encountered overlying infarcted endometrial polyps; we have seen several striking examples of this phenomenon.

A variety of curettage-related artifactual changes may be confused with endometrial hyperplasia or even carcinoma. Artifactual crowding of the endometrial glands due to excessive curettage-related fragmentation of the tissue has occasionally been misinterpreted as simple or complex hyperplasia (Fig. 47). A diagnosis of hyperplasia should rarely be

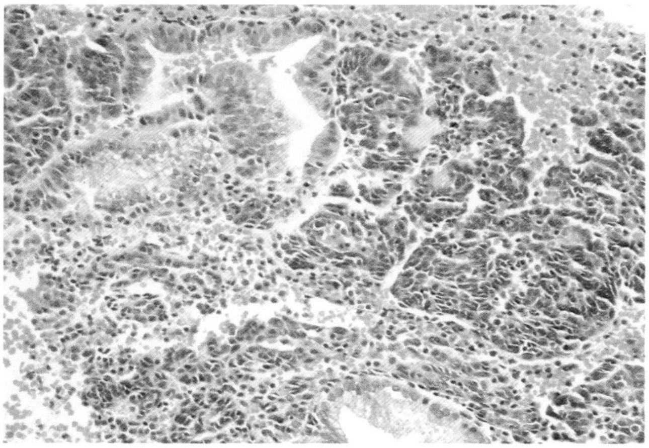

**FIG. 42.** Menstrual endometrium. The shrunken stromal cells with hyperchromatic nuclei were initially mistaken for small cell carcinoma.

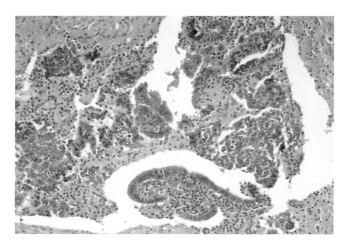

**FIG. 43.** Menstrual endometrium within a myometrial vascular lumen.

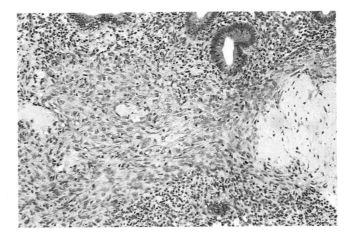

FIG. 44. Pseudosarcomatous fibroblastic proliferation in a case of simple hyperplasia. On the right, note organizing fibrin that represents a thrombosed sinusoid.

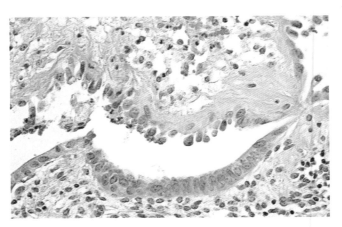

FIG. 46. Reparative surface epithelial atypia secondary to sinusoidal thrombosis and menstrual breakdown in a case of simple hyperplasia. Note hobnail cells.

made unless the glands and stroma and their relation to one another are intact and not artifactually disrupted. Similarly, curettage of an atrophic endometrium often yields strips of surface epithelium that are artifactually packed together, resulting in a crowded pseudopapillary pattern, an appearance that may be mistaken for complex hyperplasia or even carcinoma (Fig. 48). In the atrophic endometrium, the stroma may be particularly compact and dense, occasionally causing problems similar to those noted in menstrual endometrium (see above). Telescoping, in which coiled fragments of epithelium lie free within gland lumens, is another artifact that may be mistaken for hyperplasia (Fig. 47) (67).

## ADENOMYOSIS-RELATED CHANGES

Adenomyosis is a common disorder that may cause tumor-like enlargement of the uterus. Gross examination typi-

cally reveals a focally or diffusely thickened, trabeculated myometrium. Blood-filled cysts, usually <0.5 cm in diameter but occasionally larger (68), may be grossly visible within the lesions. When the process forms a discrete, leiomyoma-like mural mass, the designation adenomyoma is used, and when a polypoid mass projects into the endometrial cavity the lesion is referred to as a polypoid adenomyoma; others have formed pedunculated subserosal masses. Whether these adenomyomas represent circumscribed adenomyosis or benign mixed neoplasms is not clear. Most of the polypoid adenomyomas in the literature have had an atypical glandular component (usually with squamous metaplasia) and a stromal component of cellular smooth muscle, warranting the designation "atypical polypoid adenomyoma") (APA) (69,70).

In occasional cases of adenomyosis, especially in postmenopausal women, the glandular or the stromal component may be focally inconspicuous or absent. When the stromal

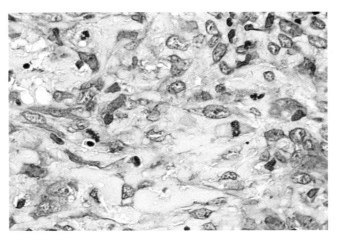

FIG. 45. Pseudosarcomatous fibroblastic proliferation in a case of simple hyperplasia. High-power view of Fig. 44.

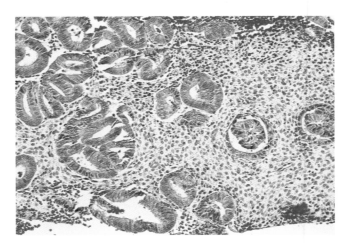

FIG. 47. Curettage-related artifact. Note focal glandular crowding and telescoping of endometrial glands.

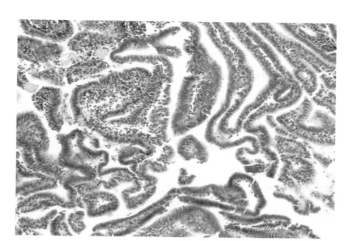

**FIG. 48.** Atrophic endometrium. A vigorous curretage has resulted in a pseudopapillary pattern that may be misconstrued as carcinoma.

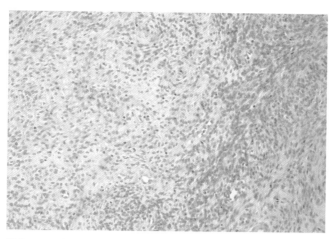

**FIG. 50.** Adenomyosis with sparse glands. Note the paler central zone on the left that is surrounded by a more cellular zone on the right. High-power view of Fig. 49.

component is atrophic, glands deep within the myometrium are surrounded directly by hyperplastic smooth muscle, a finding that should not be misinterpreted as invasive adenocarcinoma. The atrophic appearance of the adenomyotic glands, the lack of mitotic activity, the lack of a desmoplastic stroma, the usual association with more typical adenomyosis elsewhere in the myometrium, and the lack of an associated surface endometrial neoplasm facilitate the diagnosis. A more common diagnostic problem in our experience is the converse one, in which adenomyotic glands are sparse and the appearance of pure stromal elements in the myometrium can be misinterpreted as low-grade endometrial stromal sarcoma (LGESS). Goldblum et al. (71) recently reported seven such cases of "adenomyosis with sparse glands" (AWSG) (Figs. 49 and 50). In contrast to

**FIG. 49.** Adenomyosis with sparse glands. The center of the focus (which is devoid of glands) is in the upper left. Note peripheral darker zone consisting of cellular adenomyotic stroma and hyperplastic smooth muscle. The normal myometrium containing a few dilated vessels is at the extreme right.

LGESS, AWSP (a) is typically an incidental microscopic finding; (b) has a distinctive concentric zonal organization, with less-cellular pale centers surrounded by a thin rim of hypercellular stroma and/or smooth muscle, often with a thicker but ill-defined peripheral zone of hypertrophic myometrial smooth muscle; (c) is composed of atrophic stromal cells with an absence of nuclear atypia and mitotic figures; (d) lacks endometrial involvement, sclerotic areas, foam cells, sex cord–like structures, a hemangiopericytoma-like vascular pattern, prominent vascular invasion, and extrauterine extension; (e) is usually associated with typical adenomyosis with glands elsewhere in the myometrium; and (f) occurs, based on the cases reported to date, only in postmenopausal women.

Another pseudoneoplastic finding in otherwise typical adenomyosis is intravascular endometrium. Sahin et al. (72) recently demonstrated the latter in 5% of hysterectomy specimens from nonmenstruating women, all of whom had adenomyosis; approximately 18% of women with adenomyosis had intravascular endometrium. The adenomyosis in such cases was extensive and usually present in multiple foci. In eight of the 14 cases with intravascular endometrium, the latter was composed of endometrial stroma only (Fig. 51), and in the remaining cases, both glands and stroma were present. In nine cases, the vessels containing endometrial tissue were closely associated with the foci of adenomyosis, whereas in the other five cases, the involved vessels were at a distance from the adenomyosis. The vessels containing endometrium numbered up to four. In most cases, the myometrial vessels containing endometrium were thin-walled, and varied from slit-like to dilated. The authors of this report speculated that the observed findings were due to perivascular adenomyotic tissue that proliferates and protrudes into vascular spaces, eventually becoming ensheathed by endothelial cells.

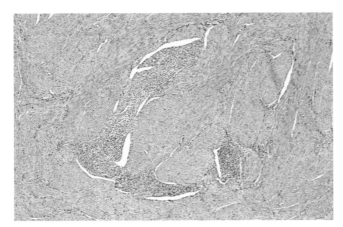

**FIG. 51.** Stroma of adenomyosis within myometrial blood vessels.

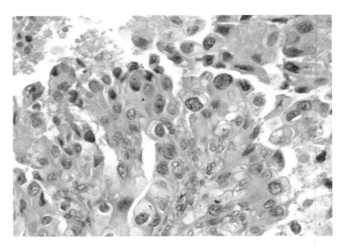

**FIG. 52.** Arias-Stella reaction of endometrium. There is an unusual degree of cellular stratification and atypia.

## ARIAS-STELLA REACTION AND CLEAR CELL CHANGE OF PREGNANCY

The Arias-Stella reaction (ASR) is a characteristic microscopic finding in endometrial glands that occurs in association with intrauterine or extrauterine pregnancy and trophoblastic disease (73–76). Similar changes also occur rarely in nonpregnant women on hormonal medication; most such patients in one recent study were postmenopausal and were being treated with progestational agents (77). The ASR can occur in sites other than eutopic endometrium, including the glands of adenomyosis (78) and endometriosis (78,79), the epithelium of the fallopian tube (78,80) and endocervix (see below), and in vaginal adenosis of the tuboendometrial type (81).

The ASR in the endometrium is typically located in the spongiosa. It may involve only a few glands or may be diffuse; the extent and intensity of the reaction do not correlate with the amount of trophoblast (74). The cells lining the glands and regular intraluminal papillae contain scanty cytoplasm and enlarged, pleomorphic, hyperchromatic nuclei, sometimes assuming a hobnail appearance; in occasional cases, these nuclear changes may be particularly conspicuous (Fig. 52). The nuclei may be smudgy or optically clear (82). Mitoses were found in 13% of cases in one recent study, but were only rarely multiple or atypical (76).

The ASR was documented in endocervical glands in 9% of gravid hysterectomy specimens in one study (83). The alteration is typically focal, involving only one or two glands in each case (Fig. 53). Involvement of superficial glands is more common than that of deep glands (83); endocervical polyps may also be affected (84).

Another endometrial alteration related to pregnancy is the presence in the glandular epithelial cells of abundant, clear, glycogen-rich cytoplasm; nuclei similar to those of the ASR may or may not be present. These cells may proliferate to the extent that they almost obliterate the lumen. Although this clear cell change is often considered a component of the ASR, it was not emphasized by Arias-Stella in his original description of the lesion bearing his name (73) or in most of the subsequent literature (75).

The ASR and clear cell change may be mistaken for clear cell carcinoma of the endometrium or cervix or cervical adenocarcinoma *in situ*, particularly in a biopsy or curettage specimen, when the pathologist is unaware that the patient is pregnant. Clear cell carcinoma, however, when it arises in the endometrium, almost always involves postmenopausal women, and in both the cervix and endometrium is often associated with symptoms and a mass. Histologic examination usually reveals features inconsistent with the ASR or clear cell change, including the presence of invasion and tubulocystic and solid patterns. When papillae are encountered in clear cell adenocarcinoma, they are not of uniform size and shape or as regularly spaced as they are in the ASR, and frequently contain hyalinized cores. The presence of decidua or

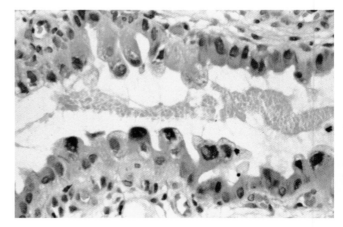

**FIG. 53.** Arias-Stella reaction in an endocervical gland.

trophoblastic tissue in some cases is an additional clue to the diagnosis of a pregnancy-related change. Cervical *in situ* adenocarcinoma, in contrast to the pregnancy changes, usually exhibits uniformly atypical stratified nuclei and relatively frequent mitotic figures, and usually lacks clear cells and hobnail cells (85).

## DECIDUA AND ECTOPIC DECIDUA

A fully developed decidual alteration of the endometrial stroma, which is almost always confined to pregnant women or those being treated with progestins, is unlikely to be confused with a neoplasm on microscopic examination. Diagnostic problems, however, may arise when the decidual reaction occurs in a woman who is neither pregnant nor on any hormonal medication, when it occurs in an ectopic site, when it causes grossly visible tumor-like nodules or masses, or when it has unusual histologic features (Figs. 54–57) (75,86).

Nuclear pleomorphism and hyperchromasia of decidual cells have been described in patients on progestin therapy (87,88). These changes, often associated with atrophy of the endometrial glands, may be misinterpreted as endometrial sarcoma. Additionally, a florid idiopathic decidual reaction of the endometrium may occur in postmenopausal women with bulky, polypoid, and necrotic tissue obtained on curettage (89). Microscopic examination in four such cases revealed diffuse decidual transformation of the endometrial stroma, but the presence of nuclear pleomorphism and hyperchromasia, signet ring–like cells (see below), focal necrosis, and focal glandular atypia raised the question of a malignant tumor in two of the cases.

Occasional cases of decidua in the endometrium and omentum, usually in pregnant women or those on progestin therapy, may contain decidual cells with one or more large

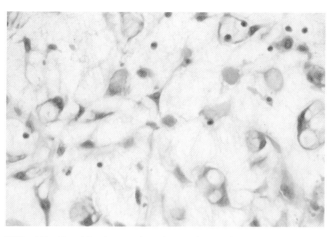

**FIG. 55.** Decidual reaction in endometrium. Note signet ring–like cells with cytoplasmic vacuoles.

cytoplasmic vacuoles that displace the nucleus, resulting in a signet ring–like appearance (Fig. 55) (75,90). In contrast to a metastatic signet ring adenocarcinoma, however, the vacuoles contain acidic material rather than neutral mucin. Ectopic decidua in the cervix (especially when accompanied by CIN) (Fig. 54) or within lymphadenectomy specimens in patients undergoing radical hysterectomy for invasive squamous cell carcinoma (75,91–94) may be mistaken for invasive or metastatic squamous cell carcinoma. Florid ectopic decidual reaction of the peritoneum, which may be associated with studding by nodules and plaques (Figs. 56 and 57) (75), should be distinguished on microscopic examination from deciduoid malignant mesothelioma (95,96). Additionally, two cases of peritoneal decidual reaction have been associated with numerous lipofuscin-laden histiocytes (see section on pigmented lesions). Awareness of the potential sites and unusual appearances of decidua, the absence of ob-

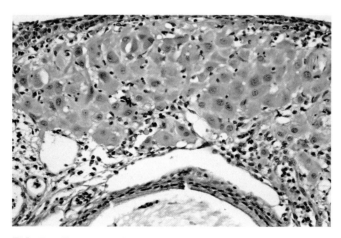

**FIG. 54.** Ectopic decidua in cervical stroma. This finding can potentially be confused with squamous cell carcinoma.

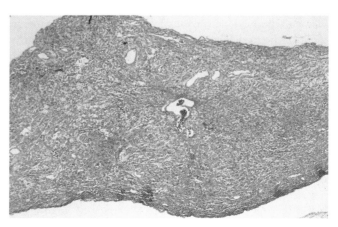

**FIG. 56.** Ectopic decidual reaction involving the peritoneum. Multiple tumor-like nodules were noted at the time of cesarean section.

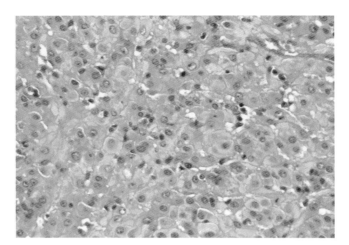

**FIG. 57.** Ectopic decidual reaction. High-power view of Fig. 56.

viously malignant nuclear features and mitotic figures, the merging with typical decidual cells, and the cytokeratin negativity of the cells should facilitate distinction from carcinoma and mesothelioma.

## HETEROTOPIC TISSUES

Heterotopic tissues (cartilage, bone, fat, glia) in a curettage specimen (97) may be confused with the heterologous elements of a malignant Müllerian mixed tumor (MMMT). Indeed, some patients have undergone unnecessary hysterectomy because an MMMT was suggested by the finding of cartilage in a curettage specimen (98). These heterotopic tissues are in most instances thought to be implanted fetal parts from a prior pregnancy, but their occasional occurrence in areas inconsistent with a fetal origin, such as the subserosal myometrium, or in cases of longstanding endometritis or pyometra suggests that some may be metaplastic, heterotopic, or dystrophic. In contrast to patients with heterotopic tissues, MMMTs typically occur in postmenopausal women who have an obvious intrauterine mass. Moreover, the heterologous elements are usually atypical or obviously malignant on histologic examination and are associated with carcinomatous and other sarcomatous elements. The usual microscopic and multifocal nature of glial tissue, its histologic maturity, its occasional association with other heterotopic elements, and its typical association with a previous instrumental abortion all aid in the distinction of the lesion from a neuroectodermal tumor with prominent glia (99) or the very rare uterine glioma (100). Fat in a curettage specimen unassociated with other heterotopic tissues may originate from a uterine lipoma or lipoleiomyoma or from traumatic uterine perforation. When a variety of heterotopic tissues are present in the same specimen, the differential diagnosis is with a mature teratoma, although many uterine "teratomas" reported as such likely represent tissue of fetal origin (101).

## PLACENTAL SITE LESIONS

### Exaggerated Placental Site

Nonneoplastic proliferations of the intermediate trophoblast (IT) of the placental site that pose diagnostic problems for the surgical pathologist, particularly in curettage specimens, are the exaggerated placental site (102) and the placental site nodule or plaque (103) (see below). The normal placental site is infiltrated by a profuse number of IT cells. On occasion, these cells extensively involve the underlying myometrium and, because of their occasional nuclear atypia and presence of giant cells, may produce a worrisome histologic appearance (Figs. 58 and 59). This process, designated "syncytial endometritis" by Ewing (104), has more recently been referred to as "exaggerated placental site reaction" (105) or, in the WHO classification, "exaggerated placental site." The cells of this lesion have the typical features of IT cells, specifically abundant eosinophilic or amphophilic cytoplasm, and irregular, often hyperchromatic, nuclei, some of which may be multiple. The trophoblast cells are admixed to varying degrees with normal myometrial cells, decidual cells, inflammatory cells, and fibrin, which is often conspicuous.

The major lesion in the differential diagnosis with this process is the placental site trophoblastic tumor (PSTT), a distinction that may be difficult in a biopsy or curettage specimen. The presence of more than an occasional mitotic figure, large confluent aggregates of trophoblast cells, massive muscle infiltration, or a combination of these findings usually warrants a diagnosis of PSTT. The presence of villi is unusual in a patient with a PSTT, although it occurs (106).

### Placental Site Nodule and Plaque (PSNP)

These terms have been recently applied to nodular or plaque-like proliferations of IT (103,107). This lesion gener-

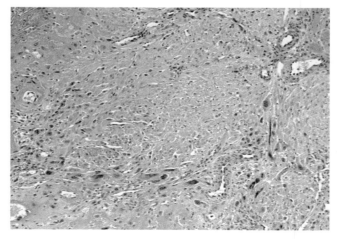

**FIG. 58.** Exaggerated placental site. Note the lack of a confluent growth of the atypical intermediate trophoblast cells.

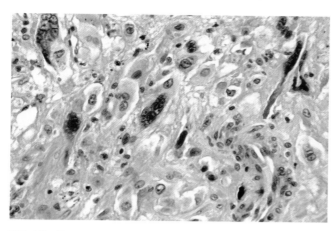

**FIG. 59.** Exaggerated placental site. High-power view of Fig. 58 showing giant cells and bizarre nuclei.

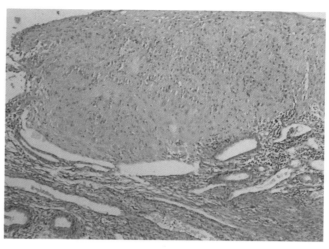

**FIG. 61.** Placental site plaque.

ally occurs in women in the reproductive age group but is occasionally discovered in the early postmenopausal years. Most of these lesions are grossly inapparent and represent incidental microscopic findings. The interval from the most recent known pregnancy ranged from 6 to 108 months (mean 29 months) in the largest series, and in the same study 35% of the patients had undergone bilateral tubal ligation 8–60 months previously (107). Although usually found in an endometrial specimen, PSNPs may be found in an endocervical specimen. From 33% to 80% of PSNPs are confined to or involve the lower uterine segment (103,107,108).

Microscopic examination (Figs. 60–65) discloses single or multiple, almost always well-circumscribed, oval or rounded nodules, sometimes with lobulated margins (Fig. 60). Less commonly, they form elongated plaque-like structures parallel to the endometrial surface (Fig. 61). PSNPs may be on the surface of the endometrium, within it or the subjacent myometrium, or in endocervical tissue. They consist of hyalinized eosinophilic material (Fig. 62) surrounding single cells, small irregular clusters of cells, or nests of cells.

Sometimes the hyalinization is most pronounced centrally and is surrounded by a cellular zone; occasional lesions are massively hyalinized. Foci of necrosis are present in almost half of cases and 10% are focally cystic (103). Although typically well-circumscribed, small pseudopods of brightly eosinophilic fibrin-like material that is immunoreactive for type IV collagen (107) often project from the periphery of the nodules (Fig. 65). The lesions are occasionally associated with evidence of a remote pregnancy in the form of necrotic or hyalinized chorionic villi.

The IT cells typically have abundant amphophilic cytoplasm, but it may be scanty or vacuolated, and may contain rounded eosinophilic hyaline bodies (Fig. 63 and 64). Nuclei may number one or more, and are irregular, often with lobulation. The chromatin may vary from hyperchromatic to pale and vesicular. Mitotic figures are either absent or (in 20% of cases) rare. Immunohistochemical stains show that the cells stain strongly and diffusely for cytokeratin and PLAP in almost every case; staining for hPL and hCG is less common and tends to be weak and focal (103,107).

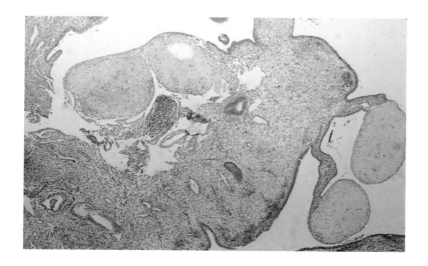

**FIG. 60.** Placental site nodules. Five small separate discrete nodules are present in the superficial endometrium, three of them forming polypoid projections.

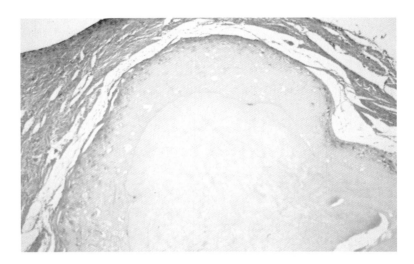

FIG. 62. Placental site nodule. The lesion is almost totally hyalinized.

Silva et al. have described cases of hydatidiform moles that were followed by PSNP-like nodules within the endometrium and myometrium (109). In contrast to most PSNPs, however, the nodules were always multiple (>15 in 4 of 7 cases), were associated with a mild elevation of the serum hCG, extended into the mid myometrium in some cases, were associated with choriocarcinoma in two cases, and did not respond well to chemotherapy. These authors considered the lesion "a mild form of nodular trophoblastic disease" (109). Its relation to PSNPs and other trophoblastic lesions remains to be fully elucidated.

The distinction of PSNPs from a PSTT is generally easy in a hysterectomy specimen because of their small size, circumscription, extensive hyalinization, and lack of mitoses. This distinction is occasionally difficult, however, in a curettage specimen because PSTTs may contain areas that closely resemble PSNPs and rarely have sharp instead of infiltrating borders. In these cases, the degenerative appearance of the cells as well as the lack or rarity of mitotic figures aid in diagnosis. The above features, and the absence of squamous differentiation, help to distinguish PSNPs from the rare hyalinizing squamous cell carcinoma of the cervix (102). Fibrin in the small pseudopods of a PSNP may mimic keratin, leading to a misdiagnosis of microinvasive squamous cell carcinoma, an error we identified in several cases (Fig. 65).

## ECTOPIC PREGNANCY

An ectopic pregnancy resulting in a hemorrhagic mass in the fallopian tube, ovary (110), or cervix (Fig. 66) (111) can

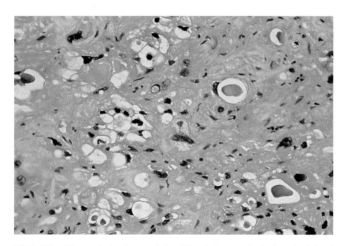

FIG. 63. Placental site nodule. The intermediate trophoblast cells are degenerate with vacuolated cytoplasm, and there is prominent stromal hyalinization.

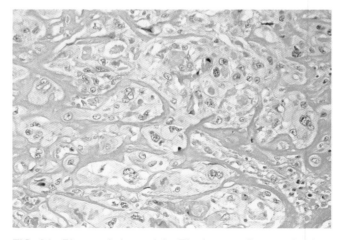

FIG. 64. Placental site nodule. The intermediate trophoblast cells in this case have conspicuous amphophilic cytoplasm and form small nests separated by hyaline material.

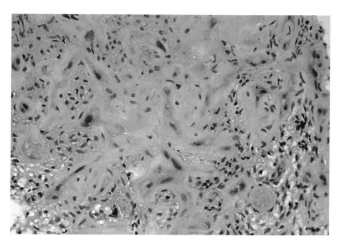

**FIG. 65.** Placental site nodule involving the endocervix. Several pseudopods are present at the periphery of the lesion and mimic microinvasive squamous cell carcinoma.

occasionally be mistaken on macroscopic examination for a malignant tumor, although the diagnosis is typically straightforward on microscopic examination. Distinction between ectopic pregnancy and the very rare examples of primary gestational trophoblastic disease in these sites is made by applying criteria similar to those used in the uterus.

## TROPHOBLASTIC DEPORTATION AND IMPLANTS

The finding of trophoblastic cells in peripheral blood (112) or in the lungs (where even villi can be seen) during or after a normal intrauterine gestation or abortion is consistent with the angioinvasive properties of normal trophoblast (113–115). Vaginal trophoblastic tissue in otherwise normal

pregnancies (116) may be due to hematogenous spread or implantation. In other cases, trophoblast implants on the pelvic or omental peritoneum follow uterine rupture during therapeutic abortion (117), or, more commonly, complicate the operative treatment of tubal pregnancy (118–121). The clinical presentation in such cases includes an initial decline in the serum hCG (associated with removal of the ectopic pregnancy) followed by a rising level, abdominal pain, and, in some cases, intra-abdominal hemorrhage (120). Microscopic examination of the implants reveals viable trophoblastic tissue that may include chorionic villi (Fig. 67). Awareness of this complication, the absence of the typical biphasic growth pattern of choriocarcinoma, and the presence of villi in some cases distinguish it from metastatic choriocarcinoma.

## CHANGES RELATED TO IN UTERO EXPOSURE TO DIETHYLSTILBESTROL (DES)

The subject of changes related to *in utero* exposure to diethylstilbestrol (DES) has been recently summarized (81). Therefore, only pseudoneoplastic findings in vaginal adenosis (and non-DES-related adenosis), most of which are rare, are noted here. Just as florid squamous metaplasia in endocervical glands can be misinterpreted as invasive squamous cell carcinoma (see page 266), so can the same process in

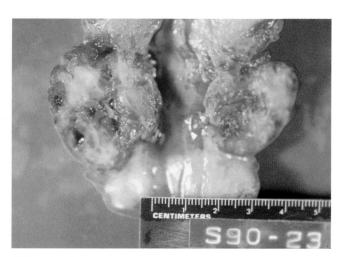

**FIG. 66.** Ectopic cervical pregnancy forming tumor-like mass.

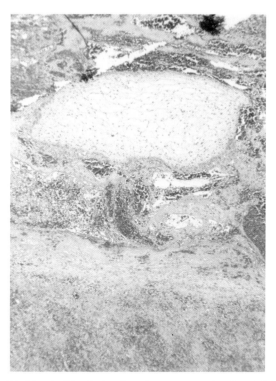

**FIG. 67.** Trophoblastic implant (on serosa of spleen) following operative removal of a tubal pregnancy.

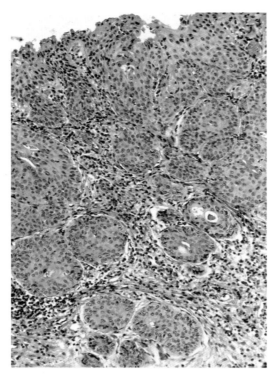

**FIG. 68.** Vaginal adenosis with florid squamous metaplasia.

vaginal adenosis (Fig. 68). The distinction from squamous cell carcinoma is based on the same criteria as those used in the cervix. Microglandular hyperplasia, similar to that occurring in the endocervix (see page 269), can also involve vaginal adenosis; all of the reported cases have occurred in women taking oral contraceptives or who were pregnant (122). As noted earlier, the Arias-Stella reaction is encountered rarely in the glands of vaginal adenosis (81). We have also seen examples of vaginal adenosis with a papillary pattern (Fig. 69). Other rare findings recently described in

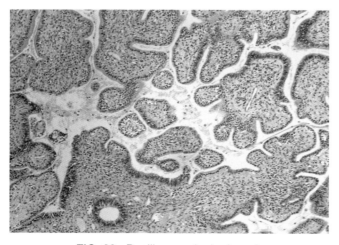

**FIG. 69.** Papillary vaginal adenosis.

adenosis have included intestinal metaplasia (123) and a pseudoinfiltrative pattern (124). In the latter case, which occurred in a patient with a negative DES history, a small biopsy revealed small glands and cords of cells haphazardly distributed through the lamina propria, raising the suspicion of an adenocarcinoma. The cells, however, had bland nuclear features, and a wider excision of the area confirmed the diagnosis of vaginal adenosis with unusual architectural features.

## FIBROEPITHELIAL POLYPS WITH STROMAL ATYPIA

Fibroepithelial polyps of the lower female genital tract with atypical stromal cells can be misdiagnosed as sarcoma botryoides, leading to their designation in some early reports as "pseudosarcoma botryoides" (125–141). They usually involve the vagina but also occur in the vulva (125,135,137) and cervix (125,126,132). In the earlier reports, the polyps occurred typically in the reproductive age group, but as many as 40% of patients in more recent series have been postmenopausal (median ages in three series 48–51 years) (128,137,141); rare polyps have been from newborn infants (125). Approximately 20% of patients have been pregnant at the time of diagnosis, and an additional 10% have given a history of hormonal treatment, either estrogen (127), oral contraceptives (135), or an unspecified hormonal agent (128). The polyps may be asymptomatic, associated with postcoital bleeding, or discovered as a mass by the patient. In one patient with multiple polyps involving the vagina and cervix during pregnancy, the polyps had regressed completely by 6 weeks postpartum (136).

The polyps may be single, are occasionally multiple, and rarely may be numerous (136). They vary from sessile to pedunculated to villiform and from soft to rubbery. Occasional vaginal lesions have had a botryoid appearance (126). They are usually 4 cm or less, but rarely as large as 12 cm in greatest dimension (126). On microscopic examination, they typically resemble fibroepithelial polyps seen elsewhere. In a minority of examples, especially in pregnant patients, the stroma is cellular and contains cells with variable amounts of granular eosinophilic cytoplasm and bizarre, hyperchromatic, multiple or multilobed nuclei that may contain prominent nucleoli (Figs. 70 and 71). Mitotic figures (MFs) may be numerous and even abnormal (125,126,131–133,136); as many as 3 MFs/10 high-power fields (HPFs) were present in one case (133).

The major differential diagnosis of polyps with bizarre stromal cells is with sarcoma botryoides. The latter, however, typically occurs in the vagina of infants and children under 5 years of age and is rare in older patients. Sarcoma botryoides of the cervix (143) occurs in an older age group (mean age 18 years) than its vaginal counterpart, so age differences are less helpful in the evaluation of cervical lesions.

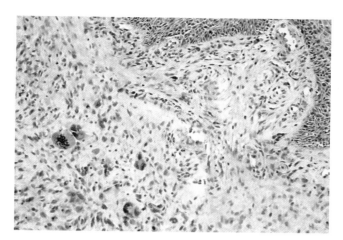

**FIG. 70.** Fibroepithelial polyp. Numerous bizarre nuclei are present in the cellular stroma.

Characteristic features of sarcoma botryoides that are lacking in fibroepithelial polyps with bizarre stromal cells are a history of rapid growth, a cellular subepithelial cambium layer composed of small, mitotically active primitive cells with scanty cytoplasm and hyperchromatic nuclei, nests of tumor cells in the overlying squamous epithelium, cells with cytoplasmic cross-striations, and cells immunoreactive for myoglobin. Fibroepithelial polyps lacking atypical stromal cells may be confused with the aggressive angiomyxoma (144,145). Although the superficial portions of angiomyxomas may protrude into the vagina as a polyp or form a vulvar swelling, pelvic examination will usually reveal a bulky mass. On microscopic examination, aggressive angiomyxomas, in contrast to fibroepithelial polyps, contain numerous blood vessels of various sizes (including thick-walled vessels), lack or have only rare multinucleated cells, and have infiltrative borders. The distinction between the two lesions, however, may occasionally be difficult in a small biopsy specimen.

## MULTINUCLEATED EPITHELIAL AND STROMAL CELLS IN LOWER FEMALE GENITAL TRACT

Multinucleated stromal giant cells identical to those occurring in fibroepithelial polyps are commonly encountered as an incidental microscopic finding in the loose subepithelial stroma of the lower female genital tract, including the cervix, vagina, and vulva (141,146–150). These giant cells are similar to those found in other parts of the body and presumably represent a reactive change in the indigenous stromal cells (150). We have also seen similar cells rarely within the stroma of endometrial polyps.

McLachlin et al. have described atypical multinucleated cells in the lower to middle layers of the vulvar epidermis in young women (151). Two of the 12 patients had a history of noncontiguous VIN that had been previously excised. None of the 12 cases contained HPV DNA. It was concluded that the cause and significance of the lesion are unclear, but the process appears to be distinct from VIN and HPV-related changes, from which it should be distinguished.

## PREGNANCY LUTEOMA

Pregnancy luteoma is a distinctive, nonneoplastic, tumor-like ovarian lesion associated with pregnancy (152–158). Eighty percent of the patients are multiparous and a similar proportion are black. The ovarian enlargement is usually incidentally discovered at term during cesarean section or at postpartum tubal ligation. In approximately 25% of the cases, hirsutism or virilization appear during the latter half of pregnancy, and female infants of masculinized mothers are also usually virilized (154–156,158).

Pregnancy luteomas vary from microscopic to 20 cm (median 6.6 cm) in diameter (153). The cut surfaces are solid, fleshy, circumscribed, red to brown, and frequently hemor-

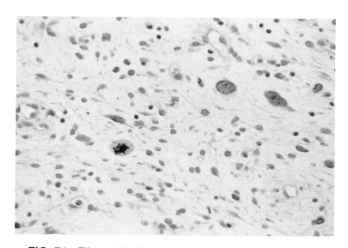

**FIG. 71.** Fibroepithelial polyp. A mitotic figure is visible.

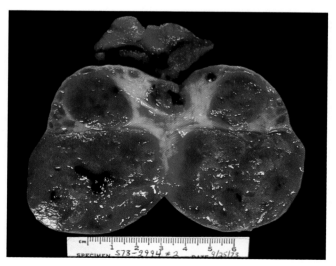

**FIG. 72.** Pregnancy luteoma. The sectioned surface of the ovary contains several discrete brown nodules.

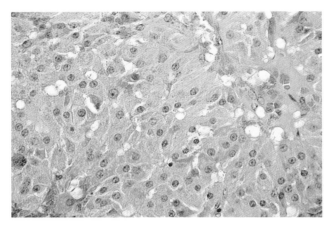

**FIG. 73.** Pregnancy luteoma. The lesional cells have abundant eosinophilic cytoplasm.

rhagic (Fig. 72). One third of the cases are bilateral and half are multiple. Microscopic examination discloses sharply circumscribed, rounded masses of cells, which are also occasionally arranged in a trabecular or follicular pattern. The cells have abundant eosinophilic cytoplasm with little or no stainable lipid (Fig. 73), and central nuclei that may exhibit slight pleomorphism and hyperchromasia; nucleoli are usually prominent. Mitotic figures, which may be frequent, are usually present, and occasionally are atypical (152,153). Examination of affected ovaries days to weeks postpartum reveals focal infarction or brown puckered scars, which on histologic examination contain degenerating lipid-filled luteoma cells with pyknotic nuclei (154); infiltration by lymphoid cells and fibrosis are also seen.

The primary lesion in the differential diagnosis is the steroid cell tumor (159); a less likely consideration is a heavily luteinized thecoma (160). Multiplicity and conspicuous mitotic activity favor pregnancy luteoma over these neoplasms, but in rare cases microscopic distinction may be impossible. In a pregnant woman a luteoma is strongly favored unless there is strong evidence to the contrary.

## HYPERREACTIO LUTEINALIS

This lesion, which is characterized by bilateral ovarian enlargement due to numerous luteinized follicle cysts, is most likely to be misdiagnosed as a neoplasm intraoperatively or on gross examination (158–171). It is most commonly associated with disorders resulting in high hCG levels, such as hydatidiform mole, choriocarcinoma, fetal hydrops, and multiple gestations, although 60% of cases unassociated with trophoblastic disease have accompanied a normal singleton pregnancy (163,166,170,171).

Hyperreactio luteinalis may be detected as a pelvic mass during any trimester, at cesarean section, or, rarely, during the puerperium (162). Symptoms are usually absent, but hemorrhage into the cysts may cause abdominal pain; rarely the involved ovary undergoes torsion or rupture, sometimes

with intraabdominal bleeding that may be fatal. In contrast to patients with the ovarian hyperstimulation syndrome (see below), ascites is rare (170). In patients with hyperreactio luteinalis secondary to trophoblastic disease, ovarian enlargement may be detected at the time of the diagnostic dilatation and curettage or postoperatively (165,167,169). In approximately 15% of cases unassociated with trophoblastic disease, there has been virilization of the patient but not the female infant (161,164,168).

On gross examination (Fig. 74), multiple, almost always bilateral, thin-walled cysts result in moderate to massive enlargement of the ovaries, which may be >35 cm in diameter; the cysts are filled with pale or hemorrhagic fluid. Microscopic examination reveals multiple luteinized follicle cysts (Fig. 75), often accompanied by marked edema of the luteinized theca layer and the intervening stroma, which may contain luteinized stromal cells.

An iatrogenic form of hyperreactio luteinalis, the ovarian hyperstimulation syndrome, can develop in women undergoing ovulation induction, typically after the administration of a follicle-stimulating hormone preparation followed by hCG, and less often after the administration of clomiphene alone (172–177). The syndrome occurs only after ovulation and is more severe in patients who conceive. In extreme cases, the ovaries can become massively enlarged and ascites, sometimes with hydrothorax (acute Meigs' syndrome), can develop due to increased serosal permeability. Elevation of serum estrogens, progesterone, and testosterone typically occurs (172,173,177). Hemoconcentration with secondary oliguria and thromboembolic phenomena is a life-threatening complication. Patients usually respond to conservative

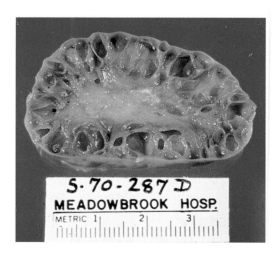

**FIG. 74.** Hyperreactio luteinalis. Numerous thin-walled cysts are present on the sectioned surface of the ovary.

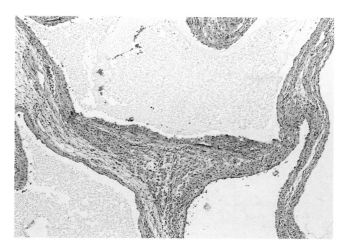

**FIG. 75.** Hyperreactio luteinalis. Several follicle cysts are lined with luteinized granulosa cells.

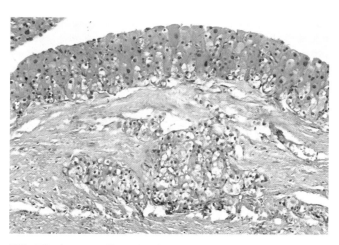

**FIG. 76.** Large solitary luteinized follicle cyst of pregnancy and puerperium. A cyst is lined with a layer of prominently luteinized granulosa cells, and similar cells are present in the cyst wall.

therapy, and the cysts typically regress within 6 weeks. Pathologic examination reveals changes identical to those seen in hyperreactio luteinalis with the additional finding of one or more corpora lutea. The differential diagnosis of hyperreactio luteinalis and the ovarian hyperstimulation syndrome is discussed in the following section.

## LARGE SOLITARY LUTEINIZED FOLLICLE CYST OF PREGNANCY AND PUERPERIUM

This rare type of follicle cyst with distinctive features occurs during pregnancy and the puerperium and may be also mistaken for a neoplasm (178–181). Because of its large size (median diameter 25 cm), the cyst may cause abdominal swelling, but it is usually an incidental finding at the time of cesarean section or on routine examination during the first postpartum visit. None of the cases reported to date have been associated with clinical evidence of an endocrine disturbance. On gross inspection, the cysts are solitary, unilocular, and thin-walled, and contain watery fluid, resembling typical follicle cysts except for their large size. On microscopic examination the cyst lining is composed of one to several layers of luteinized granulosa and theca cells, which cannot always be distinguished from one another (Fig. 76). Similar cells may be found in the fibrous cyst wall. The luteinized cells have abundant eosinophilic to vacuolated cytoplasm, vary considerably in size and shape, and in all of the reported cases have exhibited focal marked nuclear pleomorphism and hyperchromasia (Fig. 77); mitotic figures are absent.

The major differential diagnosis of the large solitary luteinized follicle cyst involves unilocular cystic granulosa cell tumors (182) of either the adult or juvenile type, both of which may rarely be indistinguishable from the luteinized cyst on gross inspection. On microscopic examination, however, the unilocular cystic adult granulosa cell tumors typi-

cally lack cells with abundant eosinophilic cytoplasm and bizarre nuclei, and usually contain foci of typical granulosa cell tumor in the cyst wall. The juvenile granulosa cell tumor may cause a greater diagnostic problem because it is characterized by cells with abundant cytoplasm that is often eosinophilic. The juvenile granulosa cell tumor demonstrates immature nuclei that may occasionally have a bizarre appearance; mitotic activity, however, is typically relatively conspicuous. Similar criteria and the bilaterality of hyperreactio luteinalis and the ovarian hyperstimulation syndrome aid in their distinction from granulosa cell tumors.

## OVARIAN GRANULOSA CELL PROLIFERATIONS

Granulosa cell proliferations that simulate small neoplasms are often an incidental finding in the ovaries of preg-

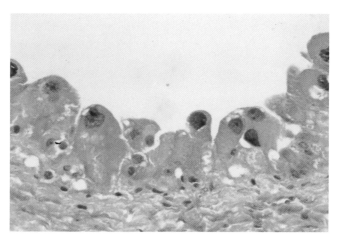

**FIG. 77.** Large solitary luteinized follicle cyst of pregnancy and puerperium. The nuclei are hyperchromatic but lack mitotic figures.

nant women (183). A few reports in the older literature have noted the presence of similar lesions in the ovaries of non-pregnant women (184,185). The lesions in pregnant patients are usually multiple and are contained in atretic follicles. The granulosa cells are typically arranged in solid, insular, micro-follicular, and trabecular patterns, mimicking similar patterns in granulosa cell tumors (Fig. 78). In one case, a prominent tubular pattern composed of cells with vacuolated cytoplasm was reminiscent of a lipid-rich Sertoli cell tumor (Fig. 79).

Although similar proliferations have been previously in-terpreted as small tumors, in our opinion these lesions more likely reflect an unusual nonneoplastic response to the hor-monal milieu of pregnancy. Their microscopic size, multifo-cality, and confinement to atretic follicles support this inter-pretation.

## NORMAL FINDINGS AND ARTIFACTS IN THE OVARY

Granulosa cells of the normal follicle may exhibit brisk mitotic activity (Fig. 80), as can the spindle cells of the nor-mal theca externa (Fig. 81). The latter may be misinterpreted as a sarcoma, particularly when only the edge of the follicle is seen microscopically. The microscopic size of the process and the bland nuclear features of the spindle cells militate against a diagnosis of sarcoma. The granulosa cells of nor-mal follicles can be artifactually introduced into tissue spaces or vascular channels during sectioning. This finding, especially when the displaced granulosa cells are shrunken or crushed, can be misinterpreted as small cell carcinoma (Fig. 82). Awareness of this artifact, the bland nuclear fea-tures of the cells, and their similarity to cells lining nearby follicles are helpful clues to the correct diagnosis. Luteinized granulosa cells on the surface of the ovary following ovula-tion may be misinterpreted as mesothelial cells, and, when numerous, a diagnosis of a mesothelial neoplasm may be suggested (Fig. 83). Finally, the degenerating corpus luteum

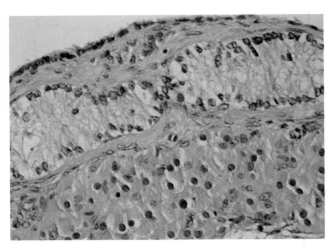

**FIG. 79.** Granulosa cell proliferation. The granulosa cells in this case have a solid tubular pattern and abundant clear cy-toplasm similar to that of a lipid-rich Sertoli cell tumor.

of late pregnancy and the puerperium may contain focal cal-cification, including psammoma bodies, a finding that can be mistaken for recurrent serous borderline tumor (Scully RE, personal communication).

A rare pseudoneoplastic alteration in surface epithelial in-clusion glands is one in which the lining cells exhibit strik-ing hydropic change, with clear cytoplasm and an eccentric nucleus, potentially mimicking a signet ring cell carcinoma, especially when the cells proliferate to form solid nests of cells (Figs. 84 and 85). Awareness of this finding, additional sections to show a relation to inclusion glands, benign nu-clear features, and negative cytoplasmic staining for mucin facilitate the correct diagnosis.

## STROMAL HYPERPLASIA AND HYPERTHECOSIS

Both stromal hyperplasia and hyperthecosis cause ovarian enlargement, usually bilateral, with each gonad measuring up

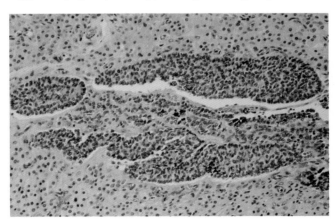

**FIG. 78.** Granulosa cell proliferation. An atretic follicle con-tains a proliferation of granulosa cells mimicking a tiny gran-ulosa cell tumor.

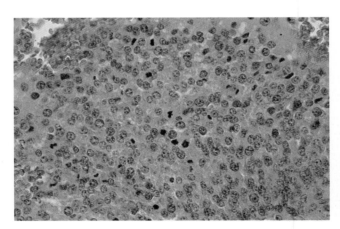

**FIG. 80.** Granulosa cells of developing follicle exhibiting brisk mitotic activity.

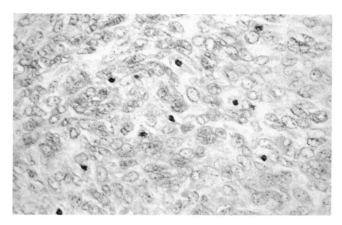

FIG. 81. Prominent mitotic activity in theca externa cells of follicle.

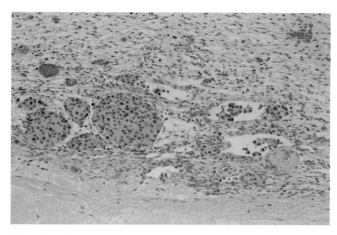

FIG. 83. Displaced luteinized granulosa cells in superficial ovarian stroma potentially simulating a mesothelial proliferation.

to 8 cm in diameter (186,187). The cut surface of the ovaries is typically homogeneous, firm, and white to yellow (Fig. 86). On microscopic examination, both the cortical and the medullary stroma may be hyperplastic. In hyperthecosis, luteinized stromal cells appear singly, in small clusters, or in nodules. They have abundant eosinophilic to vacuolated cytoplasm containing variable amounts of lipid and a round nucleus with a central small nucleolus. Confusion of these lesions with a neoplasm on histologic examination is unlikely, as the usual absence of a discrete mass, the diffuse nature of the stromal proliferation, and the entrapment of follicular derivatives are inconsistent with a neoplastic proliferation.

## MASSIVE OVARIAN EDEMA AND FIBROMATOSIS

Tumor-like enlargement of one or both ovaries secondary to an accumulation of edema fluid within the ovarian stroma

is referred to as "massive ovarian edema," whereas expansion due to a fibromatous stromal proliferation is referred to as "ovarian fibromatosis" (188). Patients are usually of reproductive age. Clinical manifestations include abdominal or pelvic pain, menstrual irregularities, and, occasionally, evidence of androgen excess. An adnexal mass is usually palpable. At operation the ovarian enlargement is unilateral in about 90% of cases. Partial or complete torsion of the involved ovary has been present in at least half of cases of massive edema and in 15% of cases of fibromatosis.

The ovary in massive edema is enlarged, soft, and fluctuant, ranging in diameter from 5.5 to 35 cm. The cut surface is tan, homogeneous, and soft, exuding a watery fluid (Fig. 87). The most superficial cortex appears white and fibrotic. In fibromatosis, the involved ovary has ranged from 6 to 12 cm in diameter, and the cut surfaces are firm, white, and solid (Fig. 88). In both disorders, residual cystic follicles may be grossly visible.

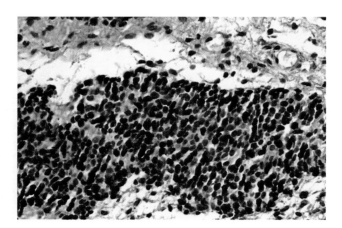

FIG. 82. Displaced granulosa cells in ovarian stroma. The small shrunken cells could be mistaken for small cell carcinoma.

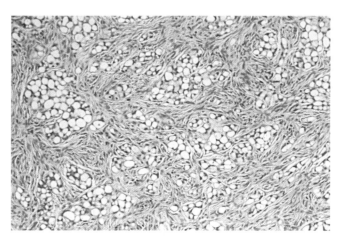

FIG. 84. Hydropic change in surface epithelial inclusion glands. Nests of cells with clear cytoplasm are scattered through the ovarian stroma.

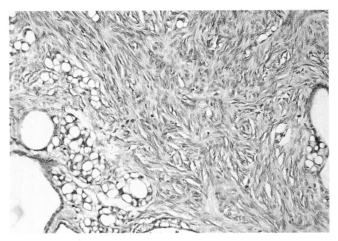

**FIG. 85.** Hydropic change in surface epithelial inclusion glands. Note relationship of clear cells to the glands.

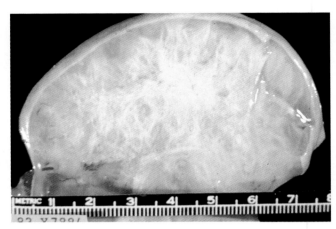

**FIG. 87.** Massive edema. The sectioned surface of the ovary is white and glistening.

In massive edema, diffuse, stromal edema surrounds follicles and their derivatives (Fig. 89), but typically spares the thickened and fibrotic superficial cortex. In approximately 40% of cases, luteinized stromal cells are present. In ovarian fibromatosis, spindle cells produce variable amounts of collagen, with the appearance varying from moderately cellular fascicles of spindle cells with a focal storiform pattern to relatively acellular bands of dense collagen (Fig. 90) (188). This process also typically surrounds normal follicular structures and produces collagenous thickening of the superficial cortex. Luteinized stromal cells and microscopic foci of sex cord cells have been seen in occasional cases.

Massive edema can be distinguished from ovarian neoplasms with an edematous or myxoid appearance, such as an edematous fibroma, a sclerosing stromal tumor, a Krukenberg tumor, a luteinized thecoma of the type associated with sclerosing peritonitis (189,190), and the rare ovarian myx-

oma, by the absence of features of those tumors as well as by the inclusion of follicular derivatives within the lesion. Ovarian fibromatosis should be distinguished from a fibroma or, if focal sex cord aggregates are present, from a fibroma with minor sex cord elements. However, these tumors usually occur in an older age group and rarely contain follicles or their derivatives.

## LEYDIG CELL HYPERPLASIA AND LEYDIG CELLS WITH BIZARRE NUCLEI

Hilus cell hyperplasia may be grossly visible as multiple, yellow, hilar nodules that, in contrast to hilus cell tumors, are usually <2 mm in diameter. On microscopic examination, the hilus cells are arranged in nodular or diffuse patterns (Fig. 91); multinucleated cells and occasional mitotic figures may be seen. In older women, the hyperplastic hilus cells may be enlarged with bizarre cellular shapes and nuclear

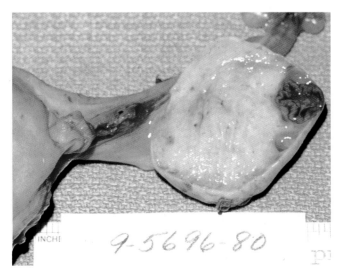

**FIG. 86.** Hyperthecosis. Most of the ovary is replaced by homogeneous white tissue, which suggests a neoplasm.

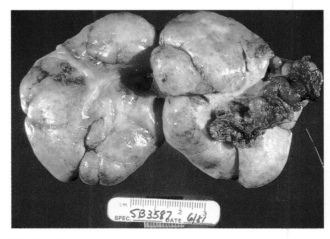

**FIG. 88.** Fibromatosis. The ovaries were lobulated and firm, causing concern for a neoplasm.

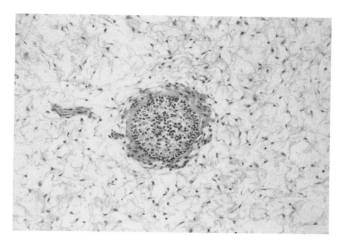

**FIG. 89.** Massive edema. Edematous tissue surrounds a follicle.

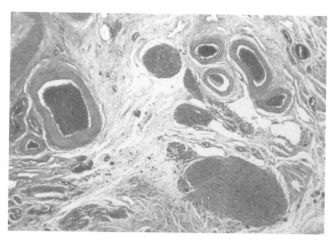

**FIG. 91.** Nodular Leydig cell hyperplasia in a pregnant woman.

hyperchromasia. The microscopic nature of this process and the usual presence of more than one nodule distinguish it from a hilus cell tumor.

## PSEUDONEOPLASTIC LESIONS OF THE FALLOPIAN TUBE

### Fallopian Tube Prolapse

Prolapse of the fallopian tube into the vagina occasionally occurs after a hysterectomy, which has been of vaginal type in approximately 80% of the reported cases (191,192). On clinical examination, a lesion simulating granulation tissue is visible at the vaginal apex and is often painful on biopsy. Microscopic examination shows glandular epithelium, sometimes with reactive atypia, surrounded by abundant inflammatory cells (Figs. 92 and 93). A villous pattern often suggests the plicae of the tube (Fig. 92) but sometimes the plicae are blunted and their tubal nature is not immediately

apparent (Fig. 93). The presence of smooth muscle of the tubal muscularis can sometimes aid in diagnosis; the latter finding will not be present in adenocarcinomas, which is the main differential diagnostic consideration.

### Metaplastic Papillary Tumor

This rare lesion of the fallopian tube has been encountered as an incidental microscopic finding in pregnant and post-partum women (193,194). The lesion involves only part of the tubal circumference (Fig. 94); small, rounded cysts may be present in the papillae. The epithelial cells are large, with abundant eosinophilic cytoplasm, which occasionally contains mucin. The nuclei are large, oval, and vesicular (Fig. 95); mitotic figures are rare. The lesion is distinguishable from primary tubal carcinoma by its microscopic size, lack of invasion, and bland or only slightly atypical nuclei. Whether this lesion is metaplastic or neoplastic is unclear,

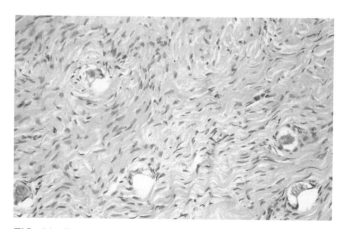

**FIG. 90.** Fibromatosis. Fibrous tissue envelops a number of primordial follicles.

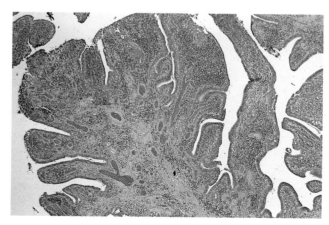

**FIG. 92.** Fallopian tube prolapse at vaginal apex. Plicae of the fallopian tube, suggesting the diagnosis, are conspicuous.

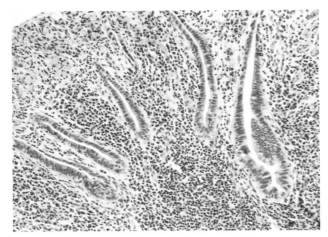

**FIG. 93.** Fallopian tube prolapse. Plicae are not conspicuous. Note prominent chronic inflammation.

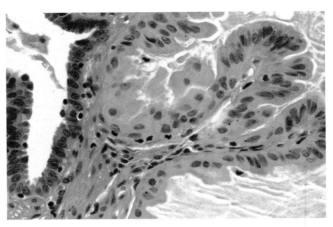

**FIG. 95.** Metaplastic papillary lesion. A high-power view shows bland cytologic features.

but it appears to bear a special relation to pregnancy, suggesting metaplasia, and has been associated with an uneventful course.

### Salpingitis Isthmica Nodosa

Salpingitis isthmica nodosa (SIN) is typically encountered in young adults (mean ages 25–36 years) (195). The lesion has a strong association with primary and secondary infertility and ectopic pregnancy. Although milder cases of SIN are often grossly inconspicuous, the presence of one or more yellow–white nodular isthmic or ampullary swellings is the hallmark of the well-developed lesion; in different studies, bilateral involvement has been noted in 35–85% of cases. Inspection of the sectioned surface of the lesion may reveal small cystic spaces scattered throughout a thickened myosalpinx (Fig. 96). On microscopic examination, glands or small cysts lined with bland tubal epithelium lie irregularly

in a hyperplastic myosalpinx, often extending to the serosa. Endometrial-type stroma surrounding some of the glands within the myosalpinx has been present in as many as 90% of the cases in some studies but has been noted only rarely or not at all in most others.

### Hyperplastic and Pseudocarcinomatous Lesions

Varying degrees of hyperplasia and atypia of the tubal epithelium may occur in response to salpingitis, both tuberculous and nontuberculous, and may simulate an *in situ* or invasive adenocarcinoma (196,197). Hyperplastic epithelial changes include the formation of papillae and cribriform spaces lined with cells with mild to moderate nuclear pleomorphism, hyperchromatism, and occasional mitoses (Figs. 97 and 98). The proliferation may involve the mucosa, muscularis, and serosa; in rare cases, epithelial papillae may be found within lymphatics (197). When associated with pseu-

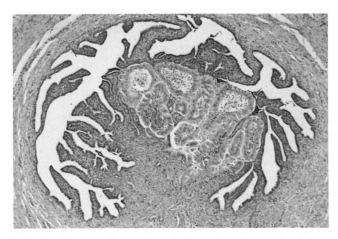

**FIG. 94.** Metaplastic papillary lesion. A portion of the fallopian tube epithelium is replaced by a papillary proliferation of cells with conspicuous eosinophilic cytoplasm.

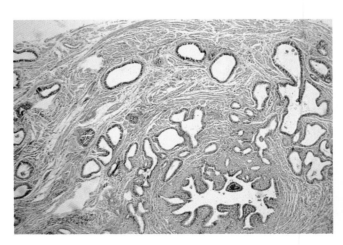

**FIG. 96.** Salpingitis isthmica nodosa. There is prominent invagination of the tubal epithelium into the muscularis.

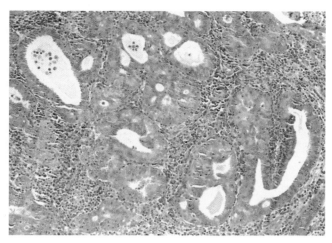

**FIG. 97.** Hyperplasia and reactive atypia of tubal epithelium in patient with pelvic inflammatory disease. There is a cribriform pattern causing concern for adenocarcinoma.

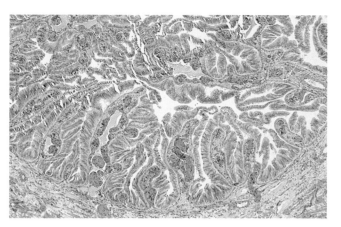

**FIG. 99.** Heat artifact of fallopian tube. This fallopian tube was subject to vigorous cautery, resulting in pseudostratification of the lining epithelium.

doglandular hyperplasia of the overlying mesothelial cells, which become incorporated within subserosal inflammatory and fibrous tissue, the combination of findings may lead to an erroneous interpretation of transmural carcinoma (197). A number of differences between carcinomas and pseudo-carcinomatous inflammatory lesions facilitate the differential diagnosis. The great majority of carcinomas are grossly evident, are not associated with significant inflammation, and exhibit severe nuclear atypia and prominent mitotic activity. Pseudocarcinomatous changes simulating carcinoma, in contrast, are incidental microscopic findings associated with overt inflammation.

Heat artifact, caused by prolonged intraoperative cautery or inadvertent heating of the specimen after surgical removal, can also simulate carcinoma by causing an appearance of marked cellular stratification (Fig. 99) (198).

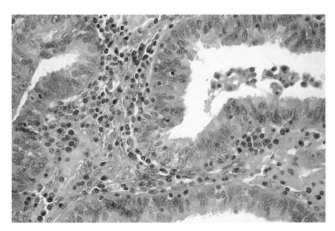

**FIG. 98.** Reactive atypia of tubal epithelium in patient with pelvic inflammatory disease. High-power view of Fig. 97. There is only mild nuclear atypia. Note the prominent inflammation.

## MESOTHELIAL HYPERPLASIA

Hyperplasia of peritoneal mesothelial cells is a common reaction to acute and chronic inflammation, chronic effusions, endometriosis, and ovarian neoplasms (199–205). Mesothelial hyperplasia may also involve a hernia sac, often secondary to trauma or incarceration (205). Although mesothelial hyperplasia can occur as solitary or multiple small nodules or plaques visible at operation, it is usually an incidental microscopic finding (199–202).

In florid examples of mesothelial hyperplasia, the hyperplastic mesothelial cells may grow in solid, trabecular, tubular, papillary, or tubulopapillary patterns (Figs. 100 and 101), in some cases accompanied by superficial extension into the underlying tissues. In such cases, the hyperplastic mesothelial cells in the ovarian stroma overlying a borderline epithelial tumor may be misinterpreted as an invasive tumor (Fig. 101) (204). A focally linear, occasionally parallel arrangement of the cells, with separation by fibrin or fibrous tissue, is common and is a helpful clue to the diagnosis (Fig. 101). Cytoplasmic vacuoles containing acid mucin (hyaluronic acid), occasional multinucleated mesothelial cells, mild nuclear atypicality, and sporadic mitotic figures are often present (Fig. 102) (199). Eosinophilic strap-shaped cells resembling rhabdomyoblasts have been rarely encountered (205). Psammoma bodies can occur, although they are more common in endosalpingiosis.

The presence of a sizable mass, necrosis, conspicuous large cytoplasmic vacuoles, more than mild nuclear atypicality, appreciable mitotic activity, and deep infiltration favors diffuse malignant mesothelioma (DMM) over mesothelial hyperplasia (199,206). These features, however, are not uniformly present or may be present only focally within a DMM. Intense cytoplasmic immunopositivity for epithelial membrane antigen is claimed by some authors to be typical of DMM but not hyperplastic mesothelial cells (207). In some cases, however, the distinction between a hyperplastic

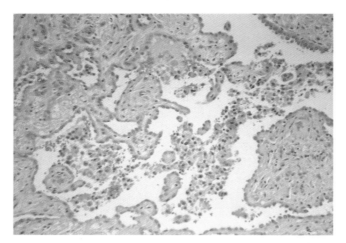

**FIG. 100.** Papillary mesothelial hyperplasia.

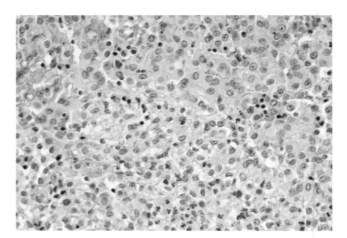

**FIG. 102.** Diffuse mesothelial hyperplasia. Note the bland cytologic features.

mesothelial lesion and a DMM may be difficult or impossible, especially in a small biopsy specimen. A DMM, however, because of its typical rapid growth, will usually reveal its nature within several months.

## PERITONEAL INCLUSION CYSTS

Although the lesions discussed here are considered neoplastic by some, we regard them as reactive. We acknowledge, however, that low-grade cystic mesotheliomas do occur rarely (see below). Peritoneal inclusion cysts (PICs) usually occur in women of reproductive age (208–217), but rarely occur in males (218–220). Many present as incidental intraoperative findings, occurring as single or multiple, small, thin-walled, translucent, unilocular cysts that are attached to the peritoneum, or can be occasionally free float-

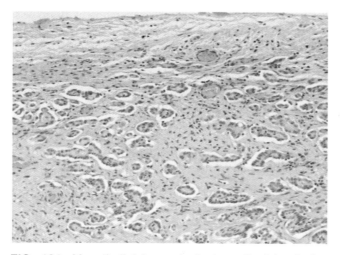

**FIG. 101.** Mesothelial hyperplasia in wall of borderline serous tumor. Note linear arrangement of mesothelial cells.

ing. Pathologic examination typically reveals a smooth lining, yellow and watery to gelatinous contents, and a single layer of flattened mesothelial cells with benign features that is easily distinguished from a neoplasm.

Multilocular peritoneal inclusion cysts (MPICs) are, however, more troublesome diagnostically (217). They form cystic masses up to 20 cm in diameter and often produce clinical manifestations, usually lower abdominal pain. The clinical picture may mimic that of an ovarian tumor. Gross examination often shows thick fibrous septa that may suggest the solid component of a cystic and solid ovarian tumor and their contents may be serosanguineous or bloody (Fig. 103).

On microscopic examination, MPICs are usually lined with a single layer of flat to cuboidal mesothelial cells with benign nuclear features (Fig. 104). A modest degree of reactive atypia, including hobnail-like nuclei, is not uncommon. The mesothelial cells may form worrisome intraluminal papillary or cribriform patterns. In some cases, mural proliferations of typical or atypical mesothelial cells, disposed singly or as glands or nests, may create an infiltrative pattern suggesting an adenocarcinoma or malignant mesothelioma (Fig. 105) (215–217). In some cases, vacuolated mesothelial cells in the stroma may raise the possibility of a signet ring carcinoma (217). The cyst walls and septa are usually composed of fibrovascular connective tissue with a sparse inflammatory infiltrate, but in other cases, severe acute and chronic inflammation, fibrin, granulation tissue, and hemorrhage are encountered and complicate the overall picture.

A history of one or more abdominal surgical procedures, pelvic inflammatory disease, or endometriosis was present in 84% of MPICs in one study (217). These findings provide support for an inflammatory pathogenesis and a benign diagnosis in individual cases of MPICs (215–217,221–223).

flammation, a frequent complication of a surgical procedure, and rarely a diagnostic problem (319). In occasional cases, however, it may difficult to differentiate between markedly reactive peritoneal fibrosis and a desmoplastic mesothelioma, particularly in a small biopsy specimen (199). Features favoring a diagnosis of mesothelioma include nuclear atypia, necrosis, the presence of organized patterns of collagen deposition (fascicular, storiform), and infiltration of adjacent tissues (199).

Sclerosing peritonitis is a rare disorder characterized by fibrous peritoneal thickening that in some instances encases the small bowel ("abdominal cocoon") causing bowel obstruction. It occurs in an idiopathic form, typically affecting adolescent girls (320,321), or it may be secondary to practolol therapy (322), chronic ambulatory peritoneal dialysis (323,324), the use of a peritoneovenous (LeVeen) shunt (325), or luteinized thecomas of the ovary (189). The intraoperative and microscopic appearance of the peritoneal lesions in several of the cases of luteinized thecoma was initially misinterpreted as metastatic thecoma (Figs. 135 and 136), the high mitotic rate of some of the thecomas contributing to the misdiagnosis. Awareness of this rare association and the differences in the histologic appearance of the peritoneal lesions and the ovarian tumors facilitates the correct diagnosis (189).

### Peritoneal Fibrous Nodules

Rarely, reactive fibrous proliferations of the peritoneum can take the form of tumor-like nodules. In one recently encountered case, three nodules were found in the cul de sac in a woman with an ovarian mucinous cystadenocarcinoma. Similar nodules involved the serosal aspect of the tumor. The nodules were composed of moderately cellular fascicles of benign-appearing spindle cells resembling fibroblasts and myofibroblasts that contained occasional mitotic figures

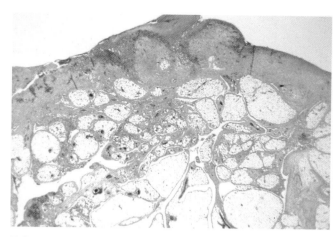

**FIG. 136.** Sclerosing peritonitis. Same case as in Fig. 135.

(Figs. 137 and 138). The spindle cells were admixed with small blood vessels, inflammatory cells, hyalinized collagen, and myxoid material. The cells were immunoreactive for vimentin, smooth muscle actin, and cytokeratin, possibly corresponding to the "multipotential subserosal cells" described by Bolen et al. (325a).

### Peritoneal Histiocytic Nodules

As noted earlier, ceroid-rich histiocytes involving the peritoneum and omentum may occur secondary to endometriosis (page 300) and in association with a peritoneal decidual reaction (page 283). Peritoneal melanin-laden histiocytes (peritoneal melanosis) are a rare complication of ovarian dermoid cysts (page 312). In addition, nonpigmented histiocytes can occasionally occur as nodular aggregates on the peritoneum that may appear as small, grossly visible nodules at operation. We are aware of one such case from a patient with a granulosa cell tumor in which the histiocytes were initially misinterpreted microscopically as metastatic granulosa cell tumor (Scully RE, personal com-

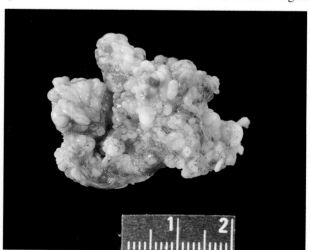

**FIG. 135.** Sclerosing peritonitis involving the omentum creates a nodular appearance. The patient had a luteinized thecoma in one ovary.

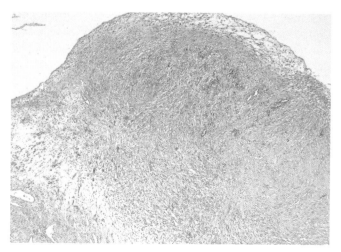

**FIG. 137.** Peritoneal fibrous nodule. The edge of one nodule, which was in the cul de sac, is seen.

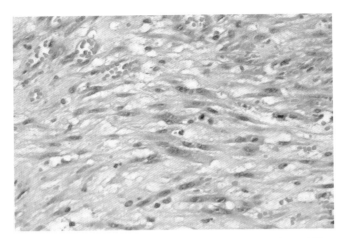

FIG. 138. Peritoneal fibrous nodule. High-power view of Fig. 137.

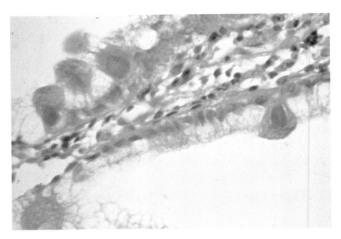

FIG. 139. Cytomegalovirus infection of the cervix.

munication). Ruffolo and Suster have described a diffuse histiocytic proliferation of the pelvic peritoneum associated with endocervicosis (264). In these cases, the histiocytes should be distinguished from mesothelial cells, a distinction that can be facilitated with the use of immunohistochemistry (264).

### Infections

As noted in the introduction to this chapter, HPV infection in the female genital tract is not considered here. Cytomegalovirus (CMV) rarely involves the vagina (326), the endocervix (327), the endometrium (328–331), and the ovaries (332–334), usually as an incidental microscopic finding, although visible foci of superficial cortical hemorrhagic necrosis that are several millimeters long have been described in the ovaries (333). Diagnosis rests on the demonstration of the characteristic large basophilic intranuclear inclusions in the infected epithelial (Fig. 139), endothelial, or stromal cells. Immunohistochemical staining for CMV antigen may be confirmatory. The intranuclear inclusions, as well as associated granular cytoplasmic inclusions, are sufficiently characteristic that confusion with a premalignant lesion or an *in situ* adenocarcinoma in the endocervix or endometrium is unlikely.

Herpes simplex virus (HSV) infection of the lower genital tract is quite common. In typical cases the clinician will often suspect the diagnosis but it is not rare for the lesion to be overlooked clinically. Herpetic endometritis is rare, and is usually associated with herpetic cervicitis, suggesting an ascending infection (335,336); some cases, however, have been found at autopsy in patients with disseminated infection. On microscopic examination, the characteristic ground-glass intranuclear inclusions (Fig. 140) should establish the diagnosis with relative ease in most cases, although occasionally misdiagnosis as a dysplastic process occurs. HSV immunoreactivity in the stromal, epithelial, or

endothelial cells may be confirmatory. The differential diagnosis in the endometrium includes glands lined with optically clear nuclei, a pregnancy-related change (82).

A variety of infections involving the female genital tract, most of which are uncommon or rare, can occasionally mimic a tumor clinically or on macroscopic examination. A neoplasm, however, is usually easily excluded on microscopic examination, the specific diagnosis in most cases requiring microscopic or cultural identification of the causative organism. Reported examples have included tuberculous cervicitis (337–339) and peritonitis (340), pelvic actinomycosis (Fig. 141) (341,342), granuloma inguinale of the cervix (343), amoebic cervicitis (344), and chlamydial salpingitis (which caused a mass and ascites) (345).

### Atypia Secondary to Radiation and Chemotherapy

Radiation to the uterus can cause markedly atypical nuclear changes that can be mistaken for a preneoplastic or neoplastic process in the endocervical or endometrial glands, particularly if the pathologist is unaware of the history

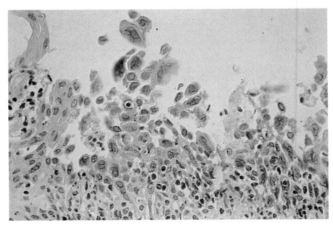

FIG. 140. Herpetic cervicitis.

(346,347). Adenomyotic glands can also exhibit radiation-induced atypia (348). In contrast to those in a neoplasm, however, the nuclear features following radiation are more variable from one cell to another, with bizarre forms and an absence of mitotic activity (Fig. 142). Radiation-induced vascular and stromal changes, including postradiation fibroblasts, may also be present. Similar criteria apply when radiation atypia in seen elsewhere in the female genital tract, although radiation atypia is primarily a problem when encountered in uterine specimens.

Changes similar to radiation-induced atypia can be associated with chemotherapeutic agents such as methotrexate, busulfan, thiotepa, chlorambucil, and cyclophosphamide (349). The squamous cells in the vulva, vagina, and cervix as well as the glandular cells of the endocervix and endometrium may be affected. The degree of the atypical changes is generally proportional to the dosage and duration of the therapy (349). As with radiation-induced changes, the distinction from a premalignant or malignant alteration depends on awareness of the drug history, the atrophic appearance of the epithelium, nuclear features (including bizarre forms) that vary markedly from one cell to another, and the absence of mitotic figures.

## PIGMENTED LESIONS

### Blue Nevi

Although technically a neoplasm, brief mention of blue nevi lesions is merited here because they are usually an inci-

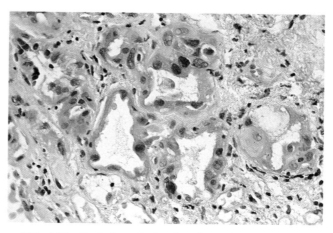

**FIG. 142.** Radiation atypia of endocervical epithelium.

dental microscopic finding and may be interpreted as a more ominous lesion. The endocervix is the most common noncutaneous site for the blue nevus (350–352); rare examples have also been described in the vagina (353). One cellular blue nevus involved the cervix, vagina, and hymenal ring (354). Until recently, only approximately 50 cervical cases had been reported (350,351), but a study from Japan in which step sections of the cervix were obtained found "stromal melanocytic foci" in 54 of 189 cases (28.6%) (352). Endocervical blue nevi are almost always an incidental gross or microscopic finding within hysterectomy or cervical biopsy specimens of adults. The vaginal lesion noted above, however, was diagnosed clinically as malignant melanoma (353). The macroscopically visible lesions have appeared as one or, occasionally, several flat, blue to black, ill-defined mucosal lesions usually <4 mm in size. The histologic appearance resembles that of cutaneous blue nevi, consisting of melanin-laden polygonal and spindle cells with dendritic processes, arranged in irregular clusters in the superficial endocervical stroma (Fig. 143). The cells are argyrophilic, argentaffinic, and immunoreactive for S-100 protein (350). They are distinguished from malignant melanoma using criteria applied to cutaneous blue nevi.

### Melanosis of Mucosal Surfaces

Occasional examples of benign melanotic pigmentation ("melanosis") of the vulva (355) or squamous epithelium of the cervix (356–360), vagina (361,362), or cervix and vagina (363) have been described. Irregular areas of mucosal pigmentation are typically seen on clinical examination, in some cases mimicking malignant melanoma. Microscopic examination usually reveals a proliferation of benign melanocytes in the basal layer, sometimes with a lentigo-like pattern (356,363), often accompanied by melanin pigmentation of the basal cells.

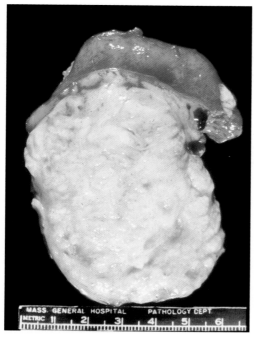

**FIG. 141.** Actinomycosis of the ovary. The ovary is replaced by a yellow–white mass.

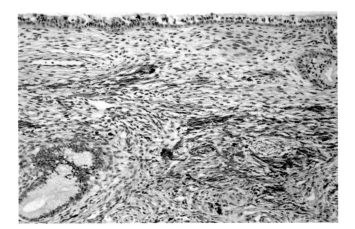

**FIG. 143.** Blue nevus of the endocervix.

## Melanosis Peritonei

The four reported cases of peritoneal melanosis (melanosis peritonei) have been associated with ovarian dermoid cysts, two cases of which had ruptured preoperatively (364–367). Tan to black, peritoneal staining or pigmented tumor-like nodules involved the pelvic peritoneum and omentum at laparotomy, raising the suspicion of metastatic tumor in several cases. Some locules in the dermoid cysts had pigmentation of their contents and lining. On microscopic examination, the ovarian and peritoneal lesions consisted of melanin-laden histiocytes in a fibrous stroma (Fig. 144). No obvious source for the pigment could be identified in any of the cases. The lesions are distinguished from malignant melanoma by noting the presence of melanin in bland histiocytes rather than in atypical melanocytes, a distinction that may be aided by immunohistochemical staining. The differential diagnosis also includes peritoneal lipofuscinosis.

### Lipofuscinosis

Lipofuscin pigment in the histiocytes ("pseudoxanthoma cells") of endometriotic lesions and pseudoxanthomatous salpingiosis has been discussed earlier in this chapter (see page 300). Lipofuscin pigment in the endometrium has also been noted earlier (see page 305) as a prominent finding in some cases of xanthogranulomatous endometritis (287,288). Two additional cases of uterine lipofuscinosis have been described. In one of them, a dark brown lesion was noted on the anterior lip of the cervix in a 59-year-old woman (368). Microscopic examination revealed an ulcer with a band-like infiltrate of ceroid-rich histiocytes. In the other case, striking dark brown pigmentation of the myometrium was observed in a 37-year-old woman with Friedrich's ataxia and the brown bowel syndrome. On microscopic examination, abundant cytoplasmic ceroid was present in the myometrial smooth muscle cells, the stromal cells of the basal endometrium, and macrophages (369).

The two reported cases of peritoneal lipofuscinosis took the form of brown pigmentation of the peritoneum observed at the time of cesarean section (370,371). In both cases, pigment-laden histiocytes were associated with ectopic decidual cells; the pigment was identified histochemically and ultrastructurally as lipofuscin. The differential diagnosis of this lesion includes melanosis peritonei (see above) and malignant melanoma.

### PSAMMOMATOUS CALCIFICATION

Two cases of psammomatous endometrial calcification associated with the use of exogenous hormones have been reported (372,373). In one, a 46-year-old woman taking combination oral contraceptives was found to have psammoma bodies on a routine cervicovaginal smear, and a subsequent endometrial biopsy revealed psammoma bodies in the glandular lumina and stroma (372). In the other case, a

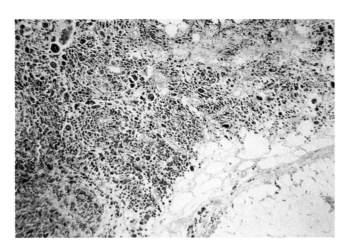

**FIG. 144.** Melanosis peritonei.

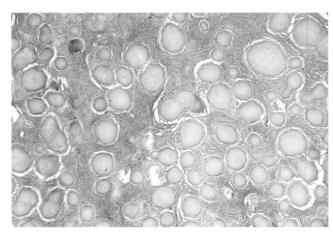

**FIG. 145.** Psammomatous calcification of ovarian stroma.

28-year-old woman, who had a history of oral contraceptive use and clomiphene treatment, underwent an endometrial curettage (373). Psammoma bodies were found in the endometrial stroma and glands, and a similar finding was present in a specimen obtained by a repeated curettage performed 5 months later.

In another case, bilateral idiopathic ovarian psammomatous calcification resulted in stone-hard but normal-sized ovaries (374). Microscopic examination showed numerous spherical laminated calcific foci without an investment of epithelial cells (Fig. 145). This process must be distinguished from a serous borderline tumor or psammocarcinoma in which at least occasional neoplastic epithelial cells are present, and from "burned-out" gonadoblastomas replaced by laminated calcific masses. In the latter cases the patient almost always has evidence of abnormal gonadal development and Y chromosome material in her karyotype, as well as residual gonadoblastoma in the same or contralateral gonad.

## VASCULAR LESIONS

Rupture of a corpus luteum can result in hemorrhage and, rarely, fatal hemoperitoneum. Although hemorrhage can occur in otherwise normal women, it is observed more often in women receiving anticoagulant therapy (375). Although torsion of an ovary on its pedicle is often associated with an ovarian neoplasm, occasionally an otherwise normal ovary, particularly in children, can undergo torsion and hemorrhagic infarction. Both hemorrhage and hemorrhagic infarc-

tion can produce a gross appearance indistinguishable from a hemorrhagic ovarian tumor (Fig. 146). Indeed, extensive microscopic examination may be required to exclude an underlying neoplasm.

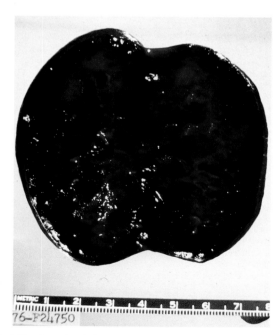

**FIG. 146.** Ovarian infarction. The ovary is completely hemorrhagic, potentially mimicking a hemorrhagic neoplasm on gross inspection.

## REFERENCES

1. Willis RA. *Pathology of tumors.* St. Louis: CV Mosby, 1949;526.
2. McLachlin CM, Devine P, Muto M, Genest DR. Pseudoinvasion of vascular spaces: report of an artifact caused by cervical lidocaine injection prior to loop diathermy. *Hum Pathol* 1994;25:208–211.
3. Munsick RA, Janovski NA. Walthard cell rest of the cervix uteri. Report of a case. *Am J Obstet Gynecol* 1961;82:909–912.
3a. Weir MM, Bell DA, Young RH. Transitional cell metaplasia of the uterine cervix and vagina: an underrecognized lesion that may be confused with high-grade dysplasia. A report of 59 cases. *Am J Surg Pathol.* In press.
3b. Egan AJM, Russell P. Transitional (urothelial) metaplasia of the uterine cervix: morphological assessment of 31 cases. *Int J Gynecol Pathol.* In press.
4. Miller N, Bedard YC, Cooter NB, Shaul DL. Histologic changes in the genital tract in transsexual women following androgen therapy. *Histopathology* 1986;10:661–669.
5. Albores-Saavedra J, Young RH. Transitional cell neoplasms (carcinoma and inverted papilloma) of the uterine cervix. A report of four cases. *Am J Surg Pathol* 1995; 19:1138–1145.
6. Young RH, Clement PB. Pseudoneoplastic lesions of the lower female genital tract. *Pathol Annu* 1989;24(2):189–226.
7. Young RH, Scully RE. Cervical papillary adenocarcinoma of villoglandular type: a clinicopathological analysis of 12 cases. *Cancer* 1989;63:1773–1779.
8. Fluhmann CF. Focal hyperplasia (tunnel clusters) of the cervix uteri. *Obstet Gynecol* 1961;17:206–214.
9. Fluhmann CF. *The cervix uteri and its diseases.* Philadelphia: WB Saunders, 1961;95–100.
10. Sherrer CW, Parmley T, Woodruff JD. Adenomatous hyperplasia of the endocervix. *Obstet Gynecol* 1977;49:65–68.
11. Segal GH, Hart WR. Cystic endocervical tunnel clusters. A clinicopathologic study of 29 cases of so-called adenomatous hyperplasia. *Am J Surg Pathol* 1990;14:895–903.
12. Gilks CB, Young RH, Aguirre P, DeLellis RA, Scully RE. Adenoma malignum (minimal deviation adenocarcinoma) of the uterine cervix: a clinicopathological and immunohistochemical analysis of 26 cases. *Am J Surg Pathol* 1989;13:1717–1729.
12a. Jones MA, Young RH. Endocervical type A (noncystic) tunnel clusters with cytologic atypia: a report of 14 cases. *Am J Surg Pathol* 1996; 20:1318–1321.
13. Anderson MC, Hartley RB. Cervical crypt involvement by intraepithelial neoplasia. *Obstet Gynecol* 1980;55:546–550.
14. Teshima S, Shimosato Y, Kishi K, Kasamatsu T, Ohmi K, Uei Y. Early stage adenocarcinoma of the uterine cervix. Histopathologic analysis with consideration of histogenesis. *Cancer* 1985;56: 167–172.
15. Noda K, Kimura K, Ikeda M, Teshima K. Studies on the histogenesis of cervical adenocarcinoma. *Int J Gynecol Pathol* 1983;1: 336–346.
16. Daya D, Young RH. Florid deep glands of the uterine cervix: another mimic of adenoma malignum. *Am J Clin Pathol* 1995;103:614–617.
17. Clement PB, Young RH. Deep Nabothian cysts of the endocervix. A possible source of confusion with minimal-deviation adenocarcinoma (adenoma malignum). *Int J Gynecol Pathol* 1989;8:340–348.
18. Taylor HB, Ivey NS, Norris HJ. Atypical endocervical hyperplasia in women taking oral contraceptives. *JAMA* 1967;202:185–187.
19. Kyriakos M, Kempson RL, Konikov NF. A clinical and pathologic study of endocervical lesions associated with oral contraceptives. *Cancer* 1968;22:99–110.
20. Candy J, Abell MR. Progestogen-induced adenomatous hyperplasia of the uterine cervix. *JAMA* 1968;203:323–326.
21. Govan ADT, Black WP, Sharp JL. Aberrant glandular polypi of the uterine cervix associated with contraceptive pills: Pathology and pathogenesis. *J Clin Pathol* 1969;22:84–89.

22. Nichols TM, Fidler HK. Microglandular hyperplasia in cervical cone biopsies taken for suspicious and positive cytology. *Am J Clin Pathol* 1971;56:424–429.

23. Wilkinson E, Dufour DR. Pathogenesis of microglandular hyperplasia of the cervix uteri. *Obstet Gynecol* 1976;47:189–195.

24. Leslie KO, Silverberg SG. Microglandular hyperplasia of the cervix: Unusual clinical and pathological presentations and their differential diagnosis. *Prog Surg Pathol* 1984;5:95–114.

25. Chumas JC, Nelson B, Mann WJ, Chalas E, Kaplan CG. Microglandular hyperplasia of the uterine cervix. *Obstet Gynecol* 1985;66:406–409.

26. Greeley C, Schroeder S, Silverberg SG. Microglandular hyperplasia of the cervix: A true "pill" lesion? *Int J Gynecol Pathol* 1995;14:50–54.

27. Young RH, Scully RE. Atypical forms of microglandular hyperplasia of the cervix simulating carcinoma: a report of five cases and review of the literature. *Am J Surg Pathol* 1989;13:50–56.

28. Young RH, Scully RE. Uterine carcinomas simulating microglandular hyperplasia. A report of six cases. *Am J Surg Pathol* 1992;16:1092–1097.

29. Jacques SM, Qureshi F, Lawrence WD. Surface epithelial changes in endometrial adenocarcinoma: Diagnostic pitfalls in curettage specimens. *Int J Gynecol Pathol* 1995; 14:191–197.

30. Steeper TA, Wick MR. Minimal deviation adenocarcinoma of the uterine cervix ("adenoma malignum"). An immunohistochemical comparison with microglandular endocervical hyperplasia and conventional endocervical adenocarcinoma. *Cancer* 1986;58:1131–1138.

31. Speers WC, Picaso LG, Silverberg SG. Immunohistochemical localization of carcinoembryonic antigen in microglandular hyperplasia and adenocarcinoma of the endocervix. *Am J Clin Pathol* 1983;79:105–107.

32. Kudo R, Sasano H, Koizumi M, Orenstein JM, Silverberg SG. Immunohistochemical comparison of new monoclonal antibody 1C5 and carcinoembryonic antigen in the differential diagnosis of adenocarcinoma of the uterine cervix. *Int J Gynecol Pathol* 1990;9:325–336.

33. Ferry JA, Scully RE. Mesonephric remnants, hyperplasia and neoplasia in the uterine cervix: a study of 49 cases. *Am J Surg Pathol* 1990;14:1100–1111.

34. Jones MA, Andrews J, Tarraza H. Mesonephric remnant hyperplasia of the cervix: A clinicopathologic analysis of 14 cases. *Gynecol Oncol* 1993;49:41–47.

35. Clement PB, Young RH, Keh P, Östör A, Scully RE. Malignant mesonephric neoplasms of the uterine cervix: A report of eight cases, including four with a malignant spindle cell component. *Am J Surg Pathol* 1995; 19:1158–1171.

36. Jones MA, Young RH, Scully RE. Diffuse laminar endocervical glandular hyperplasia: a report of seven cases. *Am J Surg Pathol* 1991;15:1123–1129.

37. Young RH, Clement PB. Tumorlike lesions of the uterine cervix. In: Clement PB, Young RH, eds. *Tumors and tumorlike lesions of the uterine corpus and cervix.* New York: Churchill Livingstone, 1993;1–50.

38. Michael H, Grawe L, Kraus FT. Minimal deviation endocervical adenocarcinoma: clinical and histologic features, immunohistochemical staining for carcinoembryonic antigen, and differentiation from confusing benign lesions. *Int J Gynecol Pathol* 1984;3:261–276.

39. Jonasson JG, Wang HH, Antonioli DA, Ducatman BS. Tubal metaplasia of the uterine cervix: a prevalence study in patients with gynecologic pathologic findings. *Int J Gynecol Pathol* 1992;11:89–95.

40. Ismail SM. Cone biopsy causes cervical endometriosis and tuboendometrioid metaplasia. *Histopathology* 1991;18:107–114.

41. Oliva E, Clement PB, Young RH. Tubal and tubo-endometrioid metaplasia of the uterine cervix: unemphasized features that may cause problems in differential diagnosis. A report of 25 cases. *Am J Clin Pathol* 1995; 103:618–623.

42. Yeh I, Bronner M, LiVolsi VA. Endometrial metaplasia of the uterine cervix. *Arch Pathol Lab Med* 1993;117:734–735.

43. Trowell JE. Intestinal metaplasia with argentaffin cells in the uterine cervix. *Histopathology* 1985;9:551–559.

44. Gloor E, Hurlimann J. Cervical intraepithelial glandular neoplasia (adenocarcinoma in situ and glandular dysplasia). A correlative study of 23 cases with histologic grading, histochemical analysis of mucins, and immunohistochemical determination of the affinity for four lectins. *Cancer* 1986;58:1272–1280.

45. Fox H, Wells M, Harris M, McWilliam LJ, Anderson GS. Enteric tumours of the lower female genital tract: a report of three cases. *Histopathology* 1988;12:167–176.

46. Michael H, Sutton G, Hull MT, Roth LM. Villous adenoma of the uterine cervix associated with invasive adenocarcinoma: a histologic, ultrastructural, and immunohistochemical study. *Int J Gynecol Pathol* 1986;5:163–169.

46a. Jones MA, Young RH. Atypical oxyphilic metaplasia of the endocervical epithelium. A report of 6 cases. *Int J Gynecol Pathol*. In press.

47. Brown LJR, Wells M. Cervical glandular atypia associated with squamous intraepithelial neoplasia: a premalignant lesion? *J Clin Pathol* 1986;39:22–28.

48. Hendrickson MR, Kempson RL. Endometrial epithelial metaplasias: proliferations frequently misdiagnosed as adenocarcinoma. Report of 89 cases and proposed classification. *Am J Surg Pathol* 1980;4:525–542.

49. Rorat E, Wallach RC. Papillary metaplasia of the endometrium: clinical and histopathologic considerations. *Obstet Gynecol* 1984;64:90S–92S.

50. Zaman SS, Mazur MT. Endometrial papillary syncytial change. A nonspecific alteration associated with active breakdown. *Am J Clin Pathol* 1993;99:741–745.

51. Gersell DJ. Endometrial papillary syncytial change (Editorial). *Am J Clin Pathol* 1993;99:756–757.

52. Clement PB. Pathology of the uterine corpus. *Hum Pathol* 1991;22:776–791.

53. Mack RJ, Liu YC, Zuzarte J. Tumor associated endometrial papillary syncytial change: an epithelial alteration frequently accompanying endometrial adenocarcinoma. *Mod Pathol* 1994;7:92A.

54. Baggish MS, Woodruff JD. The occurrence of squamous epithelium in the endometrium. *Obstet Gynecol Surv* 1967;22:69–115.

55. Crum CP, Richart RM, Fenoglio CM. Adenoacanthosis of the endometrium. A clinicopathologic study in premenopausal women. *Am J Surg Pathol* 1981;5:15–20.

56. Blaustein A. Morular metaplasia misdiagnosed as adenoacanthoma in young women with polycystic ovarian disease. *Am J Surg Pathol* 1982;6:223–228.

57. Demopoulos RI, Greco MA. Mucinous metaplasia of the endometrium: ultrastructural and histochemical characteristics. *Int J Gynecol Pathol* 1983;1:383–390.

58. Wells M, Tiltman A. Intestinal metaplasia of the endometrium. *Histopathology* 1989;15:431–433.

59. Honore LH. Benign obstructive myxometra: report of a case. *Am J Obstet Gynecol* 1979;133:227–229.

60. Baird DB, Reddick R. Extraovarian mucinous metaplasia in a patient with bilateral mucinous borderline ovarian tumors: a case report. *Int J Gynecol Pathol* 1991;10:96–103.

61. Hendrickson MR, Kempson RL. Ciliated carcinoma—a variant of endometrial adenocarcinoma: a report of 10 cases. *Int J Gynecol Pathol* 1983;2:1–12.

62. Bergeron C, Ferenczy A. Oncocytic metaplasia in endometrial hyperplasia and carcinoma. *Int J Gynecol Pathol* 1988;7:93–97.

63. Pitman MB, Young RH, Clement PB, Dickersin GR, Scully RE. Oxyphilic endometrioid carcinoma of the ovary and endometrium: a report of nine cases. *Int J Gynecol Pathol* 1994;13:290–301.

64. Picoff RC, Luginbuhl WH. The significance of foci of dense stromal cellularity in the endometrium. *Am J Obstet Gynecol* 1966;94:820–823.

65. Sampson JA. Metastatic or embolic endometriosis, due to the menstrual dissemination of endometrial tissue into the venous circulation. *Am J Pathol* 1927;3:93–109.

66. Banks ER, Mills SE, Frierson HF Jr. Uterine intravascular menstrual endometrium simulating malignancy. *Am J Surg Pathol* 1991;15:407–412.

67. Welch WR, Scully RE. Precancerous lesions of the endometrium. *Hum Pathol* 1977;8:503–512.

68. Keating S, Quenville NF, Korn GW, Clement PB. Ruptured adenomyotic cyst of the uterus—a case report. *Arch Gynecol* 1986;237:169–173.

69. Mazur MT. Atypical polypoid adenomyomas of the endometrium. *Am J Surg Pathol* 1981;5:473–482.

70. Young RH, Treger T, Scully RE. Atypical polypoid adenomyoma of the uterus. A report of 27 cases. *Am J Clin Pathol* 1986;86:139–145.

71. Goldblum J, Clement PB, Hart WR. Adenomyosis with sparse glands: a potential mimic of low-grade endometrial stromal sarcoma. *Am J Clin Pathol* 1995; 103:218–223.

72. Sahin AA, Silva EG, Landon G, Ordonez NG, Gershenson DM. Endometrial tissue in myometrial vessels not associated with menstruation. *Int J Gynecol Pathol* 1989;8:139–146.

73. Arias-Stella J. Atypical endometrial changes associated with the presence of chorionic tissue. *Arch Pathol Lab Med* 1954;58:112–128.

74. Arias-Stella J. A topographic study of uterine epithelial atypia associated with chorionic tissue: demonstration of alteration in the endocervix. *Cancer* 1959;12:782–790.

75. Clement PB, Young RH, Scully RE. Nontrophoblastic pathology of the female genital tract and peritoneum asociated with pregnancy. *Semin Diagn Pathol* 1989;6:372–406.

76. Arias-Stella J Jr, Arias-Velasquez A, Arias-Stella J. Normal and abnormal mitoses in the atypical endometrial change associated with chorionic tissue effect. *Am J Surg Pathol* 1994;18:694–701.

77. Huettner PC, Gersell DJ. Arias-Stella reaction in nonpregnant women: a clinicopathologic study of nine cases. *Int J Gynecol Pathol* 1994; 13:241–247.

78. Birch HW, Collins CG. Atypical changes of genital epithelium associated with ectopic pregnancy. *Am J Obstet Gynecol* 1961;81: 1198–1208.

79. Moller NE. The Arias-Stella phenomenon in endometriosis. *Acta Obstet Gynecol Scand* 1959;38:271–274.

80. Milchgrub S, Sandstad J. Arias-Stella reaction in fallopian tube epithelium. *Am J Clin Pathol* 1991;95:892–895.

81. Zaino RJ, Robboy SJ, Bentley R, Kurman RJ. Diseases of the vagina. In: Kurman RJ, ed. *Blaustein's pathology of the female genital tract.* 4th ed. New York: Springer-Verlag, 1994;167.

82. Mazur MT, Hendrickson MR, Kempson RL. Optically clear nuclei. An alteration of endometrial epithelium in the presence of trophoblast. *Am J Surg Pathol* 1983;7:415–423.

83. Schneider V. Arias-Stella reaction of the endocervix. Frequency and location. *Acta Cytol* 1981;25:224–228.

84. Cariani DJ, Guderian AM. Gestational atypia in endocervical polyps. The Arias-Stella reaction. *Am J Obstet Gynecol* 1966;95:589–590.

85. Cove H. The Arias-Stella reaction occurring in the endocervix in pregnancy. Recognition and comparison with an adenocarcinoma of the endocervix. *Am J Surg Pathol* 1979;3:567–568.

86. Zaytsev P, Taxy JB. Pregnancy-associated ectopic decidua. *Am J Surg Pathol* 1987;11:526–530.

87. Dockerty MB, Smith RA, Symmonds RE. Pseudomalignant endometrial changes induced by administration of new synthetic progestins. *Proc Mayo Clin* 1959;34:321–328.

88. Cruz-Aquino M, Shenker L, Blaustein A. Pseudosarcoma of the endometrium. *Obstet Gynecol* 1967;29:93–96.

89. Clement PB, Scully RE. Idiopathic postmenopausal decidual reaction of the endometrium: a clinicopathologic analysis of four cases. *Int J Gynecol Pathol* 1988;7:152–161.

90. Nogales FF, Martin F, Linares J, Naranjo R, Concha A. Myxoid change in decidualized scar endometriosis mimicking malignancy. *J Cutan Pathol* 1993;20:87–91.

91. Ashraf M, Boyd CB, Beresford WA. Ectopic decidual reaction in para-aortic and pelvic lymph nodes in the presence of cervical squamous cell carcinoma during pregnancy. *J Surg Oncol* 1984;26:6–8.

92. Burnett RA, Millan D. Decidual change in pelvic lymph nodes: a source of possible diagnostic error. *Histopathology* 1986;10: 1089–1092.

93. Yoonessi M, Satchindanand SK, Ortinez CG, Goodell T. Benign glandular elements and decidual reaction in retroperitoneal lymph nodes. *J Surg Oncol* 1982;19:81–86.

94. Cobb CJ. Ectopic decidua and metastatic squamous carcinoma: Presentation in a single pelvic lymph node. *J Surg Oncol* 1988;38: 126–129.

95. Talerman A, Montero JR, Chilcote RR, Okagaki T. Diffuse malignant peritoneal mesothelioma in a 13-year-old girl. Report of a case and review of the literature. *Am J Surg Pathol* 1985;9:73–80.

96. Nascimento AG, Keeney GL, Fletcher CDM. Deciduoid peritoneal mesothelioma. An unusual phenotype affecting young females. *Am J Surg Pathol* 1994;18:439–445.

97. Clement PB. Tumorlike lesions of the uterine corpus. In: Clement PB, Young RH, eds. *Tumors and tumorlike lesions of the uterine corpus and cervix.* New York: Churchill Livingstone, 1993;137–179.

98. Roth E, Taylor HB. Heterotopic cartilage in the uterus. *Obstet Gynecol* 1966;27:838–844.

99. Daya D, Lukka H, Clement PB. Primitive neuroectodermal tumors of the uterus: a report of four cases. *Hum Pathol* 1992;23:1120–1129.

100. Young RH, Kleinman GM, Scully RE. Glioma of the uterus. Report of a case with comments on histogenesis. *Am J Surg Pathol* 1981; 5:695–699.

101. Tyagi SP, Saxena K, Rizvi R, Langley FA. Foetal remnants in the uterus and their relation to other uterine heterotopia. *Histopathology* 1979;3:339–345.

102. Young RH, Kurman RJ, Scully RE. Proliferations and tumors of intermediate trophoblast of the placental site. *Semin Diagn Pathol* 1988; 5:223–237.

103. Young RH, Kurman RJ, Scully RE. Placental site nodules and plaques. A clinicopathologic study of 20 cases. *Am J Surg Pathol* 1990;14:1001–1009.

104. Ewing J. Chorioma. *Surg Gynecol Obstet* 1910;10:366–392.

105. Elston CW. The histopathology of trophoblastic tumours (Suppl. Royal College of Pathologists 10). *J Clin Pathol* 1976;29:111–131.

106. Collins RJ, Hgan HYS, Wong LC. Placental site trophoblastic tumor: with features between an exaggerated placental site reaction and a placental site trophoblastic tumor. *Int J Gynecol Pathol* 1990;9:170–177.

107. Huettner PC, Gersell DJ. Placental site nodule: a clinicopathologic study of 38 cases. *Int J Gynecol Pathol* 1994;13:191–198.

108. Carinelli SG, Vendola N, Zanatti F, Benzi G. Placental site nodules. A report of 17 cases (abstract). *Pathol Res Pract* 1989;185:30.

109. Silva EG, Tornos C, Lage J, Ordonez NG, Morris M, Kananagh J. Multiple nodules of intermediate trophoblast following hydatidiform moles. *Int J Gynecol Pathol* 1993;12:324–332.

110. Hallatt JG. Primary ovarian pregnancy: a report of twenty-five cases. *Am J Obstet Gynecol* 1982;143:55–60.

111. Renade V, Palmerino DA, Tronik B. Cervical pregnancy. *Obstet Gynecol* 1978;51:502–505.

112. Covone AE, Johnson PM, Mutton D, Adinolfi M. Trophoblast cells in peripheral blood from pregnant women. *Lancet* 1984;2:841–843.

113. Attwood HD, Park WW. Embolism to the lungs of trophoblast. *J Obstet Gynaecol Br Commonw* 1961;68:611–617.

114. Benirschke K, Kaufman P. *Pathology of the human placenta.* 2nd ed. New York: Springer-Verlag, 1990.

115. Tanimura A, Natsuyama H, Kawano M, Tanimura Y, Tanaka T, Kitazono M. Primary choriocarcinoma of the lung. *Hum Pathol* 1985;16: 1281–1284.

116. Maymon R, Lew S, Lotan M, Haimovich L, Zmira N, Bahary C. Normal pregnancy complicated by vaginal ectopic trophoblastic implantation; a case report. *Eur J Obstet Gynecol Reprod Biol* 1991;40: 63–66.

117. Dessouky DA. Ectopic trophoblast as a complication of first-trimester induced abortion. *Am J Obstet Gynecol* 1980;136:407–408.

118. Thatcher SS, Grainger DA, True LD, DeCherney AH. Pelvic trophoblastic implants after laparoscopic removal of a tubal pregnancy. *Obstet Gynecol* 1989;74:514–515.

119. Reich H, DeCaprio J, McGlynn F, Wilkie WL, Longo S. Peritoneal trophoblastic tissue implants after laparoscopic treatment of tubal ectopic pregnancy. *Fertil Steril* 1989;52:337.

120. Cartwright PS. Peritoneal trophoblastic implants after surgical management of tubal pregnancy. *J Reprod Med* 1991;36:523–524.

121. Cataldo NA, Nicholson M, Bihrle D. Uterine serosal trophoblastic implant after linear salpingostomy for ectopic pregancy at laparotomy. *Obstet Gynecol* 1990;76:523–525.

122. Robboy SJ, Welch WR. Microglandular hyperplasia in vaginal adenosis associated with oral contraceptives and prenatal diethylstilbestrol exposure. *Obstet Gynecol* 1977;49:430–434.

123. Merchant WJ, Gale J. Intestinal metaplasia in stilboestrol-induced vaginal adenosis. *Histopathology* 1993;23:373–376.

124. Scurry J, Planner R, Grant P. Unusual variants of vaginal adenosis: a challenge for diagnosis and treatment. *Gynecol Oncol* 1991;41: 171–177.

125. Norris HJ, Taylor HB. Polyps of the vagina. A benign lesion resembling sarcoma botryoides. *Cancer* 1966;19:227–232.

126. Elliott GB, Reynolds HA, Fidler HK. Pseudo-sarcoma botryoides of cervix and vagina in pregnancy. *J Obstet Gynaecol Br Commonw* 1967;74:728–733.

127. Burt RL, Prichard RW, Kim BS. Fibroepithelial polyp of the vagina. A report of five cases. *Obstet Gynecol* 1976;47:52S–54S.

128. Chirayil SJ, Tobon H. Polyps of the vagina: a clinicopathologic study of 18 cases. *Cancer* 1981;47:2904–2907.

129. Davies SW, Makanje HH, Woodcock AS. Pseudo-sarcomatous polyps of the vagina in pregnancy. Case report. *Br J Obstet Gynaecol* 1981;88:566–568.

130. O'Quinn AG, Edwards CL, Gallager HS. Pseudosarcoma botryoides of the vagina in pregnancy. *Gynecol Oncol* 1982;13:237–241.

131. Miettinen M, Wahlstrom T, Vesterinen E, Saksela E. Vaginal polyps with pseudosarcomatous features. A clinicopathologic study of seven cases. *Cancer* 1983;51:1148–1151.

132. Cachaza JA, Caballero JJL, Fernandez JA, Salido E. Endocervical polyp with pseudosarcomatous pattern and cytoplasmic inclusions: an electron microscopic study. *Am J Clin Pathol* 1986;85:633–635.

133. Mitchell M, Talerman A, Sholl JS, Okagaki T, Cibils LA. Pseudosarcoma botryoides in pregnancy: report of a case with ultrastructural observations. *Obstet Gynecol* 1987;70:522–526.

134. Maenpaa J, Soderstrom KO, Salmi T, Ekbad U. Large atypical polyps of the vagina during pregnancy with concomitant human papilloma virus infection. *Eur J Obstet Gynecol Reprod Biol* 1988;27:65–69.

135. Ostor AG, Fortune DW, Riley CB. Fibroepithelial polyps with atypical stromal cells (pseudosarcoma botryoides) of vulva and vagina. A report of 13 cases. *Int J Gynecol Pathol* 1988;7:351–360.

136. Tobon H, McIntyre-Seltman K, Rubino M. "Polyposis vaginalis" of pregnancy. *Arch Pathol Lab Med* 1989;113:1391–1393.

137. Mucitelli DR, Charles EZ, Kraus FT. Vulvovaginal polyps. Histologic appearance, ultrastructure, immunocytochemical characteristics, and clinicopathologic correlations. *Int J Gynecol Pathol* 1990;9:20–40.

138. Hartman C, Sperling M, Stein H. So-called fibroepithelial polyps of the vagina exhibiting an unusual but uniform antigen profile characterized by expression of desmin and steroid hormone receptors but no muscle-specific actin or macrophage markers. *Am J Clin Pathol* 1990;93:604–608.

139. Rollason TP, Byrne P, Williams A. Immunohistochemical and electron microscopic findings in benign fibroepithelial vaginal polyps. *J Clin Pathol* 1990;43:224–229.

140. Halvorsen TB, Johannesen E. Fibroepithelial polyps of the vagina: Are they old granulation tissue polyps? *J Clin Pathol* 1992;45:235–240.

141. Al-Nafussi AI, Rebello G, Hughes D, Blessing K. Benign vaginal polyp: a histological, histochemical and immunohistochemical study of 20 polyps with comparison to normal vaginal subepithelial layer. *Histopathology* 1992;20:145–150.

142. Pearl ML, Crombleholme WR, Green JR, Bottles K. Fibroepithelial polyps of the vagina in pregnancy. *Am J Perinatol* 1991;8:236–238.

143. Daya DA, Scully RE. Sarcoma botryoides of the uterine cervix in young women: a clinicopathologic study of 13 cases. *Gynecol Oncol* 1988;29:290–304.

144. Steeper TA, Rosai J. Aggressive angiomyxoma of the female pelvis and perineum. Report of nine cases of a distinctive type of gynecologic soft-tissue neoplasm. *Am J Surg Pathol* 1983;7:463–475.

145. Begin LR, Clement PB, Kirk ME, Jothy S, McCaughey WTE, Ferenczy A. Aggressive angiomyxoma of pelvic soft parts: a clinicopathological study of nine cases. *Hum Pathol* 1985;16:621–628.

146. Elliott GB, Elliott JDA. Superficial stromal reactions of lower genital tract. *Arch Pathol* 1973;95:100–101.

147. Clement PB. Multinucleated stromal giant cells of the uterine cervix. *Arch Pathol Lab Med* 1985;109:200–202.

148. Abdul-Karim FW, Cohen RE. Atypical stromal cells of lower female genital tract. *Histopathology* 1990;17:249–253.

149. Metze K, De Angelo Andrade LAL. Atypical stromal giant cells of the cervix uteri—evidence of Schwann cell origin. *Pathol Res Pract* 1991;187:1031–1035.

150. Pitt MA, Roberts ISD, Agbamu DA, Eyden BP. The nature of atypical multinucleated stromal cells: a study of 37 cases from different sites. *Histopathology* 1993;23:137–145.

151. McLachlin CM, Mutter GL, Crum CP. Multinucleated atypia of the vulva. Report of a distinct entity not associated with human papillomavirus. *Am J Surg Pathol* 1994;18:1233–1239.

152. Sternberg WH, Barclay DL. Luteoma of pregnancy. *Am J Obstet Gynecol* 1966;95:165–184.

153. Norris HJ, Taylor HB. Nodular theca-lutein hyperplasia of pregnancy (so-called "pregnancy luteoma"). A clinical and pathological study of 15 cases. *Am J Clin Pathol* 1967;47:557–566.

154. Malinak LR, Miller GV. Bilateral multicentric luteomas of pregnancy associated with masculinization of a female infant. *Am J Obstet Gynecol* 1965;91:251–259.

155. O'Malley BW, Lipsett MB, Jackson MA. Steroid content and synthesis in a virilizing luteoma. *J Clin Endocrinol* 1967;27:311–319.

156. Garcia-Bunuel R, Berek JS, Woodruff JD. Luteomas of pregnancy. *Obstet Gynecol* 1975;45:407–414.

157. Verkauf BS, Reiter EO, Hernandez L, Burns SA. Virilization of mother and fetus associated with luteoma of pregnancy: a case report with endocrinologic studies. *Am J Obstet Gynecol* 1977;129:274–279.

158. Hensleigh PA, Woodruff JD. Differential maternal-fetal response to androgenizing luteoma or hyperreactio luteinalis. *Obstet Gynecol Surv* 1978;33:262–271.

159. Hayes MC, Scully RE. Ovarian steroid cell tumors (not otherwise specified). A clinicopathological analysis of 63 cases. *Am J Surg Pathol* 1987;11:835–845.

160. Zhang J, Young RH, Arseneau J, Scully RE. Ovarian tumors containing lutein or Leydig cells (luteinized thecomas and stromal Leydig cell tumors)—a clinicopathological analysis of fifty cases. *Int J Gynecol Pathol* 1982;1:270–285.

161. Cohen DA, Daughaday WH, Weldon VV. Fetal and maternal virilization associated with pregnancy. A case report and review of the literature. *Am J Disord Child* 1982;136:353–356.

162. Barclay DL, Leverich EB, Kemmerly JR. Hyperreactio luteinalis: postpartum persistence. *Am J Obstet Gynecol* 1969;105:642–644.

163. Dick JS. Bilateral theca lutein cysts associated with apparently normal pregnancy. *J Obstet Gynecol Br Commonw* 1972;79:852–854.

164. Judd HL, Benirschke K, DeVane G, Reuter SR, Yen SSC. Maternal virilization developing during a twin pregnancy. *N Engl J Med* 1973;288:118–122.

165. Morrow CP, Kletzky OA, Disaia PJ, Townsend DE, Mishell DR, Nakamura RM. Clinical and laboratory correlates of molar pregnancy amd trophoblastic disease. *Am J Obstet Gynecol* 1977;128:424–430.

166. Barad DH, Gimovsky ML, Petrie RH, Bowe ET. Diagnosis and management of bilateral theca lutein cysts in a normal term pregnancy. *Diagn Gynecol Obstet* 1981;3:27–30.

167. Planner RS, Abell DA, Barbaro CA, Beischer NA. Massive enlargement of the ovaries after evacuation of hydatidiform moles. *Aust NZ J Obstet Gynaecol* 1982;22:96–100.

168. Berger NG, Repke JT, Woodruff JD. Markedly elevated serum testosterone in pregnancy without fetal virilization. *Obstet Gynecol* 1984;63:260–262.

169. Montz FJ, Schlaerth JB, Morrow CP. The natural history of theca lutein cysts. *Obstet Gynecol* 1988;72:247–251.

170. Wajda KJ, Lucas JG, Marsh WL Jr. Hyperreactio luteinalis. Benign disorder masquerading as an ovarian neoplasm. *Arch Pathol Lab Med* 1989;113:921–925.

171. Rosen GF, Lew MW. Severe ovarian hyperstimulation in a spontaneous singleton pregnancy. *Am J Obstet Gynecol* 1991;165:1312–1313.

172. Schumert Z, Spitz I, Diamant Y, Polishuk WZ, Rabinowitz D. Elevation of serum testosterone in ovarian hyperstimulation syndrome. *J Clin Endocrinol Metab* 1975;40:889–892.

173. Schenker JG, Weinstein D. Ovarian hyperstimulation syndrome: a current survey. *Fertil Steril* 1978;30:255–268.

174. McArdle C, Seibel M, Hann LE, Weinstein F, Taymor M. The diagnosis of ovarian hyperstimulation (OHS): the impact of ultrasound. *Fertil Steril* 1983;39:464–467.

175. Tulandi T, McInnes RA, Arronet GH. Ovarian hyperstimulation syndrome following ovulation induction with human menopausal gonadotropin. *Int J Fertil* 1984;29:113–117.

176. Chow KK, Choo HT. Ovarian hyperstimulation syndrome with clomiphene citrate. Case report. *Br J Obstet Gynaecol* 1984;91:1051–1052.

177. Haning RV Jr, Strawn EY, Nolten WE. Pathophysiology of the ovarian hyperstimulation syndrome. *Obstet Gynecol* 1985;66:220–224.

178. Albukerk JN, Berlin M. Unilateral lutein cyst in pregnancy. *N Y State J Med* 1976;76:259–261.

179. Clement PB, Scully RE. Large solitary luteinized follicle cyst of pregnancy and puerperium. *Am J Surg Pathol* 1980;4:431–438.

180. Kott MM, Schmidt WA. Massive postpartum corpus luteum cyst: a case report. *Hum Pathol* 1981;12:468–470.

181. Schuger L, Simon A, Okon E. Cytomegaly in benign ovarian cysts. *Arch Pathol Lab Med* 1986;110:928–929.

182. Nakashima N, Young RH, Scully RE. Androgenic granulosa cell tumors of the ovary. A clinicopathologic analysis of 17 cases and review of the literature. *Arch Pathol Lab Med* 1984;108:786–791.

183. Clement PB, Young RH, Scully RE. Ovarian granulosa cell proliferations of pregnancy. A report of nine cases. *Hum Pathol* 1988;19:657–662.

184. McKay DG, Hertig AT, Hickey WF. The histogenesis of granulosa and theca cell tumors of the human ovary. *Obstet Gynecol* 1953;1:125–136.

185. Norris HJ, Chorlton I. Functioning tumors of the ovary. *Clin Obstet Gynecol* 1974;17:189–228.

186. Boss JH, Scully RE, Wegner KH, Cohen RB. Structural variations in the adult ovary—clinical significance. *Obstet Gynecol* 1965;25:747–763.

187. Snowden JA, Harkin PJR, Thornton JG, Wells M. Morphometric assessment of ovarian stromal proliferation. A clinicopathological study. *Histopathology* 1989;14:369–379.

188. Young RH, Scully RE. Fibromatosis and massive edema of the ovary, possibly related entities: a report of 14 cases of fibromatosis and 11 cases of massive edema. *Int J Gynecol Pathol* 1984;3:153–178.

189. Clement PB, Young RH, Hanna W, Scully RE. Sclerosing peritonitis associated with luteinized thecomas of the ovary: a clinicopathological analysis of six cases. *Am J Surg Pathol* 1994;18:1–13.

190. Lacson AG, Alrabeeah A, Gillis DA, et al. Secondary massive ovarian edema with Meigs' syndrome. *Am J Clin Pathol* 1989;91:597–603.

191. Bilodeau B. Intravaginal prolapse of the fallopian tube following vaginal hysterectomy. *Am J Obstet Gynecol* 1982;143:970–971.

192. Wheelock JB, Schneider V, Goperlund DR. Prolapsed fallopian tube masquerading as adenocarcinoma of the vagina in a postmenopausal woman. *Gynecol Oncol* 1985;21:369–375.

193. Saffos RO, Rhatigan RM, Scully RE. Metaplastic papillary tumor of the fallopian tube—a distinctive lesion of pregnancy. *Am J Clin Pathol* 1980;74:232–236.

194. Bartnik J, Powell S, Moriber-Katz S, Amenta OS. Metaplastic papillary tumor of the fallopian tube. Case report, immunohistochemical features, and review of the literature. *Arch Pathol Lab Med* 1989;113:545–547.

195. Clement PB. Pathology of gamete and zygote transport: Cervical, endometrial, myometrial, and tubal factors in infertility. In: Kraus F, Damjanov I, eds. *Pathology of reproductive failure.* Baltimore: Williams and Wilkins, 1991;140–194.

196. Dougherty CM, Cotten NM. Proliferative epithelial lesions of the uterine tube. I. Adenomatous hyperplasia. *Obstet Gynecol* 1964;24:849–854.

197. Cheung ANY, Young RH, Scully RE. Pseudocarcinomatous hyperplasia of the fallopian tube associated with salpingitis. A report of 14 cases. *Am J Surg Pathol* 1994;18:1125–1130.

198. Cornog JL, Currie JL, Rubin A. Heat artifact simulating adenocarcinoma of fallopian tube. *JAMA* 1970;214:1118–1119.

199. McCaughey WT, Al-Jabi M. Differentiation of serosal hyperplasia and neoplasia in biopsies. *Pathol Annu* 1986;21 Pt 1:271–293.

200. Foyle A, Al-Jabi M, McCaughey WTE. Papillary peritoneal tumors in women. *Am J Surg Pathol* 1981;5:241–249.

201. Hansen RM, Caya JG, Clowry LJ Jr, Anderson T. Benign mesothelial proliferation with effusion. *Am J Med* 1984;77:887–892.

202. McCaughey WT, Kannerstein M, Churg J. Tumors and pseudotumors of the serous membranes. *Atlas of Tumor Pathology.* Armed Forces Institute of Pathology, series 2, fascicle 20, 1985.

203. Kerner H, Gaton E, Czernobilsky B. Unusual ovarian, tubal and pelvic mesothelial inclusions in patients with endometriosis. *Histopathology* 1981;5:277–282.

204. Clement PB, Young RH. Florid mesothelial hyperplasia associated with ovarian tumors: a potential source of error in tumor diagnosis and staging. *Int J Gynecol Pathol* 1993;12:51–58.

205. Rosai J, Dehner LP. Nodular mesothelial hyperplasia in hernia sacs. A benign reactive condition stimulating a neoplastic process. *Cancer* 1975;35:165–175.

206. Daya D, McCaughey WTE. Pathology of the peritoneum: a review of selected topics. *Semin Diagn Pathol* 1991;8:277–289.

207. Whitaker D, Shilkin KB. Diagnosis of pleural malignant mesothelioma in life—a practical approach. *J Pathol* 1984;143:147–175.

208. Carpenter HA, Lancaster JR, Lee RA. Multilocular cysts of the peritoneum. *Mayo Clin Proc* 1982;57:634–638.

209. Schneider V, Partridge JR, Gutierrez F, Hurt WG, Maizels MS, Demay RM. Benign cystic mesothelioma involving the female genital tract: report of four cases. *Am J Obstet Gynecol* 1983;145:355–359.

210. Katsube Y, Mukai K, Silverberg SG. Cystic mesothelioma of the peritoneum. A report of five cases and review of the literature. *Cancer* 1982;50:1615–1622.

211. Dumke K, Schnoy N, Specht G, Buse H. Comparative light and electron microscopic studies of cystic and papillary tumors of the peritoneum. *Virchows Arch A Pathol Anat* 1983;399:25–39.

212. Mennemeyer R, Smith M. Multicystic, peritoneal mesothelioma. A report with electron microscopy of a case mimicking intra-abdominal cystic hygroma (lymphangioma). *Cancer* 1979;44:692–698.

213. Miles JM, Hart WR, McMahon JT. Cystic mesothelioma of the peritoneum. Report of a case with multiple recurrences and review of the literature. *Cleve Clin Q* 1986;53:109–114.

214. Moor JH Jr, Crum CP, Chandler JG, Feldman PS. Benign cystic mesothelioma. *Cancer* 1980;45:2395–2399.

215. McFadden DE, Clement PB. Peritoneal inclusion cysts with mural mesothelial proliferation. A clinicopathological analysis of six cases. *Am J Surg Pathol* 1986;10:844–854.

216. Weiss SW, Tavassoli FA. Multicystic mesothelioma. An analysis of pathologic findings and biologic behavior in 37 cases. *Am J Surg Pathol* 1988;12:737–746.

217. Ross MJ, Welch WR, Scully RE. Multilocular peritoneal inclusion cysts (so-called cystic mesotheliomas). *Cancer* 1989;64:1336–1346.

218. Blumberg NA, Murray JF. Multicystic peritoneal mesothelioma. *S Afr Med J* 1981;59:85–86.

219. Sienkowski I, Russell AJ, Dilly SA, Djazaer B. Peritoneal cystic mesothelioma: an electron microscopic and immunohistochemical study of two male patients. *J Clin Pathol* 1986;39:440–445.

220. Kjellevold K, Nesland JM, Holm R, Johannessen JV. Multicystic peritoneal mesothelioma. *Pathol Res Pract* 1986;181:767–771.

221. Demopoulos RI, Kahn MA, Feiner HD. Epidemiology of cystic mesotheliomas. *Int J Gynecol Pathol* 1986;5:379–381.

222. Gussman D, Thickman D, Wheeler JE. Postoperative peritoneal cysts. *Obstet Gynecol* 1986;68:53S–55S.

223. Lees RF, Feldman PS, Brenbridge NAG, Anderson WA, Buschi AJ. Inflammatory cysts of the pelvic peritoneum. *AJR* 1978;131:633–636.

224. Daya D, McCaughey WTE. Well-differentiated papillary mesothelioma of the peritoneum. A clinicopathologic study of 22 cases. *Cancer* 1990;65:292–296.

225. DeStephano DB, Wesley JR, Heidelberger KP, Hutchison RJ, Blane CE, Coran AG. Primitive cystic hepatic neoplasm of infancy with mesothelial differentiation: report of a case. *Pediatr Pathol* 1985;4:291–302.

226. Clement PB. Pathology of endometriosis. *Pathol Annu* 1990;25(1):245–295.

227. Czernobilsky B, Morris WJ. A histologic study of ovarian endometriosis with emphasis on hyperplastic and atypical changes. *Obstet Gynecol* 1979;53:318–323.

228. Schuger L, Simon A, Okon E. Cytomegaly in benign ovarian cysts. *Arch Pathol Lab Med* 1986;110:928–929.

229. Rutgers JL, Scully RE. Ovarian mullerian mucinous papillary cystadenomas of borderline malignancy. A clinicopathological analysis. *Cancer* 1988;61:340–348.

230. Rutgers JL, Scully RE. Ovarian mixed-epithelial papillary cystadenomas of borderline malignancy of mullerian type. A clinicopathological analysis. *Cancer* 1988;61:546–554.

231. Clement PB, Young RH, Scully RE. Necrotic pseudoxanthomatous nodules of the ovary and peritoneum in endometriosis. *Am J Surg Pathol* 1988;12:390–397.

232. Carey M, Kirk ME. Necrotic pseudoxanthomatous nodules of the omentum and peritoneum: a peculiar reaction to endometriotic cyst contents. *Obstet Gynecol* 1993;82:650–652.

233. Seidman JD, Oberer S, Bitterman P, Aisner SC. Pathogenesis of pseudoxanthomatous salpingiosis. *Mod Pathol* 1993;6:53–55.

234. Herrera GA, Reimann BEF, Greenberg HL, Miles PA. Pigmentosis tubae, a new entity: light and electron microscopic study. *Obstet Gynecol* 1983;61:80S–83S.

235. Clement PB, Young RH, Scully RE. Stromal endometriosis of the uterine cervix. A variant of endometriosis that may simulate a sarcoma. *Am J Surg Pathol* 1990;14:449–455.

236. Hughesdon PE. The endometrial identity of benign stromatosis of the ovary and its relation to other forms of endometriosis. *J Pathol* 1976;119:201–209.

237. Clement PB, Granai CO, Young RH, Scully RE. Endometriosis with myxoid change: a case simulating pseudomyxoma peritonei. *Am J Surg Pathol* 1994;18:849–853.

238. Roth LM. Endometriosis with perineural involvement. *Am J Clin Pathol* 1973;59:807–809.

239. Abdel-Shahid RB, Beresford JM, Curry RH. Endometriosis of the ureter with vascular involvement. *Obstet Gynecol* 1974;43:113–117.

240. Zinsser KR, Wheeler JE. Endosalpingiosis in the omentum. A study of autopsy and surgical material. *Am J Surg Pathol* 1982;6:109–117.

241. Tutschka BG, Lauchlan SC. Endosalpingiosis. *Obstet Gynecol* 1980; 55:57S–60S.

242. Holmes MD, Levin HS, Ballard LA. Endosalpingiosis. *Cleve Clin Q* 1981;48:345–352.

243. Kern WH. Benign papillary structures with psammoma bodies in culdocentesis fluid. *Acta Cytol* 1969;13:178–180.

244. Sidaway MK, Silverberg SG. Endosalpingiosis in female peritoneal washings: A diagnostic pitfall. *Int J Gynecol Pathol* 1987;6:340–346.

245. Sneige M, Fernandez T, Copeland LJ, Katz RL. Mullerian inclusions in peritoneal washings. *Acta Cytol* 1986;30:271–276.

246. Hallman KB, Nahhas WA, Connolly PJ. Endosalpingiosis as a source of psammoma bodies in a Papanicolaou smear. A case report. *J Reprod Med* 1991;36:675–678.

247. Kern SB. Prevalence of psammoma bodies in Papanicolaou-stained cervicovaginal smears. *Acta Cytol* 1991;35:81–88.

248. Chen KTK. Benign glandular inclusions of the peritoneum and periaortic lymph nodes. *Diagn Gynecol Obstet* 1981;3:265–268.

249. Shen SC, Bansal M, Purrazzella R, Malviya V, Strauss L. Benign glandular inclusions in lymph nodes, endosalpingiosis, and salpingitis isthmica nodosa in a young girl with clear cell adenocarcinoma of the cervix. *Am J Surg Pathol* 1983;7:293–300.

250. Ehrmann RL, Federschneider JM, Knapp RC. Distinguishing lymph node metastases from benign glandular inclusions in low-grade ovarian carcinoma. *Am J Obstet Gynecol* 1980;136:737–746.

251. Karp LA, Czernobilsky B. Glandular inclusions in pelvic and abdominal para-aortic lymph nodes. *Am J Clin Pathol* 1969;52:212–218.

252. Kheir SM, Mann WJ, Wilkerson JA. Glandular inclusions in lymph nodes. The problem of extensive involvement and relationship to salpingitis. *Am J Surg Pathol* 1981;5:353–359.

253. Russell P, Laverty CR. Benign "mullerian" rests in pelvic lymph node. *Pathology* 1980;12:129–130.

254. Schnurr RC, Delgado G, Chun B. Benign glandular inclusions in para-aortic lymph nodes in women undergoing lymphadenectomies. *Am J Obstet Gynecol* 1978;130:813–816.

255. Schneider V, Walsh JW, Goplerud DR. Benign glandular inclusions in para-aortic lymph nodes: a cause for false positive lymphangiography. *Am J Obstet Gynecol* 1980;138:350–352.

256. Weir JH, Janovski NA. Paramesonephric lymph-node inclusions—a cause of obstructive uropathy. *Obstet Gynecol* 1963;21:363–367.

257. Kempson RL. Consultation case. *Am J Surg Pathol* 1978;2:321–325.

258. Cajigas A, Axiotis CA. Endometriosis of the vermiform appendix. *Int J Gynecol Pathol* 1990;9:291–295.

259. Bell DA, Scully RE. Serous borderline tumors of the peritoneum. *Am J Surg Pathol* 1990;14:230–239.

260. Biscotti CV, Hart WR. Peritoneal serous micropapillomatosis of low malignant potential (serous borderline tumors of the peritoneum). A clinicopathologic study of 17 cases. *Am J Surg Pathol* 1992;16:467–475.

261. Bell DA, Scully RE. Clinicopathological features of lymph node involvement with ovarian serous borderline tumors. *Mod Pathol* 1992; 5:61A.

262. Prade M, Spatz A, Bentley R, Duvillard P, Bognel C, Robboy SJ. Borderline and malignant serous tumor arising in pelvic lymph nodes: evidence of origin in benign glandular inclusions. *Int J Gynecol Pathol* 1995;14:87–91.

263. Lauchlan SC. The secondary mullerian system. *Obstet Gynecol Surv* 1972;27:133–146.

264. Ruffolo R, Suster S. Diffuse histiocytic proliferation mimicking mesothelial hyperplasia in endocervicosis of the female pelvic peritoneum. *Int J Surg Pathol* 1993;1:101–106.

265. Ferguson BR, Bennington JL, Haber SL. Histochemistry of mucosubstances and histology of mixed mullerian pelvic lymph node glandular inclusions. *Obstet Gynecol* 1969;33:617–625.

266. Clement PB, Young RH. Endocervicosis of the urinary bladder: a report of six cases of a benign mullerian lesion that may mimic adenocarcinoma. *Am J Surg Pathol* 1992;16:533–542.

267. Tavassoli FA, Norris HJ. Peritoneal leiomyomatosis (leiomyomatosis peritonealis disseminata): a clinicopathologic study of 20 cases with ultrastructural observations. *Int J Gynecol Pathol* 1982;1:59–74.

268. Walley VM. Leiomyomatosis peritonealis disseminata (letter). *Int J Gynecol Pathol* 1983;2:222–223.

269. Hsu YK, Rosenshein NB, Parmley TH, Woodruff JD, Elberfeld HT. Leiomyomatosis in pelvic lymph nodes. *Obstet Gynecol* 1981;57: 91S–93S.

270. Due W, Pickartz H. Immunohistochemical detection of estrogen and progesterone receptors in disseminated peritoneal leiomyomatosis. *Int J Gynecol Pathol* 1989;8:46–53.

271. Young RH, Harris NL, Scully RE. Lymphoma-like lesions of the lower female genital tract: a report of 16 cases. *Int J Gynecol Pathol* 1985;4:289–299.

272. Hachisuga T, Ookuma Y, Fukuda K, Iwasaka T, Sugimori H, Watanabe T. Detection of Epstein–Barr virus DNA from a lymphoma-like lesion of the uterine cervix. *Gynecol Oncol* 1992;46:69–73.

273. Harris NL, Scully RE. Malignant lymphoma and granulocytic sarcoma of the uterus and vagina. A clinicopathologic analysis of 27 cases. *Cancer* 1984;53:2530–2545.

274. Ferry JA, Harris NL, Scully RE. Uterine leiomyomas with lymphoid infiltration simulating lymphoma. A report of seven cases. *Int J Gynecol Pathol* 1989;8:263–270.

275. Hare MJ, Toone E, Taylor-Robinson D, et al. Follicular cervicitis—colposcopic appearances and association with *Chlamydia trachomatis*. *Br J Obstet Gynaecol* 1981;88:174–180.

276. Winkler B, Vrum CP. Chlamydia trachomatis infection of the female genital tract. Pathogenic and clinicopathologic correlations. *Pathol Annu* 1987;22(1):193–223.

277. Paavonen J, Vesterinen E, Meyer B, Saksela E. Colposcopic and histologic findings in cervical chlamydial infection. *Obstet Gynecol* 1982;59:712–714.

278. Winkler B, Reumann W, Mitao M, Gallo L, Richart RM, Crum CP. Chlamydial endometritis: a histological and immunohistochemical analysis. *Am J Surg Pathol* 1984;8:771–778.

279. Kiviat NB, Wolner-Hanssen P, Eschenbach DA, et al. Endometrial histopathology in patients with culture-proven upper genital tract infection and laparoscopically diagnosed acute salpingitis. *Am J Surg Pathol* 1990;14:167–175.

280. Ismail SM. Follicular myometritis. A previously undescribed component of pelvic inflammatory disease. *Histopathology* 1990;16:91–93.

281. Qizilbash AH. Chronic plasma cell cervicitis. A rare pitfall in gynecologic cytology. *Acta Cytol* 1974;18:198–200.

282. Doherty MG, Van Dinh T, Payne D, Tyring SK, Hannigan EV. Chronic plasma cell cervicitis simulating a cervical malignancy: a case report. *Obstet Gynecol* 1993;82:646–650.

283. Sirgi KE, Swanson PE, Gersell DJ. Extramedullary hematopoiesis in the endometrium. Report of four cases and review of the literature. *Am J Clin Pathol* 1994;101:643–646.

284. Ferry JA, Young RH. Malignant lymphoma, pseudolymphoma, and hematopoetic disorders of the female genital tract. *Pathol Annu* 1991; 26(1):227–263.

285. Ladefoged C, Lorentzen M. Xanthogranulomatous inflammation of the female genital tract. *Histopathology* 1988;13:541–551.

286. Russack V, Lammers RJ. Xanthogranulomatous endometritis: report of six cases and a proposed mechanism for development. *Arch Pathol Lab Med* 1990;114:929–932.

287. Shintaku M, Sasaki M, Baba Y. Ceroid-containing histiocytic granuloma of the endometrium. *Histopathology* 1991;18:169–172.

288. Buckley CH, Fox H. Histiocytic endometritis. *Histopathology* 1980; 4:105–110.

289. Strate SM, Taylor WE, Forney JP, Silva FG. Xanthogranulomatous pseudotumor of the vagina: Evidence of a local reponse to an unusual bacterium (mucoid Escherichia coli). *Am J Clin Pathol* 1983;79: 637–643.

290. Chen KTK, Hendricks EJ. Malakoplakia of the female genital tract. *Obstet Gynecol* 1985;65:84S–87S.

291. Kawai K, Fukuda K, Tsuchiyama H. Malacoplakia of the endometrium: an unusual case studied by electron microscopy and a review of the literature. *Acta Pathol Jpn* 1988;38:531–540.

292. Messim S, Heller DS, Dottino P, Deligdisch L, Gordon RE. Malakoplakia of the female genital tract causing urethral and ureteral obstruction. A case report. *J Reprod Med* 1991;36:691–694.

293. Fishman A, Ortega E, Girtanner RE, Kaplan AL. Malacoplakia of the vagina presenting as a pelvic mass. *Gynecol Oncol* 1993;49:380–382.

294. Clarke TJ, Simpson RHW. Necrotizing granulomas of peritoneum following diathermy ablation of endometriosis. *Histopathology* 1990;16: 400–402.

295. Herbold DR, Frable WJ, Kraus FT. Isolated noninfectious granuloma of the ovary. *Int J Gynecol Pathol* 1984;2:380–391.

296. Roberts JT, Roberts GT, Maudsley RF. Indolent granulomatous necrosis in patients with previous tubal diathermy. *Am J Obstet Gynecol* 1977;129:112–113.

297. Ashworth MT, Moss CI, Kenyon WE. Granulomatous endometritis following hysteroscopic resection of the endometrium. *Histopathology* 1991;18:185–187.

298. Thurrell W, Reid P, Kennedy A, Smith JHF. Necrotizing granulomas of the peritoneum (letter). *Histopathology* 1991;18:190.

299. Clark IW. Necrotizing granulomatous inflammation of the uterine body following diathermy ablation of the endometrium. *Pathology* 1992;24:32–33.

300. Ferryman SR. Necrotising granulomatous endometritis following endometrial ablation therapy. *Br J Obstet Gynaecol* 1992;99:928–930.

301. Christie AJ, Krieger HA. Indolent necrotizing granuloma of the uterine cervix, possibly related to chlamydial infection. *Am J Obstet Gynecol* 1980;136:958–960.

302. Evans CS, Klein HZ, Goldman RL, Kohout ND. Necrobiotic granulomas of the uterine cervix. A probable postoperative reaction. *Am J Surg Pathol* 1984;8:841–844.

303. Kuo T, Hsueh S. Mucicarminophilic histiocytosis. A polyvinyl-pyrrolidone (PVP) storage disease simulating signet-ring cell carcinoma. *Am J Surg Pathol* 1984;8:419–428.

304. Chen KTK, Kostich ND, Rosai J. Peritoneal foreign body granulomas to keratin in uterine adenoacanthoma. *Arch Pathol Lab Med* 1978;102:174–177.

305. Kim K, Scully RE. Peritoneal keratin granulomas with carcinomas of endometrium and ovary and atypical polypoid adenomyoma of endometrium. *Am J Surg Pathol* 1990;14:925–932.

306. Clement PB, Young RH, Scully RE. The peritoneum. In: Sternberg SS, ed. *Diagnostic surgical pathology*. 2nd ed. New York: Raven Press, 1994;2299–2328.

307. Stuart GCE, Smith JP. Ruptured benign cystic teratomas mimicking gynecologic malignancy. *Gynecol Oncol* 1983;16:139–143.

308. Proppe KH, Scully RE, Rosai J. Postoperative spindle-cell nodules of genitourinary tract resembling sarcomas. *Am J Surg Pathol* 1984;8:101–108.

309. Kay S, Schneider V. Reactive spindle cell nodule of the endocervix simulating uterine sarcoma. *Int J Gynecol Pathol* 1985;4:255–257.

310. Clement PB. Postoperative spindle-cell nodule of the endometrium. *Arch Pathol Lab Med* 1988;112:566–568.

311. Wick MR, Young RH, Mills SE, Manivel JC. Immunohistochemical features of postoperative spindle cell nodules and inflammatory pseudotumors of the genitourinary tract (abstract). *Lab Invest* 1988;58:103A.

312. Pettinato G, Manivel C, De Rosa N, Dehner LP. Inflammatory myofibroblastic tumor (plasma cell granuloma). Clinicopathologic study of 20 cases with immunohistochemical and ultrastructural observations. *Am J Clin Pathol* 1990;94:538–546.

313. Wu JP, Yunis EJ, Fetterman G, Jaeschke WF, Gilbert EG. Inflammatory pseudotumor of the abdomen: plasma cell granulomas. *J Clin Pathol* 1973;26:943–948.

314. Gilks CB, Taylor GP, Clement PB. Inflammatory pseudotumor of the uterus. *Int J Gynecol Pathol* 1987;6:275–286.

315. Allen PW. Nodular fasciitis. *Pathology* 1972;4:9–26.

316. LiVolsi VA, Brooks JJ. Nodular fasciitis of the vulva: a report of two cases. *Obstet Gynecol* 1987;69:513–516.

317. Snover DC, Phillips G, Dehner LP. Reactive fibrohistiocytic proliferation simulating fibrous histiocytoma. *Am J Clin Pathol* 1981;76:232–235.

318. Weiss SW, Enzinger FM, Johnson FB. Silica reaction simulating fibrous histiocytoma. *Cancer* 1978;42:2738–2743.

319. Weibel MA, Majno G. Peritoneal adhesions and their relation to abdominal surgery. *Am J Surg* 1973;126:345–353.

320. Dehn TCB, Lucas MG, Wood RFM. Idiopathic sclerosing peritonitis. *Postgrad Med J* 1985;61:841–842.

321. Foo KT, Ng KC, Rauff A, Foong WC, Sinniah R. Unusual small intestinal obstruction in adolescent girls: the abdominal cocoon. *Br J Surg* 1978;65:427–430.

322. Marshall AJ, Baddeley H, Barritt DW, et al. Practolol peritonitis. A study of 16 cases and a survey of small bowel function in patients taking beta adrenergic blockers. *Q J Med* 1977;46:135–149.

323. Bradley JA, McWhinnie DL, Hamilton DNH. Sclerosing obstructive peritonitis after continuous ambulatory peritoneal dialysis. *Lancet* 1983;2:113–114.

324. Wallace S, Sabto J, Pedersen J, Gurr FW. Peritoneal sclerosis in CAPD. *Pathology* 1992;24:4 (abstr).

325. Cambria RP, Shamberger RC. Small bowel obstruction caused by the abdominal cocoon syndrome: possible association with the LeVeen shunt. *Surgery* 1984;95:501–503.

325a. Bolen JW, Hammar SP, McNutt MA. Reactive and neoplastic serosal tissue. A light microscopic, ultrastructural and immunohistochemical study. *Am J Surg Pathol* 1986;10:34–47.

326. Abulafia O, DuBeshter B, Dawson AE, Sherer DM. Presence of cytomegalovirus inclusion bodies in a recurrent ulcerative vaginal lesion. *Am J Obstet Gynecol* 1993;169:1179–1180.

327. Brown S, Senekjian EK, Montag AG. Cytomegalovirus infection of the uterine cervix in a patient with acquired immunodeficiency syndrome. *Obstet Gynecol* 1988;71:489–491.

328. McCracken AW, D'Agostino AN, Brucks AB, Kingsley WB. Acquired cytomegalovirus infection presenting as viral endometritis. *Am J Clin Pathol* 1974;61:556–560.

329. Dehner LP, Askin FB. Cytomegalovirus endometritis. Report of a case associated with spontaneous abortion. *Obstet Gynecol* 1975;45:211–214.

330. Wenckebach GFC, Curry B. Cytomegalovirus infection of the female genital tract. Histologic findings in three cases and review of the literature. *Arch Pathol Lab Med* 1976;100:609–612.

331. Frank TS, Himebaugh KS, Wilson MD. Granulomatous endometritis associated with histologically occult cytomegalovirus in a healthy patient. *Am J Surg Pathol* 1992;16:716–720.

332. Evans DJ, Lampert IA. Ovarian involvement by cytomegalovirus (letter). *Hum Pathol* 1978;9:122.

333. Subietas A, Deppisch LM, Astarloa J. Cytomegalovirus oophoritis: ovarian cortical necrosis. *Hum Pathol* 1977;8:285–292.

334. Williams DJ, Connor P, Ironside JW. Pre-menopausal cytomegalovirus oophoritis. *Histopathology* 1990;16:405–407.

335. Schneider V, Behm FG, Mumaw VR. Ascending herpetic endometritis. *Obstet Gynecol* 1982;59:259–262.

336. Duncan DA, Varner RE, Mazur MT. Uterine herpes virus infection with multifocal necrotizing endometritis. *Hum Pathol* 1989;20:1021–1024.

337. Nogales-Ortiz F, Taracon I, Nogales FF. The pathology of female genital tract tuberculosis. *Obstet Gynecol* 1979;53:422–428.

338. Shobin D, Sall S, Pellman C. Genitourinary tuberculosis simulating cervical carcinoma. *J Reprod Med* 1976;17:305–308.

339. Vuong PN, Houissa-Vuong S, Bleuse B, Schoonaert M. Pseudotumoral tuberculosis of the uterine cervix. Cytologic presentation. *Acta Cytol* 1989;33:305–308.

340. Freedman LJ, Coleman B, Blasco L. Tuberculous peritonitis and endometritis mimicking a "frozen pelvis." *Am J Obstet Gynecol* 1979;134:719–721.

341. Hoffman MS, Roberts WS, Soloman P, Gunasekarin S, Cavanagh D. Advanced actinomycotic pelvic inflammatory disease simulating gynecologic malignancy. A report of two cases. *J Reprod Med* 1991;36:543–545.

342. Snowman BA, Malviya VK, Brown W, Malone JM Jr, Deppe G. Actinomyosis mimicking pelvic malignancy. *Int J Gynecol Obstet* 1989;30:283–286.

343. Hoosen AA, Draper G, Moodley J, Cooper K. Granuloma inguinale of the cervix: a carcinoma look-alike. *Genitourin Med* 1990;66:380–382.

344. Bhargava S, Tandon PL, Sant MS, Gujral MS. Amoebic cervicitis masquerading as carcinoma cervix (sic). *Ind J Pathol Microbiol* 1986;29:382–385.

345. Wallace TM, Hart WR. Acute chlamydial salpingitis with ascites and adnexal mass simulating a malignant neoplasm. *Int J Gynecol Pathol* 1991;10:394–401.

346. Kraus FT. Irradiation changes in the uterus. In: Norris HJ, Hertig AT, eds. *The uterus*. Baltimore: Williams and Wilkins, 1973;457–488.

347. Fajardo LF. *Pathology of radiation injury*. Chicago: Year Book, 1982;110–128.

348. Silverberg SG, DeGiorgi LS. Histopathologic analysis of preoperative radiation therapy in endometrial carcinoma. *Am J Obstet Gynecol* 1974;119:698–704.

349. Winkler B, Norris HJ, Fenoglio CM. The female genital tract. In: Riddell RH, ed. *Pathology of drug-induced and toxic diseases*. New York: Churchill Livingstone, 1982;297–324.

350. Patel DS, Bhagavan BS. Blue nevus of the uterine cervix. *Hum Pathol* 1985;16:79–86.

351. Casadei GP, Grigolato P, Cabibbo E. Blue nevus of the endocervix. A study of five cases. *Tumori* 1987;73:75–79.

352. Uehara T, Isumo T, Kishi K, Takayama S, Kasuga T. Stromal melanocytic foci ("blue nevus") in step sections of the uterine cervix. *Acta Pathol Jpn* 1991;41:751–756.

353. Toban H, Murphy AI. Benign blue nevus of the vagina. *Cancer* 1977; 40:3174–3176.

354. Rodriguez HA, Ackerman LV. Cellular blue nevus. Clinicopathologic study of forty-five cases. *Cancer* 1968;21:393–405.

355. Sison-Torre EQ, Ackerman AB. Melanosis of the vulva. A clinical simulator of malignant melanoma. *Am J Dermatopathol* 1985; 7:51–60 (suppl).

356. Schneider V, Zimberg S, Kay S. The pigmented portio: Benign lentigo of the uterine cervix. *Diagn Gynecol Obstet* 1981;3:269–272.

357. Deppisch LM. Cervical melanosis. *Obstet Gynecol* 1983;62:525–526.

358. Barter J, Mazur M, Holloway RW, Hatch KD. Melanosis of the cervix. *Gynecol Oncol* 1988;29:101–104.

359. Dundore W, Lamas C. Benign nevus (ephelis) of the uterine cervix. *Am J Obstet Gynecol* 1985;152:881–882.

360. Hytiroglou P, Domingo J. Development of melanosis of uterine cervix after cryotherapy for epithelial dysplasia. A case report and brief review of the literature on pigmented lesions of the cervix. *Am J Clin Pathol* 1990;93:802–805.

361. Nigogosyan G, de la Pava S, Pickren JW. Melanoblasts in vaginal mucosa. *Cancer* 1964;17:912–913.

362. Norris HJ, Taylor HB. Melanomas of the vagina. *Am J Clin Pathol* 1966;46:420–426.

363. Tsukada Y. Benign melanosis of the vagina and cervix. *Am J Obstet Gynecol* 1976;124:211–212.

364. Afonso JF, Martin GM, Nisco FS, de Alvarez RR. Melanogenic ovarian tumors. *Am J Obstet Gynecol* 1962;84:667–676.

365. Fukushima M, Sharpe L, Okagaki T. Peritoneal melanosis secondary to a benign dermoid cyst of the ovary: a case report with ultrastructural study. *Int J Gynecol Pathol* 1984;2:403–409.

366. Lee D, Pontifex AH. Melanosis peritonei. *Am J Obstet Gynecol* 1975; 122:526–527.

367. Sahin AA, Ro JY, Chen J, Ayala AG. Spindle cell nodule and peptic ulcer arising in a fully developed gastric wall in a mature cystic teratoma. *Arch Pathol Lab Med* 1990;114:529–531.

368. Al-Nafussi AI, Hughes D, Rebello G. Ceroid granuloma of the uterine cervix. *Histopathology* 1992;21:282–284.

369. Siboni A, Horn T, Christensen N. Lipofuscinosis of the human uterus. *Arch Pathol Lab Med* 1987;111:771–772.

370. White J, Chart Y-F. Lipofuscinosis peritonei associated with pregancy-related ectopic decidua. *Histopathology* 1994;25:83–85.

371. Russell P, Bannatyne P. *Surgical pathology of the ovaries*. Edinburgh: Churchill Livingstone, 1989;168–169.

372. Valicenti JF Jr, Priester SK. Psammoma bodies of benign endometrial origin in cervicovaginal cytology. *Acta Cytol* 1977;21:550–552.

373. Herbold DR, Magrane DM. Calcifications of the benign endometrium. *Arch Pathol Lab Med* 1986;110:666–669.

374. Clement PB, Cooney TP. Idiopathic multifocal calcification of the ovarian stroma. *Arch Pathol Lab Med* 1992;116:204–205.

375. Clement PB. Non-neoplastic lesions of the ovary. In: Kurman RJ, ed. *Blaustein's pathology of the female genital tract*. 4th ed. New York: Springer-Verlag, 1994;597–645.

# ADDENDUM REFERENCES

## Metaplastic Proliferations of the Uterine Cervix

Al-Saleh W, Delvenne P, Greimers R, Fridman V, Doyen J, Boniver J. Assessment of Ki-67 antigen immunostaining in squamous intraepithelial lesions of the uterine cervix: correlation with the histologic grade and human papillomavirus type. *Am J Clin Pathol* 1995;104:154–160.

Brosens JJ, de Souza NM, Barker FG. Uterine junctional zone: function and disease. *Lancet* 1995;346:558–560.

Jonasson JG, Wang HH, Antonioli DA, Ducatman BS. Tubal metaplasia of the uterine cervix: a prevalence study in patients with gynecologic pathologic findings. *Int J Gynecol Pathol* 1992;11:89–95.

Malecha MJ, Miettinen M. Patters of keratin subsets in normal and abnormal uterine cervical tissues: an immunohistochemical study. *Int J Gynecol Pathol* 1992;11:24–29.

Oliva E, Clement PB, Young RH. Tubal and tubo-endometrioid metaplasia of the uterine cervix: unemphasized features that may cause problems in differential diagnosis. A report of 25 cases. *Am J Clin Pathol* 1995;103: 618–623.

Smedts F, Ramaekers FCS, Troyanovsky S, Pruszczynski M, Robben H, Lane B, Leigh I, Plantema F, Vooijs P. Basal cell keratins in cervical reserve cells and a comparison to their expression in cervical intraepithelial neoplasia. *Am J Pathol* 1992;140:601–612.

Young RH, Clement PB. Malignant lesions of the female genital tract and peritoneum that may be underdiagnosed. *Semin Diagn Pathol* 1995;12: 14–29.

## Hyperplastic Conditions of the Uterine Cervix

Greeley C, Schroeder S, Silverberg SG. Microglandular hyperplasia of the cervix: a true "pill" lesion? *Int J Gynecol Pathol* 1995;14:50–54.

Jones MA, Andrews J, Tarraza HM. Mesonephric remnant hyperplasia of the cervix: a clinicopathologic analysis of 14 cases. *Gynecol Oncol* 1993; 49:41–47.

Jones MA, Young RH. Endocervical type A (noncystic) tunnel clusters with cytologic atypia: a report of 14 cases. *Am J Surg Pathol* 1996;20: 1312–1318.

Liao SY, Manetta A. Benign and malignant pathology of the cervix, including screening. *Curr Opin Obstet Gynecol* 1993;5:497–503.

Seidman JD, Tavassoli FA. Mesonephric hyperplasia of the uterine cervix: a clinicopathologic study of 51 cases. *Int J Gynecol Pathol* 1995;14: 293–299.

Valente PT, Schantz HD, Schultz M. Cytologic atypia associated with microglandular hyperplasia. *Diagn Cytopathol* 1994;10:326–331.

## Metaplastic Conditions of the Endometrium

Fujita M, Shroyer KR, Markham NE, Inoue M, Iwamoto S, Hyo S, Enomoto T. Association of human papillomavirus with malignant and premalignant lesions of the uterine endometrium. *Hum Pathol* 1995;26:650–658.

Jacques SM, Qureshi F, Ramirez NC, Lawrence WD. Unusual endometrial stromal cell changes mimicking metastatic carcinoma. *Pathol Res Pract* 1996;192:33–36.

Mai KT, Yazdi HM, Boone SA. "Minimal deviation" endometrioid carcinoma with oncocytic change of the endometrium. *Arch Pathol Lab Med* 1995;119:751–754.

Miranda MC, Mazur MT. Endometrial squamous metaplasia: an unusual response to progestin therapy of hyperplasia. *Arch Pathol Lab Med* 1995; 119:458–460.

Motoyama T, Tanikawa T, Watanabe H. Mixed gonadal dysgenesis: endogenous hormonal effects in the endometrium and histogenesis of germinoma. *Acta Pathol Jpn* 1993;43:423–427.

Sheth S, Hamper UM, Kurman RJ. Thickened endometrium in the postmenopausal woman: sonographic-pathologic correlation. *Radiology* 1993;187:135–139.

## Endometriosis and Adenomyosis

Donnez J, Nisolle M, Smoes P, Gillet N, Beguin S, Casanas-Roux F. Peritoneal endometriosis and "endometrioid" nodules of the rectovaginal septum are two different entities. *Fertility Sterility* 1996;66:362–368.

Goldblum JR, Clement PB, Hart WR. Adenomyosis with sparse glands: a potential mimic of low-grade endometrial stromal sarcoma. *Am J Clin Pathol* 1995;103:218–223.

Nasu K, Hayata T, Takai N, Kawano Y, Sugano T, Matsui N, Miyakawa I. Immunohistochemical study of c-erbB-2 protein expression in endometriosis. *Hum Reprod* 1995;10:935–937.

Pandis N, Karaiskos C, Bardi G, Sfikas K, Tserkezoglou A, Fotiou S, Heim S. Chromosome analysis of uterine adenomyosis: detection of the leiomyoma-associated del(7q) in three cases. *Cancer Genet Cytogenet* 1995;80:118–120.

Taskin M, Lallas TA, Shevchuk M, Barber HR. p53 expression in adenomyosis in endometrial carcinoma patients. *Gynecol Oncol* 1996;62: 241–246.

## Arias-Stella Phenomenon

Huettner PC, Gersell DJ. Arias-Stella reaction in non-pregnant women: a clinicopathologic study of nine cases. *Int J Gynecol Pathol* 1994;13: 241–247.

McCormick CJ, Menal-Williams RA. Tripolar mitotic figures occurring in an Arias-Stella reaction within an endocervical polyp. *Histopathology* 1995;39:905–908.

Mulvany NJ, Khan A, Ostor A. Arias-Stella reaction associated with cervical pregnancy: report of a case with a cytologic presentation. *Acta Cytol* 1994;38:218–222.

Rhatigan RM. Endocervical gland atypia secondary to Arias-Stella change. *Arch Pathol Lab Med* 1992;116:943–946.

### *Ectopic Decidual Tissue*

Bashir RM, Montgomery EA, Gupta PK, Nauta RM, Crockett SA, Collea JV, Al-Kawas FH. Massive gastrointestinal hemorrhage during pregnancy caused by ectopic decidua of the terminal ileum and colon. *Am J Gastroenterol* 1995;90:1325–1327.

Buttner A, Bassler R, Theele C. Pregnancy-associated ectopic decidua (deciduosis) of the greater omentum: an analysis of 60 biopsies with cases of fibrosing deciduosis and leiomyomatosis peritonealis disseminata. *Pathol Res Pract* 1993;189:352–359.

Clement PB. Tumor-like lesions of the ovary associated with pregnancy. *Int J Gynecol Pathol* 1993;12:108–115.

Massi D, Susini T, Paglierani M, Salvadori A, Giannini A. Pregnancy-associated ectopic decidua. *Acta Obstet Gynecol Scand* 1995;74:568–571.

White J, Chan YF. Lipofuscinosis peritonei associated with pregnancy-related ectopic decidua. *Histopathology* 1994;25:83–85.

### *Placental Site Nodules and Plaques*

Berkowitz RS, Goldstein DP. Gestational trophoblastic disease. *Cancer* 1995;76(Suppl 10):2079–2085.

Buettner R, Schleicher P, Schleicher B, Ruschoff J, Hofstadter F. Benign placental trophoblast nodule: case report with overview of proliferative diseases of the intermediate stage trophoblast. *Geburtsh Fruenheilk* 1996;56:257–261.

Huettner PC, Gersell DJ. Placental site nodule: a clinicopathologic study of 38 cases. *Int J Gynecol Pathol* 1994;13:191–198.

Motoyama T, Ohta T, Ajioka Y, Watanabe H. Neoplastic and non-neoplastic intermediate trophoblasts: an immunohistochemical and ultrastructural study. *Pathol Int* 1994;44:57–65.

### *Pathology of Ectopic Pregnancy*

Kutluay L, Vicdan K, Turan C, Batioglu S, Oguz S, Gokmen O. Tubal histopathology in ectopic pregnancies. *Eur J Obstet Gynecol Reprod Biol* 1994;57:91–94.

Kecuru F, Taurelle R, Bernard JP, Vilde F. Recurrent tubal pregnancy after an intratubal injection of methotrexate: analysis of a case report with a histological tubal study. *J Gynecol Obstet Biol Reprod* 1995;24:482–484.

### *Luteoma of Pregnancy, Luteinized Follicle Cyst, and Hyperreactio Luteinalis*

Chico A, Garcia JL, Matias-Guiu X, Webb SM, Rodriguez J, Prat J, Calaf J. A gonadotrophin-dependent stromal luteoma: a rare cause of postmenopausal virilization. *Clin Endocrinol* 1995;43:645–649.

Clement PB. Tumor-like lesions of the ovary associated with pregnancy. *Int J Gynecol Pathol* 1993;12:108–115.

Costa MJ, Morris R, Sasano H. Sex steroid biosynthesis enzymes in ovarian sex cord stromal tumors. *Int J Gynecol Pathol* 1993;12:108–115.

Joshi R, Dunaif A. Ovarian disorders of pregnancy. *Endocrinol Metab Clin N Amer* 1995;24:153–169.

Kainz C, Joura E. Hyperreactio luteinalis in pregnancy. *Geburtsh Frauenheilk* 1994;54:59–61.

Pezzica E, Buzzi A, Sonzogni A, Crescini C, Ruggeri E. Large solitary luteinizing follicular cysts in the puerperium. *Min Ginecol* 1992;44:201–204.

Schnorr JA Jr, Miller H, Davis JR, Hatch K, Seeds J. Hyperreactio luteinalis associated with pregnancy: a case report and review of the literature. *Am J Perinatol* 1996;13:95–97.

Seidman JD, Abbondanzo SL, Bratthauer GL. Lipid cell (steroid cell) tumor of the ovary: immunophenotype with analysis of potential pitfall due to endogenous biotin-like activity. *Int J Gynecol Pathol* 1995;14:331–338.

Thomas S, Krishnaswami H, Seshadri L. Large solitary luteinized follicle cyst of pregnancy and puerperium. *Acta Obstet Gynecol Scand* 1993;72:678–679.

### *Nonneoplastic Ovarian Stromal Cell Proliferations*

Agorastos T, Argyriadis N, Fraggidis G, Vakiani A, Zournatzi V, Bontis J. Postmenopausal virilization due to ovarian hyperthecosis. *Arch Gynecol Obstet* 1995;256:209–211.

Glaser D, Mast H. Postmenopausal virilization in thecosis of the ovaries. *Geburtsh Frauenheilk* 1992;52:65–67.

Honore LH, Chari R, Mueller HD, Cumming DC, Scott JZ. Postmenopausal hyperandrogenism of ovarian origin: a clinicopathologic study of four cases. *Gynecol Obstet Invest* 1992;34:52–56.

Mantzoros CS, Lawrence WD, Levy J. Insulin resistance in a patient with ovarian stromal hyperthecosis and the hyperandrogenism, insulin resistance, and acanthosis nigricans syndrome. Report of a case with a possible endogenous ovarian factor. *J Reprod Med* 1995;40:491–494.

### *Massive Ovarian Edema*

Eden JA. Massive ovarian edema. *Br J Obstet Gynaecol* 1994;101:456–458.

Heiss KF, Zwiren GT, Winn K. Massive ovarian edema in the pediatric patient: a rare solid tumor. *J Pediatr Surg* 1994;29:1392–1394.

Pai MR, Baliga P, Naik R. Massive edema of the ovary. *J Indian Med Assoc* 1995;93:361.

Siller BS, Gelder MS, Alvarez RD, Partridge EE. Massive edema of the ovary associated with androgenic manifestations. *South Med J* 1995;88:1153–1155.

Van den Brule F, Bourque J, Gaspard UJ, Hustin JF. Massive ovarian edema with androgen secretion: a pathologic and endocrine study with review of the literature. *Hormone Res* 1994;41:209–214.

### *Fallopian Tube Prolapse and Metaplasias*

Allen C, Johnson S. Apocrine metaplasia: a new type of mullerian metaplasia. *J Clin Pathol* 1993;46:569.

Gupta SP. Experience in 4500 cases of laparascopic sterilization. *Int Surg* 1993;78:76–78.

Hellen EA, Coghill SB, Clark JV. Prolapsed fallopian tube afer abdominal hysterectomy: a report of the cytological findings. *Cytopathology* 1993;4:181–185.

Minguillon C, Friedmann W, Vogel M, Wessel J, Lichtenegger W. Mucinous metaplasia of fallopian tube mucous membranes as a cause of pseudomyxoma peritonei. *Zentralbl Pathol* 1992;138:364–365.

Seidman JD. Mucinous lesions of the fallopian tube: a report of seven cases. *Am J Surg Pathol* 1994;18:1205–1212.

### *Salpingitis Isthmica Nodosa and Pseudocarcinomatous Hyperplasia*

Cheung AN, Young RH, Scully RE. Pseudocarcinomatous hyperplasia of the fallopian tube associated with salpingitis: a report of 14 cases. *Am J Surg Pathol* 1994;18:1125–1130.

Sathyamoorthy P. Salpingitis isthmica nodosa. *Singapore Med J* 1994;35:65–66.

Wiedemann R, Sterzik K, Gombisch V, Stuckensen J, Montag M. Beyond recanalizing proximal tube occlusion: the argument for further diagnosis and classification. *Hum Reprod* 1996;11:986–991.

### *Peritoneal Inclusion Cysts ("Multicystic Mesothelioma")*

Moran RE, Older RA, DeAngelis GA, Baghdady BH, Chrisman HB, Ciambotti JM. Peritoneal inclusion cyst in a patient with a history of prior pelvic surgery. *Am J Roentgenol* 1996;167:247–250.

Yaegashi N, Yajima A. Multilocular peritoneal inclusion cysts (benign cystic mesothelioma): a case report. *J Obstet Gynaecol Res* 1996;22:129–132.

*Pathology of Pseudoneoplastic Lesions,*
edited by M. R. Wick, P. A. Humphrey, and J. H. Ritter.
Lippincott-Raven Publishers, Philadelphia © 1997.

CHAPTER 11

# Pseudoneoplastic Pathologic Conditions of the Breast and Endocrine System

Peter A. Humphrey and Mark R. Wick

P.A. Humphrey: Lauren V. Ackerman Laboratory of Surgical Pathology, Department of Pathology, Barnes-Jewish Hospital at Washington University Medical Center, St. Louis, Missouri 63110.
M.R. Wick: Department of Pathology, Washington University School of Medicine, St. Louis, Missouri 63110.

# BREAST

There are a multitude of lesions in the breast that may be confused with mammary neoplasms. The focus of the first portion of this chapter, as in the entire book, is on those non-neoplastic entities that may be mistaken, at the gross and histopathologic levels of examination, for true neoplasms of the breast. Not discussed are purely clinical and radiologic mimics of the latter lesions. Also beyond the scope of this text is a discussion of usual or atypical epithelial hyperplasias of the breast, which constitute important conditions in the differential diagnosis of carcinomas of the breast and may be directly related to those tumors in some instances.

## Hamartoma

Hamartomas of the breast are more likely to be mistaken for a neoplasm by clinicians and radiologists than by pathologists. Indeed, pathologists may not even recognize hamartomas as representing abnormal elements in biopsies because they contain all of the constituents of normal mammary tissue. Clinically, these malformations present in women in the fifth decade are soft, sharply delineated masses that may cause significant asymmetry of the breasts (1). By mammography, they are rounded to oval and well circumscribed, with sharp demarcation from surrounding breast tissue (Fig. 1) (2,3). Accurate diagnosis often results only from efforts at combining the clinical, radiologic, and pathologic information (4–6).

At the macroscopic level, hamartomas merit consideration as pseudoneoplasms because these lesions may be confused with fibroadenomas. Most excised masses measure about 2–4 cm (7,8) but range from 1 to 17 cm, with the largest example weighing 1.4 kg (9). Typically, hamartomas are grossly well circumscribed and firm, with gray and glistening cut surfaces (9). Those examples with a prominent adipose tissue component will be softer and yellow–white such that the appearance may resemble that of normal breast tissue (8). In the presence of large amounts of fat, a gross diagnosis of lipoma might even be contemplated (3). Hamartomas may be distinguished from fibroadenomas at the macroscopic level by the lack of bulging lobular nodules (9).

Microscopically, hamartomas exhibit a spectrum of architectural patterns (8,10–14). If only a small portion of the mass is sampled by needle biopsy or incisional biopsy, and/or if the clinical and radiologic diagnoses are not provided, the sampled tissue may be difficult to recognize as histopathologically abnormal. In other words, normal breast tissue does enter into the differential diagnosis. The characteristic microscopic features of mammary hamartoma include a high density of lobular units (Fig. 2), with sparse stroma that usually (but not always) contains regions of adipose tissue (7,8). Fibrocystic alterations, including apocrine metaplasia, duct ectasia, and sclerosing adenosis, may be observed within hamartomas of the breast as well (4).

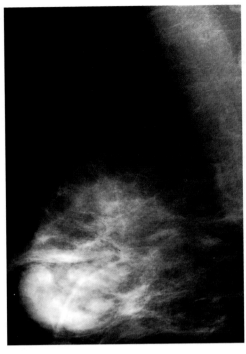

**FIG. 1.** Hamartoma. Mammographic oblique view of the right breast demonstrates a heterogeneous mass in the subareolar region. The presence of mixed fatty and glandular elements is characteristic of this lesion mammographically. (Courtesy of Dr. Fidelma Flanagan.)

Neoplastic entities in differential diagnosis include fibroadenoma, hemangioma, leiomyoma, and lipoma. Fibroadenoma is the main tumor to exclude and differs from hamartomas in the predominance of stroma over the epithelial units, a paucity of fat, and a nodular growth pattern, with attendant circumferential whorls of fibrous stroma about epithelial units and slit-like compression of epithelial spaces (13). Angioma, hemangioma, pseudoangiomatous hyperpla-

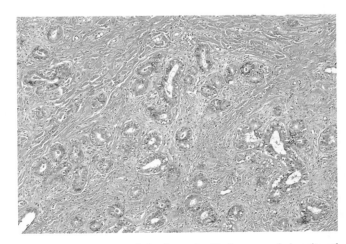

**FIG. 2.** Hamartoma of the breast with increased density of lobules.

sia, or even low-grade angiosarcoma might also be considered due to the vascular prominence in some hamartomas (13). The diagnosis of leiomyoma is entertained when a needle biopsy samples the smooth muscle stroma of a so-called muscular hamartoma (15,16). Those hamartomas with an abundance of adipose tissue, which have also been termed adenolipoma, may prompt a hasty diagnosis of lipoma, but recognition of the presence of epithelium in hamartomas of this type will resolve any diagnostic confusion. Finally, it is unsettled as to whether masses that resemble hamartomas and harbor islands of cartilage should be classified as pseudoneoplasms or neoplasms. These lesions have been previously viewed as an uncommon variant of hamartoma (11), a benign chondrolipomatous tumor (17), a benign mesenchymoma (18), a choristoma (19), and a type of myofibroblastoma.

## Lactational Change and Adenoma

Pregnancy and lactation induce profound alterations in the morphologic appearance of breast tissue (20,21). When lactational differentiation entails lobular enlargement and formation of new lobular units, the term "adenosis of pregnancy" has been used (Fig. 3). The normal physiologic characteristics of lactational change include diminution of intralobular stroma, cytoplasmic vacuolization (secondary to lipid accumulation) (Fig. 4), luminal distension, and an apical distribution of nuclei, resulting in a hobnail likeness. Lactational-like or secretory changes may also be observed in the breast tissue of women who are not pregnant or lactating (21–23) and may be noted in postmenopausal women (22). These histologic changes are correlated with the use of hormonal, antipsychotic, or antihypertensive medications. Such findings are typically incidental and focal, with no macroscopic alterations (22). Two distinct changes have been described (22). The first, termed lactational effect, refers to a predominance of secretory changes with abundant

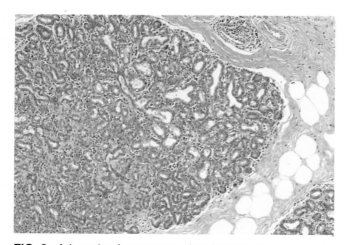

**FIG. 3.** Adenosis of pregnancy showing new and expanded lobular units.

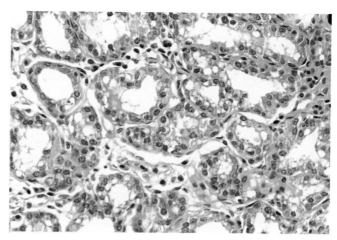

**FIG. 4.** High-power view of lactational change revealing cytoplasmic vacuolization.

cytoplasmic vacuolization and intraluminal secretions. The second major histologic abnormality is termed "clear cell change"; here the abundant lobular cell cytoplasm is clear, but not foamy or vacuolated. The nuclei in these foci are small and round. The differential diagnosis for lactational effect does not usually include a neoplastic process because it so closely resembles true lactational change (22).

However, the differential diagnosis for clear cell change does include lobular neoplasia due to the expansion of lobules by a monomorphous population of cells (22). Cytologically, the cells of atypical lobular hyperplasia and lobular carcinoma *in situ* are quite different from those of clear cell change, in having larger nuclei and a minimal amount of eosinophilic cytoplasm. They may also show intracytoplasmic lumina that may contain secretory droplets. Additional differential diagnostic considerations are glycogen-rich carcinoma, secretory carcinoma, primary clear cell carcinoma, and metastatic clear cell carcinoma (22,24). In order to distinguish pseudoneoplastic clear cell change from these malignant processes, one should appreciate the maintenance of a normal lobular architecture with two cell layers in clear cell change as opposed to effacement of tissue landmarks, with attendant mitoses, necrosis, and cytologic atypia, in malignant epithelial proliferations. For example, the abundant extracellular and intracellular secretory material and cytoplasmic vacuolization of secretory carcinoma might initially be confused with the secretory features of lactational change, particularly because of shared bland cytologic aspects. Nonetheless, secretory carcinoma lacks the orderliness of double-cell-layered acini that is seen breast tissue with lactational change (24).

Lactational change in a clinically detected breast mass may also occur in a preexisting process such as a fibroadenoma, tubular adenoma, or hamartoma, or may affect areas of nodular hyperplasia (25–29). These masses have been termed "lactating adenomas," although some undoubtedly represent exaggerated nodular hyperplasia of lobules. It is controversial whether lactating adenoma, as a neoplasm that

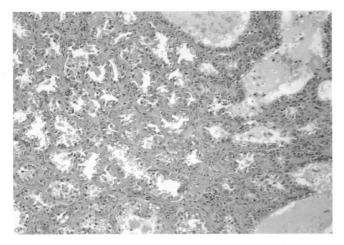

**FIG. 5.** Lactating adenoma with luminal secretions.

arises *de novo,* exists. Most reported patients with lactating adenoma were pregnant or recently pregnant, with a mean age of about 25, and clinically presented with a solitary mass diagnosed clinically as a fibroadenoma. Grossly, the resected masses were 2–3 cm in greatest dimension (range 0.8–7 cm), rubbery to firm, and lobulated, without hemorrhage or necrosis. Microscopically, lactating adenomas are nonencapsulated but sharply demarcated and in more than half of cases there is histologic evidence of an underlying fibroadenoma, tubular adenoma, or hamartoma (Fig. 5). Florid lactational change may be confused with carcinoma, particularly in fine needle aspiration specimens (22,30), but attention to a constellation of cytopathologic features, including background material and intact lobules or acini, should allow for an accurate diagnosis (30). Rare cases of carcinoma arising adjacent to lactational change have been reported (26,31) but recognition of lactational change or adenoma is not felt to represent a risk factor for concurrent and/or subsequent carcinoma.

### Fat Necrosis

Fat necrosis of the breast is most likely to be confused with carcinoma at the clinical, mammographic, and gross levels of examination (Fig. 6). Clinically, fat necrosis is uncommon, with an incidence of less than 1% of biopsied breast masses (32–34). There is often (but not always) a history of trauma or prior treatment, including lumpectomy, radiation, or breast reduction (35–40). Clinically, patients typically present in the fifth decade with an irregular palpable mass, which may also be associated with the worrisome findings of skin retraction or thickening (33,34). Mammographically, the attributes that can result in a picture indistinguishable from carcinoma include spiculated margins and branching, rod-like, or angular microcalcifications (41). This same irregular margin may be appreciated in the gross examination of fat necrosis, where in later stages a grayish-white, firm, and stellate configuration may be seen. In some cases, both mammographically and grossly, there may be single or multiple lipid-filled cysts with or without calcified walls (41), features that are readily associated with a benign process.

Fat necrosis is commonly identified as a component of postbiopsy changes in breast tissue. Grossly, in conjunction with brisk fibrosis surrounding a biopsy cavity, these changes may be difficult or impossible to discern from residual carcinoma in a reexcision or mastectomy specimen.

The histologic picture of fat necrosis is dependent on the time interval from initial insult (33,35). In the early stages, the inflammatory cell infiltrate is a mixed lymphohistiocytic one (Fig. 7) while later, there is a progression to organization with cystic change, fibrosis, hemosiderin deposition, and

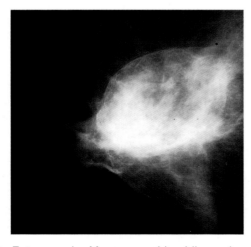

**FIG. 6.** Fat necrosis. Mammographic oblique view of the right breast in a patient 2 years following breast reduction. A moderately well-defined mass in the midbreast, with rim-like calcifications and a central lucent area, often seen with mature fat necrosis. (Courtesy of Dr. Fidelma Flanagan.)

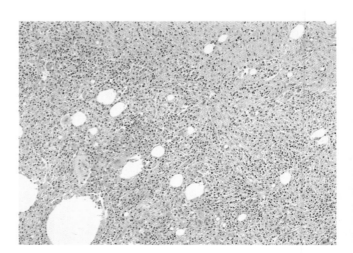

**FIG. 7.** Early phase of fat necrosis with mixed lymphoplasmacytic cellular infiltrate.

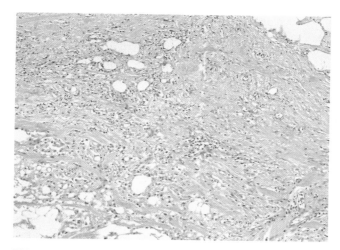

**FIG. 8.** Later phase of fat necrosis displays prominent fibrosis.

calcification (33,35) (Fig. 8). The microscopic diagnosis is usually straightforward, although fat necrosis occurring in the setting of radiation therapy may feature atypical stromal fibroblasts due to radiation effect (see section on treatment effects). Another post-treatment effect with resultant fat necrosis that may cause diagnostic concern with the microscope is that of previous excisional biopsy. With an intense fibroinflammatory response, various cell types may masquerade as neoplastic cells. For example, lymphocytes may be arranged in cords, thereby incorrectly prompting a diagnosis of lobular carcinoma (Fig. 9). Sheets of histiocytes may mimic histiocytoid or lipid-rich carcinoma (42) in that the cytoplasm is foamy but the carcinoma cells have pronounced nuclear atypia. Histiocytes with imbibed fat may assume a signet ring appearance and thereby simulate signet ring carcinoma of the breast. Similar lipid-laden signet ring histiocytes may be found in axillary lymph nodes from women who have had a previous procedure that disrupted

mammary adipose tissue (43) (Fig. 10). The differential diagnosis with metastatic carcinoma is usually resolved by careful study of hematoxylin–eosin (H&E)–stained slides. In particularly difficult cases, immunohistochemistry for CD45 and CD68 may provide reassurance of a pseudoneoplastic rather than a neoplastic entity, especially in the context of keratin negativity.

**Squamous Metaplasia**

It is likely that focal squamous metaplasia in benign mammary epithelium is not uncommon, but reported cases of extensive squamous metaplasia in the breast are rare (44,45). Similar to fat necrosis, trauma has been implicated in the genesis of some cases of squamous metaplasia of the breast (44). Squamous metaplasia of ducts and lobules may also accompany granulomatous lobular mastitis and mammary infarction (46).

Extensive squamous metaplasia of the breast does exhibit a generally lobular configuration but resembles a neoplasm because of the degree of lobular expansion by a voluminous squamous cell proliferation. This demonstrates small foci of pseudocarcinomatous invasion into adipose tissue at the periphery of the sheets of squamous cells. Additionally, a reparative response composed of a prominent lymphocytic infiltrate or fibroplasia abutting the squamous nests may cause further alarm (Fig. 11). Exclusion of a neoplasm with squamous differentiation, such as squamous cell carcinoma, ductal carcinoma with squamous differentiation, and mucoepidermoid carcinoma, may be accomplished by noting the lack of cytologic atypia and necrosis, and only rare mitoses in squamous metaplasia. Also, sharp demarcation of the metaplastic lobules of squamous cells from the reactive and fibrotic stroma is a distinctive feature. Squamous metaplasia of nonneoplastic mammary epithelium should also be separated from that associated with infarcted papillomas (45,47), papillomatosis (48), or fibroadenomas (49).

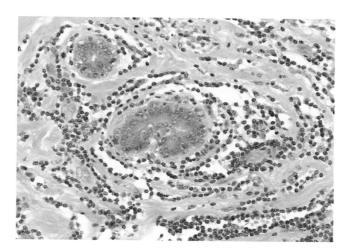

**FIG. 9.** Concentric cords of lymphocytes mimicking lobular carcinoma.

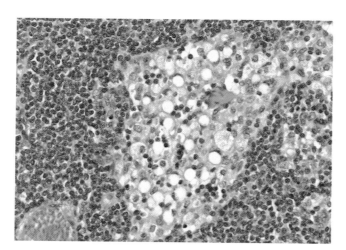

**FIG. 10.** Signet ring histiocytes mimicking signet ring carcinoma.

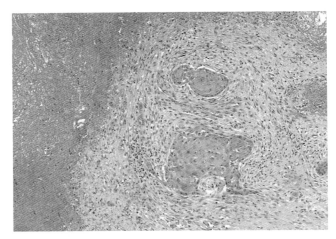

**FIG. 11.** Squamous metaplasia of breast within a fibrous background and adjacent to a biopsy cavity.

### Infarcts

Infarcts in the breast most commonly involve breast tissue also showing lactational change, including lactational adenomas, papillomas, papillomatosis, and fibroadenomas (46,47,50–52). Hemorrhagic infarcts also may occur after anticoagulant therapy (53,54). Infarcts involving both nonneoplastic and benign neoplastic tissue may produce a mass, which occasionally may be painful and exhibit an abrupt and rapid increase in size. In nonneoplastic breast tissue, the usual setting is in pregnancy or lactation (46,51,52). Grossly, these masses are usually single and well circumscribed, and they vary in size from 0.5 to 7.0 cm (46). Microscopically, zonation is usually apparent; central coagulative necrosis is surrounded by granulation tissue exhibiting variable lymphoplasmacytic infiltrates with hemosiderin-laden macrophages and fibrosis. Thrombosis has been identified in a few cases in vessels adjacent to the infarcts, but it is not clear as to whether this is a primary or secondary event. In cases of hemorrhagic necrosis induced by anticoagulant therapy, acute necrotizing arteritis and venous thrombosis are consistently found. Extensive necrosis and reactive epithelial changes at the periphery of the coagulative necrosis may raise the specter of malignant disease, but consideration of the clinical setting and careful examination of the infarcted lactational tissue (as well as adjacent, viable breast tissue with lactational change) should readily rule out a necrotic neoplasm. Similarly, a specific search should be made for viable papilloma or fibroadenoma. Usually infarction only partially involves these benign neoplasms, so they may be easily recognized as such histologically.

### Mastitis and Inflammatory Conditions

#### Duct Ectasia and Periductal Mastitis

Dilatation of mammary ducts, or duct ectasia, may suggest carcinoma to the examining physician due to a nipple discharge that may be associated with subareolar induration and mass formation, with retraction and dimpling of the skin (55–58). Grossly, the dilated ducts contain pasty creamy secretions and may be mistaken for the dilated ducts of intraductal carcinoma with comedo necrosis. Indeed, Haagensen (55) has stated the following: "A gross differentiation between carcinoma and mammary duct ectasia is impossible." However, when breast tissue with the comedo type of intraductal carcinoma is compressed, thin, solid cylinders of necrotic material are expressed. In contrast, proteinaceous secretions in duct ectasia have a more liquid consistency. Microscopic inspection of the ducts is necessary to establish the diagnosis because the lining cells in areas of duct ectasia are cytologically bland, and the intraductal material is composed of eosinophilic or amorphous proteinaceous material (Fig. 12) and cholesterol clefts. Cellular elements in the lumina are represented by foamy histiocytes and shed epithelial cells (55,56). Moreover, the lining epithelial thickness is not increased in duct ectasia, as it is in intraductal carcinoma. Duct ectasia also characteristically demonstrates a mixed inflammatory cell infiltrate (of lymphocytes, histiocytes, neutrophils, and plasma cells) that is both intraepithelial and periductal in location. Such findings are rare in intraductal carcinoma. When plasma cells are numerous, the term "plasma cell mastitis" has been applied. Periductal fibrosis accompanies the inflammation and may be particularly prominent in later stages of duct ectasia.

#### Granulomatous Mastitis

Granulomatous inflammation of the breast may occur in the varied settings of duct ectasia and periductal mastitis, infection, sarcoidosis, foreign body reaction, granulomatous lobular mastitis, and Wegener's granulomatosis (59–67). Fibroinflammatory masses produced by granulomatous inflammation are mainly a clinical diagnostic difficulty, and pathologic exclusion of a neoplasm is not usually problem-

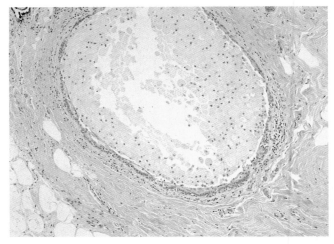

**FIG. 12.** Duct ectasia exhibits a thin, epithelial lining with intraluminal amorphous debris and foam cells.

atic (Fig. 13). The differential diagnosis between malignancy and granulomatous mastitis is rarely arduous, but a frozen section of Wegener's granulomatosis in the breast may sometimes be reported as highly suggestive of malignancy (67), and fine needle aspiration biopsy of granulomatous mastitis has posed certain obstacles in excluding neoplasia. Specifically, atypical mononuclear epithelioid histiocytes and nuclear atypia in groups of epithelial cells in granulomatous mastitis must be distinguished from the typical cytologic features of breast carcinoma cells, including singly lying malignant cells (60). Fine needle aspiration biopsies of suture granulomas of the breast may also display cells that cytologically mimic recurrent malignancy (66). In this circumstance, where typical foreign body–type giant cells are lacking, a predominance of spindle cells and dissimilarity of the atypical cells to those of the original tumor have been touted as the most helpful diagnostic clues (66).

The differential diagnosis of granulomatous mastitis also includes breast carcinoma with a prominent inflammatory cell component, including medullary carcinoma, invasive ductal carcinoma with abundant inflammatory cells, and rare mammary carcinomas with a granulomatous inflammatory response (68,69). The concern here is that the dense inflammatory infiltrate in granulomatous mastitis might obscure a neoplastic epithelial proliferation. By noting the character and distribution pattern of the inflammatory cell infiltrate, the surgical pathologist may begin to address this differential diagnosis. Most inflammatory cell infiltrates associated with invasive ductal carcinomas and medullary carcinomas of the breast are lymphoplasmacytic, as compared to the inflammation in granulomatous mastitis, where histiocytes predominate and giant cells are present. Also, the specific cytologic features of foreign body granulomas, sarcoidal granulomas, and caseating infectious granulomas, and the lobular distribution of granulomatous lobular mastitis, are significant observations in arriving at a diagnosis of a subtype of granulomatous mastitis. It should be noted that sarcoid-like granulomas may rarely be found in breast carcinomas (and in

ipsilateral axillary lymph nodes) (68,69), so that ultimately it is the nature of associated epithelial cells that obviously is most critical in deciding whether a given case is pseudoneoplastic or neoplastic. Most breast carcinomas with a striking number of tumor-infiltrating lymphocytes are poorly differentiated, and therefore the neoplastic cell population should be easily identifiable.

Lymphoproliferative disorders, including primary malignant lymphomas of the breast, are in the differential diagnosis of granulomatous mastitis. However, primary malignant lymphoma of the breast typically exhibits a monomorphous cell population that diffusely infiltrates and distorts the breast parenchyma (70–72), and is much more voluminous than the inflammation seen in atypical cases of mastitis.

### Inflammatory Myofibroblastic Pseudotumor (Plasma Cell Granuloma)

Inflammatory myofibroblastic pseudotumor (IMP) is a benign proliferation of myofibroblasts that only rarely involves the breast (73,74). Although nonmetastasizing, this proliferation generally exhibits a propensity for locally persistent growth and even recurrence (73). The true nature of IMP is uncertain, i.e., it is not clear whether it is a neoplastic or a pseudoneoplastic condition. IMP has been likened to fibromatosis (73), which is a growth considered intermediate between reactive and neoplastic fibroblastic proliferations.

Both reported patients (aged 13 and 29 years) with myofibroblastic pseudotumors of the breast presented with a mass (73,74). Grossly, these lesions were 4.0–4.5 cm in greatest dimension, well circumscribed, and slightly lobulated, with their cut surfaces showing homogeneous, fibrous, grayish-white tissue (73,74). Histologically, one case was striking for the presence of densely hyalinized collagenous tissue with large collections of plasma cells. Some stromal cells had large polygonal or multilobulated vesicular nuclei.

The differential diagnosis includes true neoplasms such as myofibroblastoma, fibrous histiocytoma, inflamed spindle cell sarcomas (73), and, in selected instances, plasma cell myeloma (74). Accurate diagnosis is contingent on awareness of the existence of IMP as a disease potentially presenting at many different anatomic sites, including the breast, and strict attention to the aggregated clinical, histopathologic, and adjunctive (immunostaining and electron microscopic) findings. Specifically, one should appreciate that IMPs have infiltrative borders and histologically display three basic patterns: (a) myxoid, vascular, and inflammatory areas resembling nodular fasciitis; (b) compact spindle cell foci with intermingled inflammatory cells (lymphocytes, plasma cells, and eosinophils) resembling fibrous histiocytoma; and (c) dense, plate-like collagenous areas resembling desmoids or scars (73). Immunohistochemistry will be of aid in demonstrating the myofibroblastic immunophenotype featuring positivity for vimentin, muscle-specific actin, and smooth muscle actin. Keratin has not been reported in the cells of mammary IMPs. For cases where plasma cell

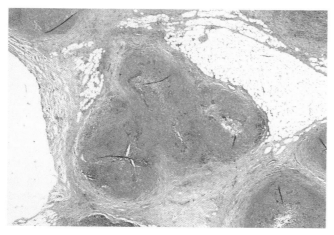

**FIG. 13.** Granulomatous lobular mastitis presents a distinctive lobulocentric image at scanning magnification.

myeloma is contemplated in differential diagnosis, immunostains for kappa and lambda light chain immunoglobulins will be of benefit in establishing a polyclonal plasma cell population in pseudotumors containing prominent plasma cells (plasma cell granulomas).

### Lymphocytic and Diabetic Mastitis (and Mastopathy)

Extensive lymphocytic infiltrates in the breast may be considered pseudoneoplastic in that a diagnosis of malignant lymphoma might be entertained in such cases, particularly in a small needle core or fine needle aspiration biopsy. Pronounced lymphocytic infiltrates may be present in lymphocytic and diabetic mastitis (mastopathy).

Lymphocytic mastitis, lymphocytic mastopathy, and sclerosing lymphocytic lobulitis are terms that have been applied to a primarily lobulocentric infiltrate of mature lymphocytes with variable density (75–79). Reported patients have all been women, usually young to middle-aged, who presented clinically with palpable breast masses. Of substantial interest, many of these patients had diabetes mellitus or other autoimmune diseases. Indeed, these disorders may constitute one segment in the spectrum of autoimmune breast disease (75–79).

Grossly, lymphocytic mastitis presents as an ill-defined to nodular fibrous mass varying from 1 to 6 cm in greatest dimension, with grayish-white cut surfaces (76,79). The designation of fibrous mastopathy refers to the fibrous component of these masses.

Microscopically, lymphocytic mastitis, mastopathy, and lobulitis exhibit dense lobulocentric permeation by mature lymphocytes (Fig. 14), and direct migration by lymphocytes into the epithelium is found (75,76,79). In addition to small, mature lymphocytes, a lesser number of plasma cells, histiocytes, and neutrophils can be identified. The infiltrate is not restricted to the lobules and may also be seen in perilobular, periductal, and perivascular locations. Additionally, lym-

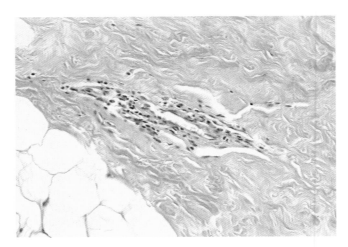

**FIG. 15.** A hallmark of lymphocytic mastitis is lymphocytic vasculitis.

phocytic vasculitis is a hallmark of lymphocytic mastitis (Fig. 15), but this does not include fibrinoid necrosis of vessel walls. Stromal changes entail dense lobular sclerosis of a nonspecific type that is identical to lobular involution, and extensive interlobular fibrosis with diminished adipose tissue (75,76,79). The differential diagnosis of the dense lymphoid infiltrate includes malignant lymphoma, a distinctly uncommon neoplasm of the breast (70–72). In larger (incisional) specimens, the lobulocentric lymphoid infiltrate of lymphocytic mastitis and lobulitis does not display the typical image of mammary lymphoma (see above), which tends to efface the normal architecture of the breast. Such a microanatomic distribution may not, of course, be evident in small needle cores or fine needle aspiration biopsy specimens, occasionally necessitating adjunctive analysis for confident diagnosis. The lymphocytes are small and mature in lymphocytic mastitis, whereas in comparison, most mammary lymphomas are intermediate to high grade (70,72) and feature a substantial population of large lymphoid cells.

The presence of germinal centers, albeit usually focal in lymphocytic mastitis/mastopathy (75), is also helpful in arriving at a diagnosis of benignancy. Immunohistochemistry for lymphocyte subsets is not particularly helpful because both lymphocytic mastitis/mastopathy and mammary lymphoma are composed mainly of B cells. Immunohistologic evidence of restricted light chain immunoglobulin expression (to either kappa or lambda) is important information in support of a malignant rather than a pseudoneoplastic proliferation. One limitation of this analysis is that frozen tissue must be used because kappa and lambda light chain immunostains are unreliable in formalin-fixed, paraffin-embedded tissue sections. Also unhelpful diagnostically are so-called lymphoepithelial lesions (intraepithelial lymphoid infiltrates), which may be observed in both benign and malignant lymphoid proliferations in the breast. Lastly, it should be noted that a putative relationship between lymphocytic lobulitis/mastitis and a risk for development of lymphoma is controversial (70,71,80,81).

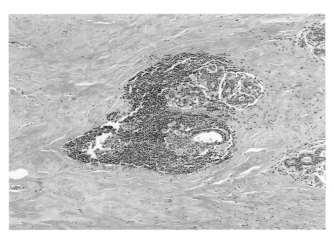

**FIG. 14.** Lymphocytic lobulitis shows mature lymphocytes in the lobule and in epithelium.

Another element of lymphocytic mastitis that must be deemed pseudoneoplastic is the epithelioid stromal population (79). These large, rounded, mononuclear fibroblast derivatives are dispersed in a fibrous stroma, singly and in long rows. The cells have an abundant amount of granular cytoplasm and centrally located round nuclei. No mitotic figures are apparent. In several reported cases, experienced pathologists have seriously considered diagnoses of infiltrating carcinoma because of such cells, and one lesion was originally classified as a granular cell tumor (79). Employment of immunohistochemical stains is worthwhile diagnostically in this setting, as the epithelioid stromal cells show an immunophenotype consistent with myofibroblastic differentiation and featuring muscle-specific actin and CD68 immunoreactivity (79). In conjunction with histologic findings, negative immunostains for keratin and S-100 protein can be used to argue against an epithelial neoplasm and a granular cell tumor, respectively.

Many of the features of lymphocytic mastitis are also identified in diabetic mastopathy, including keloidal fibrosis, epithelioid fibroblasts, periductal/lobular lymphocytic infiltration, and perivascular lymphocytic infiltration (82–84). However, these histologic traits are not specific for diabetes (79) and may be more of a general indicator of possible autoimmune breast diseases. As in lymphocytic mastitis, the lymphoid infiltrates and epithelioid stromal cells in diabetic mastopathy may mimic the elements of lymphoid and epithelial malignancies, respectively.

### Pseudolymphoma

Hyperplastic lymphoid proliferations in the breast may be so florid as to histologically mimic lymphoma; these infiltrates have been designated lymphoid pseudotumors (85) or pseudolymphomas (86–91). The term pseudolymphoma of the breast was apparently first applied in 1975 by Lauren V. Ackerman (92).

Pseudolymphoma is a rare cause of a clinically detected breast mass, with an incidence of 0.06% (87). Many patients present with a dull, aching sensation, although several have experienced no symptoms or signs other than a mass. Because a history of trauma has been elicited in some cases, it has been proposed that mammary pseudolymphoma may represent an exaggerated local response to injury (87). Mammographic study of pseudolymphomas has usually revealed smooth to spherical, nodular or lobulated masses (86,88,89); shaggy borders have been described in only one case (90). The clinical diagnosis in most cases is usually that of fibroadenoma (87). Follow-up ranging from 2 to 8 years has shown no untoward outcomes.

Grossly, the masses have been described as soft to firm, circumscribed, round to ovoid nodules of 2.2–4.5 cm in size (86,87), although one 11-cm lesion has been reported (91). Coloration was homogeneously tan, with small areas of yellow flecking, representing fat necrosis.

Histologically, the dense lymphoid proliferation is mainly composed of mature lymphocytes, with scattered, admixed plasma cells and histiocytes and a few eosinophils. Nodularity and circumscription of the infiltrate are characteristic, with occasional germinal centers being formed. Focal extension of the process into fat may, however, be seen (86). Immunophenotyping performed in some cases demonstrated a mixed population of lymphocytes with expression of both kappa and lambda light chain immunoglobulins (86,89).

The main differential diagnostic consideration in the neoplastic realm is that of malignant lymphoma. Those features favoring pseudolymphoma over lymphoma include sharp demarcation, cellular polymorphism, lymphocytic maturity, the presence of germinal centers, and the lack of effacement of the normal breast architecture. Fresh tissue for frozen section immunohistochemistry and flow cytometry may be invaluable in arriving at a definitive diagnosis, and should be specifically sought if a prominent, atypical, lymphoid cell population is identified in breast tissue.

### Sinus Histiocytosis with Massive Lymphadenopathy (Rosai–Dorfman Disease)

Sinus histiocytosis with massive lymphadenopathy, also known as Rosai–Dorfman disease, is a rare, idiopathic, histiocytic, proliferative disorder that may represent an immunologic disturbance with mass formation in lymph nodes or extranodal sites (93). Rare cases involving the parenchyma of the breast (93), an intramammary lymph node (94), and the skin overlying the breast (95) have been reported. In the two cases of direct involvement of breast tissue the women averaged 22 years of age and presented with a breast mass (93). In the first case, multiple bilateral masses were detected by mammogram, with the largest measuring 1.8 cm in greatest dimension. Excision revealed a lesion with a gross appearance similar to that of a fibroadenoma (93). Histologically, a definitive diagnosis of extranodal Rosai–

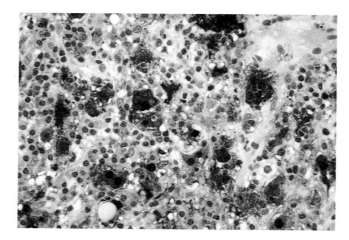

**FIG. 16.** S-100 protein immunopositivity in the histiocytes of Rosai–Dorfman disease.

Dorfman disease requires a large number of the distinctive histiocytes and easily detectable lymphocytic phagocytosis (93).

The differential diagnosis does include a number of neoplasms, including melanoma, carcinoma, and Hodgkin's disease. Breast carcinoma, melanoma, and the histiocytes of Rosai–Dorfman disease may all be positive for S-100 protein (Fig. 16) but the distinctive histiocytes often react with antibodies directed against the lymphoid antigens CD43 and LN-1 (96). On the other hand, malignant melanocytes are positive with immunostains for HMB-45, and epithelial markers such as cytokeratin will be found in carcinoma cells. Usually the histiocytes are recognizable as such by conventional morphology, with immunostains providing confirmation of the diagnostic impression of extranodal Rosai–Dorfman disease.

## Extramedullary Hematopoiesis

Extramedullary hematopoiesis (myeloid metaplasia) of the breast is rare and is usually clinically detectable in the form of a breast mass in elderly women with myelofibrosis (97,98). There may be a significant time interval between the initial diagnosis of myelofibrosis and the development of a breast mass; in one case (98), this time span was 16 years. A clinical diagnosis of malignancy may be made because of the presence of a breast mass with regional lymph node enlargement (97). Grossly, reported masses have ranged from 1.8 to 6 cm in greatest dimension and were firm, gray–white, and irregular. Microscopically, the low-power view is that of a densely fibrotic background with numerous interspersed megakaryocytes. Eosinophilic myelocytes are numerous but erythroid elements are rare (97) or absent (98). As is typical of extramedullary hematopoiesis, the hematopoietic elements cluster within and about blood vessels. A naphthol-AS-D-chloroacetate esterase (Leder) stain was employed in one case to better distinguish the myeloid cells.

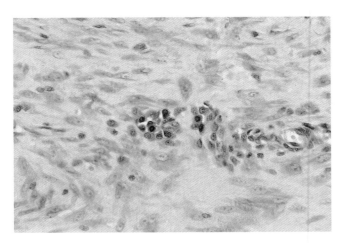

FIG. 18. Myeloid metaplasia in the breast (Leder stain).

Myeloid metaplasia may mimic several neoplasms, including sarcoma, leukemic infiltrates (including granulocytic sarcoma), non-Hodgkin's lymphoma, Hodgkin's disease, and sarcomatoid carcinoma. Identification of multiple hematopoietic cell types is important in excluding those lesions. A panel of special stains, including a Leder reaction and immunostains for myeloperoxidase, hemoglobin, and glycophorin, may be helpful in confirming the identity of the myeloid and erythroid elements.

Extramedullary hematopoiesis may also occur as an incidental finding in the breast. Recently, we reviewed a case of a mastectomy done for ductal carcinoma of the breast, where extramedullary hematopoiesis was identified in the healing surgical wound at the previous biopsy site. The myeloid precursors were occasionally aligned in linear arrays, similar to those seen in lobular carcinoma (Fig. 17). A Leder stain (Fig. 18) and a myeloperoxidase immunostain (Fig. 19) confirmed the myeloid nature of these cells. The presence of clusters of orthochromic normoblasts was also helpful in establishing the diagnosis.

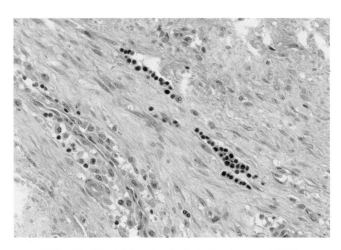

FIG. 17. Myeloid metaplasia in the breast (H&E).

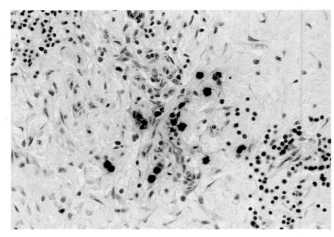

FIG. 19. Myeloid metaplasia in the breast (myeloperoxidase immunostain).

## Adenosis

Adenosis has been defined as an elongation of the terminal ductules of the mammary lobule resulting in a caricature of the lobule (99). Another view is that adenosis is purely a descriptive term, denoting a benign condition of glandular elements that may assume profiles reminiscent of the acini or ductules that are normally found in the breast (100). Its diagnostic importance resides in possible confusion with invasive carcinoma. Different patterns of adenosis include sclerosing adenosis, adenosis tumor, microglandular adenosis, apocrine adenosis, tubular adenosis, and blunt duct adenosis, or columnar alteration of lobules. The last entity is more likely to be misdiagnosed as hyperplasia rather than as a neoplasm and so is not discussed here.

### Sclerosing Adenosis

Sclerosing adenosis may present clinically as a palpable mass or it may be an incidental histologic finding (103,104). This lesion is a relatively common entity, occurring in 2–18% of surgical excisions (103–107). It is far more likely to be an incidental finding than a dominant, palpable abnormality (103,107). In fact, in two large series (105,107) of more than 1000 patients each, clinically evident sclerosing adenosis was seen at an incidence of 0.8% (11/1450) to 1.2% (12/1010). Affected women are typically 20–50 years of age (103–109). When palpable, the mass, which is usually solitary, is usually freely mobile and is associated with pain or tenderness in about half of cases. Sclerosing adenosis may be misdiagnosed as a malignancy both clinically and by mammography (109).

Sclerosing adenosis or other forms of adenosis that produce a grossly visible mass have been termed adenosis tumor (110) (Fig. 20). Macroscopically, these tumefactions are variable in appearance, but are usually of a rubbery to firm

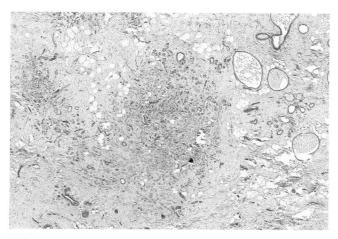

**FIG. 21.** Sclerosing adenosis with lobulocentric growth pattern.

consistency and are most often irregular and ill defined (110). Even when they are more discrete, they are not smooth and globoid or elliptical as fibroadenomas are (103). Cut surfaces are grayish-white and, of critical importance, a gross lobularity (or fine nodularity) of 1 mm to 1 cm may be observed (103). These nodular structures have been likened to closely apposed or coalescing, expanded lobules or minute fibroadenomas (103). Confusion with carcinoma may arise at the gross level if more irregular peripheral outlines and a firmer consistency are evident. However, necrosis, hemorrhage, and the characteristic chalky streaks of carcinoma are lacking (103,110).

The microscopic picture of sclerosing adenosis has long been recognized as the benign breast lesion most commonly misinterpreted as invasive carcinoma (105,107,111,112). This is particularly true in frozen sections (113,114). In one series of 359 frozen sections of the breast, the only two false positives were both cases of florid sclerosing adenosis (114).

The key diagnostic feature of sclerosing adenosis should be visualized at low-power magnification. That is, sclerosing adenosis is fundamentally a lobulocentric process (Fig. 21). A circumscribed ductular and myoepithelial cell proliferation is associated with stromal fibrosis. The process is commonly multifocal. It is the often-striking degree of gland density, in conjunction with gland distortion, that results in a pseudoinfiltrative architectural pattern. One should note that the constituent glands often possess an oval to elongated contour and that ducts at the periphery of the lesion are often dilated, compared to the luminal compression that may be observed in the center of the lesion (99). The myoepithelial cell population very frequently includes a spindle cell component, and this proliferation contributes further to lobular distortion and apparently infiltrative ductular growth (Fig. 22). Microcalcifications are common in sclerosing adenosis but this finding has no diagnostic value (Table 1). A final pseudoneoplastic characteristic of sclerosing adenosis is its capacity to involve nerves (Fig. 23). This finding was present in 20 of 1000 cases (2%) of sclerosing adenosis (115).

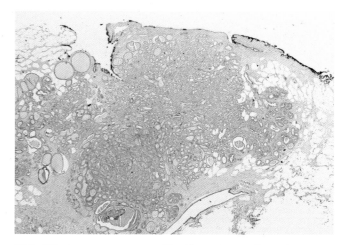

**FIG. 20.** Low-power magnification of an adenosis tumor. This mass of adenotic glands was grossly visible and measured 6 mm in greatest dimension.

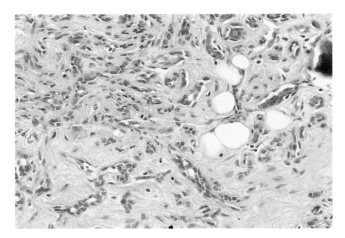

**FIG. 22.** Sclerosing adenosis with spindled myoepithelial and compressed tubular elements.

The myoepithelial cells of sclerosing adenosis also may resemble nerves themselves (116). The presence of glands in sclerosing adenosis has also been reported in blood vessel walls (117).

The differential diagnosis of sclerosing adenosis as a pseudoneoplasm versus true neoplasms centers on its distinction from tubular carcinoma (118) (see Table 1); uncommonly, a diagnosis of lobular carcinoma or myoepithelioma might likewise be entertained. Important features that should readily allow a diagnostic separation of sclerosing adenosis from tubular carcinoma include the multifocality and lobulocentricity of sclerosing adenosis, and the presence of a two-cell population in sclerosing adenosis. Additionally, as discussed above, the gland profiles of sclerosing adenosis are distinctive and quite different from those of tubular carcinoma, which often displays angulated or teardrop glandular profiles. Also, elastosis is unusual and sparse in sclerosing adenosis but elastotic clumps are often found in tubular carcinoma.

A diagnosis of invasive lobular carcinoma may be contemplated when the dominant elements in sclerosing adenosis are elongated tubules with compressed and inapparent lumina. Invasive carcinoma may also be suggested when carcinoma *in situ* involves sclerosing adenosis (119-121). Sclerosing adenosis with a prominent spindle cell myoepithelial component should be diagnostically partitioned from cytologically similar variants of adenomyoepithelioma including myoepithelioma. That lesion represents the end of the spectrum of differentiation in adenomyoepithelioma where myoepithelial differentiation is dominant. To make

**TABLE 1.** *Differential diagnosis of adenosis and tubular carcinoma*

| Feature | Normal lobule | Sclerosing adenosis | Microglandular adenosis | Apocrine adenosis | Tubular adenosis | Tubular carcinoma |
|---|---|---|---|---|---|---|
| Gross outline | Normal | Irregular | Ill defined | Irregular | Unknown | Irregular |
| Gross consistency | Not palpable | Rubbery to firm | Firm | Firm | Unknown | Hard |
| Gland distribution | Multifocal | Commonly multifocal | Haphazard | Multifocal | Haphazard | Usually unifocal |
| Lobulocentric | + | + | − | + | − | − |
| Gland profile | Rounded | Distorted | Rounded | Distorted to rounded | Rounded, elongated | Angulated |
| Elastosis | − | Unusual, sparse | − | − | − | + |
| Basal lamina[a] | + | + | + | + | + | − |
| Two-cell layer | + | + | − | + | + | − |
| Intermingled intraductal carcinoma | − | Rare | − | − | + | + |
| Extension into fat | + | + | + | + | + | + |
| Microcalcifications | − | 50% + | + | 32–83% + | + | 50% + |
| Perineural extension | − | + | − | − | − | + |
| Intraluminal secretion | Sparse | Sparse | Colloid-like | Eosinophilic granular | Eosinophilic to basophilic | Eosinophilic to amphophilic |
| Lumina | Open | Open or closed | Open | Open or closed | Collapsed to dilated | Open |
| Apical snouts | − | ± | − | + | − | + |
| Cytologic atypia | − | − | − | +[b] | − | mild |
| Mitoses | − | rare | rare | rare | − | rare |

[a] Demonstrable by histochemical stains (periodic acid–Schiff or reticulin), immunostains for type IV collagen and laminin, and electron microscopy.
[b] Cytologic atypia manifested as cells with nuclear enlargement and prominent nucleoli but with abundant cytoplasm, typical of apocrine change.

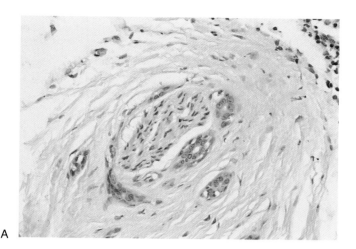

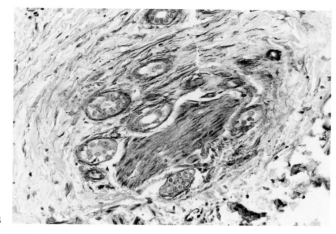

**FIG. 23. A:** Perineural involvement by sclerosing adenosis. **B:** Identification of immunoreactive collagen type IV as a circumferential rim around the small glands substantiates the benign diagnosis.

this separation, one must remember that adenomyoepithelioma typically represents a solitary, intraductal proliferation whereas sclerosing adenosis is often multicentric and is a lobular process. Myoepitheliomas have bundles of interlacing spindle cells that most closely resemble a smooth muscle neoplasm, whereas the spindle cell myoepithelial cell population in sclerosing adenosis is often focal and more disorganized. Finally, sclerosing adenosis with prominent spindle cells should be readily distinguished from the exceedingly rare malignant myoepithelioma (myoepithelial carcinoma) (122) and spindle cell carcinoma of the breast (123), both of which are overtly malignant with an invasive growth pattern, cytologic atypia, and mitoses. Sarcomatoid carcinomas of the breast often show squamous differentiation as well (123).

Most diagnoses of sclerosing adenosis may be rendered based on examination of H&E-stained sections alone. In particularly difficult cases, such as the interpretation of a needle biopsy of sclerosing adenosis, where the lobulocentric qualities are entirely lost, special studies to document the presence of myoepithelial cells and basal lamina may be helpful.

For example, muscle-specific actin immunolabeling has been used to substantiate the existence of myoepithelial cells (Fig. 24) (124), whereas antibodies directed against laminin, type IV collagen, and basement membrane proteoglycan may verify a continuous and intact basement membrane around the glands of sclerosing adenosis; tubular carcinomas lack such staining (125). As always, such stains should be interpreted in the context of the constellation of histologic findings. Negative results do not necessarily equate a diagnosis of carcinoma because absence of proof is not proof of absence. Recently, image analysis (126) and a neural network (127) have been applied in attempts to provide diagnostic aids in distinguishing sclerosing adenosis from tubular carcinoma.

Sclerosing adenosis has not been shown to be a precursor proliferation for carcinoma, but some data suggest that it does impart roughly a twofold increased risk of subsequent development of breast cancer (111,128).

### Microglandular Adenosis

Microglandular adenosis is a rare, benign entity that shares selected histologic features with both well-differentiated (tubular) carcinoma and sclerosing adenosis (129–141) (see Table 1). It is vital to recognize microglandular adenosis as such and to separate it from carcinoma. Most patients are in the sixth decade of life, with a mean age of 51–53 (129,131,136), although a wide age range of 28–82 has been noted. Microglandular adenosis usually presents as a painless, palpable mass, although in some cases the tumefaction may be due to associated fibrocystic changes (129). It may also present as a mammographic (136) or histologic incidental finding. There are no distinctive radiologic abnormalities (129). Increased density and vascularity have both been reported, and several mammograms of microglandular adenosis have been interpreted as suspicious for carcinoma (129,131,140).

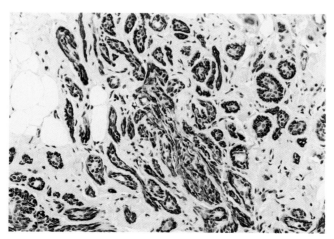

**FIG. 24.** Immunohistochemical reactivity for muscle-specific actin in sclerosing adenosis, a diagnostic aid in small needle biopsies.

Gross examination usually reveals an ill-defined induration in gray–white fibrofatty tissue (131) or a firm, nodular mass (136). In many cases a discrete lesion is not obvious. Concern for carcinoma grossly may be heightened by unusual cases with irregular outlines or gritty cut surfaces (136). Reported sizes vary from 0.3 to 20 cm with most measuring 2–4 cm (129,132,138). However, gross measurement of microglandular adenosis often underestimates its extent (138).

Microscopically, this proliferation exhibits a haphazard dispersion of small, rounded glands embedded within a fibrotic stroma or fat (Fig. 25). A disturbing finding is the presence of a single-cell layer in constituent glands. The cytoplasmic tinctorial character may be amphophilic, pale and eosinophilic, or lucent. There is often a distinctive colloid-like, eosinophilic intraluminal secretion, which may calcify. Neoplasms in the differential diagnosis mainly include tubular adenoma, tubular carcinoma (see Table 1), and carcinoma developing in microglandular adenosis (138). Tubular adenomas are well circumscribed and have densely packed tubules, while the acini of microglandular adenosis are randomly scattered throughout the breast stroma. Rounded gland profiles with colloid-like intraluminal secretions argue for microglandular adenosis, whereas angulated glands with a degree of nuclear atypia, luminal cytoplasmic protrusions (apical snouts), and associated intraductal carcinoma (often of cribriform and micropapillary types) favor a diagnosis of tubular carcinoma (see Table 1). Glands in fat and a single-cell layer may be observed in both entities and are therefore not diagnostic. Immunohistochemical assessment of a myoepithelial cell population in microglandular adenosis using muscle-specific actin antibodies has provided mixed results. In some cases, microglandular adenosis may harbor a detectable myoepithelial cell layer (136); these cases have also been termed "secretory adenosis" (102,141) and "adenomyoepithelial adenosis" (142,143). Immunohistochemical identification of circumferential type IV collagen deposition is an important diagnostic procedure because this immuno-

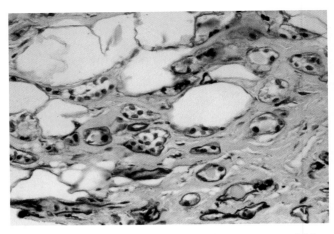

**FIG. 26.** Microglandular adenosis. Collagen type IV immunolabeling is helpful in the differential diagnosis with tubular carcinoma.

staining pattern is uniform in microglandular adenosis (Fig. 26) and absent in tubular carcinoma. Staining for laminin reveals a similar reactivity pattern (140). An ultrastructural study has confirmed the presence of a thick basement membrane around individual tubules of microglandular adenosis (133).

The differential diagnosis of benign microglandular adenosis also includes atypical microglandular adenosis and carcinoma in microglandular adenosis (134,138,142,143). Carcinoma was identified in association with microglandular adenosis in 14 of 60 cases (23%) in one series (138). In 13 examples microglandular adenosis reportedly showed a morphologic transition to carcinoma (138). These cases demonstrated cellular crowding, glandular complexity with tubules having two or more lumina, and cytologic atypia as manifested by nuclear enlargement, irregular nuclear membranes, and clumped chromatin. Continuity of these areas with clear-cut carcinoma *in situ* and invasive carcinoma was present. In other published papers (129,132,136), however, microglandular adenosis was not associated with carcinoma and it did not constitute a risk for subsequent breast cancer.

### Apocrine Adenosis

Apocrine change or metaplasia is common in the breast. When acini of adenosis are lined with apocrine cells, the designation apocrine adenosis has been applied (140, 144–146) (Fig. 27). Clinically, it may be detected due to microcalcifications on mammography or it may appear as an incidental histologic finding. Apocrine adenosis has been identified in 3% of benign breast biopsies (144,145).

This form of adenosis may be particularly provocative because of nuclear atypia in the adenotic glands. The nuclear irregularities seen in apocrine changes in the breast commonly feature nuclear enlargement with prominent nucleoli. The cytoplasm of the cells may be either eosinophilic and granular or focally clear and vacuolated.

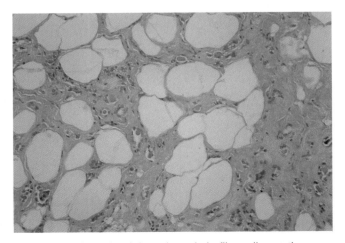

**FIG. 25.** Microglandular adenosis in fibroadipose tissue.

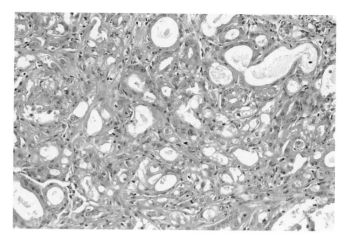

**FIG. 27.** Apocrine adenosis. Jumbled aggregate of tubules lined with apocrine cells.

The differential diagnosis includes tubular carcinoma, ductal apocrine carcinoma *in situ*, and invasive apocrine carcinoma. The potential difficulty of this diagnosis is highlighted by the fact that in one series of 55 consultation cases, most had been referred because of a suspicion of malignancy (144). Moreover, apocrine adenosis has been reported as the cause of a false-positive fine needle aspiration biopsy (147). The most valuable diagnostic findings in apocrine adenosis include identification of a background of typical microglandular or sclerosing adenosis, the lobulocentricity of this alteration, the presence of a myoepithelial cell layer (which may be demonstrated by immunohistochemical staining with antibodies reactive with smooth muscle–specific actin), and the presence of a basal lamina, as determined by immunohistochemical staining for laminin (see Table 1).

The risk of the patient developing carcinoma subsequent to a diagnosis of apocrine adenosis has not been established. However, this condition does appear to be associated with concurrent atypical ductal hyperplasia (144), which itself is a marker of four- to fivefold increased relative risk (148). In a second series of 51 patients, none of the women with apocrine adenosis (termed atypical apocrine metaplasia in this study) developed breast cancer during a follow-up period that averaged about 3 years (145). Clinical follow-up and observation has been recommended (145).

### Tubular Adenosis

This variant pattern of adenosis is quite uncommon; in one series, only four cases were identified in a 10-year period (149). All patients were women with a median age of 62 years (range 40–82 years). They presented with a mass, although in only one case was the lesion composed solely of adenosis. In this example, which lacked an associated epithelial abnormality, the mass measured 3 cm. Histologically, tubular adenosis is characterized by a haphazard proliferation of elongated and interdigitating tubules of fairly

uniform size (99,149). It differs from sclerosing adenosis in lacking a whorled, lobulocentric arrangement of glands. In similarity to other patterns of adenosis (and tubular carcinoma), extension into fat is common (see Table 1). Like sclerosing adenosis, tubular adenosis exhibits two cell layers, which may be accentuated by immunohistochemical stains for muscle-specific actin and S-100 protein expression in myoepithelial cells. In three of four of the reported cases, ductal carcinoma *in situ* was found to extend into tubular adenosis, but whether tubular adenosis itself constitutes a risk factor for subsequent development of carcinoma is unknown (149). The differential diagnosis, as is true of other forms of adenosis, converges on tubular carcinoma (149). The most important feature favoring tubular adenosis is the finding of a myoepithelial cell population (149). Minor criteria in support of a diagnosis of tubular adenosis over tubular carcinoma include absence of angular-shaped tubules, lack of prominent apical luminal snouts, and acellular collagenous stroma rather than a desmoplastic matrix (149).

### Radial Scar/Complex Sclerosing Lesion

These sclerosing lesions of the breast are composed of both an epithelial proliferation and stromal sclerosis (150–169). Because of the variable contribution of these elements to individual lesions, a variety of terms have been appended to them, including sclerosing papillary proliferation (150), nonencapsulated sclerosing lesions (151), infiltrating epitheliosis (152), indurative mastopathy (153), benign sclerosing ductal proliferation (154), rosette-like lesions (155), complex compound, heteromorphic lesions (156), obliterative mastopathy (157), radial sclerosing lesion (158), scleroelastic lesion (159), radial scar (157,160), and radial scar/complex sclerosing lesion (161,162). The term radial scar has achieved fairly widespread usage (161–164). Radial scars are distinguished from complex sclerosing lesions based on size, where radial scars are 1 cm and smaller, with complex sclerosing lesions ranging upward from that dimension (160,161).

Radial scars/complex sclerosing lesions are fairly common in the breast, with a reported incidence of 2–28% (164–166). The incidence is no doubt dependent on sampling because the highest figures stem from extensively sampled breast tissue in autopsy series (164). In a screening study, 24 cases were identified among 54,407 women for an overall detection rate of 0.04%. Of the 392 subjects who were biopsied, the incidence was 24/392, or 6%. Currently, the clinical presentation is usually of a middle-aged woman with a mammographic abnormality, although radial scars may be palpable (149,166). Most common of all are small radial scars that are impalpable and not detectable by mammograms but that are seen as incidental histologic findings in biopsies done for other reasons. The mammographic appearance of a radial scar is indistinguishable from that of a small carcinoma because both are spiculated lesions with or without a central fibrous core and calcifications (169).

Most radial scars/complex sclerosing lesions are 1–17 mm in size (164,165,167). Not surprisingly, those detected by mammography (mean size 11.5 mm, range 6–17 mm) are larger than those detected as an incidental histologic finding (mean 3.7 mm, range 1–13 mm) (167). Multicentricity (44–67% of cases) and bilaterality (43%) are common (164,165). The gross appearance of most radial scars may also be indiscernible from carcinoma. Classically, the majority have a stellate outline and resemble a contracted scar. However, up to 33% of cases may have an oval peripheral margin (165). Punctate and linear white chalky streaks, which represent elastosis, and which are also commonly seen in tubular carcinomas, may be present and create further consternation ("a state of paralyzing dismay") (153).

Microscopically, radial scar/complex sclerosing lesion has a characteristic zonation at scanning magnification, with a central sclerotic domain merging into a peripheral zone with a prominent epithelial proliferation, including hyperplasia and adenosis (Fig. 28). Centrally, there is often abundant sclerosis and elastosis, although the amount of sclerosis is variable and likely depends on the age of the lesion. Early forms exhibit little fibroelastosis and older ones have densely hyalinized sclerosis. This central sclerosing mechanism causes distortion of entrapped tubules and ducts, simulating invasive carcinoma (Fig. 29). These tubules possess two cell layers, and the lining cells lack cytologic pleomorphism. At the periphery of sclerosing lesions epithelial processes may be found, including epithelial hyperplasia of the usual type, papillomas, cystic change, and apocrine metaplasia.

Diagnostic difficulty at the microscope may arise if one focuses only on the center of the lesion, if the center of a radial scar/complex sclerosing lesion is sampled by a needle core biopsy, or if fine needle aspiration biopsy is performed (168). In one series, 5 of 54 cases (9%) of radial scar/complex sclerosing lesions were misdiagnosed as carcinoma and major surgery was performed (150). In a series of 22 cases sampled by fine needle aspiration biopsy, 1 (5%) was diag-

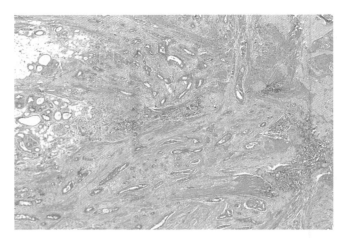

**FIG. 29.** Radial scar. Compressed tubules and elastosis may cause concern for tubular carcinoma.

nosed as malignant and 8 (36%) were interpreted as suspicious (168). The major neoplastic disease in the differential diagnosis is tubular carcinoma (Table 2). Close attention to the overall configuration, the two-cell populations, the sclerotic rather than loose myxoid stroma, and the lack of extension of tubules into fat (see Table 2) should allow one to make the correct histopathologic diagnosis of radial scar/complex sclerosing lesion. Definite proof of a two-cell layer may be obtained by immunohistochemical identification of myoepithelial cells, as accomplished by binding of anti-smooth muscle-specific actin antibodies (170), although this is not usually necessary. In fine needle aspiration, over-reliance on abnormally shaped groups of epithelial cells, including tubular structures, in establishing a cytologic diagnosis of malignancy may lead to misdiagnosis of radial scar/complex sclerosing lesion as carcinoma (168).

One may observe atypical hyperplasia and carcinoma in radial scar/complex sclerosing lesions (167), but the association of those proliferations and carcinoma is generally viewed as weak. Some have postulated that these sclerosing lesions might be precursors for tubular carcinomas (151,160), but the more likely natural history of the former would be progression to sclerosis.

### Collagenous Spherulosis

Collagenous spherulosis is a rare mixed epithelial and myoepithelial proliferative abnormality of the breast that may be confused at the microscopic level with adenoid cystic carcinoma and intraductal carcinoma (171,172).

The patients are women between the ages of 25 and 55 (mean 40) who present with a palpable mass or mammographic abnormality (171,172). However, collagenous spherulosis is usually an incidental histologic finding and only rarely produces a mass itself (172). It is commonly multifocal and usually quite small (1 mm or smaller) (171) but rarely may range up to 3.5 cm (172). The one documented

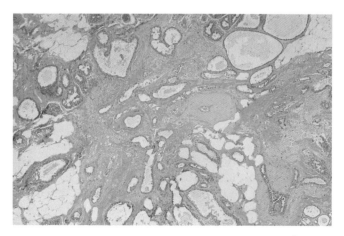

**FIG. 28.** Radial scars often harbor a sclerotic center and dilated and hyperplastic glands at the periphery.

**TABLE 2.** *Differential diagnosis of radial scar (complex sclerosing lesion) and tubular carcinoma*

| Feature | Radial scar/complex sclerosing lesion | Tubular carcinoma |
|---|---|---|
| Gross outline | Irregular to stellate | Irregular to stellate |
| Gross consistency | Firm and indurated | Hard |
| Gross distribution | Often (44–67%) multicentric | Usually unifocal |
| Gland profile at center | Angulated | Angulated |
| Gland profile at periphery | Dilated, with epithelial hyperplasia and/or adenosis | Angulated |
| Intermingled carcinoma *in situ* | Uncommon to rare | + |
| Central stroma | Sclerotic | Loose, myxoid |
| Elastosis | + | + |
| Basal lamina[a] | + | − |
| Two-cell layer | + | − |
| Perineural extension | Entrapment possible | + |
| Extension into fat | − | + |
| Cytologic atypia | − | Mild |
| Mitoses | Rare | Rare |

[a] Demonstrable by immunostains for type IV collagen and laminin.

case of extensive collagenous spherulosis was grossly unremarkable, with the breast tissue being described as irregular and yellow–white.

Microscopically, the basic finding is of intraluminal clusters of eosinophilic spherules (Fig. 30) that exhibit arresting concentric and radiating fibrillar patterns (171). These are composed of basement membrane proteins, including type IV collagen (172). Collagenous spherulosis is normally found adjacent to, or intermingled with, other benign epithelial proliferations, including papilloma, sclerosing adenosis, and radial scar (171).

Collagenous spherulosis may, as mentioned, simulate adenoid cystic carcinoma, but the former is almost always a minute, incidental histologic abnormality whereas adenoid cystic carcinoma produces a palpable mass. Although adenoid cystic carcinoma may have a prominent cribriform component with basement membrane production, it also typically exhibits other growth patterns, including solid, tubular, trabecular, and irregularly invasive arrangements.

Also in the differential diagnosis is the common intraductal carcinoma of cribriform type but that proliferation lacks

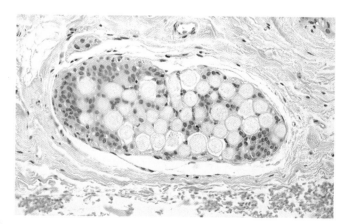

**FIG. 30.** Collagenous spherulosis. An incidental benign intraductal epithelial proliferation.

myoepithelial cells surrounding the luminal spaces as well as intraluminal basement membrane deposition. The rare intraductal carcinoma of signet ring cell type (174) should also be excluded (172) but in these proliferations there are true signet ring cells with malignant nuclear features. Moreover, the signet ring spaces lack immunoreactive collagen type IV. Intraductal (172) and invasive ductal carcinoma (171) and phyllodes tumor (171) have been found in association with collagen spherulosis, but all follow-up data to date suggest that these associations were coincidental (171).

### Multinucleated Stromal Giant Cells

Stromal giant cells may be observed as an incidental, focal, but sometimes multicentric histologic finding in 4.5% of cases (175). The average age of women with this finding is 51 years. This was determined in a series of 200 mastectomies performed for carcinoma, but giant cells may also be found in noncancerous breast tissue (175,176).

Microscopically, atypical stromal giant cells are visible at low power (10×) and are dispersed in the interlobular matrix (175). The nuclei are multiple and hyperchromatic and may show a florette-like arrangement (177). Cytoplasm is scanty. These giant cells resemble fibrohistiocytic cells seen normally in stromal tissue at several other anatomic sites, including the vagina, uterine cervix, and bladder. The immunophenotype of these cells is suggestive of mesenchymal differentiation, as they are often positive for vimentin, $\alpha_1$-antitrypsin, and $\alpha_1$-antichymotrypsin, and negative for cytokeratin, von Willebrand's factor, and S-100 protein (178). Ultrastructurally, the cells have features of fibroblasts (176).

The potential exists to misinterpret atypical stromal giant cells, mainly due to hyperchromasia and high nuclear/cytoplasmic ratio, as neoplastic mesenchymal cells or malignant epithelial cells (175). The giant cells have also been identified in the stroma of fibroadenomas and phyllodes tumors (178) and could be confused with those of fibrous histiocytomas in those settings. In all of these instances the overall architectural and histologic configuration must be considered. Infiltrating carcinomas, particularly those with giant cell features, such as sarcomatoid carcinomas (179) and mammary carcinomas with osteoclast-like giant cells (180), should be readily excluded because they have clearly malignant areas and do not show merely isolated, dispersed giant cells. Moreover, mammary stromal giant cells are morphologically different from the osteoclast-like elements that have been described in mammary carcinoma (180).

The histogenesis of atypical giant cells is not settled, although fibrohistiocytic differentiation is generally accepted (176,177). The clinical significance is that they should not be confused with neoplastic cells; it is doubtful that they constitute any risk factor whatever for future malignancy (177).

## Pseudoangiomatous Stromal Hyperplasia

Pseudoangiomatous stromal hyperplasia (PSH) (181–184) should be separated from vascular and epithelial neoplasms, including hemangiomas, low-grade angiosarcomas, pseudoangiosarcomatous carcinomas, and phyllodes tumors. Clinically, this entity may produce a palpable mass, although it is most often encountered as an incidental histologic finding. It is quite common, with an estimated incidence of 23% (183). The mean patient age is 37–40 years, with a wide range of 14–76 years (181,183). When presenting as palpable masses, PSH was described as firm, nontender, and unilateral (180). Mammographic evaluation often revealed a discrete, dense, homogeneous area indistinguishable from a fibroadenoma (181). Indeed, the most common clinical diagnosis was the latter tumor (181). Rarely, a peau d'orange appearance of the overlying skin may cause clinical concern for inflammatory carcinoma (183,184).

Incidental lesions were seen in 40% of cases in only one microscopic focus but were often multifocal (183). In contrast, mass-producing PSH had a mean size of 6 cm (range 1.2–12 cm) and the lesions were, in general, well-circumscribed, nonencapsulated, firm, lobulated nodules with tan–pink to yellow cut surfaces (181). This appearance has been likened to that of edematous fibroadenoma (135).

Microscopically, PSH manifests a spectrum of mesenchymal tissue alterations (181–184). Typical pseudoangiomatous hyperplasia is characterized by an interanastomosing network of slit-like spaces, which may expand the intralobular stroma and diffusely involve the interlobular regions as well. These spaces are histologic artifacts and represent the separation of stromal collagen from myofibroblasts; therefore, they are not truly vascular channels but rather are mimics thereof. The myofibroblasts lining the numerous spaces are small and devoid of nuclear atypia. The intervening collagen is dense and hyalinized (181,184). More proliferative lesions demonstrate increased stromal cellularity, with an increase in nuclear size and hyperchromasia. At the extreme end of this continuum the cases show fascicular stroma with small bundles of myofibroblastic cells and compression of

the narrow spaces. Keloidal-like fibrosis separates the groups of myofibroblasts.

Differential diagnostic considerations are linked to the cellularity and size of the lesions. With small or microscopic PSH, perilobular hemangioma should also be considered, but the latter lesion most closely resembles a cavernous hemangioma with open rather than narrow spaces. It likewise lacks a prominent intralesional stroma (185,186).

The tumorous form of pseudoangiomatous hyperplasia should be discriminated from hemangiomas, angiosarcomas, myofibroblastomas, phyllodes tumors, and pseudoangiosarcomatous carcinomas. By far the most serious and common mistake is to incorrectly diagnose PSH as a low-grade angiosarcoma. To avoid this problem one should recall that mammary angiosarcoma is a highly infiltrative and permeative growth that has open vascular channels. Pseudoangiomatous stromal hyperplasia shows narrow spaces grouped in a lobulocentric pattern and does not invade the mammary fat. Necrosis, hemorrhage, papillary endothelial growth, and solid spindle cell areas clearly favor a diagnosis of angiosarcoma (183).

Cellular areas of the fascicular type of PSH may bear a histologic likeness to myofibroblastoma, but it has been pointed out that pseudoangiomatous stromal hyperplasia does not have the homogeneous, organized, densely cellular pattern divided by collagen bands that characterizes myofibroblastoma (181). The cellular variant of pseudoangiomatous hyperplasia may also bring phyllodes tumor to mind (181), but PSH lacks a leaf-like growth pattern and the stromal overgrowth seen in phyllodes tumors. Finally, carcinomas of the breast mimicking angiosarcoma (123,187,188) are easily excluded because they are poorly differentiated malignancies and the angiosarcoma-like regions compose only a portion of the neoplasms.

Pseudoangiomatous hyperplasia may complicate fibroadenomas and may be seen adjacent to invasive carcinoma (183). It has been postulated that PSH is a microscopic, exaggerated physiologic response associated with the menstrual cycle but that the tumorous form may acquire a capacity for autonomous growth such as that of a neoplasm (181). This hypothesis awaits confirmation.

## Mucocele-like Lesion (Tumor)

Rupture of mucinous cysts of the breast, with extrusion of mucin and detached benign epithelial fragments in the stroma, may masquerade as mucinous or colloid carcinoma of the breast (189–192). Clinically, patients with such lesions are women between the ages of 25 and 70 (189–192). Most patients present with a mass, although mammographic (192) and incidental (189) detection is also possible. Mammograms done to evaluate tumefactions in this context showed ill-defined masses and scattered calcifications in two of three cases (191). The one incidentally detected mucocele-like lesion measured 0.5 cm.

cytomas. Lastly, the close anatomic relationship with Rathke's cleft cysts and salivary rests speaks for itself in regard to diagnostic importance.

## Rathke's Cleft Cysts

These cysts are usually incidental findings at postmortem examination, where 13–22% of pituitary glands are seen to harbor such expansions of the hypophyseal cleft (224–227). Most incidental cysts are less than 2 mm in size (226). When they achieve sufficient dimensions (usually >1 cm), clinical symptoms such as visual disturbances, hypopituitarism, headache, diabetes insipidus, and diplopia may occur (228). Histologically, Rathke's cleft cysts may be lined with a single layer of a multitude of different epithelial cells, including cuboidal, columnar, ciliated, mucinous, squamous, and adenohypophyseal elements (Fig. 38). Usually, ciliated columnar epithelial cells predominate. True neoplasms do not usually enter into differential diagnosis, but one should be cognizant of the occurrence of pituitary adenomas in conjunction with Rathke's cleft cysts (214).

## Epidermoid Cysts

Intrasellar epidermoid cysts are rare (229,230). Histologically, they contain laminated keratin and are lined with mature, stratified squamous epithelium. A small biopsy may create difficulty in the differential diagnosis with craniopharyngioma, particularly when the latter tumor has a biphasic growth pattern as seen in some cysts (213). The relationship of epidermoid cysts and craniopharyngioma is controversial; some believe that such cysts represent a form of the neoplasm in question (214,219), but most authors consider epidermoid cysts to be malformations (214). Hence, the continued distinction between epidermoid cysts and craniopharyngioma has been recommended (229). Metastatic squamous cell carcinoma and the exceedingly rare primary squamous cell carci-

noma of the pituitary (231) can also be distinguished from epidermoid cysts of the pituitary because of differing degrees of nuclear atypia and architectural disorder in the former two lesions.

## Choristomas and Hamartomas (Gangliocytomas)

Ganglion cell lesions in the pituitary are rare (214,216,217,232–236). The presence of hypothalamic neurons in the hypophysis has been variably thought of as choristomatous, hamartomatous, or neoplastic in nature. Using rigorous terminology, ganglion cells in the normal adenohypophysis constitute sufficient evidence for a choristoma (214). They may be found as minute, asymptomatic foci at autopsy, but more commonly they are discovered in association with an adenoma, and here the designation of adenohypophyseal neuronal choristoma has been applied (214). When associated but not admixed with hyperplastic or adenomatous pituitary tissue, these masses, many of which result in clinical symptoms (usually precocious puberty or acromegaly), have been alternately viewed as either hamartomas or neoplasms (236). In the first of these eventualities, it has been proposed that the neurons express hormone-releasing factors that induce development of the adenoma (233,235), whereas in the second, the postulate is that the neuron-like elements may actually represent transformed adenoma cells (236). One important neoplasm in the differential diagnosis is the ganglioglioma, which, in contrast to gangliocytomas, harbors astroglial elements.

## Hemorrhage and Infarction

Hemorrhagic and necrotic pituitary tissue should be studied in detail to exclude an infarcted pituitary neoplasm. In particular, pituitary adenoma is prone to such alterations (237–240). Hemorrhage into pituitary adenomas has been reported in 10–17% of cases (237–240). Extensive hemorrhage or infarction of an adenoma may result in the clinical syndrome known as pituitary apoplexy, which is characterized by sudden headache, visual impairment, and ophthalmoplegia (240). Between 1% and 10% of patients with pituitary adenomas experience this complication (240). However, hemorrhage and necrosis should not be construed as immutably indicative of a neoplasm (226, 242). They may be seen in many conditions other than infarction of an adenoma, including postpartum hypovolemia, diabetes mellitus, systemic hypertension, hypoparathyroidism, tuberculosis, tetanus, cardiac failure, hemolytic crises, meningitis, temporal arteritis, and intracranial hypertension (240,243). A reticulin stain may be helpful in determining the type of necrotic tissue that is seen (213).

Another potential diagnostic pitfall is represented by squamous metaplasia that may develop adjacent to pituitary necrosis in the postpartum period (241). The squamous metaplastic cells in this setting show reactive cytologic

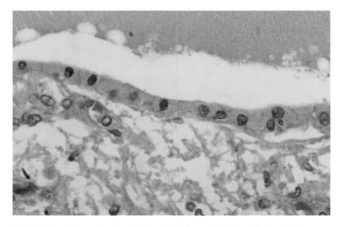

**FIG. 38.** Ciliated cuboidal cell lining of a Rathke's cleft cyst. (Courtesy of Dr. Daniel McKeel.)

atypia and mitotic figures, which should not be taken as evidence of squamous cell carcinoma. Craniopharyngioma should also be excluded in such a case. Finally, cystic change in the pituitary may occur secondary to progressive intermittent infarction, hemorrhage, and necrosis (244). Grossly, three reported cases with this alteration were all initially thought to represent craniopharyngiomas because of brownish black to yellow motor oil–like fluid contents (244). Microscopically, the cysts had a dense connective tissue wall with many hemosiderin-laden macrophages, and adenohypophyseal cells were located immediately adjacent to the lesions. This type of cystic change should be differentiated from that seen in craniopharyngioma and adenoma with secondary cystification.

## Lymphocytic Hypophysitis

Benign lymphocytic infiltrates in the pituitary (lymphocytic hypophysitis) may be mistaken for leukemia or lymphoma involving the pituitary. Lymphocytic hypophysitis is a rare disorder almost always affecting women, usually during pregnancy or immediately postpartum. These patients present with a pituitary mass and variable, progressive loss of corresponding endocrine function (245–251). An autoimmune etiologic basis is suspected because patients may have circulating autoantibodies, thyroiditis, adrenalitis, atrophic gastritis/pernicious anemia, parathyroiditis, or retroperitoneal fibrosis.

Clinical and magnetic resonance imaging (MRI) findings may be suggestive of adenohypophysitis (246) but biopsy is often necessary to establish a firm diagnosis. Most patients have undergone partial pituitary resections or biopsies alone for lymphocytic hypophysitis, but some have had total hypophysectomy when frozen sections were not diagnostic. Grossly, the pituitary tissue in hypophysitis has been described as firm and dull white, gray, yellow, or purple (249). Histologically, the anterior pituitary is involved by a diffuse but variably dense, predominantly lymphocytic infiltrate (Fig. 39). A few admixed plasma cells and eosinophils may be identified. Germinal center formation is present in a few cases. Attendant edema and fibrosis are variable (249). The morphologic differential diagnosis includes a clinically nonfunctional pituitary adenoma with a dense lymphocytic infiltrate, another neoplasm adjacent to lymphocytic hypophysitis (243,250), and secondary leukemia/lymphoma. At autopsy, chronic lymphocytic leukemia (CLL) has been identified in the pituitary in one third of cases (251), but these infiltrates are usually clinically silent and nontumefactive. An exceedingly rare case of CLL with pituitary mass formation (clinically simulating pituitary adenoma) has been reported (252). If confronted with the question of lymphocytic hypophysitis versus a neoplastic lymphocytic infiltrate, immunohistochemistry should be performed on frozen sections to evaluate T- and B-lymphocytic markers and restricted kappa or lambda light chain immunoglobulin ex-

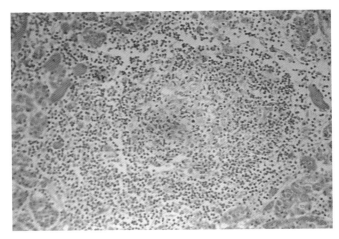

**FIG. 39.** Lymphocytic hypophysitis showing a dense infiltrate of small, bland lymphocytes. (Courtesy of Dr. Daniel McKeel.)

pression as an indicator of clonality. Most examples of lymphocytic hypophysitis show a predominance of T cells in the infiltrate.

## Fibrosclerosing Pseudotumor

Rare cases of fibroinflammatory masses involving the pituitary have been reported (253–256). In two instances (253,254), the pituitary was involved by direct extension of a sphenoidal mass. In all documented cases the patient had a fibrosclerosing mass elsewhere (orbit, mediastinum, retroperitoneum, or testis). Two patients were women aged 54 and 62 years, and two were men aged 26 and 29. One woman presented with symptoms of intermittent meningeal irritation and hypopituitarism, whereas the second had a past medical history of an orbital fibrosing pseudotumor that had been stable for 8 years. She was admitted to the hospital with acute anterior pituitary failure and a 4-day history of anorexia, lethargy, and hypersomnia. Both men complained only of unilateral visual loss. Histologically, the biopsies in each of these cases were remarkable for dense fibrosis and lymphoplasmocytic infiltrates. Scattered eosinophils and neutrophils were seen in two examples. Calcification was present in a single case. In one, there were scattered poorly formed granulomas, raising the possibility of an undetected infection. In fact, it is crucial to exclude both infections and neoplasms before diagnosing an idiopathic fibrosclerosing process, be it of the pituitary, orbit, mediastinum, or retroperitoneum. Morphologically, these multifocal fibrosclerosing lesions may resemble neoplasms because of infiltrative and destructive growth. One should specifically look for malignant cells in the fibrous background, especially malignant lymphoma with sclerosis and metastatic carcinomas with an exuberant fibrogenic response. Again, immunostains may be helpful in this context. A predominance of B lymphocytes is worrisome for bona fide lymphoma, and reactivity for keratin points to a diagnosis of occult carcinoma.

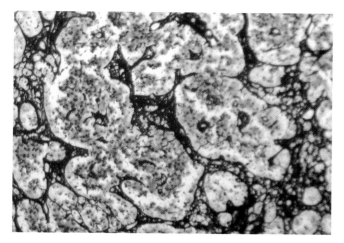

**FIG. 40.** Adenohypophyseal hyperplasia demonstrates a reticulin network around cell clusters. (Courtesy of Dr. Daniel McKeel.)

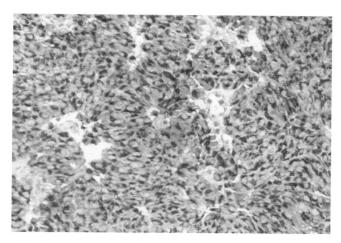

**FIG. 42.** Detection of diffuse prolactin immunoreactivity in a prolactinoma. (Courtesy of Dr. Daniel McKeel.)

## Hyperplasia

Sometimes it is exceedingly difficult to distinguish pituitary hyperplasia from a neoplasm, i.e., adenoma (213,218, 236,257–260). This dilemma derives from several factors, including the regional distribution of some adenohypophyseal cell types, often fragmented and diminutive surgical specimens, and the lack of generally accepted morphologic criteria for use in this setting (259).

Uncommonly, hyperplasia of the pituitary might, even in the absence of adenoma, cause clinical symptoms of pituitary hyperfunction (257). Acromegaly is usually caused by a solitary growth hormone–producing adenoma, but it may also result from synthesis of growth hormone–releasing factor by another endocrine neoplasm with secondary hyperplasia of pituitary growth hormone cells (257). Similarly, most

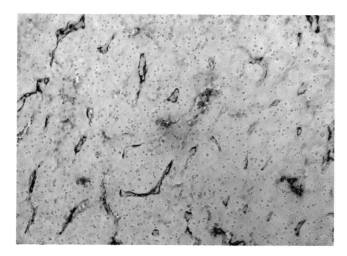

**FIG. 41.** Absence of reticulin staining of pituitary adenoma except for around blood vessels. (Courtesy of Dr. Daniel McKeel.)

cases of Cushing's disease are caused by an adenoma but rare cases show only pituitary hyperplasia or hyperplasia admixed with an adenoma (257). Interestingly, clinically silent prolactin cell hyperplasia is a common incidental finding at autopsy (261).

Histologically, adenohypophyseal hyperplasia may be diffuse or nodular. The former pattern of proliferation is often the normal response to a physiologic stimulation such as pregnancy, lactation, or declining circulating levels of gonadal steroids with aging (259). Somatotroph cell and corticotroph cell hyperplasia typically manifests mixed diffuse and nodular patterns (259). Nodules of hyperplasia tend not to compress surrounding pituitary tissue, whereas sufficiently large adenomas do so. Microadenomas may not cause such compression. Overall, the differential diagnosis of nodular hyperplasia and microadenoma can be difficult or even impossible in small biopsies. Reticulin stains and immunohistochemistry can be most rewarding in making such a distinction (218). In hyperplasia, expanded acini show preserved, continuous reticulin investment of the cell groups (Fig. 40), whereas the reticulin pattern is fragmented and discontinuous to absent in pituitary adenomas (Fig. 41). By immunohistochemical analysis, hyperplasia exhibits the presence of several different hormone-producing cells, with one cell type being most numerous. Adenomas are composed of only one or two types of hormone-producing cells (Fig. 42).

## PARATHYROID

### Variants of Normal Anatomy

The number and location of normal parathyroid glands are variable (262,263). Nonneoplastic parathyroid tissue, if found in an unusual site, may be erroneously diagnosed as a neoplasm, in particular one that is metastatic. Therefore, it is important to be aware that parathyroid tissue might be found, due to embryologic migration pathways, in the superior mediastinum, in the thymus, in the thyroid, in the retropharynx, in a retroesophageal location, in esophageal submucosa, in soft tissue of the neck, and even in the vagus nerve (262–276). The diagnostic criteria for distinguishing non-neoplastic from neoplastic parathyroidal epithelial proliferations in these unusual locations are the same as those applied to proliferations in the usual anatomic sites (see section on hyperplasia). When they are intrathyroidal, nodules of parathyroid hyperplasia could be grossly confused with a primary thyroid tumor.

A rare condition featuring many small nests of cytologically bland hyperplastic parathyroid cells (mostly chief cells) in the soft tissue of the neck and mediastinum and outside hyperplastic glands has been referred to as parathyromatosis. Although the haphazard arrangement of epithelial cell nests in adipose tissue might initially suggest a malignancy, it appears that this condition is merely another form of parathyroid tissue ectopia, with superimposed hyperplasia (277). Similar nests may be seen after previous surgery; here tissue spillage with implantation has been invoked as a mechanism to explain the presence of many histologically benign nests in soft tissue (277–281) (see section on treatment effects). Clinical follow-up on all patients with a diagnosis of parathyromatosis has revealed no evidence of malignant disease.

## Cysts

Clinically detected cysts are uncommon in the parathyroid (282–289). Some are pseudoneoplastic, and represent either congenital, embryologic abnormalities with cystic change in the third or fourth branchial cleft remnants, or acquired cystic change in normal or hyperplastic glands. Other examples represent parathyroid adenomas with secondary cystic alteration, which occurs in 9% of such lesions (284). Yet other cases are indeterminate, where it may not be possible to clinically or morphologically ascertain the original nature of parathyroid tissue that has undergone cystification.

Clinically, parathyroid cysts usually present in patients of either sex in the fifth or sixth decade of life (age range 27–72), as either asymptomatic neck masses or with hypercalcemia, hypophosphatemia, and elevated levels of serum parathyroid hormone (286). This has led to a clinical classification of parathyroid cysts as functional or nonfunctional. Large cysts may cause dyspnea, hoarseness, or dysphagia. Hemorrhage into such lesions has been reported as a rare cause of sudden severe pain, with attendant increase in the cyst size (283). The preoperative clinical diagnosis is often that of a thyroid nodule or adenoma, an impression that is buttressed by radiologic findings (285,288).

Intraoperatively, most parathyroid cysts are located in the neck near the lower pole of thyroid and appear loosely attached to it or to the thymic tongue, but with a definite cleav-

age plane. A few cysts have also been found in the mediastinum.

Grossly, nonneoplastic cysts qualify as pseudoneoplasms because their distinction from a parathyroid adenoma with cystic change may not be possible. Parathyroid cysts vary in size from 1 to 10 cm, with an average size of 3.9 cm in one series (286). They typically have a smooth and fluctuant outer surface, with a grayish-white translucent cyst wall. The contents are characteristically clear and serous, although rare cysts contain bloody fluid due to the above-mentioned complication of hemorrhage. The inner surface of the wall is smooth; one should specifically search for solid nodules that could represent adenomatous tissue.

Microscopically, the cyst wall is composed of fibrous tissue with embedded, diagnostic islands of parathyroid cells. An inner lining of cuboidal parathyroid cells may be evident as well. If elements of thymic tissue are present, with neither parathyroid nor thymic tissue predominating, a diagnosis of third pharyngeal pouch cyst may be made (287).

The main differential diagnostic problem is exclusion of a parathyroid adenoma with cystic change. Minute foci of cystification occur in up to 50% of normal parathyroid glands (290,291), but this change is of insufficient magnitude to attract clinical attention. Also, these are not hyperfunctioning glands. Cystic change in adenomas occurs in 9% (284) to many (263) cases. Such lesions are smaller than those reported for nonadenomatous cysts, with a range of 0.1–1.0 cm in diameter. The distinction between normal or hyperplastic parathyroidal epithelium from an adenoma may be particularly difficult in the setting of epithelial distortion and compression secondary to pressure effects from the cyst. The separation must be made at the clinicopathologic level, as discussed below in the section on hyperplasia.

## Hamartoma

Those cases designated in the past as hamartoma of the parathyroid (292,293) actually represent a type of adenoma, i.e., lipoadenoma, of the parathyroid gland (294–299). When benign thymic tissue is admixed, the term "lipothymoadenoma" has been employed (300).

## Chronic Parathyroiditis

Incidentally detected, perivascular, lymphocytic infiltrates in the parathyroid are found in up to 10% of glands at postmortem examination (301). However, dense infiltrates with coexisting hyperplasia and resultant clinical hyperparathyroidism are rare (302–304). An intriguing speculation is that the etiologic basis for this condition may be an autoimmune one. Histologically, the infiltrate is lymphoplasmocytic with lymphoid follicles and germinal centers. A small biopsy might result in concern over a lymphoid malignancy, but the mixed infiltrate with true germinal center formation should allow the histopathologist to exclude involvement of the parathyroid gland by leukemia or lymphoma (305), which is usually an incidental finding in the context of clinically obvious, widely disseminated disease. Further support for a benign diagnosis may be sought by immunohistochemical demonstration of a mixed population of T (CD45RO+) and B (CD20+) lymphocytes (304).

## Hyperplasia

Hyperplasia of the parathyroid may closely resemble an adenoma. Historically, diagnostic separation of these two entities has been challenging for surgeons and pathologists alike (263,264,305–311). The diagnosis of parathyroid hyperplasia is a clinicopathologic one, with a description of intraoperative findings by the surgeon essential (262,263). The clinical presentations of parathyroid hyperplasia and adenoma with glandular hyperfunction are similar. Both chief cell hyperplasia and adenoma may occur in the setting of multiple endocrine neoplasia (MEN) syndrome (263), but clear cell hyperplasia is not typically associated with MEN.

Grossly, a distinction between hyperplasia and adenoma based on glandular size, shape, color, or consistency is not possible (305). The intraoperative assessment of the number of enlarged glands is a key diagnostic requirement. The vast majority of adenomas involve a single gland, whereas the presence of two or more enlarged glands suggests hyperplasia. As noted 26 years ago (307), this pattern of involvement is not always clear. Large, nodular, hyperplastic parathyroids may be accompanied by smaller yet hyperplastic glands in a pseudoadenoma pattern (307). In an occult group of hyperplasia cases, all glands seem relatively small (307). Grossly, glands with chief cell hyperplasia vary from minimally enlarged to expansive masses with smooth contours or large, firm, irregular, and nodular dark tan glands with occasional pseudopodial extensions (309). Clear cell hyperplasia has a similar macroscopic image but usually exhibits a marked increase in the size of all glands, with preferential enlargement of the upper parathyroids (263,309,312). Cut surfaces in the latter condition usually are homogeneous and yellow–brown to red, and nodularity and cystic change are often seen (307).

Microscopically, two types of hyperplasia are recognized, i.e., chief cell and clear cell types (263,305–312). Chief cell hyperplasia classically shows nodular (more often) or diffuse arrangement of cords, sheets, and follicles, with replacement of stromal fat cells microscopically. Because the nodular expansion may be similar to the configuration of an adenoma (Fig. 43), the term "pseudoadenomatous hyperplasia" has also been applied. Chief cells may be seen as a pure population but there is also commonly a mixture of oxyphil cells and transitional cells (309). The rare clear cell hyperplasia exhibits a diffuse and uniform distribution of large cells, 8–40 μm in diameter, with distinct intercellular borders and lucent cytoplasm (Fig. 44) (263,309). Stromal fat

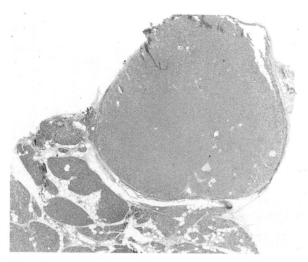

**FIG. 43.** Nodular hyperplasia of the parathyroid, with large nodule composed of oxyphilic cells and smaller nodules of chief cells.

and oxyphil cells are absent. Focal nuclear enlargement (Fig. 45) should not be equated with neoplastic transformation.

The microscopic differences between parathyroid hyperplasia and adenoma in a single gland may be difficult or impossible to discern. One important observation is that of a normal rim of compressed normal parathyroid tissue adjacent to adenomas (291,306,308), but this cap is not present in all adenomas (291), particularly larger ones (263). Moreover, compressed hyperplastic tissue adjacent to nodular hyperplasia may closely mimic a compressed rim of normal parathyroid (309). The use of intraoperative fat stains has been recommended as a means to discriminate between hyperplasia and adenoma (313). In one study (313), examination of two complete glands, with a modified oil red O stain for fat led to accurate classification in 92% of cases. The fat stain was reported to be particularly helpful in identifying

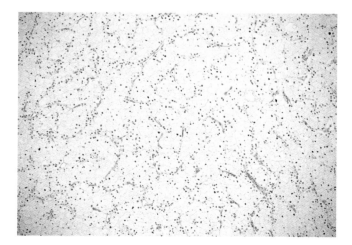

**FIG. 44.** Clear cell hyperplasia of the parathyroid. Out of context, clear cell neoplasms such as renal cell carcinoma might be diagnosed.

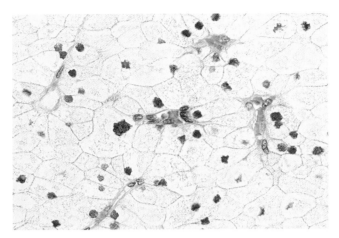

**FIG. 45.** Focal nuclear atypia in clear cell hyperplasia of the parathyroid.

remnants of normal parathyroid tissue adjacent to adenomas (313). Given the variability in the fat content of normal glands (314), however, caution is advised in interpretation of these stains.

Currently, adjunctive techniques do not contribute diagnostic information to this area of differential diagnosis. For example, DNA content (315), cellular proliferation markers (315), and determinations of clonality (317) do not reliably separate hyperplasia from adenoma. It remains to be determined whether molecular genetic findings (318) will be useful in this setting.

### Treatment Effects

Implantation of parathyroid tissue may occur after spillage of benign cells at surgery, resulting in parathyromatosis, or the presence of multiple nodules of hyperfunctioning parathyroid tissue in the neck and mediastinum (see above) (277–281). The rare reported cases of this phenomenon have usually occurred after operative removal of an adenoma, although a few cases were of hyperplasia (see literature review in ref. 280). Because of the multifocal nature of such nodules with an infiltrative growth pattern into soft tissue, the question of parathyroid carcinoma may be raised. Histologically, however, parathyromatosis shows bland morphologic features without evidence of angiolymphatic invasion or numerous mitoses, which are expected in locally recurrent parathyroid carcinomas (263). Clinical follow-up of parathyromatosis cases has revealed a benign course, whereas 30% of patients with parathyroid carcinoma suffer metastatic disease (263,319).

Lastly, hyperplastic parathyroid tissue may histologically resemble malignancy after it is autotransplanted into the forearm (320). Nests of parathyroid cells may be found at a distance from the main mass of the allograft and may exhibit an infiltrative pattern of growth into skeletal muscle (321). In sum, the pathologic findings in that specific context are much like those of parathyromatosis.

### THYROID GLAND

#### Variants of Normal Anatomy

As is true of the parathyroid, identification of thyroid tissue outside its normal location may prompt consideration of neoplastic disease. An understanding of the variation in the anatomic distribution of thyroid tissue is based on knowledge of the embryologic development of the thyroid gland (322–325). Ectopic locations of thyroid tissue may be traced to failure of descent or overdescent during normal development. Maldescent can lead to the presence of thyroid tissue anywhere along the pathway of the thyroglossal duct, i.e., from the oropharynx along the midline to the thyroid isthmus (323,326). The base of the tongue is the most common ectopic location (327–331), followed by sublingual and perihyoid localization (326). Lingual thyroid tissue is present in 10% of routine necropsies (327,328), but symptomatic expression of that finding is uncommon or rare.

The most common presenting symptoms are those of dysphagia, dysphonia, and dyspnea (329). Biopsy of these clinically significant nodules may reveal normal thyroid tissue, thyroiditis, hyperplasia, adenoma, or, rarely, carcinoma (328). Histologically, nonneoplastic thyroidal follicles may simulate malignancy because of dispersion between muscle fibers of the tongue (326,330,331). Furthermore, no capsule is present. It has been emphasized that in comparison to the profiles of carcinoma, benign follicles interdigitating between the skeletal muscle fibers of the tongue do not elicit a demoplastic response (325). Ectopic thyroid tissue can also be found in other locations, including the trachea, heart, pericardium, retroesophageal soft tissue, thymic territory, aortic arch, diaphragm, gallbladder, common bile duct, retroperitoneum, vagina, sella turcica, inguinal region, and duodenum (326,332–338). It is difficult to explain the presence of thyroid tissue outside of the head, neck, and mediastinum on an embryologic basis; some of these implants could be teratomatous in nature (325).

Ectopic thyroid tissue in the midline can also be found in up to 45% of thyroglossal duct abnormalities, such as ducts, cysts, or fistulas (339). These lesions could grossly cause concern over a metastatic thyroid carcinoma with cystic change or carcinoma developing in a thyroglossal abnormality. In this instance, macroscopically solid areas or papillary excrescences should be well sampled because these could represent carcinoma (usually of the papillary type) in a thyroglossal duct abnormality. This is an uncommon finding, seen in only 2% of thyroglossal abnormalities (339,341). Microscopically, the distinction between benign thyroid tissue and carcinoma involving a thyroglossal duct cyst should be straightforward because carcinomas tend to invade adjacent tissue (339).

Ectopic thyroid tissue lateral to the jugular vein, when *unassociated* with a lymph node, may represent dissociated nonneoplastic thyroid tissue that has become detached from the gland by inflammation, fibrosis, trauma, or surgery (see below sections on thyroiditis and treatment effects). When found in a lymph node in the same region, normal-appearing thyroid tissue invariably represents metastatic follicular-variant papillary carcinoma (323). Previously, the term "aberrant lateral thyroid" had been used for all thyroid tissues, benign or malignant, that were located lateral to the thyroid gland. This terminology is imprecise and should be abandoned.

Solid cell nests of the thyroid represent remnants of ultimobranchial bodies (343–350). They are incidental, microscopic structures found in anywhere from 3% to 61% of thyroid glands, depending on the extent of sampling (345). These inclusions are usually single, but may be multiple (345,349), and range from 0.08 to 1.0 mm in maximal diameter (349). Most measure about 0.1 mm (324) and are usually located in the middle or occasionally the upper third of the lateral thyroid lobes (345). Histologically, the nests are positioned between thyroid follicles and are composed of squamoid or basaloid polygonal cells with eosinophilic cytoplasm, round, oval or fusiform nuclei, and scant cytoplasm (Fig. 46). At the periphery of solid cell nests, cells with cleared cytoplasm and rounded nuclei are often evident (345). Intercellular bridges are lacking. Although the aggregates are usually solid, microcystic change and formation of true lumina with mucinous (Alcian blue/mucicarmine-positive) cells and secretions are common. Some solid cell nests are directly connected with follicles and are termed mixed follicles. By immunohistochemistry, low molecular keratin, carcinoembryonic antigen (CEA), and somatostatin have been localized to the epidermoid-like cells (so-called main cells), whereas the cells with clear cytoplasm (C cells) have exhibited positivity for calcitonin, chromogranin, and calcitonin gene–related peptide (343,345–347). Thyroglobulin is usually absent.

Solid cell nests should be distinguished from papillary microcarcinoma, medullary carcinoma, and micrometastases to the thyroid, particularly metastatic basaloid squamous cell carcinoma (345). Papillary microcarcinomas, like solid cell

nests, are common incidental findings (in 4–37% of thyroid glands) (324,351) but, in contrast to the latter lesions, they harbor the typical nuclear alterations of papillary carcinoma (optical clearing and grooving), with or without psammoma bodies and obvious papillae. At one time, solid cell nests were postulated to be a latent form of medullary carcinoma (352), but this premise is currently regarded as untrue. Metastatic squamous carcinoma cells in the thyroid show vascular invasion and cytologic atypia, whereas solid cell nests do not.

Rarely, mature benign adipose tissue, skeletal muscle, or cartilage may be discovered in the thyroid gland (324, 326,343,353,354). This heterotopia should not be confused with a mesenchymal neoplasm or mesenchymal differentiation in an epithelial neoplasm such as an adenoma or a sarcomatoid carcinoma (355). An association with solid cell nests suggests a mechanism of embryologic maldevelopment for the appearance of these mesenchymal tissues in the thyroid (343).

**Hamartoma and Teratoma**

Hamartomas and teratomas are rarities in the thyroid gland. Lipomatous and chondromatous hamartomas have been described (356,357) but may instead represent adipose metaplasia of interfollicular mesenchyme (354) and teratomatous lesions (325), respectively.

Teratomas of the thyroid occur most often in children under the age of 1 year (358–360). Most are present in the fetus *in utero* and may be associated with polyhydramnios. Due to their large size, they can cause interference with breathing or swallowing at birth (359). Many of these are huge midline masses that presumably involve the thyroid only due to their general anatomic location, but microscopic evidence of thyroid tissue is lacking (358–360). Regardless of whether these lesions are classified as thyroidal teratomas or cervical teratomas, the biological behavior is the same, i.e., benign (360). Thyroidal teratomas of childhood are typically cystic and multiloculated with only focally solid areas. Microscopically, an admixture of all three germ layers, with mature elements, allows for a confident diagnosis of teratoma and the exclusion of another neoplasm.

Teratomas of the thyroid in adulthood are different from those of infancy because malignant neoplasms have been identified therein in most cases. Although these have been reported as malignant germ cell neoplasms, it seems that many, and perhaps most, of these cases are not germinal in nature at all (324) but rather represent other tumor types such as malignant primitive neuroepithelial neoplasms and spindle cell epithelial tumors with thymus-like differentiation (SETTLE) (361).

**Thyroiditis**

Certain inflammatory and fibrosing diseases of the thyroid may assume pseudoneoplastic morphologic guises. Fore-

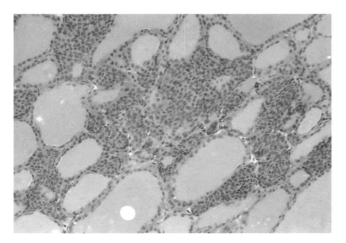

**FIG. 46.** Solid cell nests of the thyroid are remnants of ultimobranchial bodies.

most among these are granulomatous thyroiditis, lymphocytic thyroiditis, Hashimoto's thyroiditis, and Riedel's thyroiditis (362–366).

Granulomatous (also known as de Quervain's or subacute [painful]) thyroiditis occurs in middle-aged women (in 80% of cases) who present with the abrupt onset of significant, unilateral, anterior neck pain, typically after a viral prodrome (362). On physical examination, the thyroid is enlarged, exquisitely tender, and firm in the acute phase. The clinical manifestations of this transient, probably virally induced inflammatory disease vary widely (367,370). A tissue diagnosis is rarely necessary, unless a nodule raises the possibility of a neoplasm. Grossly, granulomatous thyroiditis may bear a resemblance to carcinoma (371), particularly when adhesions to adjacent structures are present (370–372). However, this degree of adherence is not like that of Riedel's thyroiditis, which often exhibits extraglandular infiltration and loss of tissue planes. Grossly, the thyroid in granulomatous thyroiditis is moderately enlarged, and involvement may be unilateral or bilateral. The affected regions are tough to firm or even hard and gritty, and cut surfaces are white to yellow–white (370,371). The microscopic appearance depends on the age of the lesion. Early, a neutrophilic infiltrate of the epithelium is accompanied by necrosis. Later multi-nucleated giant cells ring and then replace follicles and engulf colloid, with eventual progression to scarification (370–373). The authors have seen at least one case in which late-stage de Quervain's disease resembled a fibrohistiocytic neoplasm histologically.

Both lymphocytic and Hashimoto's thyroiditis are manifestations of autoimmune thyroiditis (322,324–326, 374–376). Focal lymphocytic thyroiditis is a common incidental finding at autopsy, with an incidence of 38% when the entire thyroid is available for histologic examination (377). Interestingly, the degree of inflammation correlates directly with the presence and titer of microsomal autoantibodies in that disease (377). Clinically, lymphocytic thyroiditis can present in children as an asymptomatic goiter (374) or in middle-aged adults, predominantly women, with mild signs and symptoms of hyperthyroidism (375). Needle biopsies of the former, so-called juvenile form have revealed lymphoplasmocytic infiltrates with follicular atrophy, fibrosis, and variable oxyphilic change and lymphoid follicle formation (325–375). Biopsies of the latter variant of lymphocytic thyroiditis, also termed silent or painless thyroiditis with hyperthyroidism, are similar but show focal oxyphilic change and follicular hyperplasia rather than atrophy (324,375). The prominent lymphocytic infiltrate may stimulate differential diagnostic consideration of lymphoma (see below).

Hashimoto's thyroiditis, also known as struma lymphomatosa, chronic lymphocytic thyroiditis with oxyphilia, or classic autoimmune thyroiditis, most commonly affects middle-aged women and usually leads to goiter formation. There is often a progression from a euthyroid to a hypothyroid state. In this clinical setting, high titers of antithyroid peroxidase (formerly antimicrosomal) or antithyroglobulin

antibodies strongly suggests a diagnosis of Hashimoto's thyroiditis. Usually a biopsy is necessary only if a neoplasm is suspected, based on rapid enlargement of the gland with a hard nodule or fixation. Grossly, Hashimoto's thyroiditis is not likely to masquerade as carcinoma. The gland is diffusely enlarged and firm, and is actually most reminiscent of a hyperplastic lymph node (326). The capsule is intact with or without adhesions. Only rarely is there a solitary, dominant nodule (378). Microscopically, the paramount findings are those of a dense lymphoplasmocytic infiltrate with germinal center formation and diffuse oxyphilic change in the follicular epithelial cells (Fig. 47).

Several diagnostic pitfalls attend this disorder. First, it is possible to confuse, both grossly and microscopically, thyroid glands that are involved by Hashimoto's thyroiditis with lymph nodes. In this instance the thyroid follicles may be misinterpreted as metastatic carcinoma! Second, further diagnostic complications may ensue if one notices that the epithelial cell nuclei are focally optically clear and overlapping (326), thereby raising the specter of follicular variant papillary carcinoma. Third, islands of squamous metaplasia in fibrous tissue may be mistaken for foci of carcinoma in the fibrous variant of Hashimoto's thyroiditis (379). Fourth, the widespread oxyphilic cytoplasmic change in follicular epithelial cells may be perceived as a Hurthle cell neoplasm (380) (Fig. 48). Fifth, because of the degree of lymphoid infiltration, lymphoma may be misdiagnosed, particularly in small biopsy samples (380). Indeed, a lymphoma-like variant of Hashimoto's thyroiditis has been described (381). True reactive germinal centers, a mixed cell population, and lack of effacement of thyroidal architecture aid in the diagnosis of a benign lymphoid infiltrate. In some cases in which fine needle aspiration biopsy has been done, the cytologic distinction between lymphoma and the lymphocytic infiltrate of Hashimoto's thyroiditis may, however, be impossible (380). Immunophenotypic (CD2, CD4, CD20, CD8, kappa and lambda light chain immunoglobulins) and molec-

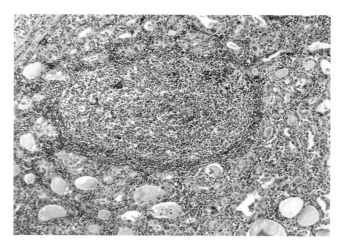

**FIG. 47.** Hashimoto's thyroiditis with characteristic germinal center formation and diffuse oxyphilic cell alteration.

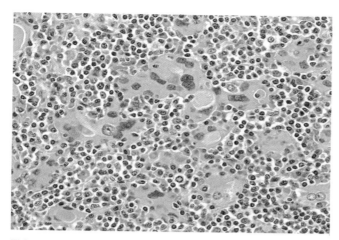

**FIG. 48.** Cytologic atypia in oxyphilic cells in Hashimoto's thyroiditis should not be interpreted as a neoplastic condition.

ular genetic (immunoglobulin and T-cell receptor [B chain] gene rearrangement) analyses of fresh tissue have shown that the lymphocytes in Hashimoto's thyroiditis are polyclonal, whereas lymphomas involving the thyroid demonstrate monotypism (382). A final potential pitfall is that psammoma bodies have been identified in fine needle aspiration biopsies of Hashimoto's thyroiditis (383). These structures are an important indicator of the existence of papillary carcinoma and have only rarely been found in benign thyroid glands. In cytologic material, they are highly suggestive, but not diagnostic, of papillary carcinoma in the absence of additional morphologic features such as fibrovascular cores, optically clear nuclei, and intranuclear cytoplasmic inclusions (383).

Yet another level of diagnostic complexity is introduced when excluding a neoplasm in the setting of Hashimoto's thyroiditis. This statement refers to the increased risk these patients have for developing thyroid lymphoma and epithelial malignancies alike, including papillary carcinoma, Hurthle cell carcinoma, and sclerosing mucoepidermoid thyroid carcinoma (384–390).

Riedel's thyroiditis, also known as invasive fibrous thyroiditis, sclerosing thyroiditis, or Riedel's struma, is an extremely rare inflammatory and fibrosclerosing disease that may be associated with other fibroinflammatory processes. The latter include mediastinal fibrosis, retroperitoneal fibrosis, sclerosing cholangitis, and orbital pseudotumor (368, 391–396). Most patients are middle-aged (mean 48 years, range 23–77) women (66–83% of patients) who present with a gradually or rapidly increasing goiter (368,395). The mass produced may cause dyspnea or dysphagia (368,395). Most patients are euthyroid but some eventually become hypothyroid due to destruction of thyroid tissue. Clinically and grossly, there may be profound concern over malignancy because the mass is stony hard and fixed to adjacent structures, such as strap muscles, the carotid sheaths, the trachea, and the nerves. Usually the process involves only a portion of the thyroid gland and breaches the thyroid capsule. Microscopi-

cally, there is extensive destruction and replacement of follicular tissue by hyalinized fibrous tissue, sometimes keloid-like, with a patchy lymphoplasmocytic infiltrate (Fig. 49). This disorder extends into the perithyroidal soft tissue and splays skeletal muscle fibers. A supportive diagnostic finding is that of vasculitis (mainly phlebitis). Although the gross findings are more worrisome than the histologic features, one should be certain to exclude lymphoma and carcinoma with extensive sclerosis, just as for the allied disorders of mediastinal and retroperitoneal fibrosis. It is additionally notable that a markedly fibrous stroma is a common feature of papillary carcinoma (324).

### Hyperplasia

C-cell hyperplasia and follicular cell hyperplasia, with both nodular and papillary growth patterns, may be confused with and difficult to separate from epithelial neoplasia. It is associated with a number of conditions, including multiple endocrine neoplasia (MEN) types 2A and 2B, hypercalcemia (principally caused by hyperparathyroidism), hypergastrinemia (as in Zollinger–Ellison syndrome), Hashimoto's thyroiditis, estrogen ingestion, cimetidine treatment, solid cell nests, follicular tumors, and papillary neoplasms (397,398). In the MEN syndromes it is diffuse and multifocal, and considered preneoplastic. At the same time, one must realize that C-cell hyperplasia, including large nodules of C-cells (defined as aggregates of 85-343 C cells) (399), may be an incidental finding at autopsy (399–401). This process is not grossly apparent. Microscopically, peak concentrations of C cells are found near the junction of the middle and upper thirds of the lateral lobes (400). These cells are large and polygonal, and are disposed as intrafollicular clusters that may encircle the follicles without disruption of the follicular epithelium (Fig. 50). Nodular C-cell hyperplasia is characterized by complete obliteration of the follicular spaces (402). C cells may be difficult to identify and distinguish

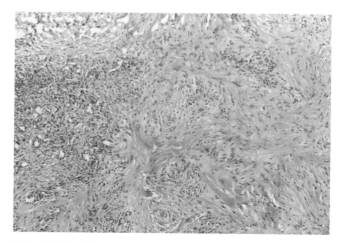

**FIG. 49.** Riedel's thyroiditis is an inflammatory and fibrosclerosing disease.

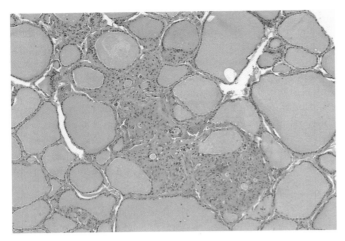

**FIG. 50.** C-cell hyperplasia of the thyroid in a patient with multiple endocrine neoplasia syndrome.

from tangentially cut follicular epithelium in H&E-stained sections (323). Immunostaining for calcitonin or CEA is then invaluable in the definitive identification of these elements and in their quantitation.

The differential diagnosis of C-cell hyperplasia versus minute medullary carcinoma may be a challenging one. Disruption or loss of the basal lamina is a key feature for diagnosis of microinvasive medullary carcinoma involving the interstitium (402,403). Assessment of this structural boundary may be accomplished by either electron microscopy (402) or immunostaining for collagen type IV (Fig. 51) (403). The latter technique allows for a larger tissue survey in a more cost-effective fashion (403).

Follicular hyperplasia may be either diffuse or nodular, and may or may not possess a papillary component. Three major clinicopathologic types of hyperplasia are recognized: dyshormogenetic goiter, Graves' disease, and nodular hyperplasia (326). Another approach to classification of these follicular lesions is to segregate hyperplastic goiter (which is

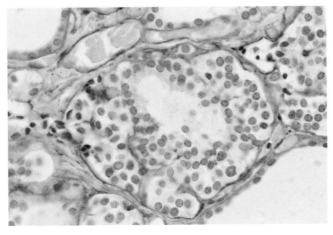

**FIG. 51.** Complete collagen IV investment of hyperplastic C-cell aggregates, as revealed by immunohistochemistry.

associated with dyshormonogenesis, Graves' disease, trophoblastic disease, and pituitary disease) from nodular goiter of the toxic and nontoxic types (325).

Follicular hyperplasia in dyshormonogenetic goiter may be caused by a number of different hereditary genetic errors in thyroid hormone metabolism, including constitutive activation of the thyrotropin receptor caused by a mutation in the thyrotropin receptor gene (404), an iodine transport defect, an organification abnormality, a coupling defect, a thyroglobulin aberration, a deiodinase deficiency, and abnormalities of thyroid hormone transport (325). Grossly, the glands in this condition are enlarged and usually nodular, with microcysts often being noted on inspection of the cut surfaces (405). Most glands are multinodular with degenerative changes such as hemorrhage and cystic alteration, but uncommon cases are diffusely hyperplastic with a single dominant nodule (405). Histologically, the usual pattern in the nodules is trabecular/microfollicular. Papillary areas are, however, also common. As discussed subsequently, solitary hyperplastic nodules and papillary hyperplasia (as may be observed in dyshormonogenetic goiter) constitute common pseudoneoplastic changes in the thyroid. Only rarely is dyshormonogenetic goiter associated with the development of carcinoma (405,406).

Graves' disease (diffuse toxic goiter, Basedow's disease, thyrotoxicosis) is one of the most common causes of hyperthyroidism, which typically produces complaints of nervousness, heat intolerance, weight loss (despite an increased appetite), sweating, palpitations, and diarrhea (407,408). The clinical faces of hyperthyroidism are many (407,408). The surgical pathologist most commonly examines thyroid tissues showing Graves' disease after a subtotal thyroidectomy is performed (408). Grossly, there is a little cause for concern for a neoplasm because the gland is diffusely enlarged without nodules (322). Histologically, however, there is a variable degree of diffuse papillary hyperplasia (Fig. 52), with focal oxyphilic cells, colloid depletion, potential micronodularity, minimal inflammation, and occasional germinal centers (409,410). Most commonly, the patient will have undergone treatment prior to surgical excision. $^{131}$I therapy produces adenomatous nodules, inflammation, cystic change, and oxyphilic cell change with nuclear atypia (411). The last-cited of these changes should not be mistaken for a neoplasm.

Graves' disease may also present the false front of a neoplasm because of the presence of hyperplastic thyroidal tissue in skeletal muscle near the thyroid (326). In distinguishing papillary hyperplasia (as a pseudoneoplasm) from papillary carcinoma, the diagnostician should pay attention to both architectural and cytologic properties (412–414). Hyperplastic papillae evolve by an exaggeration of follicular hyperplasia into papillary change, where infoldings of tall columnar cells are produced without true fibrovascular cores, although there may be centrally edematous or paucicellular stroma (412). In contrast, truly neoplastic papillae contain fibrovascular cores mantled by crowded, oval nuclei

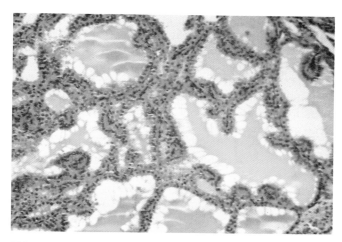

**FIG. 52.** Papillary hyperplasia and colloid depletion in Graves' disease.

(412). Papillae are seen in thyroidal epithelial hyperplasia in Graves' disease, Hashimoto's disease, and nodular hyperplasia. Features of those structures that distinguish them from the papillae of papillary carcinoma include a short length and stubby appearance, lack of branching, and a tendency for the papillary tips to be oriented toward the centers of cystic spaces (414). The lining epithelial cells in hyperplasia have basal, round, and uniform nuclei that are nonoverlapping and generally lack optical clearing, nuclear grooving, and pseudoinclusions. It should be remembered that these traits, while reliable, are not absolutely specific for malignancy (414–417). For example, focally and sometimes extensively lucent nuclei, also termed "ground glass nuclei" or "Orphan Annie eye nuclei," may be observed in Graves' disease, Hashimoto's thyroiditis, and nodular hyperplasia (414). It is important to discriminate truly clear nuclei from pseudoclear nuclei (415). Nuclear grooves, although usually less abundant, may still be seen in nonneoplastic diseases of the thyroid (416,417). Alcian blue histochemical staining and epithelial membrane antigen immunostaining have been forwarded as means to distinguish benign from malignant papillary thyroidal proliferations (418), but ultimately this decision must be based on a constellation of morphologic findings.

Nodular hyperplasia (adenomatous hyperplasia, adenomatoid goiter, nodular or multinodular goiter) has the potential to be confused with follicular and papillary neoplasms of the thyroid. As discussed above, papillary hyperplasia may occur in that condition. In this context, the presence of the above-cited nuclear alterations as well as the occasional presence of psammoma bodies (419) may create movement down an incorrect diagnostic pathway.

The differential diagnosis of a solitary hyperplastic nodule versus a follicular neoplasm may be a formidable one (325,326). Grossly, thyroid glands with nodular hyperplasia are usually enlarged and multinodular with evidence of degenerative changes, including hemorrhage, fibrosis, calcification, and cystic change (326,420). Microscopically, the

hyperplastic nodules tend to have an incomplete capsule, and the follicles resemble those seen in the internodular thyroidal tissue, although this is not always the case (Fig. 53). In contrast, follicular adenomas have a propensity for uninodularity, complete encapsulation, compression of surrounding thyroidal tissue, and uniform follicles that are frequently smaller than those of the surrounding normal thyroid (326). Compared to adenomas, hyperplastic nodules have a lower proliferation index (421), and lower adenylate cyclase activity (422), and are more likely to be polyclonal (423). Whether such tests will become practical diagnostic tools will require further investigation.

Physicians should be aware that in rare cases, nodules of hyperplastic thyroid tissue have been identified *without* associated lymph node tissue, in the lateral neck of patients with multinodular goiter (424). This phenomenon has been termed "sequestered nodular goiter." The operant mechanism here may well be mechanical separation of benign nodules from the multinodular goiter (424). Careful clinical exclusion of metastatic carcinoma is obviously well advised in this setting.

Finally, one should not make an erroneous diagnosis of vascular neoplasia or angiomatoid carcinoma (425) when confronted with reactive endothelial cell hyperplasia in nodular hyperplasia, a process that is present in about 2% of multinodular goiters (426).

## Inflammatory Myofibroblastic Pseudotumor (Plasma Cell Granuloma)

Plasma cell granuloma, now known as inflammatory myofibroblastic pseudotumor (73), occurs rarely in the thyroid (427–429). Three patients, aged 35–70 years, have been reported with an enlarging neck mass. In one case (429), it was sufficiently large to produce dyspnea. Grossly, the masses measured 3–9 cm in greatest dimension and were firm, ho-

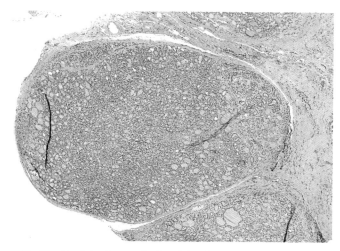

**FIG. 53.** Nodular hyperplasia of the thyroid with microfollicular proliferation.

mogeneous, and gray to white. Histologically, they were plasma cell–rich lesions with cellular fibrous tissue also being described in one case (427). These masses could present the facade of a plasmacytic neoplasm, and immunohistochemical studies for immunoglobulins IgG, IgA, IgM, and kappa and lambda light chains are helpful in excluding that possibility. In all cases of thyroidal plasma cell granuloma, a polyclonal plasma cell population was present.

### Malakoplakia

A single case of malakoplakia of the thyroid has been reported in a 50-year-old Japanese woman who presented initially with fever and abdominal pain and was later found to have a neck mass (430). Grossly, a right thyroid lobectomy specimen contained a 1.5-cm, well-demarcated, yellow–white mass with a central cystic cavity. Light microscopic examination showed sheets of van Hansemann's histiocytes with Michaelis–Guttmann bodies. Electron microscopy revealed characteristic bacilliform bodies. The histiocytes of malakoplakia may superficially resemble areas in one of the many thyroidal neoplasms with clear cell features, such as oncocytic neoplasms, follicular neoplasms, papillary neoplasms, and even metastatic renal cell carcinoma (324). Nevertheless, negative keratin stains in malakoplakia would exclude these other possibilities.

### Sinus Histiocytosis with Massive Lymphadenopathy (Rosai–Dorfman Disease)

Sinus histiocytosis with massive lymphadenopathy (Rosai–Dorfman disease) has been rarely reported in the thyroid gland (431). As noted earlier in the section on Rosai–Dorfman disease in the breast, melanoma, carcinoma, and Hodgkin's disease are all diagnostic alternatives in this setting. The proper approach to their exclusion is discussed above.

### Treatment Effects

Irradiation of the thyroid causes a spectrum of epithelial proliferations, from hyperplasia to adenoma to carcinoma (432–434), as well as lymphoid infiltration and fibrosis (433). Cytologic atypia, including nuclear enlargement, nuclear membranous irregularities, nuclear crowding, and single, prominent nucleoli, has been observed in adenomatous nodules in the thyroid after cervical irradiation for lymphoma (435). In each reported case, pathologic consultation had been requested to rule out carcinoma.

## PANCREAS

### Variants of Normal Anatomy

Heterotopic pancreatic tissue may be found in the stomach, duodenum, jejunum, ileum (including Meckel's diverticula), gallbladder, umbilicus, fallopian tube, mediastinum, and hilum of the spleen (436–445). The first three sites are by far the most common. The incidence at autopsy is 1–14% (443,444) and at abdominal surgery roughly 0.2% of cases (436,443). Many of these ectopias are incidental findings, and while a firm causal relationship to symptoms may be difficult to establish (440), anywhere from 12% to 44% of patients experienced some complaints, often abdominal or epigastric pain. Most patients are in the fourth to sixth decades, although a wide age range of 1–77 has been reported (436,438,443). A preoperative diagnosis of heterotopic pancreatic tissue is not usually suspected. Because most of these ectopias involve the submucosa of the gut or deeper layers of the stomach and intestines, endoscopic biopsy does not often sample the abnormal tissue (12.5% of patients in one series) (439). A frozen section is often requested at the time of surgery. Thus, the pathologist should be aware of the anatomic distribution of heterotopic pancreatic tissue so as not to immediately assume that it must represent a metastatic tumor. Accurate interpretation will result in an appropriately conservative resection (439). Grossly, heterotopic pancreatic tissue typically presents as a single, firm, yellow–white, and lobulated or rounded nodule (443). Most examples measure roughly 2 cm, with a range of 0.2–5.5 cm. Histologic sections reveal a variable cellular composition, most often in the submucosa of the gastrointestinal tract (54%), with the second most common location being the muscularis propria (23%). In 11% of cases, the subserosa or serosa is involved; this may cause considerable concern over metastatic disease, but one should recall that the heterotopic tissues usually occupy a solitary site. Using Heinrich's classification for ectopic pancreatic tissue (445), most cases are either type I (acini, ducts, and islets of Langerhans) or type II (acini and ducts), whereas type III (ducts only) is uncommon (436, 437). Microscopic identification of islets of Langerhans obviously greatly facilitates the diagnosis, but this is not possible in every case; the reported range is approximately 33% to 84% (436–438,445). Heterotopic pancreatic tissue is subject to those alterations that are also seen in the main gland, including cystic change, acute and chronic inflammation, hemorrhage, necrosis, and neoplasia (443). Changes observed in adjacent tissues include fat necrosis, inflammation, hemorrhage, ulceration, and diverticular formation (443). When nests of endocrine cells are present, associated pancreatic ducts and acini should help in excluding a carcinoid tumor. Apparent infiltration of such tissues into the muscularis propria tissue, in the absence of islets, could also be misinterpreted as a carcinoma.

Another anatomic variation that may obfuscate the correct diagnosis is the accessory pancreatic ductal system of the major duodenal papilla, which appears to invade smooth muscle of the duodenal wall (446). In difficult cases, serial sections cut more deeply from paraffin blocks may help clarify the situation.

An increase in adipose tissue in the pancreas, or lipomatosis (447–449), could be misjudged as a lipomatous neoplasm. Nonetheless, the intrapancreatic fat in this condition is mature, and it does not displace parenchymal tissue but rather is intimately intermingled with it. Features of acinar atrophy, with only residual islets remaining, are present in the most extreme examples (447–449). The extent of fatty change in the pancreas has been linked to age, obesity (449), and antecedent adult onset diabetes mellitus (450).

Lastly, occasional mitotic figures, and nuclear enlargement in islet cells, with associated polyploid DNA content (452), is of no clinical consequence and should not be equated with incipient neoplasia.

### Hamartomas and Teratomas

Hamartomas of the pancreas are exceedingly rare (453–455). Isolated pediatric and adult cases have been reported. One reported tumor in a 25-year-old man was quite large at 10.6 cm in greatest dimension (453). This mass was well–circumscribed, solid, and cystic. Microscopically, there were ectactic ducts of varying size, surrounded by fibrous connective tissue. A second case has been reported as a multicystic pancreatic hamartoma, found in a 20-month-old with abdominal pain and distension (455). The 9-cm mass in that example consisted of cystically dilated ducts and large irregular lobules of acini admixed with fibrous tissue and fat. Cystic neoplasms, including mucinous cystadenoma, microcystic adenoma, and papillary and solid epithelial neoplasms (papillary-cystic neoplasm), should be excluded in differential diagnosis.

Teratomas of the pancreas are likewise exceptionally rare, with 12 reported cases (456–458). Eight of those individuals were women with a mean age of 26.1 (range 2–57 years). Almost all patients presented with abdominal or lumbar pain. One underwent fine needle aspiration biopsy, which revealed mature squamous cells with neutrophils and abundant keratin debris (457). Grossly, the surgically removed masses were cystic and typically contained hair. They ranged up to 20 cm in greatest dimension (456,457). Microscopic recognition of differentiation along all three germinal lines, including the presence of smooth muscle, hyaline, cartilage, hair, bone, fat, and neural and endodermal tissues, will prevent the diagnosis of a neoplasm.

### Cystic Disease

Nonneoplastic, benign pancreatic cysts should be set apart from cystic neoplasms of the pancreas. Most cysts in that gland are actually *pseudocysts* (459–463), which are cystic spaces lined with a fibrinofibrous wall without an epithelial lining. In surgical specimens, pseudocysts are not likely to be diagnosed by pathologists as neoplasms. Preoperatively, cyst fluid amylase isoenzyme analysis may be helpful in differentiating between those possibilities (465). Other nonneoplastic cystic lesions are rare and include congenital dysgenetic cysts, enteric duplication cysts, retention cysts, dyschylic cysts of cystic fibrosis, infectious cysts, and lymphoepithelial cysts (464). In regard to congenital dysgenetic

cysts, it has been emphasized that, in contrast to cystic pancreatic neoplasms, epithelial tufting and significant mucin production should be absent (464).

### Chronic Pancreatitis

Among the most treacherous of all diagnostic straits to be navigated by the surgical pathologist is the interpretation, particularly at frozen section, of pancreatic needle biopsies. Typically, the diagnoses being contemplated are those of chronic pancreatitis versus adenocarcinoma of the pancreas (466–470). Here the prognostic implications and therapeutic consequences of a diagnosis of cancer are profound. As an incidental finding, chronic pancreatitis is seen in 13% of individuals (472). Chronic pancreatitis has been defined as an irreversible, irregular scarring of glandular parenchyma due to duct changes subsequent to necrotic-inflammatory processes in the pancreas (471). It is principally a disease of young to middle-aged men (25–50 years of age), most of whom are alcoholics (471,472). Many patients report recurrent attacks of upper abdominal pain with nausea and vomiting (472). Grossly, there is nodular fibrosis, often with associated pseudocysts or necrosis.

The microscopic changes of pancreatitis are dependent on the stage of the disease (471,473). At an early time point, interlobular (perilobular) fibrosis is most prominent, with a lymphoplasmacytic and histiocytic infiltrate. Fat necrosis and pseudocysts may be present as well. Later, the fibrosis becomes more extensive and involves the lobules themselves. The architectural arrangement of ducts, atrophic acini, residual islets, blood vessels, and nerves becomes highly disordered. It is the distorted ductal profiles and disorganized ducts and acini, in conjunction with inflammatory and reactive cytologic atypia of epithelial lining cells (Figs. 54 and 55), that may create the greatest indecision in diagnosis. The stromal background of reactive fibrosis and inflammation is characteristic of either chronic pancreatitis or infiltrating ductal carcinomas, and therefore is unhelpful in

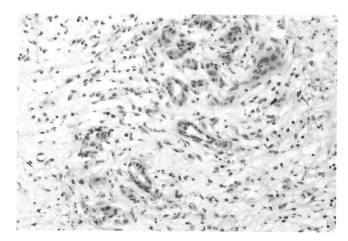

**FIG. 54.** Atypical glandular profiles in a frozen section of chronic fibrosing pancreatitis.

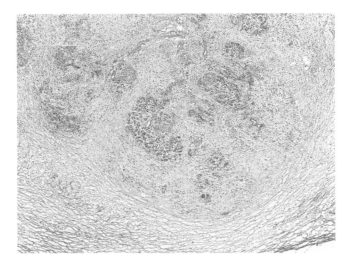

**FIG. 55.** The lobular configuration of the atypical glands depicted in Fig. 51 is appreciated at scanning magnification. However, the architectural outlines seen in this incisional biopsy might not be apparent in a needle core biopsy.

diagnostic decision making. In general, the most useful criteria favoring the diagnosis of a neoplastic over a pseudoneoplastic ductal proliferation are a disorganized ductal distribution, incomplete ductal lumina, and a nuclear size variation of 4:1 or greater among the ductal epithelial cells (467). Abnormal glandular shapes may also be helpful (466). Minor criteria that are valuable in the diagnosis of pancreatic carcinoma include huge, irregular epithelial nucleoli, necrotic glandular debris, glandular mitoses, and perineural invasion (467). However, caution is warranted in this regard because benign pancreatic acini and islet cells have also been seen in and around nerves (474,475).

The role of special studies in the diagnostic discrimination between chronic pancreatitis and ductal pancreatic carcinoma is unsettled. Morphometric analysis using image analyzers holds promise (476–478), but it is expensive, time-consuming, and labor-intensive. Differences in mucin expression have been reported (479) but overlap limits the practical diagnostic usefulness of histochemistry. Similarly, tumor markers detected by immunohistochemistry have to date not been proven to show sufficient specificity to warrant routine application in daily practice (480–483).

A most unusual form of pancreatitis that should be distinguished from a neoplasm is that of lymphoplasmacytic sclerosing pancreatitis with cholangitis (484). While radiologic studies of this variant of primary sclerosing cholangitis may suggest carcinoma, histologic evaluations are more likely to provoke concern over a lymphoid neoplasm.

### Pseudoneoplastic Proliferation of Endocrine Cells in Pancreatic Fibrosis

In the setting of exocrine duct obstruction, fibrosis and atrophy of exocrine acini may ensue, sometimes with neofor-

mation of neuroendocrine tissue (475,485). The presence of a nesting pattern or cords of endocrine cells in an intensely fibrotic background yields images suggesting stromal invasion by a neoplasm. Further difficulty may arise when the proliferating cells are identified in perineural spaces (475). Although most of these cases appear to represent regenerative and hyperplastic proliferations of neuroendocrine cells, for a few cases the boundaries between exuberant hyperplasia and neoplasia are not easily defined. In order to render a definitive diagnosis of a pancreatic endocrine neoplasm in such cases, it is preferable to observe either significant extension of the lesion into regional tissues or metastatic disease (475). Immunohistochemistry for pancreatic hormones (insulin, glucagon, somatostatin, and pancreatic polypeptide) is not diagnostically helpful because the types of hormone-producing cells that are present in normal, regenerative and neoplastic pancreatic endocrine cell proliferations may be surprisingly similar in scope (475,486).

### Hyperplasia

It has been postulated that ductal hyperplasia of the pancreas is a proliferative response to exogenous agents that injure that gland (487). In chronic pancreatitis, a spectrum of ductal epithelial abnormalities has been described (488). The premise that some of the proliferations designated as hyperplasias might actually be *preneoplastic* is indicated by a high mutation rate of c-Ki-ras (489), an oncogene that is activated by point mutations in 75–100% of pancreatic carcinomas. Furthermore, abnormal DNA content (490) and p53 protein accumulation (491) have also been demonstrated in pancreatic duct hyperplasia. Given the uncertainty regarding the preneoplastic or even incipient neoplastic nature of ductal hyperplasia of the pancreas, we do not consider this entity further.

It is important to be cognizant of other pancreatic hyperplasias that could masquerade as neoplasms, such as nesidioblastic endocrine hyperplasia and acinar adenomatous hyperplasia.

Nesidioblastosis is a term initially used to define a diffuse or disseminated proliferation of islet cells (492). At the histopathologic level it is viewed as a somewhat elusive entity, since the characteristic morphologic alterations of nesidioblastosis have been observed in the *normal* pancreas as well as in the clinical scenario of intractable neonatal or infantile hypoglycemia secondary to insulin excess (464). The main feature is an increase in the total volume of pancreatic endocrine cells (464), which are focally or diffusely arranged (493). Focal nesidioblastosis features nodular hyperplasia of islet-like cell clusters, with hypertrophied insulin-containing cells containing giant nuclei and ductuloinsular complexes (493). The latter are small aggregates of ductular and endocrine cells in which nests of neuroendocrine cells surround and indent the ducts (464). In diffuse nesidioblastosis the entire pancreas demonstrates irregularly sized islets

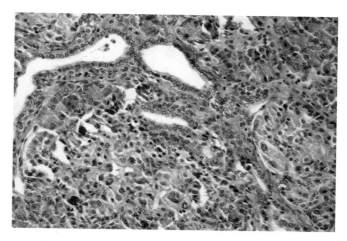

**FIG. 56.** Ductuloinsular complex in nesidioblastosis.

and ductuloinsular complexes (Fig. 56), which often possess giant and bizarre nuclei. Immunohistochemical staining (for synaptophysin, chromogranin, or neuron-specific enolase) is helpful in determining the total number of neuroendocrine cells and the number of insulin-synthesizing cells (464). This type of endocrine cell proliferation should be distinguished from a discrete islet cell tumor, which would be distinctly uncommon in infants. In adults, ductuloinsular lesions and hyperplastic islets are common in multiple endocrine neoplasia, type 1. In such patients, nodules of hyperplasia may be difficult or impossible to segregate from microscopic neoplasms.

Acinar adenomatous hyperplasia is a microscopic, incidental finding that is typified by nonencapsulated, well-demarcated foci of cells arranged in irregular sheets or clumps, with acinar formations (494). Mass-forming neoplastic acinar cell nodules are usually grossly apparent and readily distinguished from hyperplasia.

## Pseudolymphoma

A single case of localized pancreatic lymphoid hyperplasia, or pseudolymphoma, has been reported in a 57-year-old woman who complained of malaise and icterus (495). Grossly, there was a circumscribed 2-cm, soft, yellow–white nodule in the head of the pancreas. Microscopically, numerous lymphoid follicles with reactive germinal centers were present. Follow-up at 3 years was uneventful, although immunohistologic and genotypic data on the case were not provided.

## Inflammatory Myofibroblastic Pseudotumor

Six cases of inflammatory myofibroblastic pseudotumor (formerly known as inflammatory pseudotumor or plasma cell granuloma) have been reported in the pancreas (496–501). All but two patients with that disorder were adults (age range 8–52). The mode of clinical presentation was variable and included right upper quadrant pain, obstructive jaundice, an abdominal mass, and weight loss with epigastric pain. Grossly, the masses ranged from 3 to 13 cm in greatest dimension, were generally firm to hard and gray–white, and were variably well circumscribed. Microscopically, the lesion was typically fibroinflammatory with a prominent population of fibroblasts and a mixed inflammatory cell infiltrate comprised of lymphocytes, mature plasma cells, eosinophils, and histiocytes. Immunostaining revealed vimentin, desmin, muscle-specific actin, $\alpha_1$-antitrypsin, $\alpha_1$-antichymotrypsin, and HAM-56 positivity in the spindle cells, a polyclonal population of plasma cells, and a mixed population of T and B lymphocytes (499,501). As in other anatomic sites, one must specifically rule out lymphoma, plasmacytoma, sarcomatoid carcinoma, and mesenchymal neoplasms.

## ADRENAL TISSUE

### Variants of Normal Anatomy

It has long been known that adrenal tissue (mainly cortical tissue) may be found in extraadrenal locations. Indeed, in 1740 Morgagni described accessory adrenal tissue near the normal glands. As is true of other tissue heterotopias, it is important not to interpret normal adrenal tissue in aberrant locations as a neoplasm or as metastases.

Adrenal tissue heterotopias are usually seen along the pathway of migration and descent of the sex organs (502–523), including the celiac plexus area (502), broad ligament (505), kidneys (503–505), retroperitoneum (523), inguinal canal and spermatic cord (505,508,510,513,514,516, 517,519), testes and scrotum (505,507,511,512,517), ovaries (524), and periappendiceal soft tissue (515). Unusual locations include the gallbladder wall (509), liver (520), cranial cavity (506), cranial nerves (522), and lungs (521).

The incidence of heterotopic adrenal tissue is dependent on the anatomic site. Adrenal rests have been identified in 32% of individuals in the celiac-plexus region (502). At autopsy, 0.1% of all subjects have subcapsular intrarenal adrenal tissue (503). In surgical series, adrenal tissue was found in 7.5% of cases in the testes or peritesticular tissues (507), along the spermatic cord in 9.3% of cases (508), and in hernia sacs in 1–3% of cases (510,519).

Almost invariably, adrenal heterotopias are incidental and microscopic findings, usually measuring only a few millimeters in greatest dimension. However, 1- to 2-cm masses have been reported as well (515,517). Grossly, these nodules are rounded to oval, well circumscribed, firm, and yellow to orange. Microscopically, most cases are well-circumscribed nodules of adrenal cortical tissue. Further evidence of adrenal cortical differentiation may be obtained by frozen section immunostaining for cytoplasmic p450scc, an enzyme involved in steroid synthesis (520). Adrenal medullary tissue may be identified, though, in a significant percentage (up to 50%) of heterotopias near the normal gland (502).

In the differential diagnosis one must consider true clear cell neoplasms, including such tumors as renal cell carcinoma. The solitary, small, well-encapsulated nature of heterotopic adrenal tissue and its bland cytologic features should allow the observer to arrive at the correct diagnosis. Rarely, however, true neoplasms may arise within heterotopic adrenal tissue (525).

One should be aware that, in extraordinarily rare cases, ectopic inclusions of nonadrenal tissues might also be encountered in the adrenal glands (526,527). Single examples of an intraadrenal hepatocellular nodule (526) and renal tissue (complete with renal tubules and glomeruli) (527) have been documented. In these cases, one should rule out metastatic disease because the adrenal is a well-known site for secondary carcinomatous deposits. Ovarian thecal metaplasia is another example of an incidental finding in the adrenal gland (428).

Foci of large atypical cells in the fetal and neonatal adrenal cortex, known as adrenal cytomegaly (521,529–532), and similar changes in the normal adrenal medulla (533 should not be a cause for alarm. Adrenal cytomegaly is thought to represent a degenerative change in selected adrenal cortical cells (531), with nuclei that exhibit enlargement (often to 20 microns) (529), hyperchromasia, and intranuclear cytoplasmic invaginations (pseudoinclusions). There is an association between that condition and Beckwith's syndrome, but there is no evidence of a viral etiology or of malignant potential. Similar nuclear atypia may be seen in adrenal medullary cells, most commonly at the corticomedullary junction (Fig. 57). Ordinarily, no more than one atypical cell is found per medium-power microscopic field (533).

## Hamartoma

Several cases of adrenal hamartoma have been reported in patients with tuberous sclerosis (534). Angiomyolipomatous components were present in one case, with HMB-45-posi-

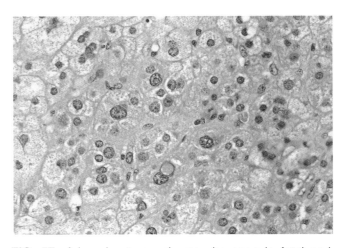

**FIG. 57.** Adrenal cytomegaly may be seen in fetal and neonatal adrenal cortex and in adult medullary cells at the corticomedullary junction.

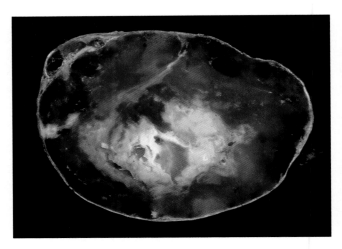

**FIG. 58.** Adrenal pseudocyst with abundant hemorrhage.

tive and muscle-specific actin-reactive cells identified by immunohistochemistry (534). Angiomyolipomas, depending on the predominant histologic components, can be confused with lipomas or spindle cell neoplasms such as sarcomatoid carcinomas or sarcomas. Diagnostic synthesis of the clinical setting, characteristically tripartite differentiation, and the immunohistochemical profile should lead to the correct diagnosis.

## Cysts

Most adrenal cysts are incidental findings at autopsy; they are uncommon, with an incidence of less than 0.1% (535). There are no typical clinical symptoms associated with adrenal cysts, and patients may present with abdominal pain, gastrointestinal symptoms, and constitutional complaints (especially with large cysts) (541). Accurate classification of the nature of the cyst is important because both benign and malignant diseases of the adrenal might exhibit cystic change. Adrenal cysts have been classified into four general categories: pseudocysts, cystic neoplasms, true cysts, and infectious cysts (536,547).

Pseudocysts are cystic lesions with a fibrous wall and no epithelial lining (542,544,547). Grossly, the cysts measure from 1.8 to 20 cm in greatest dimension (542,544,548). There is a 0.1- to 0.3-cm-thick cyst wall with a smooth inner lining. The cysts contain red–brown, thrombotic, and hemorrhagic material (Fig. 58); calcification of the cyst wall, and the contents also might be identified. Histologically, the fibrous wall is composed of densely hyalinized fibrous tissue. Nests of adrenal cortical cells in this fibrocollagenous matrix (Fig. 59) and in the cyst lumen (Fig. 60) should not be perceived as neoplastic. The contents of the pseudocyst include necrotic material, histiocytes laden with hemosiderin, thrombotic debris, islands of adrenal cortical cells (see Fig. 60) (547), and even adipose and myelolipomatous tissues (544).

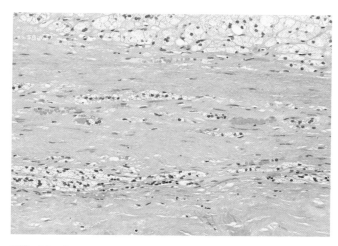

**FIG. 59.** Cords of entrapped benign adrenal cortical epithelial cells within the wall of an adrenal pseudocyst.

Vascular structures (dilated sinusoids) may be found adjacent to or within the inner pseudocyst wall, and even within the cystic space itself (542,544,548). It has been proposed that some, and perhaps the majority of, adrenal pseudocysts originate as endothelial lesions (542,548) Diagnostic considerations may include vascular neoplasms because of this feature; cortical epithelial neoplasms or pheochromocytomas; or metastatic carcinomas. In that context, it has been stressed that residual tumor is easily identified in most cystic true neoplasms of the adrenal gland tissues (542,547). Because the residual tumor cells may, in certain exceptional cases, be present only focally (544,545), thorough gross sampling and a careful histologic search through hemorrhagic and necrotic material in cystic adrenal lesions is warranted (544,547).

True epithelial cysts of the adrenals are rare (543). Some of these may actually be mesothelial cysts (546). In either case, the single lining layer of bland cuboidal or squamoid cells is highly characteristic and easily distinguished from a cystic neoplasm.

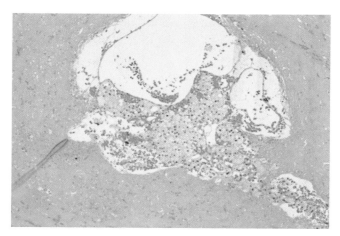

**FIG. 60.** Nests of benign adrenal epithelial cells may be found in the contents of an adrenal pseudocyst.

## Lymphocytic Infiltrates

Scattered lymphocytic infiltrates are common as incidental histologic findings in the adrenal cortex (549). Most of these are composed of CD3+, CD4+ T cells, which may be a manifestation of subclinical, autoimmune adrenalitis (549). Small, bland lymphocytic aggregates are not likely to be mistaken for destructive, lymphomatous involvement of the adrenal gland, which is common in systemic lymphoma but extremely rare as a primary disease of the adrenal (547).

## Myelolipoma

Myelolipomas are uncommon, usually unilateral, benign, nonfunctioning admixtures of mature adipose tissue and variable numbers of myeloid, erythroid, and megakaryocytic elements (534,547,550–574). They are not truly neoplastic (547) but rather may be viewed as a hyperplasia of a choristomatous or metaplastic lesion (559). In some cases, these masses may be related to hormonal stimulation (550,559, 566,567,571) and the concurrent presence of cortical adenomas and endocrinopathies including Cushing's and Addison's diseases. There is also an epidemiologic linkage with chronic diseases such as diabetes mellitus, hypertension, and severe atherosclerosis (559). In the past, myelolipomas were usually incidental discoveries at autopsy, but increasingly, they are being detected clinically as incidentalomas by radiologic evaluation done for other reasons (570). The autopsy incidence of myelolipomas is 0.03–0.4% (552,553,557,559) but only approximately 40 patients have presented with symptoms attributable to the adrenal mass (572). The most common complaint was abdominal pain. Rarely, large masses might rupture, producing hemorrhage in the retroperitoneum. The diagnosis may be suspected preoperatively when CT scans show nonenhancing fatty adrenal masses.

Grossly, myelolipomas vary tremendously in size, with a reported range of microscopic dimensions to 34 cm (559). The masses are usually well demarcated, and may compress the remaining normal adrenal gland. Yellow adipose tissue and mottled dark brown areas are present. Microscopically, either the fatty or hematopoietic component may predominate (Fig. 61). Hemorrhage, hemosiderin deposition, and calcification are common.

Adrenal myelolipomas should be distinguished from fatty neoplasms, including lipomas and retroperitoneal liposarcomas (547). These tumors lack the hematopoietic elements of myelolipoma. Granulocytic sarcoma should also be incorporated into the differential diagnosis but differs in the presence of blasts and lack of intrinsic fat.

## Hyperplasia

Adrenal hyperplasia may be subdivided into cortical hyperplasia of congenital and acquired types, and medullary hyperplasia.

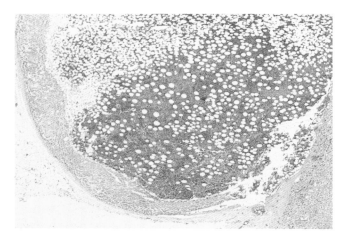

**FIG. 61.** Adrenal myelolipoma displaying adipose tissue and hematopoietic cell elements.

Congenital adrenal hyperplasia in the setting of inborn errors of metabolism results from an abnormality in any of the five enzymatic steps that are required to synthesize cortisol from cholesterol (575). 90 to 95 percent of cases are due to a deficiency of 21-hydroxylase (575). The resulting high levels of circulating androgens cause virilization; in some cases there are electrolyte imbalances as well (575). Pathologically, one sees diffuse cortical hyperplasia, which is not likely to be confused with a neoplasm.

Acquired adrenal cortical hyperplasia, which is usually due to an adrenocorticotropic hormone–secreting tumor (pituitary or ectopic), is most often bilateral and diffuse. In a minority of patients, there is bilateral nodular hyperplasia (576), and mixed diffuse and nodular patterns also occur. Hyperplasia of the adrenal cortex is associated with a wide variety of clinical syndromes, including Addison's disease, Waterhouse–Friedrichsen syndrome, Cushing's syndrome, virilization, feminization, and Conn's syndrome (577).

The nodules of adrenal cortical hyperplasia assume pseudoneoplastic status when their size and apparent monomorphism cause difficulty in morphologic differential diagnosis with adrenal cortical adenoma or carcinoma. Usually the distinction is readily made; hyperplastic nodules are usually multiple and bilateral with hyperplastic intervening cortical tissue, whereas adenomas tend to be solitary, unilateral, and well encapsulated, sometimes with atrophy of the nonnodular tissue. There is a degree of overlap in size, with hyperplastic nodules ranging from 1 mm to 2.5 cm and adenomas usually measuring between 1 and 7 cm in greatest dimension (576). However, some cortical nodules interpreted as adenomas may be as small as 3 mm (578), and, conversely, bilateral 0.5- to 7-cm adrenal nodules have been seen in macronodular adrenal hyperplasia (576,579,580). Microscopically, adrenal cortical hyperplasia is composed of variable proportions of clear and amphophilic cells corresponding, respectively, to the zona fasciculata and zona reticularis (Fig. 62). In Conn's syndrome, hyperplasia mainly affects the zona glomerulosa. A rare type of adrenal cortical hyperplasia, which is associated with Carney's syndrome, exhibits bilateral, small, pigmented (brown to black) adrenal nodules and has been termed "primary pigmented nodular adrenal hyperplasia" (576,581). Microscopically, the nodules in that condition are composed of enlarged, globular cells with granular, eosinophilic cytoplasm, often containing lipofuscin (581).

Adrenal medullary hyperplasia is most often seen in association with multiple endocrine neoplasia (MEN) types 2a or 2b (582–587), where it is considered the precursor of pheochromocytomas (582,583,585). The increase in total medullary mass in adrenal medullary hyperplasia results from diffuse and multifocal nodular proliferation in the head and body of the gland (586). Interpretative separation of nodular or diffuse adrenal medullary hyperplasia from pheochromocytoma has been regarded as an arbitrary process (582). In fact, some cases originally diagnosed as pheochromocytoma in patients with MEN are now viewed as exaggerated forms of hyperplasia (582). One proposal for the separation of adrenal medullary hyperplasia and pheochromocytomas is based on the size of the nodules, where medullary nodules of 1 cm or greater are classified as pheochromocytoma and those <1 cm are designated as nodular medullary hyperplasia (583). DNA analysis has also been forwarded as a means to discriminate between medullary hyperplasia and pheochromocytoma (588). DNA content has likewise been used, in conjunction with morphometrically determined nuclear shape and adrenal weight, to classify lesions as adrenal cortical hyperplasia or cortical neoplasms (589). These approaches are currently experimental and will require further investigation before consideration of their routine implementation. Microscopically, atypical nuclei, including giant and hyperchromatic forms, may be seen in hyperplasia (582, 586); these should not be equated with neoplasia.

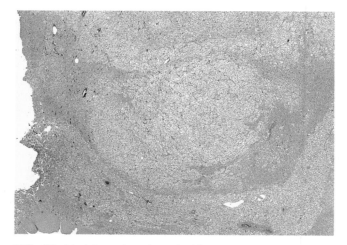

**FIG. 62.** Nodular adrenal cortical hyperplasia composed of clear cells.

## Inflammatory Myofibroblastic Pseudotumor (Plasma Cell Granuloma)

A single case of inflammatory myofibroblastic pseudotumor of the adrenal gland has been reported in a 17-year-old female, who presented with complaints of amenorrhea, fatigue, faintness, and weight loss (590). CT scans demonstrated a 10-cm adrenal mass, which, after excision, was noted to be well delineated and firm with grayish-white cut surfaces. The sections were remarkable for fibrous connective tissue and a pronounced plasma cell infiltrate, along with a few lymphocytes and histiocytes. The plasma cells were polyclonal, as determined by immunopositivity for kappa and lambda light chain immunoglobulins (590). Neoplasms such as fibrous histiocytoma, sarcoma, sarcomatoid carcinoma, and plasma cell myeloma entered into the differential diagnosis of this pseudoneoplastic condition.

## REFERENCES

1. Ljungqvist U, Andersson I, Hidell J, Linell F. Mammary hamartoma, a benign breast lesion. *Acta Chir Scand* 1979;145:227–230.
2. Andersson I, Hidell J, Linell F, Ljungqvist U. Mammary hamartomas. *Acta Radiol Diagn* 1979;20:712–720.
3. Hessler C, Schnyder P, Ozzello L. Hamartoma of the breast: Diagnostic observation of 16 cases. *Radiology* 1978;126:95–98.
4. Jones MW, Norris HJ, Wargotz ES: Hamartoma of the breast. *Surg Gynecol Obstet* 1991;173:54–56.
5. Davies JD, Kulka J, Mumford AD, Armstrong JS, Wells CA. Hamartomas of the breast: six novel diagnostic features in three-dimensional thick sections. *Histopathology* 1994;24:161–168.
6. Evers K, Yeh I-T, Troupin RH, Patterson EA, Friedman AK. Mammary hamartomas: the importance of radiologic-pathologic correlation. *Breast Dis* 1992;5:35–43.
7. Fehner RE. Fibroadenoma and related lesions. In: Page DL, Anderson TJ, eds. *Diagnostic histopathology of the breast*. New York: Churchill Livingstone, 1987;79–80.
8. Oberman HA. Hamartomas and hamartoma variants of the breast. *Semin Diagn Pathol* 1989;6:135–145.
9. Linell R, Ostberg G, Soderstrom J, Andersson I, Hidell J, Ljungqvist U. Breast hamartomas. An important entity in mammary pathology. *Virchows Arch A Path Anat* 1979;383:253–264.
10. Arrigoni MG, Dockerty MB, Judd ES. The identification and treatment of mammary hamartoma. *Surg Gynecol Obstet* 1991;133:577–583.
11. Rosen PP, Oberman HA. Hamartoma and variant lesions. In: Rosai J, Sobin LK, eds. *Tumors of the mammary gland*. Washington, DC: Armed Forces Institute of Pathology, 1993;350–352.
12. Altermatt HJ, Gebbers JO, Laissue JA. Multiple hamartomas of the breast. *Appl Pathol* 1989;7:145–148.
13. Fisher CJ, Hanby AM, Robinson L, Millis RR. Mammary hamartoma: a review of 35 cases. *Histopathology* 1992;20:99–106.
14. Daya D, Trus T, D Souza TJ, Minuk T, Yemen B. Hamartoma of the breast, an underrecognized breast lesion. A clinicopathologic and radiographic study of 25 cases. *Am J Clin Pathol* 1995;103:685–689.
15. Davies JD, Riddell RH. Muscular hamartomas of the breast. *J Pathol* 1973;111:209–211.
16. Huntrakoon M, Lin F. Muscular hamartoma of the breast. An electron microscopic study. *Virchows Arch A Path Anat* 1984;403:307–312.
17. Kaplan L, Walts AE. Benign chondrolipomatous tumor of the human female breast. *Arch Pathol Lab Med* 1977;101:149–151.
18. Benisch B, Peison B, Sarno J. Benign mesenchymoma of the breast. *Mt Sinai J Med* 1976;43:530–533.
19. Metcalf JS, Ellis B. Choristoma of the breast. *Hum Pathol* 1985;16:739–740.
20. McCarty KS , Tucker JA. Breast. In: Sternberg SS, ed. *Histology for pathologists*. New York: Raven Press, 1992;900–901.
21. McFarland J. Residual lactation acini in the female breast: their relation to chronic cystic mastitis and malignant disease. *Arch Surg* 1992;5:1–64.
22. Tavassoli FA, Yeh IT. Lactational and clear cell changes of the breast in nonlactating nonpregnant women. *Am J Clin Pathol* 1987;87:23–24.
23. Mills SE, Fechner RE. Focal pregnancy-like change of the breast. *Diagn Gynecol Obstet* 1980;2:67-70.
24. Tavassoli FA, Norris HJ. Secretory carcinoma of the breast. *Cancer* 1980;45:2404–2413.
25. O'Hara MF, Page DL. Adenomas of the breast and ectopic breast under lactational influences. *Hum Pathol* 1985;16:707–712.
26. Hertel BF, Zaloudek C, Kempson RL. Breast adenomas. *Cancer* 1976;37:2891–2905.
27. Slavin JL, Billson VR, Ostor AG. Nodular breast lesions during pregnancy and lactation. *Histopathology* 1993;22:481–485.
28. Le Gal Y. Adenomas of the breast. Relationship of adenofibromas to pregnancy and lactation. *Am J Surg* 1961;27:14–22.
29. James K, Bridges J, Anthony PP. Breast tumor of pregnancy (lactating adenoma). *J Pathol* 1988;156:37–44.
30. Grenko RT, Lee KP, Lee KR. Fine needle aspiration cytology of lactating adenoma of the breast. A comparative light microscopic and morphometric study. *Acta Cytol* 1990;34:21–26.
31. Geschickler CF, Lewis D. Pregnancy and lactation changes in fibroadenoma of the breast. *Br Med J* 1938;1:499–504.
32. Menville J. Fatty tissue tumors of the breast. *Am J Cancer* 1935;24:797–806.
33. Meyer JE, Silverman P, Gandbhir L. Fat necrosis of the breast. *Arch Surg* 1978;113:801–805.
34. Adair FE, Manzer JT. Fat necrosis of the female breast. *Am J Surg* 1947;74:117–128.
35. Boyages J, Bilous M, Barraclough B, Langlands AO. Fat necrosis of the breast following lumpectomy and radiation therapy for early breast cancer. *Radiother Oncol* 1988;13:69–74.
36. Mandrekas AD, Assimakopoulos GI, Mastorakos DP, Pantzalis K. Fat necrosis following breast reduction. *Br J Plast Surg* 1994;47:560–562.
37. Rostom AY, El-Sayed ME. Fat necrosis of the breast. An unusual complication of lumpectomy and radiotherapy in breast cancer. *Clin Radiol* 1987;38:31.
38. Girling AC, Hanby AM, Millis RR. Radiation and other pathological changes in breast tissue after conservative treatment for carcinoma. *J Clin Pathol* 1980;43:152–156.
39. Clarke D, Curtis JL, Martinez A, Fajardo L, Goffinet D. Fat necrosis of the breast simulating recurrent carcinoma after primary radiotherapy in the management of early stage breast carcinoma. *Cancer* 1983;52:442–445.
40. Lee BJ, Adair F. Traumatic fat necrosis of the female breast and its differentiation from carcinoma. *Ann Surg* 1920;72:188–195.
41. Bassett LW, Gold RH, Core HC. Mammographic spectrum of traumatic fat necrosis. The fallibility of pathognomic signs of carcinoma. *AJR* 1978;130:119–122.
42. van Bogaert LJ, Maldague P. Histologic variants of lipid-secreting carcinoma of the breast. *Virchows Arch A Path Anat* 1977;375:345–353.
43. Frost AR, Shek YH, Lack EE. Signet ring sinus histiocytosis mimicking metastatic adenocarcinoma. Report of two cases with immunohistochemical and ultrastructural study. *Mod Pathol* 1992;5:497–500.
44. Hurt M, Diaz-Arias AA, Rosenholtz MJ, Harvey AD, Stephenson HE. Post traumatic lobular squamous metaplasia of breast. An unusual pseudocarcinomatous metaplasia resembling squamous (necrotizing) sialometaplasia of the salivary gland. *Mod Pathol* 1988;1:385–390.
45. Reddick RL, Jennette JC, Askin FB. Squamous metaplasia of the breast. An ultrastructural and immunologic evaluation. *Am J Clin Pathol* 1985;84:530–533.
46. Lucey JJ. Spontaneous infarction of the breast. *J Clin Pathol* 1975;28:937–943.
47. Flint A, Oberman HA. Infarction and squamous metaplasia of intraductal papilloma. A benign breast lesion that may simulate carcinoma. *Hum Pathol* 1984;15:764–767.
48. Soderstrom KO, Toikkanen S. Extensive squamous metaplasia simu-

lating squamous cell carcinoma in benign breast papillomatosis. *Hum Pathol* 1983;14:1081–1082.

49. Salm R. Epidermoid metaplasia in mammary fibro-adenoma with formation of keratin cysts. *J Pathol Bacteriol* 1957;74:221–223.

50. Newman J, Kahn LB. Infarction of fibro-adenoma of the breast. *Br J Surg* 1973;60:738–740.

51. Rickert RR, Rajan S. Localized breast infarcts associated with pregnancy. *Arch Pathol* 1974;97:159–161.

52. Hasson J, Pope CH. Mammary infarcts associated with pregnancy presenting as breast tumors. *Surgery* 1961;49:313–316.

53. Hermann G, Schwartz IS, Slater G. Breast mass in a 69-year-old woman. *JAMA* 1986;255:939–940.

54. Lopez Valle CA, Hebert G. Warfarin-induced complete bilateral breast necrosis. *Br J Plast Surg* 1992;45:600–609.

55. Haagensen CD. Mammary-duct ectasia: a disease that may simulate carcinoma. *Cancer* 1951;4:749–761.

56. Tice GI, Dockerty MB, Harrington SW. Comedomastitis: a clinical and pathologic study of data in 172 cases. *Surg Gynecol Obstet* 1984;87:525–540.

57. Dixon JM, Anderson TJ, Lumsden AB, Elton RA, Roberts MM, Forrest APM. Mammary duct ectasia. *Br J Surg* 1983;70:601–603.

58. Sweeney DJ, Wylie EJ. Mammographic appearances of mammary duct ectasia that mimic carcinoma in a screening programme. *Australasian Radiol* 1995;39:18–23.

59. Shinde SR, Chandawarkar RY, Deshmakh SP. Tuberculosis of the breast masquerading as carcinoma. A study of 100 patients. *World J Surg* 1995;19:379–381.

60. Farmer C, Stanley MW, Bardales RH, Korourian S, Shah H, Bradsher R, Klimberg VS. Mycoses of the breast. Diagnosis by fine-needle aspiration. *Diagn Cytopathol* 1995;12:51–55.

61. Donn W, Rebbeck P, Wilson C, Gilks B. Idiopathic granulomatous mastitis. A report of three cases and review of the literature. *Arch Pathol Lab Med* 1994;118:822–825.

62. Kessler E, Wolloch Y. Granulomatous mastitis: a lesion clinically simulating carcinoma. *Am J Clin Pathol* 1972;58:642–646.

63. Jorgensen MB, Nielsen DM. Diagnosis and treatment of granulomatous mastitis. *Am J Med* 1992;93:97–101.

64. Fitzgibbons DL, Smiley DF, Kern WJ. Sarcoidosis presenting initially as breast mass: report of two cases. *Hum Pathol* 1985;16:851–852.

65. Osborne DM. Granulomatous mastitis caused by histoplasma and mimicking inflammatory breast carcinoma. *Hum Pathol* 1989;20:47–52.

66. Maygarden SJ, Novotny DB, Johnson DE, Powers CN, Frable WJ. Fine-needle aspiration cytology of suture granulomas of the breast. A potential pitfall in the cytologic diagnosis of recurrent breast cancer. *Diagn Cytopathol* 1994;10:175–179.

67. Gobel U, Kettritz R, Kettritz U, Thieme U, Schneider W, Luft FC. Wegener's granulomatosis masquerading as breast cancer. *Arch Intern Med* 1995;155:205–207.

68. Bassler R, Birke F. Histopathology of tumor associated sarcoid-like stromal reaction in breast cancer. Analysis of 5 cases with immunohistochemical investigations. *Virchows Arch A Path Anat* 1988;412:231–239.

69. Oberman HA. Invasive carcinoma of the breast with granulomatous response. *Am J Clin Pathol* 1987;88:718–721.

70. Arber DA, Simpson JF, Weiss LM, Rappaport H. Non-Hodgkin's lymphoma involving the breast. *Am J Surg Pathol* 1994;18:288–295.

71. Mattia AR, Ferry JA, Harris NL. Breast lymphoma. A B-cell spectrum including the low grade B-cell lymphoma of mucosa associated lymphoid tissue. *Am J Surg Pathol* 1993;17:574–587.

72. Lin Y, Govindan R, Hess J. Lymphoma mimicking carcinoma: a clinicopathologic study of primary breast lymphoma. *Mod Pathol* 1996;9:19A (abstract).

73. Coffin CM, Watterson J, Priest JR, Dehner LP. Extrapulmonary inflammatory myofibroblastic tumor (inflammatory pseudotumor). *Am J Surg Pathol* 1995;19:859–872.

74. Pettinato G, Manivel JC, Insalato L, De Chiara A, Petrella G. Plasma cell granuloma (inflammatory pseudotumor) of the breast. *Am J Clin Pathol* 1988;90:627–632.

75. Schwartz IS, Strauchen JA. Lymphocytic mastopathy. An autoimmune disease of the breast? *Am J Clin Pathol* 1990;93:725–730.

76. Lammie GA, Bohrow LG, Staunton MDM, Levison DA, Page G, Millis RR. Sclerosing lymphocytic lobulitis of the breast: evidence for an autoimmune pathogenesis. *Histopathology* 1991;19:13–20.

77. Mills SE. Lymphocytic mastopathy, a new autoimmune disease? *Am J Clin Pathol* 1990;93:834–835.

78. Davies JD. Sclerosing lymphocytic lobulitis and autoimmune mastitides. *Histopathology* 1992;21:397.

79. Ashton MA, Lefkowitz M, Tavassoli FA. Epithelioid stromal cells in lymphocytic mastitis—a source of confusion with invasive carcinoma. *Mod Pathol* 1994;7:49–54.

80. Rooney N, Snead D, Goodman S, Webb AJ. Primary breast lymphoma with skin involvement arising in lymphocytic lobulitis. *Histopathology* 1994;24:81–84.

81. Aozasa K, Ohsawa M, Seki K, Horiuchi K, Kawano K, Tagushi T. Malignant lymphoma of the breast. Immunologic type and association with lymphocytic mastopathy. *Am J Clin Pathol* 1992;97:699–704.

82. Tomaszewski JE, Brooks JSJ, Hicks D, LiVolsi VA. Diabetic mastopathy. A distinctive clinicopathologic entity. *Hum Pathol* 1992;23:780–786.

83. Seidman JD, Schnaper LA, Phillips LE. Mastopathy in insulin-requiring diabetes mellitus. *Hum Pathol* 1994;25:819–824.

84. Morgan MC, Weaver MG, Crowe JP, Abdul-Karim FW. Diabetic mastopathy. A clinicopathologic study in palpable and nonpalpable breast lesions. *Mod Pathol* 1995;8:349–354.

85. Oberman HA. Primary lymphoreticular neoplasms of the breast. *Surg Gynecol Obstet* 1966;121:1047–1051.

86. Fisher ER, Palekar AS, Paulson JD, Golinger R. Pseudolymphoma of breast. *Cancer* 1979;44:258–263.

87. Lin JJ, Farha GJ, Taylor RJ. Pseudolymphoma of the breast. I. In a study of 8,654 consecutive tylectomies and mastectomies. *Cancer* 1980;45:973–978.

88. Nakano A, Hamada Y, Hirono M, Hattori T. Differentiation between pseudo- and malignant lymphoma of the breast. A case report. *Jpn J Surg* 1982;12:76–78.

89. Maldonado ME, Sierra RD. Pseudolymphoma of the breast. Case report and literature reivew. *Military Med* 1994;159:469–471.

90. Mendelson EB, Doshi N, Grabb BC, Goldfarb WI. Pseudolymphoma of the breast. Imaging findings. *Am J Radiol* 1994;162:617–619.

91. Chang DW, Weiss PR. Pseudolymphoma of the breast. *Plast Reconst Surg* 1995;95:145–147.

92. Ackerman LV. *Tumor of the breast.* 6th Annual Seminar. Nassau Academy of Medicine, 1975; 6:15–16.

93. Foucar E, Rosai J, Dorfman R. Sinus histiocytosis with massive lymphadenopathy (Rosai–Dorfman disease). Review of the entity. *Semin Diagn Pathol* 1990;7:19–73.

94. Tavassoli FA. Miscellaneous Lesions. In: *Pathology of the breast.* Norwalk, CT: Appleton and Lange, 1992;627–630.

95. Lai FM-M, Lam WY, Chin CW, Ng WL. Cutaneous Rosai–Dorfman disease presenting as a suspicious breast mass. *J Cutan Pathol* 1994;21:377–382.

96. Eisen RN, Buckley PJ, Rosai J. Immunophenotypic characterization of sinus histiocytosis with massive lymphadenopathy (Rosai–Dorfman disease). *Semin Diagn Pathol* 1990;7:74–82.

97. Martinelli G, Santini D, Bazzocchi F, Pileri S, Cosanova S. Myeloid metaplasia of the breast. A lesion which clinically mimics carcinoma. *Virchows Arch A Path Anat* 1983;401:203–207.

98. Brooks, JJ, Krugman DT, Damjanov I. Myeloid metaplasia presenting as a breast mass. *Am J Surg Pathol* 1980;4:281–285.

99. Rosen PP, Oberman HA. Benign proliferative lesions. In: Rosai J, Sobin LK, eds. *Tumors of the mammary gland.* Washington, DC: Armed Forces Institute of Pathology, 1993;50–58.

100. Page DL, Anderson TJ. Adenosis. In: Page DL, Anderson TJ, eds. *Diagnostic histopathology of the breast.* New York: Churchill Livingstone, 1987;51–61.

101. Fechner RE, Mills SE. Radial scar, sclerosing adenosis and adenosis tumor. In: *Breast pathology, benign proliferations, atypias and in situ carcinmas.* Chicago: ASCP Press, 1990;53–66.

102. Tavassoli FA. Benign lesions. In: *Pathology of the breast.* Norwalk, CT: Appleton and Lange, 1992;91–100.

103. Foote FW, Stewart FW. Comparative studies of cancerous versus noncancerous breast. *Ann Surg* 1945;121:6–53.

104. Preece PE. Sclerosing adenosis. *World J Surg* 1989;13:721–725.

105. Urban JA, Adair FE. Sclerosing adenosis. *Cancer* 1949;2:625–634.

106. Heller EL, Fleming JC. Fibrosing adenomatosis of the breast. *Am J Clin Pathol* 1950;20:141–146.

107. Sandison AT. A study of surgically removed specimens of breast, with special reference to sclerosing adenosis. *J Clin Pathol* 1958;11:101–109.

108. Dawson EK. Fibrosing adenosis. A little recognized mammary picture. *Edinb Med J* 1954;61:391–401.
109. MacErlean DP, Nathan BE. Calcification in sclerosing adenosis simulating malignant breast calcification. *Br J Radiol* 1972;45:944–945.
110. Nielsen BB. Adenosis tumour of the breast: a clinicopathological investigation of 27 cases. *Histopathology* 1987;11:1259–1275.
111. Jensen RA, Page DL, Dupont WD, Rogers LW. Invasive breast cancer risk in women with sclerosing adenosis. *Cancer* 1989;64:1977–1983.
112. Haagensen CD. In: *Diseases of the breast*. 3rd ed. Philadelphia: WB Saunders, 1986;102–117.
113. Ackerman LV. In: *Surgical pathology*. St. Louis: CV Mosby, 1953;591.
114. Tinnemans JGM, Wobbes T, Holland R, Hendriks JHCL, van der Sluis RF, Lubbers E-JC, de Boer HHM. Mammographic and histopathologic correlation of nonpalpable lesions of the breast and the reliability of frozen section diagnosis. *Surg Gynecol Obstet* 1987;165:523–529.
115. Taylor HB, Norris HJ. Epithelial invasion of nerves in benign diseases of the breast. *Cancer* 1967;20:2245–2249.
116. Michal M. Nerve-like myxoid differentiation in sclerosing adenosis of breast. A diagnostic pitfall. *Zentralbl Pathol* 1993;139:89–90.
117. Eusebi V, Azzopardi JG. Vascular infiltration in benign breast disease. *J Pathol* 1976;118:9–16.
118. McDivitt RW, Boyce W, Gersell D. Tubular carcinoma of the breast. Clinical and pathological observations concerning 135 cases. *Am J Surg Pathol* 1982;6:401–411.
119. Fechner RE. Lobular carcinoma in situ in sclerosing adenosis. *Am J Surg Pathol* 1981;5:233–239.
120. Eusebi V, Collina G, Bussolati G. Carcinoma in situ in sclerosing adenosis of the breast. An immunocytochemical study. *Semin Diagn Pathol* 1989;6:146–152.
121. Oberman HA, Markey BA. Noninvasive carcinoma of the breast presenting in adenosis. *Mod Pathol* 1991;4:31–35.
122. Tavassoli FA. Myoepithelial lesions of the breast. Myoepitheliosis, adenomyoepithelioma, and myoepithelial carcinoma. *Am J Surg Pathol* 1991;15:554–568.
123. Gersell DJ, Katzenstein AA. Spindle cell carcinoma of the breast. A clinicopathologic and ultrastructural study. *Hum Pathol* 1981;12:550–560.
124. Gottlieb C, Raju U, Greenawald KA. Myoepithelial cells in the differential diagnosis of complex benign and malignant breast lesions. An immunohistochemical study. *Mod Pathol* 1990;3:135–140.
125. Ekblon P, Miettinen M, Forsman L, Andersson LC. Basement membrane and apocrine epithelial antigens in differential diagnosis between tubular carcinoma and sclerosing adenosis of the breast. *J Clin Pathol* 1984;37:357–363.
126. Becker RL, Mikel UV, O'Leary TJ. Morphometric distinction of sclerosing adenosis from tubular carcinoma of the breast. *Pathol Res Pract* 1992;188:847–851.
127. O'Leary TJ, Mikel UV, Becker RL. Computer-assisted image interpretation. Use of neural network to differentiate tubular carcinoma from sclerosing adenosis. *Mod Pathol* 1992;5:402–405.
128. Dupont WD, Page DL. Risk factors for breast cancer in women with proliferative breast disease. *N Engl J Med* 1985;312:146–151.
129. Tavassoli FA, Norris HJ. Microglandular adenosis of the breast. A clinicopathologic study of 11 cases with ultrastructural observations. *Am J Surg Pathol* 1983;7:731–737.
130. McDivitt RW, Stewart FW, Berg JW. In: *Tumors of the breast*. Washington, DC: Armed Forces Institute of Pathology, 1968;91.
131. Rosen PP. Microglandular adenosis. A benign lesion simulating invasive mammary carcinoma. *Am J Surg Pathol* 1983;7:137–144.
132. Clement PB, Azzopardi JG. Microglandular adenosis of the breast—a lesion simulating tubular carcinoma. *Histopathology* 1983;7:169–180.
133. Kay S. Microglandular adenosis of the female mammary gland: study of a case with ultrastructural observations. *Hum Pathol* 1985;16:637–640.
134. Rosenblum MK, Purrazzella R, Rosen PP. Is microglandular adenosis a precancerous disease? A study of carcinoma arising therein. *Am J Surg Pathol* 1986;10:237–245.
135. Weidner N. Benign breast lesions that mimic malignant tumors: analysis of five distinct lesions. *Semin Diagn Pathol* 1990;7:90–101.
136. Diaz NM, McDivitt RW, Wick MR. Microglandular adenosis of the breast. An immunohistochemical comparison with tubular carcinoma. *Arch Pathol Lab Med* 1991;115:578–582.
137. Gherardi G, Bernardi C, Marveggio C. Microglandular adenosis of the breast. Fine-needle aspiration biopsy of two cases. *Diagn Cytopathol* 1993;9:72–76.
138. James BA, Cranor ML, Rosen PP. Carcinoma of the breast arising in microglandular adenosis. *Am J Clin Pathol* 1993;100:507–513.
139. Linell F, Ljungberg O, Andersson I. Breast carcinoma. Aspects of early stages, progression and related problems. *Acta Pathol Microbiol Scand A* 1980;272S:123–128.
140. Eusebi V, Foschini MP, Betts CM, Gherardi G, Millis RR, Bussolati G, Azzopardi JG. Microglandular adenosis, apocrine adenosis, and tubular carcinoma of the breast. *Am J Surg Pathol* 1993;17:99–109.
141. Tavassoli FA, Bratthauer GL. Immunohistochemical profile and differential diagnosis of microglandular adenosis. *Mod Pathol* 1993;6:318–322.
142. Kiner H, Nielsen B, Paulsen S, Sorensen IM, Dyreborg U, Blichert-Toft M. Adenomyoepithelial adenosis and low-grade malignant adenomyoepithelioma of the breast. *Virchows Arch A Path Anat* 1984;405:55–67.
143. Tsuda H, Mukai K, Fukutomi T, Hirohashi S. Malignant progression of adenomyoepithelial adenosis of the breast. *Pathol Int* 1994;44:475–479.
144. Simpson JF, Page DL, Dupont WD. Apocrine adenosis—a mimic of mammary carcinoma. *Surg Pathol* 1990;3:289–299.
145. Carter DJ, Rosen PP. Atypical apocrine metaplasia in sclerosing lesions of the breast. A study of 51 patients. *Mod Pathol* 1991;4:1–5.
146. Raju U, Zarbo RJ, Kubus J, Schultz DS. The histologic spectrum of apocrine breast proliferations. A comparative study of morphology and DNA control by image analysis. *Hum Pathol* 1993;24:173–181.
147. Makunura CN, Curling OM, Yeomans P, Perry N, Wells CA. Apocrine adenosis within a radial scar: a case of false positive cytodiagnosis. *Cytopathology* 1994;5:123–128.
148. Page DL, Dupont WD, Rogers LW, Rados MS. Atypical hyperplastic lesions of the female breast. A long-term follow-up study. *Cancer* 1985;55:2698–2708.
149. Lee K-C, Chan JKC, Gwi E. Tubular adenosis of the breast. A distinctive benign lesion mimicking invasive carcinoma. *Am J Surg Pathol* 1996;20:46–54.
150. Fenoglio C, Lattes R. Sclerosing papillary proliferations in the female breast. A benign lesion often mistaken for carcinoma. *Cancer* 1974;33:691–700.
151. Fisher ER, Palekar AS, Kotwal N, Lipana N. A nonencapsulated sclerosing lesion of the breast. *Am J Clin Pathol* 1979;71:240–246.
152. Azzopardi JG. In: *Problems in breast pathology*, Philadelphia: WB Saunders, 1979;174–188.
153. Rickert RR, Kalisher L, Hutter RVP. Indurative mastopathy. A benign sclerosing lesion of breast with elastosis which may simulate carcinoma. *Cancer* 1981;47:561–571.
154. Tremblay G, Ruell RH, Seemayer TA. Elastosis in benign sclerosing ductal proliferations of the female breast. *Am J Surg Pathol* 1977;1:1155–1158.
155. Semb C. Fibroadenomatosis cystica mammae. *Acta Chir Scand* (suppl) 1928;10:1–484.
156. Wellings SR, Jensen HM, Marcam RG. An atlas of subgross pathology of the human breast with special reference to possible precancerous lesions. *JNCI* 1975;55:231–273.
157. Hamperl H. Strahlinge narben und obliterierende mastopathie. *Virchows Arch A Path Anat* 1975;361:55–68.
158. Rosen PP, Oberman HA. Benign proliferative lesions. In: Rosai J, Sobin LK, eds. *Tumors of the mammary gland*. Washington, DC: Armed Forces Institute of Pathology, 1993;59–63.
159. Eusebi V, Grassigli A, Grosso F. Lesioni focali scleroelastotiche mammarie simulanti il carcinoma infiltrante. *Pathologica* 1976;68:507–518.
160. Linell F, Ljungberg O, Andersson I. Breast carcinoma. Aspects of early stages, progression and related problems. *Acta Pathol Microbiol Scand A* (Suppl) 1980;272S:14–62.
161. Andersen JA, Carter D, Linell F. A symposium on sclerosing duct lesions of the breast. *Pathol Ann* 1986;21:145–179.
162. Page DL, Anderson TJ. Radial scars and complex sclerosing lesions. In: *Diagnostic histopathology of the breast*. New York: Churchill Livingstone, 1987;89–103.
163. Tavassoli FA. Benign lesions. In: *Pathology of the breast*. Norwalk, CT: Appleton and Lange, 1992;107–114.

164. Andersen JA, Gram JB. Radial scar in the female breast. A long-term follow-up study of 32 cases. *Cancer* 1984;53:2557–2560.

165. Nielsen M, Jensen J, Andersen JA. An autopsy study of radial scar in the female breast. *Histopathology* 1985;9:287–295.

166. Wallis MG, Devakumar R, Hosie KB, James KA, Bishop HM. Complex sclerosing lesions (radial scars) of the breast can be palpable. *Clin Radiol* 1993;48:319–320.

167. Sloane JP, Mayers MM. Carcinoma and atypical hyperplasia in radial scars and complex sclerosing lesions: importance of lesion size and patient age. *Histopathology* 1993;23:225–231.

168. Lamb J, McGoogan E. Fine needle aspiration cytology of breast in invasive carcinoma of tubular type and in radial scar/complex sclerosing lesions. *Cytopathology* 1994;5:17–26.

169. Frouge C, Tristant H, Guinebretiere J-M, Meunier M, Contesso G, Di Paola R, Blery M. Mammographic lesions suggestive of radial scars. Microscopic findings in 40 cases. *Radiology* 1995;195:623–625.

170. Hijazi YM, Lessard JL, Weiss MA. Use of anti-actin and S-100 protein antibodies in differentiating benign and malignant sclerosing breast lesions. *Surg Pathol* 1989;2:125–135.

171. Clement PB, Young RH, Azzopardi JG. Collagenous spherulosis of the breast. *Am J Surg Pathol* 1987;11:411–416.

172. Grignon DJ, Ro JY, Mackay BN, Ordonez NG, Ayala AG. Collagenous spherulosis of the breast. Immunohistochemical and ultrastructural studies. *Am J Clin Pathol* 1989;91:386–392.

173. Rosen PP. Adenoid cystic carcinoma of the breast. A morphologically heterogeneous neoplasia. *Pathol Annu* 1989;24:237–254.

174. Fisher ER, Brown R. Intraductal signet ring carcinoma. A hitherto undescribed form of intraductal carcinoma of the breast. *Cancer* 1985;55:2533–2537.

175. Rosen PP. Multinucleated mammary stromal giant cells. A benign lesion that simulates invasive carcinoma. *Cancer* 1979;44:1305–1308.

176. Campbell AP. Multinucleated stromal giant cells in adolescent gynecomastia. *J Clin Pathol* 1992;45:443–444.

177. Tavassoli FA. Mesenchymal lesions. In: *Pathology of the breast.* Norwalk, CT: Appleton and Lange, 1992;517–518.

178. Powell CM, Cranor ML, Rosen PP. Multinucleated stromal giant cells in mammary fibroepithelial neoplasms. A study of 11 patients. *Arch Pathol Lab Med* 1994;118:912–916.

179. Foschini MP, Dina RE, Eusebi V. Sarcomatoid neoplasms of the breast: proposed definitions for biphasic and monophasic mammary carcinomas. *Semin Diagn Pathol* 1993;10:128–136.

180. Agnatis NT, Rosen PP. Mammary carcinoma with osteoclast like giant cells. *Am J Clin Pathol* 1979;72:383–389.

181. Powell CM, Cranor ML, Rosen PP. Pseudoangiomatous stromal hyperplasia (PASH). A mammary stromal tumor with myofibroblastic differentiation. *Am J Surg Pathol* 1995;19:270–277.

182. Seidman JD, Borkowski A, Aisner SC, Sun C-CJ. Rapid growth of pseudoangiomatous hyperplasia of mammary stroma in axillary gynecomastia in an immunosuppressed patient. *Arch Pathol Lab Med* 1993;117:736–738.

183. Ibrahim RE, Sciotto CG, Weidner N. Pseudoangiomatous hyperplasia of mammary stroma: some observations regarding its clinicopathologic spectrum. *Cancer* 1989;63:1154–1160.

184. Vuitch MF, Rosen PP, Erlandson RA. Pseudoangiomatous hyperplasia of mammary stroma. *Hum Pathol* 1986;17:185–191.

185. Rosen PP, Ridolfi RL. The perilobular hemangioma. A benign microscopic vascular lesion of the breast. *Am J Clin Pathol* 1977;68:21–23.

186. Jozefczyk MA, Rosen PP. Vascular tumors of the breast. II. Perilobular hemangiomas and hemangiomas. *Am J Surg Pathol* 1985;9:491–503.

187. Banerjee SS, Eyden BP, McWilliam LJ, Harris M. Pseudoangiosarcomatous carcinoma: a clinicopathological study of seven cases. *Histopathology* 1992;21:13–23.

188. Wargotz ES, Deos PH, Norris HJ. Metaplastic carcinomas of the breast. II. Spindle cell carcinomas. *Hum Pathol* 1989;20:732–740.

189. Rosen PP. Mucocele-like tumors of the breast. *Am J Surg Pathol* 1986;10:464–469.

190. Bhargava V, Miller TR, Cohen MB. Mucocele-like tumors of the breast. Cytologic findings in two cases. *Am J Clin Pathol* 1991;95:875–877.

191. Kirk IR, Schultz DS, Katz RL, Libshitz HI. Mucocele of the breast (letter). *Am J Radiol* 1991;156:199–220.

192. Ro JY, Sneige N, Sahin AA, Silva EG, del Junco GW, Ayala AG. Mucocele-like tumor of the breast associated with atypical ductal hyperplasia or mucinous carcinoma. A clinicopathologic study of seven cases. *Arch Pathol Lab Med* 1991;115:137–140.

193. Rosen PP, Scott M. Cystic hypersecretory duct carcinoma of the breast. *Am J Surg Pathol* 1984;8:31–41.

194. Lee KC, Chan JKC, Lo LC. Histologic changes in the breast after fine-needle aspiration. *Am J Surg Pathol* 1994;18:1039–1047.

195. Youngson BJ, Liberman L, Rosen PP. Displacement of carcinomatous epithelium in surgical breast specimens following stereotaxic core biopsy. *Am J Clin Pathol* 1995;103:598–602.

196. Tabbara SO, Frierson HF Jr, Fechner RE. Diagnostic problems in tissues previously sampled by fine-needle aspiration. *Am J Clin Pathol* 1991;96:76–80.

197. Boppana S, May M, Hoda S. Does prior fine-needle aspiration cause diagnostic difficulties in histologic evaluation of breast carcinomas? *Lab Invest* 1994;70:13A (abstract).

198. Youngson DJ, Cranor M, Rosen PP. Epithelial displacement in surgical breast specimens following needling procedures. *Am J Surg Pathol* 1994;18:896–903.

199. Schnitt SJ, Connolly JL, Harris JR, Cohen RB. Radiation-induced changes in the breast. *Hum Pathol* 1984;15:545–550.

200. Bondeson L. Aspiration cytology of radiation-induced changes of normal breast epithelium. *Acta Cytol* 1987;31:309–310.

201. Peterse JL, Thunnissen FBJM, van Heerde P. Fine needle aspiration cytology of radiation-induced changes in nonneoplastic breast lesions. Possible pitfalls in cytodiagnosis. *Acta Cytol* 1989;33:176–180.

202. Chaudary MM, Girling A, Girling S, Habib F, Millis RR, Hayward JL. New lumps in the breast following conservative treatment of early breast cancer. *Br Cancer Treat Res* 1988;11:51–58.

203. Stromper PC, Recht A, Berenberg AL, Jochelson MS, Harris JR. Mammographic detection of recurrent cancer in the irradiated breast. *AJR* 1987;148:39–43.

204. Vilcoq JR, Calle R, Stacey P, Ghossein WA. The outcome of treatment by tumorectomy and radiotherapy of patients with operable breast cancer. *Int J Radiat Oncol Biol Phys* 1981;7:1327–1332.

205. Dornfeld JM, Thompson SK, Sharbaji MS. Radiation-induced change in the breast. A potential diagnostic pitfall on fine-needle aspiration. *Diagn Cytopathol* 1992;8:79–81.

206. Lumb G. Changes in carcinoma of the breast following irradiation. *Br J Surg* 1950;38:82–93.

207. Pinedo F, Vargas J, de Agustin P, Garzon A, Perez-Barrios A, Ballestin C. Epithelial atypia in gynecomastia induced by chemotherapeutic drugs. A possible pitfall in fine needle aspiration biopsy. *Acta Cytol* 1991;35:229–233.

208. Kennedy S, Merino MJ, Swain SM, Lippman ME. The effects of hormonal and chemotherapy on tumoral and nonneoplastic breast tissue. *Hum Pathol* 1990;21:192–198.

209. Pernicone PJ, Scheithauer BW, Horvath E, Kovacs K. Pituitary and sellar region. In: Sternberg SS, ed. *Histology for pathologists.* New York: Raven Press, 1992;296–297.

210. Sano T, Kovacs KT, Scheithauer BW, Young WF Jr. Aging and the human pituitary gland. *Mayo Clin Proc* 1993;68:971–977.

211. Luse SA, Kernohan JW. Squamous-cell nests of the pituitary gland. *Cancer* 1955;8:623–628.

212. Asa SL, Kovacs K, Bilbao JM. The pars tuberalis of the human pituitary: a histologic, immunohistochemical, ultrastructural and immunoelectron microscopic analysis. *Virchows Arch A Path Anat* 1983;399:49–59.

213. Scheithauer BW. The pituitary and sellar region. In: Sternberg SS, ed. *Diagnostic surgical pathology.* New York: Raven Press, 1994;493–522.

214. Scheithauer BW. Pathology of the pituitary and sellar region. Exclusive of pituitary adenoma. In: Sommers SC, Rosen PP, Fechner RE, eds. *Pathology annual.* part 1. Norwalk, CT: Appleton-Century-Crofts, 1985;67–155.

215. Stoffer SS, McKeel DW Jr, Randall RV, Laws ER Jr. Pituitary prolactin cell hyperplasia with autonomous prolactin secretion and primary hypothyroidism. *Fertil Steril* 1981;36:682–685.

216. Luse SA, Kernohan JW. Granular cell tumors of the stalk and posterior lobe of the pituitary gland. *Cancer* 1955;8:616–622.

217. Shanklin WM. The origin, histology and senescence of tumorettes in the human neurohypophysis. *Acta Anat* 1953;18:1–20.

218. Asa SL. Diseases of the pituitary. *Neurosurg Clin North Am* 1994;5:71–95.

219. Shanklin WM. On the origin of tumorettes in the human neurohypophysis. *Anat Rec* 1947;99:297–327.

220. Popovitch ER, Sutton CH, Becker NH, Zimmerman HM. Fine structure and histochemical studies of choristomas of the neurohypophysis. *J Neuropathol Exp Neurol* 1970;29:155–156 (abstract).

221. Schlachter LB, Tindall GT, Pearl GS. Granular cell tumor of the pituitary gland associated with diabetes insipidus. *Neurosurgery* 1980; 8:418–421.
222. Waller RR, Riley FC, Sundt TM Jr. A rare cause of the chiasmal syndrome. *Arch Ophthalmol* 1972;88:269–272.
223. Schochet SS, McCormick WF, Halmi NS. Salivary gland rests in the human pituitary. *Arch Pathol* 1974;98:193–200.
224. McGrath P. Cysts of sellar and pharyngeal hypophyses. *Pathology* 1971;3:123–131.
225. Bayoumi ML. Rathke's cleft and its cysts. *Edinb Med J* 1948;55: 745–749.
226. Teramoto A, Hirakawa K, Sanno N, Osamura Y. Incidental pituitary lesions in 1,000 unselected autopsy specimens. *Radiology* 1994;193: 161–164.
227. Shanklin WM. On the presence of cysts in the human pituitary. *Anat Rec* 1949;104:379–407.
228. Yoshida J, Kobayashi T, Kageyama W, Kanzaki M. Symptomatic Rathke's cleft cysts. Morphological study with light and electron microscopy and tissue culture. *J Neurosurg* 1977;47:451–458.
229. Boggan JE, Davis RL, Zorman G, Wilson CB. Intrasellar epidermoid cyst. Case report. *J Neurosurg* 1983;58:411–415.
230. Verkijk A, Bots GTAM. An intrasellar cyst with both Rathke's cleft and epidermoid charcteristics. *Acta Neurochir* 1980;51:203–207.
231. Salyer D, Carter D. Squamous carcinoma arising in the pituitary gland. *Cancer* 1973;31:713–718.
232. Ule G, Waidelich FW. Neurosekretorisches ganglienzell-choristom is der adenohypophyse. *Acta Neuropathol (Berl)* 1976;36:81–84.
233. Puchner MJA, Ludecke DK, Valdueza JM, Saeger W, Willig RP, Stalla GK, Odink RJ. Cushing's disease in a child caused by a corticotropin-releasing hormone-secreting intrasellar gangliocytoma associated with an adrenocorticotropic hormone–secreting pituitary adenoma. *Neurosurgery* 1993;33:920–925.
234. Rhodes RH, Dusseau JJ, Boyd AS Jr, Knigge KM. Intrasellar neural-adenohypophyseal choristoma. A morphological and immunocytochemical study. *J Neuropathol Exp Neurol* 1982;41:267–280.
235. Iwase T, Nishizawa S, Baba S, Hinokuma K, Sugimura H, Nakamura S-I, Uemura K-I, Shirasawa H, Kino I. Intrasellar neuronal choristoma associated with growth hormone-producing pituitary adenoma containing amyloid deposits. *Hum Pathol* 1995;26:925–928.
236. Bilbao JM. Pituitary gland. In: Rosai J, ed. *Ackerman's surgical pathology.* 8th ed. St. Louis: CV Mosby, 1996;2435.
237. Wakai S, Fukushima T, Teramoto A, Sano K. Pituitary apoplexy. Its incidence and clinical significance. *J Neurosurg* 1981;55:187–193.
238. Lazaro CM, Guo WY, Sami M, Hindmarsh T, Ericson K, Hutting AL, Wersall J. Haemorrhagic pituitary tumours. *Neuroradiology* 1994;36: 111–114.
239. Mohr G, Hardy J. Hemorrhage, necrosis, and apoplexy in pituitary adenomas. *Surg Neurol* 1982;18:181–189.
240. Cardoso ER, Peterson EW. Pituitary apoplexy: a review. *Neurosurgery* 1984;14:363–373.
241. Kepes JJ, Sayler J, Hiszczynskyj R. Squamous metaplasia following necrosis of the adenohypophysis and of a chromophobe adenoma of the pituitary. *Virchows Arch A Path Anat* 1982;395:69–76.
242. Kovacs K. Adenohypophysial necrosis in routine autopsies. *Endokrinologie* 1972;60:309–316.
243. Asa SL, Kovacs K. Histological classification of pituitary disease. *Clin Endocrinol Metab* 1983;12:567–596.
244. Weber EL, Vogel FS, Odom GL. Cysts of the sella turcica. *J Neurosurg* 1970;33:48–53.
245. Jenkins PJ, Chew SL, Lowe DG, Afshart F, Charlesworth M, Besser GM, Wass JAH. Lymphocytic hypophysitis: unusual features of a rare disorder. *Clin Endocrinol* 1995;42:529–534.
246. Ahmadi J, Meyers GS, Segall HD, Sharma OP, Hinton DR. Lymphocytic adenohypophysitis: contrast-enhanced MR imaging in five cases. *Radiology* 1995;195:30–34.
247. Thodou E, Asa SL, Kontogeorgos G, Kovacs K, Horvath E, Ezzat S. Clinical case seminar. Lymphocytic hypophysitis: clinicopathologic findings. *J Clin Endocrinol Metab* 1995;80:2302–2311.
248. Pestell RG, Best JD, Alford FP. Lymphocytic hypophysitis. The clinical spectrum of the disorder and evidence for an autoimmune pathogenesis. *Clin Endocrinol* 1990;33:457–466.
249. Cosman F, Post KD, Holub DA, Wardlaw SL. Lymphocytic hypophysitis. Report of 3 cases and review of the literature. *Medicine* 1989;68:240–256.
250. Puchner MJA, Ladecke DK, Saeger W. The anterior pituitary lobe in patients with craniopharyngiomas. Three cases of associated lymphocytic hypophysitis. *Acta Neurochir (Wien)* 1994;126:38–43.
251. Buchmann E, Schwesinger G. Hypophyse and hamoblastosen. *Zentralbl Neurochir* 1979;40:35–42.
252. Nemoto K, Ohnishi Y, Tsukada T. Chronic lymphocytic leukemia showing pituitary tumor with massive leukemic cell infiltration, and special reference to clinicopathological findings of CLL. *Acta Pathol Jpn* 1978;28:797–805.
253. Gartman JJ Jr, Powers SK, Fortune M. Pseudotumor of the sellar and parasellar areas. *Neurosurgery* 1989;24:896–901.
254. Olmos PR, Falko JM, Rea GL, Boesel CP, Chakeres DW, McGhee DB. Fibrosing pseudotumor of the sella and parasellar area producing hypopituitarism and multiple cranial nerve palsies. *Neurosurgery* 1993;32:1015-1021.
255. Brazier DJ, Sanders MD. Multifocal fibrosclerosis associated with suprasellar and macular lesions. *Br J Ophthalmol* 1983;67:292–296.
256. Grossman A, Gibson J, Stanfield AG, Besser GM. Pituitary and testicular fibrosis in association with retroperitoneal fibrosis. *Clin Endocrinol (Oxf)* 1980;12:371–374.
257. Saeger W, Ladecke DK. Pituitary hyperplasia. Definition, light and electron microscopical structures and significance in surgical specimens. *Virchows Arch A Path Anat* 1983;399:277–287.
258. Scheithauer BW, Kovacs K, Randall RV, Ryan N. Pituitary gland in hypothyroidism. Histologic and immunocytologic study. *Arch Pathol Lab Med* 1985;109:499–504.
259. Horvath E. Pituitary hyperplasia. *Pathol Res Pract* 1988;113: 623–625.
260. Bloodworth JMB Jr. Assessment of the pituitary hyperplasia/neoplasia interface. *Pathol Res Pract* 1988;183:626–630.
261. McKeel DW Jr, Fowler M, Jacobs LS. The high prevalence of prolactin cell hyperplasia in the human adenohypophysis. *Proc Endocr Soc* 1978;60:353 (abstract).
262. LiVolsi VA, Hamilton R. Intraoperative assessment of parathyroid gland pathology. *Am J Clin Pathol* 1994;102:365–373.
263. DeLellis RA. In: Rosai J, Sobin LH, eds. *Tumors of the parathyroid gland.* 3rd series. Fascicle 6. Washington, DC: Armed Forces Institute of Pathology, 1993.
264. Spiegel AM, Marx SJ, Doppman JL, Beazley RM, Ketcham AS, Kasten B, Aurbach GD. Intrathyroidal parathyroid adenoma or hyperplasia. An occasionally overlooked cause of surgical failure in primary hyperparathyroidism. *JAMA* 1975;234:1029–1033.
265. Sawady J, Mendelsohn G, Sirota R, Taxy JB. The intrathyroidal hyperfunctioning parathyroid gland. *Mod Pathol* 1989;2:652–657.
266. Wang C-A. The anatomic basis of parathyroid surgery. *Ann Surg* 1976;183:271–275.
267. Lack EE, Delay S, Linnoila I. Ectopic parathyroid tissue within the vagus nerve. Incidence and possible clinical significance. *Arch Pathol Lab Med* 1988;112:304–306.
268. Harach HR, Vujanic GM. Intrathyroidal parathyroid. *Pediatr Pathol* 1993;13:71–74.
269. Vellar ID, Shaw J, Brosnan G. Glandula in glandula. The intrathyroid parathyroid. *Aust NZ J Surg* 1973;42:257–259.
270. Sloane JA, Moody HC. Parathyroid adenoma in submucosa of esophagus. *Arch Pathol Lab Med* 1978;102:242–243.
271. Edis AJ, Purnell DC, van Heerden JA. The undescended parathymus. An occasional cause of failed neck exploration for hyperparathyroidism. *Ann Surg* 1979;190:64–68.
272. Russell CF, Edis AJ, Scholz DA, Sheedy PF, van Heerden JA. Mediastinal parathyroid tumors. Experience with 38 tumors requiring mediastinotomy for removal. *Ann Surg* 1981;193:805–809.
273. Nathaniels EK, Nathaniels AM, Wang C-A. Mediastinal parathyroid tumors. A clinical and pathologic study of 84 cases. *Ann Surg* 1970; 171:165–170.
274. Feliciano DV. Parathyroid pathology in an intrathyroid position. *Am J Surg* 1992;164:496–500.
275. Russell CF, Grant CS, van Heerden JA. Hyperfunctioning supernumerary parathyroid glands. An occasional case of hyperparathyroidism. *Mayo Clin Proc* 1982;57:121–124.
276. Tsuchiya M, Kamegaya K, Shimabukuro K, Takagi K, Yoshimatsu H. Intrathymic parathyroid tissue in man: clinical significance and report of a case of intrathymic parathyroid adenoma. *Keio J Med* 1971;20: 91–102.
277. Reddick RL, Costa JC, Marx SJ. Parathyroid hyperplasia and parathyromatosis. *Lancet* 1977;1:549.
278. Palmer JA, Brown WA, Keer WH, Rosen IB, Watters NA. The surgical aspects of hyperparathyroidism. *Arch Surg* 1975;110:1004–1007.

279. Fitko R, Roth SI, Hines JR, Roxe DM, Cahill E. Parathyromatosis in hyperparathyroidism. *Hum Pathol* 1990;21:234–237.

280. Sokol MS, Kavolius J, Schaaf M, D Avis J. Recurrent hyperparathyroidism from benign neoplastic seeding. A review with recommendations for management. *Surgery* 1993;113:456–461.

281. Rattner DW, Marrone GC, Kasdon E, Silen W. Recurrent hyperparathyroidism due to implantation of parathyroid tissue. *Am J Surg* 1985;149:745–748.

282. Shields TW, Staley CJ. Functioning parathyroid cysts. *Ann Surg* 1961; 82:175–180.

283. Haid SP, Method HL, Beal JM. Parathyroid cysts. Report of two cases and a review of the literature. *Arch Surg* 1967;94:421–426.

284. Rogers LA, Fetter BF, Peete WPJ. Parathyroid cyst and cystic degeneration of parathyroid adenoma. *Arch Pathol* 1969;87:476–479.

285. Calandra DB, Shah KH, Prinz RA, Sullivan H, Hofmann C, Oslapas R, Ernst K, Lawrence AM, Paloyan E. Parathyroid cysts. A report of eleven cases including two associated with hyperparathyroid crisis. *Surgery* 1983;94:887–891.

286. Wang C-A, Vickery AL Jr, Maloof F. Large parathyroid cysts mimicking thyroid nodules. *Ann Surg* 1972;175:448–453.

287. Wick MR. Mediastinal cysts and intrathoracic thyroid tumors. *Semin Diagn Pathol* 7:285–294.

288. Hughes CR, Kanmaz B, Isitman AT, Akansel G, Lawson T, Collier BD. Misleading imaging results in the diagnosis of parathyroid cysts. *Clin Nucl Med* 1994;19:422–425.

289. Clark OH. Hyperparathyroidism due to primary cystic hyperplasia. *Arch Surg* 1978;113:748–750.

290. Black BM, Watts CF. Cysts of parathyroid origin: report of two cases and study of incidence and pathogenesis of cysts in parathyroid glands. *Surgery* 1949;25:941–949.

291. Castleman B, Mallory TB. Pathology of parathyroid gland in hyperparathyroidism. A study of 25 cases. *Am J Pathol* 1935;11:1–72.

292. Ober WB, Kaiser GA. Hamartoma of the parathyroid. *Cancer* 1958; 11:601–606.

293. Legolvan DP, Moore BP, Nishiyama RH. Parathyroid hamartoma. Report of two cases and review of the literature. *Am J Clin Pathol* 1977;67:31–35.

294. Geelhoed GW. Parathyroid adenolipoma. Clinical and morphologic features. *Surgery* 1982;92:806–810.

295. Perosio P, Brooks JJ, LiVolsi VA. Orbital brown tumor as the initial manifestation of parathyroid lipoadenoma. *Surg Pathol* 1988;1: 77–82.

296. Wolff M, Goodman EW. Functioning lipoadenoma of a supernumerary parathyroid gland in the mediastinum. *Head Neck Surg* 1980; 2:302–307.

297. Daroca PJ, Landau RL, Reed RJ, Kappelman MD. Functioning lipoadenoma of the parathyroid gland. *Arch Pathol Lab Med* 1977; 101:28–30.

298. Weiland LH, Garrison RC, ReMine WH, Scholz DA. Lipoadenoma of the parathyroid gland. *Am J Surg Pathol* 1978;2:3–7.

299. Abul-Haj SK, Conklin H, Hewitt WC. Functioning lipoadenoma of the parathyroid gland. Report of a unique case. *N Engl J Med* 1962; 266:121–123.

300. van Hoeven KH, Brennan MF. Lipothymoadenoma of the parathyroid. *Arch Pathol Lab Med* 1993;117:312–314.

301. Reiner L, Klayman MJ, Cohen RB. Lymphocytic infiltration of the parathyroid glands. *Jewish Mem Hosp Bull* 1962;7:103–118.

302. Boyce BF, Doherty VR, Mortimer G. Hyperplastic parathyroiditis—a new autoimmune disease? *J Clin Pathol* 1982;35:812–814.

303. Bondeson A-G, Bondeson L, Ljungberg O. Chronic parathyroiditis associated with parathyroid hyperplasia and hyperparathyroidism. *Am J Surg Pathol* 1984;8:211–215.

304. Sinha SN, McArdle JP, Shepherd JJ. Hyperparathyroidism with chronic parathyroiditis in a multiple endocrine neoplasia patient. *Aust NZ J Surg* 1993;63:981–982.

305. Horwitz CA, Myers WP, Foote FW Jr. Secondary malignant tumors of the parathyroid glands. Report of two cases with associated hyperparathyroidism. *Am J Med* 1972;52:797–808.

306. Roth SI. Pathology of the parathyroids in hyperparathyroidism. *Arch Pathol* 1962;73:75–90.

307. Black WC, Haff RC. The surgical pathology of parathyroid chief cell hyperplasia. *Am J Clin Pathol* 1970;53:565–579.

308. Black WC III, Utley JR. The differential diagnosis of parathyroid adenoma and chief cell hyperplasia. *Am J Clin Pathol* 1968;49:761–775.

309. Castleman B, Schantz A, Roth SI. Parathyroid hyperplasia in primary hyperparathyroidism. *Cancer* 1976;38:1668–1675.

310. Lawrence DA. A histological comparison of adenomatous and hyperplastic parathyroid glands. *J Clin Pathol* 1978;31:626–632.

311. Yong JLC, Vrga L, Warren BA. A study of parathyroid hyperplasia in chronic renal failure. *Pathology* 1994;26:99–109.

312. Cope O, Keynes M, Roth SI, Castleman B. Primary chief-cell hyperplasia of the parathyroid glands. A new entity in the surgery of hyperparathyroidism. *Ann Surg* 1958;148:375–388.

313. Bondeson A-G, Bondeson L, Ljungberg O, Tibblin S. Fat staining in parathyroid disease—diagnostic value and impact on surgical strategy: clinicopathologic analysis of 191 cases. *Hum Pathol* 1985; 16:1255–1263.

314. Dufour DR, Wilkerson SY. The normal parathyroid revisited. Percentage of stromal fat. *Hum Pathol* 1982;13:717–721.

315. Bowlby LS, DeBault LE, Abraham SR. Flow cytometric DNA analysis of parathyroid glands. *Am J Pathol* 1987;128:338–344.

316. Loda M, Lipman J, Cukor B, Bur M, Kwan P, DeLellis RA. Nodular foci in parathyroid adenomas and hyperplasias. An immunohistochemical analysis of proliferative activity. *Hum Pathol* 1994; 25:1050–1056.

317. Arnold A, Brown MF, Urena P, Gaz RD, Sarfati E, Draeke TB. Monoclonality of parathyroid tumors in chronic renal failure and in primary parathyroid hyperplasia. *J Clin Invest* 1995;95:2047–2053.

318. Arnold A. Molecular mechanisms of parathyroid neoplasia. *Endocrinol Metab Clin North Am* 1994;23:93–107.

319. Schantz A, Castleman B. Parathyroid carcinoma. A study of 70 cases. *Cancer* 1973;31:600–605.

320. Klempa I, Frei U, Rottger P, Schneider M, Koch KM. Parathyroid autografts—morphology and function: six years experience with parathyroid autotransplantation in uremic patients. *World J Surg* 1984;8:540–546.

321. Rosai J. Parathyroid glands. In: *Ackerman's surgical pathology*. St. Louis: CV Mosby, 1996;574–576.

322. LiVolsi VA. The thyroid and parathyroid. In: Sternberg SS, ed. *Diagnostic surgical pathology*. 2nd ed. New York: Raven Press, 1994;523–543.

323. LiVolsi VA. Thyroid. In: Sternberg SS, ed. *Histology for pathologists*. New York: Raven Press, 1992;301–310.

324. Rosai J, Carcangiu ML, DeLellis RA. In: Rosai J, Sobin LH, eds. *Tumors of the thyroid gland*. 3rd series. Fascicle 5. Washington, DC: Armed Forces Institute of Pathology, 1992.

325. LiVolsi VA. *Surgical pathology of the thyroid*. (Major problems in pathology. vol 22.) Philadelphia: WB Saunders, 1990.

326. Rosai J. Thyroid gland. In: *Ackerman's surgical pathology*. St. Louis: CV Mosby, 1996;493–567.

327. Sauk JR Jr. Ectopic lingual thyroid. *J Pathol* 1970;102:239–243.

328. Baughman RA. Lingual thyroid and lingual thyroglossal tract remnants. A clinical and histopathologic study with review of the literature. *Oral Surg* 1972;34:781–799.

329. Montgomery ML. Lingual thyroid. A comprehensive review. *West J Surg Obstet Gynecol* 1935;43:559–661.

330. Larochelle D, Arcand P, Belzile M, Gagnon N-B. Ectopic thyroid tissue—a review of the literature. *J Otolaryngol* 1979;8:523–530.

331. Noyek AM, Friedberg J. Thyroglassal duct and ectopic thyroid disorders. *Otolaryngol Clin North Am* 1981;14:187–201.

332. Myers EW, Pantangco IP Jr. Intratracheal thyroid. *Laryngoscope* 1975;85:1833–1840.

333. Al-Hajjaj MS. Ectopic intratracheal thyroid presenting as bronchial asthma. *Respiration* 1991;58:329–331.

334. Polvani GL, Antona C, Porqueddu M, Pompilio G, Cavoretto D, Gherli T, Sala A, Biglioli P. Intracardiac ectopic thyroid: conservative surgical treatment. *Ann Thorac Surg* 1993;55:1249–1251.

335. Kantelip B, Lusson JR, De Riberolles C, Lamaison D, Bailly P. Intracardiac ectopic thyroid. *Hum Pathol* 1986;17:1293–1296.

336. Arriaga MA, Myers EN. Ectopic thyroid in the retroesophageal superior mediastinum. *Otolaryngol Head Neck Surg* 1988;99:338–340.

337. Spinner RJ, Moore KL, Gottfried MR, Lowe JE, Sabiston DC Jr. Thoracic intrathymic thyroid. *Ann Surg* 1994;220:91–96.

338. Takahashi T, Ishikura H, Kato H, Tanabe T, Yoshiki T. Ectopic thyroid follicles in the submucosa of the duodenum. *Virchows Arch A Path Anat* 1991;418:547–550.

339. LiVolsi VA, Perzin KH, Savetsky L. Carcinoma arising in median ectopic thyroid (including thyroglossal duct tissue). *Cancer* 1974; 34:1303–1315.

340. Joseph TJ, Komorowski RA. Thyroglossal duct carcinoma. *Hum Pathol* 1975;6:717–729.

341. Weiss SD, Orlich CC. Primary papillary carcinoma of a thyroglossal duct cyst: report of a case and literature review. *Br J Surg* 1991;78:87–89.

342. Grabowska H. Papillary carcinoma arising from ectopic thyroid gland in the wall of a thyroglossal duct cyst. *Pathol Res Pract* 1993;189:1228–1229.

343. Camesselle-Teijeiro J, Varela-Duran J, Sambade C, Villanueva JP, Varela-Nunez R, Sobrinho-Simoes M. Solid cell nests of the thyroid. Light microscopy and immunohistochemical profile. *Hum Pathol* 1994;25:684–693.

344. Ozaki O, Ito K, Fujisawa T, Kawano M, Iwabuchi H, Kitamura Y, Sugino K, Mimura T. Solid cell nests of the thyroid in medullary thyroid carcinoma. *Histopathology* 1994;24:77–80.

345. Harach HR. Solid cell nests of the thyroid. *J Pathol* 1988; 155:191–200.

346. Mizukami Y, Nonomura A, Michigishi T, Noguchi M, Hashimoto T, Nakamura S, Ishizaki T. Solid cell nests of the thyroid. A histologic and immunohistochemical study. *Am J Clin Pathol* 1994;101: 186–191.

347. Autelitano F, Santeusanio G, di Tondo U, Constantino AM, Renda F, Autelitano M. Immunohistochemical study of solid cell nests of the thyroid gland found from an autopsy study. *Cancer* 1987;59:477–483.

348. Harach HR. Solid cell nests of the thyroid. An anatomical survey and immunohistochemical study for the presence of thyroglobulin. *Acta Anat* 1985;122:249–253.

349. Yamaoka Y. Solid cell nest (SCN) of the human thyroid gland. *Acta Pathol Jpn* 1973;23:493–506.

350. Beckner ME, Schultz JJ, Richardson T. Solid and cystic ultramobranchial body remnants in the thyroid. *Arch Pathol Lab Med* 1990;114:1049–1052.

351. Kaleem Z, Dehner LP. Papillary microcarcinoma of the thyroid: a pathologist cancer. *Mod Pathol* 1996;9:102A (abstract).

352. Fukunaga FH, Lockett LJ. Thyroid carcinoma in the Japanese in Hawaii. *Arch Pathol* 1971;92:6–13.

353. Visona A, Pea M, Bozzola L, Stracca-Pansa V, Meli S. Follicular adenoma of the thyroid gland with extensive chondroid metaplasia. *Histopathology* 1991;18:278–279.

354. Schroder S, Bocker W. Lipomatous lesions of the thyroid gland. A review. *Appl Pathol* 1985;3:140–149.

355. Finkle HI, Goldman RL. Heterotopic cartilage in the thyroid. *Arch Pathol* 1973;95:48–49.

356. Asirwatham JE, Barcos M, Shimaoka K. Hamartomatous adiposity of thyroid gland. *J Med* 1979;10:197–206.

357. Chahal AS, Subramanyam CSV, Bhattacharjea AK. Chondromatous hamartoma of the thyroid gland. Report of a case. *Aust NZ J Surg* 1975;45:30–31.

358. Bale GF. Teratoma of the neck in the region of the thyroid gland. A review of the literature and report of four cases. *Am J Pathol* 1950;26:565–580.

359. Silberman R, Mendelson IR. Teratoma of the neck. Report of two cases and review of the literature. *Arch Disord Child* 1960;35:159–170.

360. Fisher JE, Cooney DR, Voorhess ML, Jewett TC Jr. Teratoma of thyroid gland in infancy. Review of the literature and two case reports. *J Surg Oncol* 1982;21:135–140.

361. Chan JK, Rosai J. Tumors of the neck showing thymic or related branchial pouch differentiation: a unifying concept. *Hum Pathol* 1991;22:349–367.

362. Singer PA. Thyroiditis. Acute, subacute and chronic. *Med Clin North Am* 1991;75:61–77.

363. Mizukami Y, Michigishi T, Nonomura A, Nakamura S, Ishizaki T. Pathology of chronic thyroiditis. A new clinically relevant classification. *Pathol Annu* 1994;29:135–158.

364. Volpe R. Etiology, pathogenesis and clinical aspects of thyroiditis. *Pathol Annu* 1978;13:399–413.

365. Volpe R. The pathology of thyroiditis. *Hum Pathol* 1978;9:429–438.

366. Hazard JB. Thyroiditis. A review. *Am J Clin Pathol* 1955;25:289–298.

367. Volpe R. The management of subacute (DeQuervain s) thyroiditis. *Thyroid* 1993;3:253–255.

368. Volpe R. Subacute and sclerosing thyroiditis. In: DeGroot LJ, Besser M, Burger HG, Jameson JL, Loriaux DL, Marshall JC, Odell WD, Potts JT Jr, Rubenstein AH, eds. *Endocrinology*. Philadelphia: WB Saunders, 1995;742–751.

369. Furszyfer J, McConahey WM, Wahner HW, Kurland LT. Subacute (granulomatous) thyroiditis in Olmsted County, Minnesota. *Mayo Clin Proc* 1970;45:396–404.

370. Lindsay J, Dailey ME. Granulomatous or giant cell thyroiditis. A clinical and pathologic study of thirty-seven patients. *Surg Gynecol Obstet* 1954;98:197–212.

371. Woolner LB, McConahey WM, Beahrs OH. Granulomatous thyroiditis (de Quervain's thyroiditis). *J Clin Endocrinol Metab* 1957;17: 1202–1221.

372. Stein AA, Hernandez I, McClintock JC. Subacute granulomatous thyroiditis. A clinicopathologic review. *Ann Surg* 1961;153:149–156.

373. Meachim G, Young MH. De Quervain's subacute granulomatous thyroiditis: histological identification and incidence. *J Clin Pathol* 1963;16:189–199.

374. Greenberg AH, Czernichow P, Hung W, Shelley W, Winship T, Blizzard RM. Juvenile chronic lymphocytic thyroiditis. Clinical, laboratory and histological correlations. *J Clin Endocrinol* 1970;30: 293–301.

375. Nikolai TF, Brosseau J, Kettrick MA, Robert R, Beltaos E. Lymphocytic thyroiditis with spontaneously resolving hyperthyroidism (silent thyroiditis). *Arch Intern Med* 1980;140:478–482.

376. Rapoport B. Pathophysiology of Hashimoto's thyroiditis and hypothyroidism. *Annu Rev Med* 1991;42:91–96.

377. Mitchell JD, Kirkham N, Machin D. Focal lymphocytic thyroiditis in Southampton. *J Pathol* 1984;144:269–273.

378. Bialis P, Marks S, Dekker A, Field JB. Hashimoto's thyroiditis presenting as a solitary functioning thyroid nodule. *J Clin Endocrinol Metab* 1976;43:1365–1369.

379. Katz SM, Vickery AL Jr. The fibrous variant of Hashimoto's thyroiditis. *Hum Pathol* 1974;5:161–170.

380. Nunez C, Mendelsohn G. Fine-needle aspiration and needle biopsy of the thyroid gland. *Pathol Annu* 1989;24:161–198.

381. Woolner LB, McConahey WM, Beahrs OH. Stroma lymphomatosa (Hashimoto's thyroiditis) and related thyroidal disorders. *J Clin Endocrinol Metab* 1959;19:53–83.

382. Ben-Ezra J, Wu A, Sheibani K. Hashimoto's thyroiditis lacks detectable clonal immunoglobulin and T cell receptor gene rearrangements. *Hum Pathol* 1988;19:1444–1448.

383. Dugan JM, Atkinson BF, Avitabile A, Schimmel M, LiVolsi VA. Psammoma bodies in fine needle aspirate of the thyroid in lymphocytic thyroiditis. *Acta Cytol* 1987;31:330–333.

384. Aozasa K. Hashimoto's thyroiditis as a risk factor of thyroid lymphoma. *Acta Pathol Jpn* 1990;40:459–468.

385. Chan JKC, Albores-Saavedra J, Battifora H, Carcangiu ML, Rosai J. Sclerosing mucoepidermoid thyroid carcinoma with eosinophils. A distinctive low-grade malignancy arising from the metaplastic follicles of Hashimoto's thyroiditis. *Am J Surg Pathol* 1991;15:438–446.

386. Dailey ME, Lindsay S, Skahen R. Relation of thyroid neoplasms to Hashimoto's disease of the thyroid gland. *Arch Surg* 1955; 70:291–297.

387. Holm L-E, Blomgren H, Lowhagen T. Cancer risks in patients with chronic lymphocytic thyroiditis. *N Engl J Med* 1985;312:601–604.

388. Hyjek E, Isaacson PG. Primary B cell lymphoma of the thyroid and its relationship to Hashimoto's thyroiditis. *Hum Pathol* 1988;19: 1315–1326.

389. Ott RA, McCall AR, McHenry C, Jarosz H, Armin A, Lawrence AM, Paloyan E. The incidence of thyroid carcinoma in Hashimoto's thyroiditis. *Am Surg* 1987;53:442–445.

390. Segal K, Ben-Bassat M, Avraham A, Har-El G, Sidi J. Hashimoto's thyroiditis and carcinoma of the thyroid gland. *Int Surg* 1985; 70:205–209.

391. Woolner LB, McConahey WM, Beahrs OH. Invasive fibrous thyroiditis (Riedel's struma). *J Clin Endocrinol Metab* 1957;17:201–220.

392. Comings DE, Skubi KD, Van Eyes J, Motulsky AG. Familial multifocal fibrosclerosis. Findings suggesting that retroperitoneal fibrosis, mediastinal fibrosis, sclerosing cholangitis, Riedel's thyroiditis, and pseudotumor of the orbit may be different manifestations of a single disease. *Ann Intern Med* 1967;66:884–892.

393. Meyer S, Hausman R. Occlusive phlebitis in multifocal fibrosclerosis. *Am J Clin Pathol* 1976;65:274–283.

394. Harach HR, Williams ED. Fibrous thyroiditis—an immunopathological study. *Histopathology* 1983;7:739–751.

395. Schwaegerle SM, Bauer TW, Esselstyn CB Jr. Riedel's thyroiditis. *Am J Clin Pathol* 1988;90:715–722.

396. Malotte MJ, Chonkich GD, Zuppan CW. Riedel's thyroiditis. *Arch Otolaryngol Head Neck Surg* 1991;117:214–217.

397. Albores-Saavedra J, Monforte H, Nadji M, Morales AR. C-cell hyperplasia in thyroid tissue adjacent to follicular cell tumors. *Hum Pathol* 1988;19:795–799.

398. Tomita T, Millard DM. C-cell hyperplasia in secondary hyperparathyroidism. *Histopathology* 1992;21:469–474.

399. Gibson WCH, Peng T-C, Croker BP. C-cell nodules in adult human thyroid. A common autopsy finding. *Am J Clin Pathol* 1981; 75:347–350.

400. Gibson WGH, Peng T-C, Croker BP. Age-associated c-cell hyperplasia in the human thyroid. *Am J Pathol* 1982;106:388–393.

401. O'Toole K, Fenoglio-Preiser C, Pushparaj N. Endocrine changes associated with the human aging process. III. Effect of age in the number of calcitonin immunoreactive cells in the thyroid gland. *Hum Pathol* 1985;16:991–1000.

402. DeLellis RA, Nunnemacher G, Wolfe HJ. C-cell hyperplasia. An ultrastructural analysis. *Lab Invest* 1977;31:237–248.

403. McDermott MB, Swanson PE, Wick MR. Immunostains for collagen type IV discriminate between C-cell hyperplasia and microscopic medullary carcinoma in multiple endocrine neoplasia, type 2. *Hum Pathol* 1995;26:1308–1312.

404. Kopp P, van Sande J, Parma J, Duprez L, Gerber H, Joss E, Jameson JL, Dumont JE, Vassart G. Brief report. Congenital hyperthyroidism caused by a mutation in the thyrotropin-receptor gene. *N Engl J Med* 1995;332:150–154.

405. Kennedy JS. The pathology of dyshormonogenetic goiter. *J Pathol* 1969;99:251–264.

406. Cooper DS, Axelrod L, DeGroot LJ, Vicker AL Jr., Maloof F. Congenital goiter and the development of metastatic follicular carcinoma with evidence for a leak of nonhormonal iodide. Clinical, pathological, kinetic, and biochemical studies and a review of the literature. *J Clin Endocrinol Metab* 1981;52:294–306.

407. Spaulding SW, Lippes H. Hyperthyroidism. Causes, clinical features, and diagnosis. *Med Clin North Am* 1985;69:737–750.

408. McKenzie JM, Zakarija M. Hyperthyroidism. In: DeGroot LJ, Besser M, Burger HG, Jameson JL, Loriaux DL, Marshall JC, Odell WD, Butts JT Jr, Rubenstein AH, eds. *Endocrinology*. Philadelphia: WB Saunders, 1995;742–751.

409. Spjut HJ, Warren WD, Ackerman LV. A clinical-pathological study of 76 cases of recurrent Graves' disease, toxic (non-exophthalmic) goiter, and non-toxic goiter. *Am J Clin Pathol* 1957;27:367-392.

410. Takamatsu J, Takeda K, Katayama S, Sakane S, Morita S, Kuma K, Ohsawa N. Epithelial hyperplasia and decreased colloid content of the thyroid gland in triiodothyronine-predominant Graves' disease. *J Clin Endocrinol Metab* 1992;75:1145–1150.

411. Mizukami Y, Michigishi T, Nonomura A, Hashimoto T, Noguchi M, Ohmura K, Matsubara F. Histologic changes in Graves' thyroid gland after [131]I therapy for hyperthyroidism. *Acta Pathol Jpn* 1992;42: 419–426.

412. LiVolsi VA. Papillary neoplasms of the thyroid. Pathologic and prognostic features. *Am J Clin Pathol* 1992;97:426–434.

413. Carcangiu ML, Zampi G, Rosai J. Papillary thyroid carcinoma. A study of its many morphologic expressions and clinical correlates. *Pathol Annu* 1985;20:1–44.

414. Rosai J, Carcangiu ML. Pitfalls in the diagnosis of thyroid neoplasms. *Pathol Res Pract* 1987;182:169–179.

415. Hapke MR, Dehner LP. The optically clear nucleus. A reliable sign of papillary carcinoma of the thyroid? *Am J Surg Pathol* 1979;3:31–38.

416. Gould E, Watzak L, Chamizo W, Albores-Saavedra J. Nuclear grooves in cytologic preparations. A study of the utility of this feature in the diagnosis of papillary carcinoma. *Acta Cytol* 1989;33:16–20.

417. Rupp M, Ehya H. Nuclear grooves in the aspiration cytology of papillary carcinoma of the thyroid. *Acta Cytol* 1989;33:21–26.

418. Damiani S, Fratamico F, Lapertosa G, Dina R, Eusebi V. Alcian blue and epithelial membrane antigen are useful markers in differentiating benign from malignant papillae in thyroid lesions. *Virchows Arch A Path Anat* 1991;419:131–135.

419. Fiorella RM, Isley W, Miller LK, Kragel PJ. Multinodular goiter of the thyroid mimicking malignancy. Diagnostic pitfalls in fine-needle aspiration biopsy. *Diagn Cytopathol* 1993;9:351–357.

420. Ramelli F, Studer H, Bruggisser D. Pathogenesis of thyroid nodules in multinodular goiter. *Am J Pathol* 1982;109:215–223.

421. Katoh R, Bray CE, Suzuki K, Komiyama A, Hemmi A, Kawaoi A, Oyama T, Sugai T, Sasou S. Growth activity in hyperplastic and neoplastic human thyroid determined by an immunohistochemical staining procedure using monoclonal antibody MIB-1. *Hum Pathol* 1995;26:139–146.

422. Thomas CG Jr., Combest W, McQuade R, Jordan H, Reddick R, Nayfeh SN. Biological characteristics of adenomatous nodules, adenomas, and hyperfunctionng nodules as defined by adenylate activity and TSH receptors. *World J Surg* 1984;8:445–451.

423. Hicks DG, LiVolsi VA, Neidich JA, Puck JM, Kant JA. Clonal analysis of solitary follicular nodules in the thyroid. *Am J Pathol* 1990;137:553–562.

424. Sisson JC, Schmidt RW, Beierwaltes WH. Sequestered nodular goiter. *N Engl J Med* 1964;270:927–932.

425. Mills SE, Gaffey MJ, Watts JC, Swanson PE, Wick MR, LiVolsi VA, Nappi O, Weiss LM. Angiomatoid carcinoma and angiosarcoma of the thyroid gland. A spectrum of endothelial differentiation. *Am J Clin Pathol* 1994;102:322–330.

426. Sapino A, Papotti M, Macri L, Satolli MA, Bussolati G. Intranodular reactive endothelial hyperplasia in adenomatous goiter. *Histopathology* 1995;26:457–462.

427. Chan KW, Poon GD, Choi CH. Plasma cell granuloma of the thyroid. *J Clin Pathol* 1986;39:1105–1107.

428. Yapp R, Linder J, Schenken JR, Karrer FW. Plasma cell granuloma of the thyroid. *Hum Pathol* 1985;16:848–850.

429. Holck S. Plasma cell granuloma of the thyroid. *Cancer* 1981; 48:830–832.

430. Katoh R, Ishizaki T, Tomichi N, Yagawa K, Kurihara H. Malacoplakia of the thyroid gland. *Am J Clin Pathol* 1989;92:813–820.

431. Larkin DF, Dervan PA, Munnelly J, Finucane J. Sinus histiocytosis with massive lymphadenopathy simulating subacute thyroiditis. *Hum Pathol* 1986;17:321–324.

432. DeGroot LJ. Effects of irradiation on the thyroid gland. *Endocrinol Metab Clin North Am* 1993;22:607–615.

433. Hanson GA, Komorowski RA, Cerletty JM, Wilson SD. Thyroid gland morphology in young adults. Normal subjects versus those with prior low-dose neck irradiation in childhood. *Surgery* 1993;94: 984–988.

434. Favus MJ, Schneider AB, Stachura ME, Arnold JE, Ryo UY, Pinsky SM, Colman M, Arnold MJ, Frohman LA. Thyroid cancer occurring as a late consequence of head and neck irradiation. Evaluation of 1056 patients. *N Engl J Med* 1976;294:1019–1025.

435. Carr RF, LiVolsi VA. Morphologic changes in the thyroid after irradiation for Hodgkin's and non-Hodgkin's lymphoma. *Cancer* 1989;64:825–829.

436. Tanaka K, Tsunoda T, Eto T, Yamada M, Tajima Y, Shimogama H, Yamaguchi T, Matsuo S, Izawa K. Diagnosis and management of heterotopic pancreas. *Int Surg* 1993;78:32–35.

437. Yamagiwa H, Onishi N, Nishii M. Heterotopic pancreas of the stomach. Histogenesis and immunohistochemistry. *Acta Pathol Jpn* 1992;42:249–254.

438. Pang L-C. Pancreatic heterotopia. A reappraisal and clinicopathologic analysis of 32 cases. *South Med J* 1988;81:1264–1275.

439. Lai ECS, Tompkins RK. Heterotopic pancreas. Review of 26 year experience. *Am J Surg* 1986;151:697–700.

440. Dolan RV, ReMine WH, Dockerty MB. The fate of heterotopic pancreatic tissue. *Arch Surg* 1974;109:762–765.

441. Busard JM, Walters W. Heterotopic pancreatic tissue. Report of a case presenting symptoms of ulcer and review of the recent literature. *Arch Surg* 1950;60:674–682.

442. Hara M, Tsutsumi Y. Immunohistochemical studies of endocrine cells in heterotopic pancreas. *Virchows Arch A Path Anat* 1986;408: 385–394.

443. De Castro Barbosa JJ, Dockerty MB, Waugh JM. Pancreatic heterotopia. Review of the literature and report of 41 authenticated surgical cases of which 25 were clinically significant. *Surg Gynecol Obstet* 1946;82:527–542.

444. Feldman M, Weinberg T. Aberrant pancreas. A case of duodenal syndrome. *JAMA* 1952;148:893–898.

445. Nickels J, Laasonen EM. Pancreatic heterotopia. *Scand J Gastroenterol* 1970;5:639–640.

446. Loquvam GS, Russell WO. Accessory pancreatic ducts of the major duodenal papilla. Normal structures to be differentiated from cancer. *Am J Clin Pathol* 1950;20:305–313.

447. Robson HN, Scott GBD. Lipomatous pseudohypertrophy of the pancreas. *Gastroenterology* 1953;23:74–81.

448. Bartholomew LG, Baggenstoss AH, Morlock CG, Comfort MW. Primary atrophy and lipomatosis of the pancreas. *Gastroenterology* 1959;36:563–572.

449. Olsen TS. Lipomatosis of the pancreas in autopsy material and its relation to age and overweight. *Acta Pathol Microbiol Scand A* 1978;86:367–373.

450. Stamm BH. Incidence and diagnostic significance of minor pathologic changes in the adult pancreas at autopsy. A systemic study of 112 autopsies in patients without known pancreatic disease. *Hum Pathol* 1984;15:677–683.

451. LeCompte PM, Merriam JC Jr. Mitotic figures and enlarged nuclei in the islands of Langerhans in man. *Diabetes* 1962;11:35–39.

452. Ehrie MG, Swartz FJ. Diploid, tetraploid and octaploid beta cells in the islets of Langerhans of the normal human pancreas. *Diabetes* 1974;23:583–588.

453. Izbicki JR, Knoefel WT, Muller-Hocker J, Mandelkow HK. Pancreatic hamartoma. A benign tumor of the pancreas. *Am J Gastroenterology* 1994;89:1261–1262.

454. Burt TB, Condon VR, Matlak ME. Fetal pancreatic hamartoma. *Pediatr Radiol* 1983;13:287–289.

455. Flaherty MJ, Benjamin DR. Multicystic pancreatic hamartoma. A distinctive lesion with immunohistochemical and ultrastructural study. *Hum Pathol* 1992;23:1309–1312.

456. Mester M, Trajber HJ, Compton CC, de Camargo HSA Jr, Cardoso de Almeida PC, Hoover HC Jr. Cystic teratomas of the pancreas. *Arch Surg* 1990;125:1215–1218.

457. Markovsky V, Russin VL. Fine-needle aspiration of dermoid cyst of the pancreas. A case report. *Diagn Cytopathol* 1993;9:66–69.

458. Jacobs JE, Dinsmore BJ. Mature cystic teratoma of the pancreas. Sonographic and CT findings. *Am J Radiol* 1993;160:523–524.

459. Howard JM. Cystic neoplasms and true cysts of the pancreas. *Surg Clin North Am* 1989;69:651–665.

460. Elliott DW. Pancreatic pseudocysts. *Surg Clin North Am* 1975;55:339–362.

461. Bourliere M, Sarles H. Pancreatic cysts and pseudocysts associated with acute and chronic pancreatitis. *Dig Dis Sci* 1989;34:343–348.

462. D'Egidio A, Schein M. Pancreatic pseudocysts. A proposed classification and its management implications. *Br J Surg* 1991;78:981–984.

463. Kloppel G, Maillet B. Pseudocysts in chronic pancreatitis. A morphological analysis of 57 resection specimens and 9 autopsy pancreata. *Pancreas* 1991;6:266–274.

464. Compton CC. Diseases of the pancreas. In: Weidner N, ed. *The difficult diagnosis in surgical pathology.* Philadelphia: WB Saunders, 1996;258–283.

465. Lewandrowski KB, Southern JF, Pins MR, Compton CC, Warshaw AL. Cystic fluid analysis in the differential diagnosis of pancreatic cysts. A comparison of pseudocysts, serous cystadenomas, mucinous cystic neoplasms, and mucinous cystadenocarcinoma. *Ann Surg* 1993;217:41–47.

466. Seifert G, Kloppel G. Diagnostic value of pancreatic biopsy. *Pathol Res Pract* 1979;164:357–384.

467. Hyland C, Kheir SM, Kashlan MB. Frozen section diagnosis of pancreatic carcinoma. A prospective study of 64 biopsies. *Am J Surg Pathol* 1981;5:179–191.

468. Beazley RM. Needle biopsy diagnosis of pancreatic cancer. *Cancer* 1981;47:1685–1687.

469. Lee, Y-TN(M). Tissue diagnosis for carcinoma of the pancreas and periampullary structures. *Cancer* 1982;49:1035–1039.

470. Weiland LH. Frozen section diagnosis in tumors of the pancreas. *Semin Diagn Pathol* 1984;1:54–58.

471. Kloppel G. Maillet B. Pathology of acute and chronic pancreatitis. *Pancreas* 1993;8:659–670.

472. Steer ML, Waxman I, Freedman S. Chronic pancreatitis. *N Engl J Med* 1995;332:1482–1490.

473. Singh SM, Reber HA. The pathology of chronic pancreatitis. *World J Surg* 1990;14:2–10.

474. Costa J. Benign epithelial inclusions in pancreatic nerves. *Am J Clin Pathol* 1977;67:306–307.

475. Bartow S, Mukai K, Rosai J. Pseudoneoplastic proliferation of endocrine cells in pancreatic fibrosis. *Cancer* 1981;47:2627–2633.

476. Rickaert F, Gelin M, van Gansbeke D, Lambilliotte J-P, Verhest A, Pasteels J-L, Kloppel G, Kiss R. Computerized morphonuclear characteristics and DNA content of adenocarcinoma of the pancreas, chronic pancreatitis, and normal tissues. Relationship with histopathologic grading. *Hum Pathol* 1992;23:1210–1215.

477. Weger AR, Lindholm JL. Discrimination of pancreatic adenocarcinomas from chronic pancreatitis by morphometric analysis. *Pathol Res Pract* 1992;188:44–48.

478. Linder S, Weger A-R, Lindholm J, Jui H, Blasjo M, Sundelin P, von Rosen A. Morphometric characteristics in adenocarcinoma of the pancreas and chronic pancreatitis. *Scand J Gastroenterol* 1994;29:764–768.

479. Xerri L, Payan M-J, Choux R, Gros N, Figarella-Branger D, Sarles H. Predominance of sialomucin secretion in malignant and premalignant pancreatic lesions. *Hum Pathol* 1990;21:927–931.

480. Shimizu M, Saitoh Y, Itoh H. Immunohistochemical staining of Ha-ras oncogene product in normal, benign, and malignant human pancreatic tissues. *Hum Pathol* 1990;21:607–612.

481. Shimizu M, Saitoh Y, Ohyanagi H, Itoh H. Immunohistochemical staining of pancreatic cancer with CA19-9, KMO1, unabsorbed CEA, and absorbed CEA. A comparison with normal pancreas and chronic pancreatitis. *Arch Pathol Lab Med* 1990;114:195–200.

482. Loy TS, Springer D, Chapman RK, Diaz-Arias AA, Bulatao IS, Bickel JT. Lack of specificity of monoclonal antibody B72.3 in distinguishing chronic pancreatitis from pancreatic adenocarcinoma. *Am J Clin Pathol* 1991;96:684–688.

483. Haglund C, Roberts PJ, Nordling S, Ekblom P. Expression of laminin in pancreatic neoplasms and in chronic pancreatitis. *Am J Surg Pathol* 1984;8:669–676.

484. Kawaguchi K, Koike M, Tsuruta K, Okamoto A, Tabata I, Fujita N. Lymphoplasmacytic sclerosing pancreatitis. *Hum Pathol* 1991;22:387–395.

485. Suda K, Tsukahara M, Miyake T, Hirai S. A morphologic analysis of naked islets of Langerhans in lobular atrophy of the pancreas. *Pathol Int* 1994;44:618–623.

486. Oertel JE, Heffess CS, Oertel YC. Pancreas. In: Sternberg SS, ed. *Histology for pathologists*. New York: Raven Press, 1992;657–668.

487. Allen-Mersh TG. Pancreatic ductal mucinous hyperplasia: distribution within the pancreas, and effect of variation in ampullary and pancreatic duct anatomy. *Gut* 1988;29:1392–1396.

488. Volkholz P, Stolte M, Becker V. Epithelial dysplasia in chronic pancreatitis. *Virchows Arch A Path Anat* 1982;396:331–348.

489. Yanagisawa A, Ohtake K, Ohashi K, Hori M, Kitagawa T, Sugano H, Kato Y. Frequent c-Ki-ras oncogene activation in mucous cell hyperplasias of pancreas suffering from chronic inflammation. *Cancer Res* 1993;53:953–956.

490. Kozuka S, Nagasawa S, Tsubone M, Taki T. DNA content of pancreatic duct hyperplasia and carcinoma. *Jpn J Cancer Res* 1982;73:119–123.

491. Boschman CR, Stryker S, Reddy JK, Rao MS. Expression of p53 protein in precursor lesions and adenocarcinoma of human pancreas. *Am J Pathol* 1994;145:1291–1295.

492. Laidlaw GF. Nesidioblastoma. The islet tumor of pancreas. *Am J Pathol* 1938;14:125–139.

493. Goosens A, Gepts W, Saudubray J-M, Bonnefont JP, Nihoul-Fekete, Heitz PhU, Kloppel G. Diffuse and focal nesidioblastosis. A clinicopathologic study of 24 patients with persistent neonatal hyperinsulinemic hypoglycemia. *Am J Surg Pathol* 1989;13:766–775.

494. Glenner GG, Mallory GK. The cystadenoma and related nonfunctional tumors of the pancreas. Pathogenesis, classification, and significance. *Cancer* 1956;9:980–996.

495. Nakashiro H, Tokunaga O, Wantanabe T, Ishibashi K, Kuwaki T. Localized lymphoid hyperplasia (pseudolymphoma) of the pancreas presenting with obstructive jaundice. *Hum Pathol* 1991;22:721–726.

496. Johnson RL, Page DL, Dean RH. Pseudotumor of the pancreas. *South Med J* 1983;76:647–649.

497. Abrebanel P, Sarfaty S, Gal R, Chaimoff C, Kessler E. Plasma cell granuloma of the pancreas. *Arch Pathol Lab Med* 1984;108:531–532 (letter).

498. Remberger K, Weiss M, Gokel JM, Landgraf R, Illner WD, Land W. Pancreatic inflammatory pseudotumor with persistent hyperinsulinemia hypoglycemia following long term pancreatic transplantation. *Verh Dtsch Ges Pathol* 1987;71:328–332.

499. Uzoaru I, Chou P, Reyes-Mugica M, Shen-Schwarz S, Gonzalez-Crussi F. Inflammatory myofibroblastic tumor of the pancreas. *Surg Pathol* 1993;5:181–188.

500. Dudiak KM. Abdominal case of the day. Inflammatory pseudotumor of the pancreas. *Am J Radiol* 1993;160:1324–1325.

501. Palazzo JP, Chang CD. Inflammatory pseudotumor of the pancreas. *Histopathology* 1993;23:475–477.

502. Graham LS. Celiac accessory adrenal glands. *Cancer* 1953;6:149–152.

503. Mitchell N, Angrist A. Adrenal rests in the kidney. *Arch Pathol* 1943;35:46–52.

504. Culp OS. Adrenal heterotopia. A survey of the literature and report of a case. *J Urol* 1939;41:303–309.

505. Nelson AA. Accessory adrenal cortical tissue. *Arch Pathol* 1939;27:955–965.

506. Wiener MF, Dallgaard SA. Intracranial adrenal gland. A case report. *Arch Pathol* 1959;67:228–233.

507. Dahl EV, Bahn RC. Aberrant adrenal cortical tissue near the testis in human infants. *Am J Pathol* 1962;40:587–598.

508. Mares AJ, Shkolnik A, Sacks M, Feuchtwanger MM. Aberrant (ectopic) adrenocortical tissue along the spermatic cord. *J Pediatr Surg* 1980;15:289–292.

509. Busuttil A. Ectopic adrenal within the gall-bladder wall. *J Pathol* 1974;113:231–233.

510. Michowitz M, Schujman E, Solowiejczyk M. Aberrant adrenal tissue in the wall of a hernial sac. *Am Surg* 1979;45:67–69.

511. Czaplicki M, Bablok L, Kuzaka B, Janczewski Z. Heterotopic adrenal tissue. *Int Urol Nephrol* 1985;17:177–181.

512. Burke EF, Gilbert E, Uehling DT. Adrenal rest tumors of the testes. *J Urol* 1973;109:649–652.

513. Feldman AE, Rosenthal RS, Shaw JL. Aberrant adrenal tissue. An incidental finding during orchiopexy. *J Urol* 1975;113:706–708.

514. Gutowski WT III, Gray GF Jr. Ectopic adrenal in inguinal hernia sacs. *J Urol* 1979;121:353–354.

515. Anderson JR, McLean Ross AH. Ectopic adrenal tissue in adults. *Postgrad Med J* 1980;56:806–808.

516. Schechter DC. Aberrant adrenal tissue. *Ann Surg* 1968;167:421–426.

517. Habuchi T, Mizutani Y, Miyakawa M. Ectopic aberrant adrenals with epididymal abnormality. *Urology* 1992;34:251–253.

518. Chin L, Brody RI, Morales P, Black VH. Immunocytochemical characterization of intrarenal adrenal tissue. *Urology* 1994;44:429–432.

519. MacLennan A. On the presence of adrenal rests in the walls of hernial sacs. *Surg Gynecol Obstet* 1919;29:387–388.

520. Vestfrid MA. Ectopic adrenal cortex in neonatal liver. *Histopathology* 1980;4:669–672.

521. Armin A, Castelli M. Congenital adrenal tissue in the lung with adrenal cytomegaly. *Am J Clin Pathol* 1984;82:225–228.

522. Meyer AW. A congenital intracranial intradural adrenal. *Anat Rec* 1917;23:43–50.

523. Jaffe HL. The suprarenal glands. *Arch Pathol* 1927;3:414.

524. Symonds DA, Driscoll SG. An adrenal cortical rest within the fetal ovary: report of a case. *Am J Clin Pathol* 1973;60:562–564.

525. Nguyen GK,Vriend R, Ronaghan D, Lakey WK. Heterotopic adrenocortical oncocytoma. A case report with light and electron microscopic studies. *Cancer* 1992;70:2681–2684.

526. Honore LH. Intra-adrenal hepatic heterotopia. *J Urol* 1985;133: 652–654.

527. Milliser RV, Greenberg SR, Neiman BH. Heterotopic renal tissue in the human adrenal gland. *J Urol* 1969;102:280–284.

528. Fidler WJ. Ovarian thecal metaplasia in adrenal glands. *Am J Clin Pathol* 1977;67:318–323.

529. Kampmeier OF. Giant epithelial cells of the human fetal adrenal. *Anat Rec* 1927;37:95–102.

530. Oppenheimer EH. Adrenal cytomegaly. Studies by light and electron microscopy. Comparison with the adrenal in Beckwith's and virilism syndromes. *Arch Pathol* 1979;90:57–64.

531. Nakamura H, Yano H, Nakashima T. False intranuclear inclusions in adrenal cytomegaly. *Arch Pathol Lab Med* 1981;105:358–360.

532. Borit A, Kosek J. Cytomegaly of the adrenal cortex. Electron microscopy in Beckwith's syndrome. *Arch Pathol* 1969;88:58–64.

533. Carney JA. Adrenal Gland. In: Sternberg SS, ed. *Histology for pathologists*. New York: Raven Press, 1992;321–346.

534. Lam KY. Lipomatous tumors of the adrenal gland. Clinicopathologic study of eight cases. *J Urol Pathol* 1995;3:95–106.

535. Wahl HR. Adrenal cysts. *Am J Pathol* 1951;27:758.

536. Hodges FV, Ellis FR. Cystic lesions of the adrenal glands. *Arch Pathol* 1958;60:53–58.

537. Foster DG. Adrenal cysts. *Arch Surg* 1966;92:131–143.

538. Kearney GP, Mahoney EM, Maher E, Harrison JH. Functioning and nonfunctioning cysts of the adrenal cortex and medulla. *Am J Surg* 1977;134:363–368.

539. Incze JS, Lui PS, Merriam JC, Austen G, Widrich WC, Gerzof SG. Morphology and pathogenesis of adrenal cysts. 1979;95:423–428.

540. Ghandur-Mnaymneh L, Slim M, Muakassa K. Adrenal cysts. Pathogenesis and histological identification with a report of 6 cases. *J Urol* 1979;122:87–91.

541. Cheema P, Cartagena R, Staubitz W. Adrenal cysts. Diagnosis and treatment. *J Urol* 1981;126:396–399.

542. Medeiros LJ, Lewandowski KB, Vickery AL Jr. Adrenal pseudocyst. A clinical and pathological study of eight cases. *Hum Pathol* 1989; 20:660–665.

543. Medeiros LJ, Weiss LM, Vickery AL Jr. Epithelial-lined (true) cyst of the adrenal gland: a case report. *Hum Pathol* 1989;20:491–492.

544. Gaffey MJ, Mills SE, Medeiros LJ, Weiss LM. Unusual variants of adrenal pseudocysts with intracystic fat, myelolipomatous metaplasia, and metastatic carcinoma. *Am J Clin Pathol* 1990;94:706–713.

545. Melicow MM. One hundred cases of pheochromocytoma (107 tumors) at the Columbia-Presbyterian Medical Center, 1926–1976: a clinicopathologic analysis. *Cancer* 1977;40:1987–2004.

546. Fukushima N, Oonishi T, Yamaguchi K, Fukayama M. Mediastinal cyst of the adrenal gland. *Pathol Int* 1995;45:156–159.

547. Medeiros LJ, Weiss LM. Adrenal gland. Tumors and tumor-like lesions. In: Weidner N, ed. *The difficult diagnosis in surgical pathology*. Philadelphia: WB Saunders, 1996;377–407.

548. Gaffey MJ, Mills SE, Fechner RE, Berthoff MF, Allen MS Jr. Vascular adrenal cysts. A clinicopathologic and imunohistochemical study of endothelial and hemorrhagic (pseudocystic) variants. *Am J Surg Pathol* 1989;13:740–747.

549. Hayashi Y, Hiyoshi T, Takemura T, Kurashima C, Hirokawa K. Focal lymphocytic infiltrates in the adrenal cortex of elderly: immunohistological analysis of infiltrating lymphocytes. *Clin Exp Immunol* 1989;77:101–105.

550. Selye H, Stone H. Hormonally induced transformation of adrenal into myeloid tissue. *Am J Pathol* 1950;23:211–233.

551. Richardson JC. A tumour of the adrenal gland composed of the elements of bone marrow tissue. *Am J Cancer* 1935;25: 746–752.

552. McDonnell WV. Myelolipoma of adrenal. *Arch Pathol* 1956;61: 416–419.

553. Plaut A. Myelolipoma in the adrenal cortex (myeloadipose structures). *Am J Pathol* 1958;34:487–502.

554. Whittaker LD. Myelolipoma of the adrenal gland. Surgical removal. *Arch Surg* 1968;97:628–631.

555. Newman PH, Silen W. Myelolipoma of the adrenal gland. Report of the third case of a symptomatic tumor and review of the literature. *Arch Surg* 1968;97:637–647.

556. Tulcinsky DB, Deutsch V, Bubis JJ. Myelolipoma of the adrenal gland. *Br J Surg* 1970;57:465–467.

557. Olsson CA, Krane RJ, Klugo RC, Selikowitz SM. Adrenal myelolipoma. *Surgery* 1973;73:665–670.

558. Rubin HB, Hirose F, Benfield JR. Myelolipoma of the adrenal gland. Angiographic findings and review of the literature. *Am J Surg* 1975;130:354–358.

559. Boudreaux D, Waisman J, Skinner DG, Low R. Giant adrenal myelolipoma and testicular interstitial cell tumor in a man with congenital 21-hydroxylase deficiency. *Am J Surg Pathol* 1979;3: 109–123.

560. Ayyat F, Fosslin E, Kent R, Hudson HC. Myelolipoma of adrenal gland. *Urology* 1980;16:415–418.

561. Wilhelmus JL, Schrodt GR, Alberhasky MT, Alcorn MO. Giant adrenal myelolipoma. *Arch Pathol Lab Med* 1981;532–535.

562. Ishikawa H, Tachibana M, Hata M, Tazaki H, Akatsuka S, Iri H. Myelolipoma of the adrenal gland. *J Urol* 1981;126:777–779.

563. Fernandez-Sanz J, Galera H, Garcia-Donas A, Gonzalez-Campora RG, Llamas R, Matilla A. Adrenal myelolipoma simulating a retroperitoneal malignant neoplasm. *J Urol* 1981;126:780–782.

564. Noble MJ, Montague DK, Levin HS. Myelolipoma. An unusual surgical lesion of the adrenal gland. *Cancer* 1982;49:952–958.

565. Medeiros LJ, Wolf BC. Traumatic rupture of an adrenal myelolipoma. *Arch Pathol Lab Med* 1983;107:500 (letter).

566. Condom E, Villabona CM, Gomez JM, Carrera M. Adrenal myelolipoma in a woman with congenital 17-hydroxylase deficiency. *Arch Pathol Lab Med* 1985;109:1116–1117.

567. Vyberg M, Sestoft L. Combined adrenal myelolipoma and adenoma associated with Cushing's syndrome. *Am J Clin Pathol* 1986; 86:541–545.

568. Bennett BD, McKenna TJ, Hough AJ, Dean R, Page DL. Adrenal myelolipoma associated with Cushing's disease. *Am J Clin Pathol* 1980;73:443–447.

569. Seniuta P, Cazenave-Mahe J-P, Le Treut A, Trojani M. (Adrenal myelolipoma and Castleman's pseudotumor. A case of association in a retroperitoneal tumor.) *J d'Urol* 1989;95:511–514.

570. Kraimps JL, Marechaud R, Levillain P, Lacour JF, Barbier J. Bilateral symptomatic adrenal myelolipoma. *Surgery* 1992;111:114–117.

571. Goetz SP, Neimann TH, Robinson RA, Cohen MB. Hematopoietic elements associated with adrenal glands. A study of the spectrum of change in nine cases. *Arch Pathol Lab Med* 1994;118:895–896.

572. Sanders R, Bissada N, Curry N, Gordon B. Clinical spectrum of adrenal myelolipoma. Analysis of 8 tumors in 7 patients. *J Urol* 1995;153:1791–1793.

573. Reynard JM, Newman ML, Pollock L, Lord MG. Giant adrenal myelolipoma. *Br J Urol* 1995;75:795–803.

574. Goldman HB, Howard RC, Patterson AL. Spontaneous retroperitoneal hemorrhage from a giant adrenal myelolipoma. *J Urol* 1996;155:639.

575. White PC, New MI, Dupont B. Congenital adrenal hyperplasia. *N Engl J Med* 1987;316:1519–1524, 1580–1586.

576. Samuels MH, Loriaux DL. Cushing's syndrome and the nodular adrenal gland. *Endocrinol Metab Clin North Am* 1994;23:555–569.

577. DeLellis RA. The adrenal glands. In: Sternberg SS, ed. *Diagnostic surgical pathology*. 2nd ed. New York: Raven Press, 1994;575–583.

578. Petersen RO. Adrenal gland. In: *Urologic pathology*, Philadelphia: JB Lippincott, 1992;726–759.

579. Smals AGH, Pieters GFFM, van Haelst UJG, Kloppenborg PWC. Macronodular adrenocortical hyperplasia in long-standing Cushing's disease. *J Clin Endocrinol Metab* 1984;58:25–31.

580. Doppman JL, Miller DL, Dwyer AJ, Loughlin T, Nieman L, Cutler GB, Chrousos GP, Oldfield E, Loriaux DL. Macronodular adrenal hyperplasia in Cushing's disease. *Radiology* 1988;166:347–352.

581. Shenoy BV, Carpenter DC, Carney JA. Bilateral primary pigmented nodular adrenocortical disease. Rare cause of the Cushing syndrome. *Am J Surg Pathol* 1984;8:335–344.

582. Lack EE. Adrenal medullary hyperplasia and pheochromocytoma. In: *Pathology of adrenal and extra-adrenal paraganglia*. Philadelphia: WB Saunders, 1994;220–272.

583. Carney JA, Sizemore GW, Sheps SG. Adrenal medullary disease in multiple endocrine neoplasia, type 2. Pheochromocytoma and its precursors. *Am J Clin Pathol* 1976;66:279–290.

584. Visser JW, Axt R. Bilateral adrenal medullary hyperplasia. A clinicopathological entity. *J Clin Pathol* 1975;28:298–304.

585. Carney JA, Sizemore GW, Tyre GM. Bilateral adrenal medullary hyperplasia in multiple endocrine neoplasia, type 2. The precursor of bilateral pheochromocytoma. *Mayo Clin Proc* 1975;50:3–10.

586. DeLellis RA, Wolfe HJ, Gagel RF, Feldman ZT, Miller HH, Gang DL, Reichlin J. Adrenal medullary hyperplasia. A morphometric analysis in patients with familial medullary thyroid carcinoma. *Am J Pathol* 1976;83:177–196.

587. Rudy FR, Bates RD, Cimorelli AJ, Hill GS, Engelman K. Adrenal medullary hyperplasia. A clinicopathologic study of four cases. *Hum Pathol* 1980;11:650–657.

588. Padberg B-C, Garbe E, Achilles E, Dralle H, Bressel M, Schroder S. Adrenomedullary hyperplasia and phaeochromocytoma. DNA cytophotometric findings in 47 cases. *Virchows Arch A Path Anat* 1990;416:443–446.

589. Diaz-Cano S, Gonzalez-Campora R, Rios-Martin JJ, Lerma-Puertas E, Jorda-Heras M, Vazquez-Ramirez F, Bibbo M, Galera-Davidson H. Nuclear DNA patterns in adrenal cortex proliferative lesions. *Virchows Arch A Path Anat* 1993;423:323–328.

590. De Mascarel A, Vergier B, Merlino J-P, Goussot JF, Coindre J-M. Plasma cell granuloma of the adrenal gland and the thyroid: report of two cases. *J Surg Oncol* 1989;41:139–142.

## ADDENDUM REFERENCES

### *Hamartomas of the Breast*

Charpin C, Mathoulin MP, Andrac L, Barberis J, Boulat J, Sarradour B, Bonnier P, Piana L. Reappraisal of breast hamartomas: a morphological study of 41 cases. *Pathol Res Pract* 1994;190:362–371.

Reck T, Dworak O, Thaler KH, Kockerling F. Hamartoma of aberrant breast tissue in the inguinal region. *Chirurg* 1995;66:923–926.

Rohen C, Caselitz J, Stern C, Wanschura S, Schoenmakers EF, Van de Ven WJ, Bartnitzke S, Bullerdiek J. A hamartoma of the breast with an aberration of 12q mapped to the MAR region by fluorescence in situ hybridization. *Cancer Genet Cytogenet* 1995;84:82–84.

Testempassi E, Ishi C, Yamada T, Fukuda K, Tada S, Nikaido T. Breast hamartoma: MR findings. *Radiat Med* 1995;13:187–189.

Williams NP, Williams E. Mammary hamartoma: an under-recognized breast lesion. *W Ind Med J* 1996;45:67–69.

### *Mammary Fat Necrosis*

Hogge JP, Robinson RE, Magnant CM, Zuurbier RA. The mammographic spectrum of fat necrosis of the breast. *Radiographics* 1995;15:1347–1356.

Willis SL, Ramzy I. Analysis of false results in a series of 835 fine needle aspirates of breast lesions. *Acta Cytol* 1995;39:858–864.

### *Mammary Squamous Metaplasia*

Fiorica JV. Special problems: Mondor's disease, macrocysts, trauma, squamous metaplasia, & miscellaneous disorders of the nipple. *Obstet Gynecol Clin N Amer* 1994;21:479–485.

### *Tumefactive Mastitis*

Bisceglia M, Nirchio V, Carosi I, Cappucci U, Decata A, Paragone T, DiMattia AL. Tumor and tumor-like benign mesenchymal lesions of the breast. *Pathologica* 1995;87:20–41.

### *Rosai-Dorfman Disease of the Breast*

Perez-Guillermo M, Sola-Perez J, Rodriguez-Bermejo M. Malacoplakia and Rosai-Dorfman disease: two entities of histiocytic origin infrequently localized in the female breast— the cytologic aspect in aspirates obtained via fine needle aspiration cytology. *Diagn Cytopathol* 1993;9:698–704.

### *Mammary Adenosis*

Cardillo MR, Stamp GW, Pignatelli M. Proliferating cell nuclear antigen in benign breast diseases. *Eur J Gynaecol Oncol* 1995;16:476–481.

Prabhakar BR. Multiple intraductal papillomas and sclerosing adenosis in the male breast. *Ind J Pathol Microbiol* 1994;37(Suppl):S9–S10.

Rasbridge SA, Millis RR. Carcinoma in situ involving sclerosing adenosis: a mimic of invasive breast carcinoma. *Histopathology* 1995;27:269–273.

Seidman JD, Ashton M, Lefkowitz M. Atypical apocrine adenosis of the breast: a clinicopathologic study of 37 patients with 8.7 year followup. *Cancer* 1996;77:2529–2537.

Visscher DW, Wallis TL, Crissman JD. Evaluation of chromosome aneuploidy in tissue sections of preinvasive breast carcinomas using interphase cytogenetics. *Cancer* 1996;77:315–320.

Wells CA, McGregor IL, Makunura CN, Yeomans P, Davies JD. Apocrine adenosis: a precursor of aggressive breast cancer? *J Clin Pathol* 1995;48:737–742.

### *Radial Scar of the Breast*

De la Torre M, Lindholm K, Lindgren A. Fine needle aspiration cytology of tubular breast carcinoma and radial scar. *Acta Cytol* 1994;38:884–890.

Makunura CN, Curling OM, Yeomans P, Perry N, Wells CA. Apocrine adenosis within a radial scar: a case of false positive breast cytodiagnosis. *Cytopathology* 1994;5:123–128.

Orel SG, Evers K, Yeh IT, Troupin RH. Radial scar with microcalcifications: radiologic-pathologic correlation. *Radiology* 1992;183:479–482.

Ruiz-Sauri A, Almenar-Medina S, Callaghan RC, Calderon J, Llombart-Bosch A. Radial scar versus tubular carcinoma of the breast: a comparative study with quantitative techniques (morphometry, image- and flow cytometry). *Pathol Res Pract* 1995;191:547–554.

### *Collagenous Spherulosis of the Breast*

Cardesi E, Cera G, Campione D, Macario-Gioia M, Mariscotti G, Mariatti M. Collagenous spherulosis of the breast. *Pathologica* 1994;86:656–658.

Rey A, Redondo E, Servent R. Collagenous spherulosis of the breast diagnosed by fine needle aspiration biopsy. *Acta Cytol* 1995;39:1071–1073.

Sgroi D, Koemer FC. Involvement of collagenous spherulosis by lobular carcinoma in situ: potential confusion with cribriform ductal carcinoma in situ. *Am J Surg Pathol* 1995;19:1366–1370.

Stephenson TJ, Hird PM, Laing RW, Davies JD. Nodular basement membrane deposits in breast carcinoma and atypical ductal hyperplasia: mimics of collagenous spherulosis. *Pathologica* 1994;86:234–239.

### *Pseudoangiomatous Stromal Hyperplasia of the Breast*

Badve S, Sloane JP. Pseudoangiomatous hyperplasia of male breast. *Histopathology* 1995;26:463–466.

Cohen MA, Morris EA, Rosen PP, Dershaw DD, Liberman L, Abramson

AF. Pseudoangiomatous stromal hyperplasia: mammographic, sonographic, and clinical patterns. *Radiology* 1996;198:117–120.

Polger MR, Denison CM, Lester S, Meyer JE. Pseudoangiomatous stromal hyperplasia: mammographic and sonographic appearance. *Am J Roentgenol* 1996;166:349–352.

### *Mucocele of the Breast*

Hamele-Bena D, Cranor ML, Rosen PP. Mammary mucocele-like lesions: benign and malignant. *Am J Surg Pathol* 1996;20:1081–1085.

Mesonero CE, Tabbara S. Fine needle aspiration cytology of ductal adenoma: report of a case associated with a mucocele-like lesion. *Diagn Cytopathol* 1995;13:252–256.

Weaver MG, Abdul-Karim FW, Al-Kaisi N. Mucinous lesions of the breast: a pathological continuum. *Pathol Res Pract* 1993;189:873–876.

### *Rathke Cleft Cysts of the Pituitary*

Kleinschmidt-DeMasters BK, Lillihei KO, Stears JC. The pathologic, surgical, and MR spectrum of Rathke cleft cysts. *Surg Neurol* 1995;44:19–27.

Naylor MF, Scheithauer BW, Forbes GS, Tomlinson FH, Young WF. Rathke cleft cyst: CT, MR, and pathology of 23 cases. *J Comput Asst Tomogr* 1995;19:853–859.

### *Pituitary Choristomas*

Horvath E, Kovacs K, Scheithauer BW, Lloyd RV, Smyth HS. Pituitary adenoma with neuronal choristoma (PANCH): composite lesion or lineage infidelity? *Ultrastruct Pathol* 1994;18:565–574.

Oka H, Kameya T, Sasano H, Aiba M, Kovacs K, Horvath E, Yokota Y, Kawano N, Yada K. Pituitary choristoma composed of corticotroph and adrenocortical cells in the sella turcica. *Virchows Arch A* 1996;427:613–617.

Siegel SF, Ahdab-Barmada M, Arslanian S, Foley TP Jr. Ectopic posterior pituitary tissue and paracentric inversion of the short arm of chromosome 1 in twins. *Eur J Endocrinol* 1995;133:87–92.

### *Pituitary and Hypothalamic Hamartomas*

Chamouilli JM, Razafimahefa B, Pierron H. Precocious puberty and hypothalamic hamartoma: treatment with triptorelin during eight years. *Arch Pediatr* 1995;2:438–441.

### *Pituitary "Gangliocytoma"*

Puchner MJ, Ludecke DK, Saeger W, Riedel M, Asa SL. Gangliocytomas of the sellar region: a review. *Exp Clin Endocrinol Diabetes* 1995;103:129–149.

Saeger W, Puchner MJ, Ludecke DK. Combined sellar gangliocytoma and pituitary adenoma in acromegaly or Cushing's disease. A report of 3 cases. *Virchows Arch A* 1994;425:93–99.

### *Pseudotumoral Pituitary Infarction*

Goel A, Deogaonkar M, Desai K. Fatal postoperative "pituitary apoplexy": its cause and management. *Br J Neurosurg* 1995;9:37–40.

Masago A, Ueda Y, Kanai H, Nagai H, Umemura S. Pituitary apoplexy after pituitary function test: a report of two cases and review of the literature. *Surg Neurol* 1995;43:158–165.

### *Lymphocytic Hypophysitis*

Beressi N, Cohen R, Beressi JP, Dumas JL, Legrand M, Iba-Zizen MT, Modigliani E. Pseudotumoral lymphocytic hypophysitis successfully treated by corticosteroid alone: first case report. *Neurosurgery* 1994;35:505–508.

Cohen R, Beressi N, Modigliani E. Lymphocytic hypophysitis. *Clin Endocrinol* 1995;43:769.

Jenkins PJ, Chew SL, Lowe DG, Afshart F, Charlesworth M, Besser GM, Wass JA. Lymphocytic hypophysitis: unusual features of a rare disorder. *Clin Endocrinol* 1995;42:529–534.

McDonald MA, Brophy BP, Raymond W. Lymphocytic hypophysitis: a rare cause of hyperprolactinemia. *Austr NZ J Surg* 1995;65:538–539.

Nishioka H, Ito H, Sano T, Ito Y. Two cases of lymphocytic hypophysitis presenting with diabetes insipidus: a variant of lymphocytic infundibuloneurohypophysitis. *Surg Neurol* 1996;46:285–291.

Patel MC, Guneratne N, Haq N, West TE, Weetman AP, Clayton RN. Peripartum hypopituitarism and lymphocytic hypophysitis. *Q J Med* 1995;88:571–580.

Prager D, Braunstein GD. Pituitary disorders during pregnancy. *Endocrinol Metab Clin N Amer* 1995;24:1–14.

Pressman EK, Zeidman SM, Reddy UM, Epstein JI, Brem H. Differentiating lymphocytic adenohypophysitis from pituitary adenoma in the peripartum patient. *J Reprod Med* 1995;40:251–259.

Proust F, Hannequin D, Bellow F, Langlois O, Tadie M, Creissard P, Freger P. Stress-induced pituitary apoplexy in 2 phases. *Neurochirurgie* 1995;41:372–376.

Sautner D, Saeger W, Ludecke DK, Jansen V, Puchner MJ. Hypophysitis in surgical and autoptical specimens. *Acta Neuropathol* 1995;90:637–644.

Virally-Monod ML, Barrou Z, Basin C, Thomopoulos P, Luton JP. Lymphocytic hypophysitis: a reality. *Presse Med* 1996;25:933–938.

### *Parathyroid Cysts*

Cooper KJ, Hill AD, Sangwan Y, Al-Adnani M, Menzies-Gow N, Darzi A. Hypercalcemia associated with a parathyroid cyst. *Ulster Med J* 1994;63:246–247.

Lydiatt DD, Byers RM, Khouri KG, Whitworth PW, Sellin RV. Functional parathyroid cyst and hypocalciuric hypercalcemia. *Ear Nose Throat J* 1995;74:713–716.

McCluggage WG, Russell CF, Toner PG. Parathyroid cyst of the thymus. *Thorax* 1995;50:913–914.

Patel KD, Rege JD, Varthakavi PK, Desai SA, Nihalani KD. Fine needle aspiration of an unsuspected parathyroid cyst. *J Assoc Phys India* 1995;43:791.

Spitz AF. Management of a functioning mediastinal parathyroid cyst. *J Clin Endocrinol Metab* 1995;80:2866–2868.

Wakabayashi K, Takahashi T, Tejima S. Parathyroid cyst. *Jpn J Clin Med* 1995;53:1004–1007.

### *Parathyroid Hyperplasia*

Calender A, Cougard P. Primary hyperparathyroidism: genetic heterogeneity suggesting different pathogenesis in sporadic and familial forms of parathyroid hyperplasia and tumors. *Eur J Endocrinol* 1996;134:263–266.

Duh QY, Ciulla TA, Clark OH. Primary parathyroid hyperplasia associated with thyroid hemiagenesis and agenesis of the isthmus. *Surgery* 1994;115:257–263.

Sloan DA, Schwartz RW, McGrath PC, Kenady DE. Diagnosis and management of thyroid and parathyroid hyperplasia and neoplasia. *Curr Opin Oncol* 1995;7:47–55.

### *Malakoplakia of the Thyroid*

Larsimont D, Hamels J, Fortunati D. Thyroid gland malakoplakia with autoimmune thyroiditis. *Histopathology* 1993;23:491–494.

### *Pancreatic "Teratoma"*

Kohzaki S, Fukuda T, Fujimoto T, Kirao K, Matsunaga N, Hayashi K, Irie J, Kondo N. Ciliated foregut cyst of the pancreas mimicking teratomatous tumor. *Br J Radiol* 1994;67:601–604.

Perez-Ordonez B, Wesson DE, Smith CR, Asa SL. A pancreatic cyst of the anterior mediastinum. *Mod Pathol* 1996;9:210–214.

Resnick JM, Manivel JC. Immunohistochemical characterization of teratomatous and fetal neuroendocrine pancreas. *Arch Pathol Lab Med* 1994;118:155–159.

### *Pancreatic Hyperplasias and Pseudoneoplastic Lymphocytic Infiltrates*

Hatzitheoklitos E, Buchler MW, Friess H, DiSebastiano P, Poch B, Beger HG, Mohr W. Pseudolymphoma of the pancreas mimicking cancer. *Pancreas* 1994;9:668–670.

Kimura W, Nagai H, Kuroda A, Muto T, Esaki Y. Analysis of small cystic lesions of the pancreas. *Int J Pancreatol* 1995;18:197–206.

Tada M, Ohashi M, Shiratori Y, Okudaira T, Komatsu Y, Kawabe T, Yoshida H, Machinami R, Kishi K, Omata M. Analysis of K-*ras* gene mutation in hyperplastic duct cells of the pancreas without pancreatic disease. *Gastroenterology* 1996;110:227–231.

### *Pancreatic Inflammatory Pseudotumors*

Chutaputti A, Burrell MI, Boyer JL. Pseudotumor of the pancreas associated with retroperitoneal fibrosis: a dramatic response to corticosteroid therapy. *Am J Gastroenterol* 1995;90:1155–1158.

Eckstein RP, Hollings RM, Martin PA, Katelaris CH. Pancreatic pseudotumor arising in association with Sjogren's syndrome. *Pathology* 1995;27: 284–288.

Kroft SH, Stryker SJ, Winter JN, Ergun G, Rao MS. Inflammatory pseudo-tumor of the pancreas. *Int J Pancreatol* 1995;18:277–283.

## Adrenal Cysts

Bastounis E, Pikoulis E, Leppaniemi A, Cyrochristos D. Hydatid disease: a rare cause of adrenal cyst. *Am Surg* 1996;62:383–385.

Jagusch CR, Adickes ED, Neal PM. Lymphangiomatous cyst of the adrenal gland: an unusual cause of flank pain. *Nebr Med J* 1996;81:186–190.

Kloos RT, Gross MD, Francis IR, Korobkin M, Shapiro B. Incidentally dis-covered adrenal masses. *Endocrine Rev* 1995;16:460–484.

Moons P, Oyen RH, Baert AL, Baert L. Symptomatic adrenal pseudocyst. *J Belge Radiol* 1996;79:23–25.

Trauffer PM, Malee MP. Adrenal pseudocyst in pregnancy: a case report. *J Reprod Med* 1996;41:195–197.

## Tumefactive Adrenalitis

Pozilli P, Carotenuto P, Delitala G. Lymphocytic traffic and homing into target tissue and the generation of endocrine autoimmunity. *Clin En-docrinol* 1994;41:545–554.

## Adrenal Myelolipoma

Feldberg E, Guy M, Eisenkraft S, Czernobilsky B. Adrenal cortical ade-noma with extensive fat cell metaplasia. *Pathol Res Pract* 1996;192: 62–66.

Moran RE, Older RA, DeAngelis GA, Baghdady BH, Chrisman HB, Ciambotti JM. Giant myelolipoma. *Am J Roentgenol* 1996;167:246–248.

Sekido N, Kawai K, Takeshima H, Uchida K, Akaza H, Koiso K. Adrenal myelolipoma associated with hereditary spherocytosis. *Int J Urol* 1996; 3:61–63.

*Pathology of Pseudoneoplastic Lesions,*
edited by M. R. Wick, P. A. Humphrey, and J. H. Ritter.
Lippincott-Raven Publishers, Philadelphia © 1997.

CHAPTER 12

# Pseudoneoplastic Lesions of Deep Somatic Soft Tissue and the Skeletal System

Michael B. McDermott and Paul E. Swanson

---

**Pseudoneoplastic Lesions of Deep Soft Tissue**
    Pseudoneoplastic Proliferations of (Myo)fibroblasts
    Tumefactive Fibroinflammatory Lesions
    Myositis Ossificans
    Noninfectious Histiocytic Proliferations Resembling
        Neoplasms
    Infectious Processes Simulating Neoplasms
    Pseudoneoplastic Vascular Proliferations
    Hamartomatous Lesions in Soft Tissue

    Stroma-Predominant Fibroproliferative Processes
        Mimicking Soft Tissue Neoplasms
    Pseudoneoplastic Processes Affecting Peritoneum and
        Peritonealized Soft Tissues
**Pseudoneoplastic Lesions of Bone**
    Fibrous and Fibro-osseous Proliferations of Bone
    Fibroinflammatory and Reactive/Reparative Lesions
    Aneurysmal Bone Cyst
**References**

---

## PSEUDONEOPLASTIC LESIONS OF DEEP SOFT TISSUE

Clinical evaluation of the deep soft tissues, despite advances in imaging techniques, remains an inexact science. As a result, most mass lesions in soft tissue, whether they are palpable or incidentally encountered, typically evoke a clinical differential diagnosis that includes neoplasia. The range of proliferations in somatic and visceral soft tissues that may still be mistaken for neoplasms after gross morphologic and histologic examination is appreciably less diverse but no less problematic for the pathologist and clinician alike.

In soft tissue, proliferations of (myo)fibroblasts—with or without a conspicuous inflammatory component—constitute the overwhelming majority of lesions that meet the general criteria for pseudoneoplasia espoused in the first chapter. However, most mesenchymal elements, and the hematolymphoid cells that they harbor, may participate in some manner in surreptitious efforts by human cells to confuse the surgical pathologist.

For some readers, the absence of the (myo)fibromatoses in the following discussion may be regarded as a serious over-

sight. However, as other authors have repeated in this text, most lesions commonly included in the spectrum of fibromatosis are in fact neoplastic in nature. Hence, apart from the histopathologic settings in which true pseudoneoplasms are associated with fibromatosis-like lesions, neoplastic proliferations of myofibroblasts are not discussed in any detail in this chapter.

Extranodal hematolymphoid proliferations that mimic lymphoma/leukemia, plasmacytoma, and mastocytoma are discussed in detail elsewhere in this text (see Chapter 13); however, pseudoneoplastic histiocytic lesions that reside primarily in soft tissue are reviewed here. The soft tissue pseudoneoplasms that are described in this chapter are listed in Table 1.

### Pseudoneoplastic Proliferations of (Myo)fibroblasts

#### *Nodular Fasciitis*

Perhaps more than any other lesion described in this book, nodular fasciitis should be considered the prototypical pseudotumor. Despite the publication of several large series documenting the typical clinical presentation and varied histopathologic appearances of this lesion (1–8), it continues to confound both clinicians and pathologists. A recently pub-

---

M. B. McDermott and P. E. Swanson: Washington University School of Medicine, St. Louis, Missouri 63110.

**TABLE 1.** *Pseudoneoplastic lesions in soft tissue*

I. Pseudoneoplastic proliferations of (myo)fibroblasts
　Nodular fasciitis
　Intravascular fasciitis
　Fasciitis ossificans
　Parosteal fasciitis
　Cranial fasciitis
　Proliferative myositis
　Proliferative fasciitis
　Ischemic fasciitis
　Other fasciitides
　　Plantar fasciitis
　　Necrotizing fasciitis
　　Eosinophilic fasciitis
　　Palmar fasciitis
　Focal myositis
II. Tumefactive fibroinflammatory lesions
　Inflammatory myofibroblastic tumor
　Calcifying fibrous pseudotumor
　Wegener's granulomatosis
III. Myositis ossificans
IV. Noninfectious histiocytic proliferations resembling neoplasms
　Extranodal Rosai–Dorfman disease
　Other nonneoplastic histiocytic infiltrates
　　Crystal storing histiocytosis
　　Granular cell reaction
　　Silica reaction
　　Postimmunization injection site reaction
　　Polyvinylpyrrolidone granuloma
V. Infectious processes simulating neoplasms
　Histoid leprosy
　"Retroperitoneal xanthogranuloma"
　Malakoplakia
　Mesenchymal lesions due to infection in immunocompromised patients
　　Mycobacterial spindle cell tumor
　　Bacillary angiomatosis
VI. Pseudoneoplastic vascular proliferations
　Vegetant intravascular papillary endothelial hyperplasia
　Angiomatosis/lymphangiomatosis
　Spindle cell hemangioendothelioma
VII. Hamartomatous lesions in soft tissue
　Fibrous hamartoma of infancy
　Fibrolipomatous hamartoma of nerve
　Neuromuscular hamartoma
　Angiomyolipoma
VIII. Stroma-predominant fibroproliferative processes mimicking neoplasms
　Elastofibroma
　Myxoma
IX. Pseudoneoplastic processes affecting peritoneum and peritonealized soft tissues

lished series recorded a 51% error rate in diagnosis at initial pathologic interpretation (6). More significantly, 21% were read as malignant lesions, in one case leading to unnecessarily radical surgery (6). Such diagnostic inaccuracy may also have dire consequences for the pathologist (9).

Nodular fasciitis was first described by Konwaler in 1953 under the designation "spontaneous pseudosarcomatous fibromatosis" (fasciitis) (10). The term nodular fasciitis is credited to Shuman in 1961 (7), but this lesion has also been referred to as nodular fibrositis, subcutaneous fibromatosis, and infiltrative fasciitis (5,7). Typically, it presents in young

adults, with the peak incidence in the third or fourth decade (2–7). However, cases in children have been reported (11,12) and the elderly may also be affected (5). There is no predilection for either sex.

Pain and local tenderness are recorded at presentation in 10–35% of patients, although in a Japanese series from Shimizu et al. these complaints were reported in 76% of cases (3). A small number of patients describe limited loss of function of the involved extremity (7). However, the almost universal presenting complaint is that of a mass or nodule (5,7). Characteristically, the duration of such symptoms is short, with 37–50% of patients undergoing surgery <1 month and 80% within 3 months of first noticing the swelling (2,4). Smaller numbers of patients report a more slowly growing or stable mass and occasionally a history of 3 or more years is documented (2,3). Rapid clinical enlargement is one of the most alarming features of nodular fasciitis, but to the experienced clinician this should be a source of some comfort; malignant soft tissue lesions rarely, if ever, exhibit such prodigious growth.

There is no consistent association with laboratory abnormalities (5), and despite the assertion that nodular fasciitis represents an abnormal healing response to injury, <10% of patients give a history of trauma to the site (2,7,13). The vast majority of patients are otherwise in excellent health, with no underlying illness or disability (5,14) (see section on ischemic fasciitis).

Although in practice any site may be involved (e.g., we have recently seen an otherwise typical example in the eyelid), the most common location for nodular fasciitis is the upper limb and, in particular, the forearm. This predilection appears to be true for both adults and children, although in a recent series, Coffin et al. reported a somewhat higher frequency of pediatric lesions in the head and neck region (12). A summary of the distribution of lesions in seven large series is presented in Table 2.

Topographically, the majority of cases arise in the subcutaneous tissues (4) and appear centered on the superficial fascia, remnants of which may be visible within or adjacent to the lesion (7). The proliferation may be confined to the fascial planes but more commonly extends into adjacent soft tissue on either side (2). However, cases associated with deep fascia may extend into contiguous fat or skeletal muscle, and such cases accounted for 10% in Allen's series (4). Rarely, nodular fasciitis may arise in the dermis (15). Some authors additionally describe a parosteal location for nodular fasciitis; we have addressed this issue separately in this chapter (4) (see section on parosteal fasciitis).

Multiple lesions are only infrequently reported. Only 1 of 250 cases in the series by Shimizu et al. (3) was multifocal at diagnosis, whereas Hutter et al. (14) described six patients with multiple tumors in a smaller series of 70 cases. The former of these authors also documented a single case in which a patient developed 8–10 nodules simultaneously over the body, one of which was biopsy-proven (3).

A consistent and diagnostically useful feature of nodular fasciitis is its small size (Fig. 1), with the average dimension

**TABLE 2.** *Distribution of nodular fasciitis in published series*

| Location | Stout (11) n = 123 | Bernstein and Lattes (8) n = 116 | Kleinstiver and Rodriguez (5) n = 45 | Meister et al. (2) n = 97 | Shimizu et al. (3) n = 250 | Price et al. (7) n = 65 |
|---|---|---|---|---|---|---|
| Upper extremity | 46 | 41[a] | 54 | 50[a] | 44 | 44[a] |
| Arm | 13 | 11 | 27 | 14 | 12 | 22 |
| Forearm | 32 | 25 | 27 | 32 | 27 | 22 |
| Hand | <1 | | | 4 | | |
| Elbow | | 5 | | | | |
| Lower extremity | 20 | 15[a] | 6 | 23[a] | | |
| Thigh | 15 | 6 | 4 | 16 | 17 | 12 |
| Leg | 5 | 5 | 2 | 5 | 8 | |
| Foot | <1 | | | 1 | | |
| Knee | | 3 | | | | |
| Trunk | 20 | 24[a] | | 21 | | |
| Shoulder/axilla | | 8 | 9 | | | 8 |
| Chest wall | | 6 | 11 | | 9 | 17 |
| Back | | 7 | | | | 9 |
| Abdomen | | 3 | 4 | | | |
| Head and neck | 9 | 15 | 9 | 6 | 7 | 12 |
| Breast | 2 | <1 | | | | |
| Others | 2 | 3 | 4 | | | |

in several reported series being about 2 cm, and a typical range of 0.4–3.5 cm (2–6,12). Occasionally, larger examples have been documented, some of which have attained sizes up to 10 cm (4). Clearly, one cannot exclude the diagnosis of nodular fasciitis on the basis of size alone. However, when faced with a lesion >5 cm, great caution must be exercised before rendering such an interpretation.

Operatively, these lesions are usually described as well-circumscribed or localized masses. Some authors even report a connective tissue pseudocapsule or true capsule, with the latter perhaps being derived from the fascia itself in a small percentage of cases (4,5,7). However, nodular fasciitis may also demonstrate irregular projections into adjacent tissue and occasionally adheres to nearby structures (5,11). Macroscopically, the lesions may exhibit a variety of patterns, from a firm, white–gray appearance to a softer, slimy or gelati-

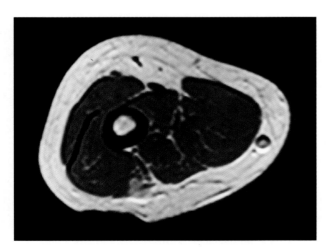

**FIG. 1.** Nodular fasciitis. The origin of these typically small lesions in fascia is depicted in this magnetic resonance image.

nous character (8). Frequently, more than one configuration may be appreciated in a single tumor.

The histologic appearance of nodular fasciitis is similarly variable. Price et al. (7), in the most often quoted and easily applied classification of these lesions, described myxoid (type I), intermediate or cellular (type II), and fibromatous or fibrous (type III) variants. However, Bernstein and Lattes suggested four different subtypes, and Allen has discussed as many as 12 (4,8). Fortunately, for those of us who prefer things to be as simple as possible, there is no proven clinical significance to any of the published classifications, and therefore no reason to adopt a categorization that is more complex than that suggested by Price et al.

Histologically, nodular fasciitis is characterized by a proliferation of spindle cells in a variably myxoid or collagen-rich background. Distinction among types 1, 2, and 3 is largely based on the relative proportions of these elements because in practice more than one pattern is typically identified in each individual lesion. Somewhat counterintuitively, there appears to be no correlation between the degree of fibrosis and duration of lesional growth (14).

The spindle cell population may vary from plump and ovoid to thin and elongated with long cytoplasmic processes. Frequently, the cells exhibit a more stellate appearance, particularly in association with an edematous or myxoid background when multidirectional cytoplasmic extensions are more readily visualized (6). The cytoplasm is usually eosinophilic and featureless, but pale and vacuolated cells typify some lesions, whereas rare examples appear granular (4). Occasional cells may show longitudinally oriented, intracytoplasmic fibrillar structures (16). Cell borders are typically indistinct. The nuclei are bland with a regular outline and a fine vesicular chromatin pattern (4,5). These nuclear features are relatively constant, showing little variation from area to area, despite potential variability in cytologic appear-

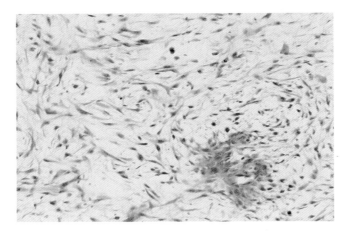

**FIG. 2.** Nodular fasciitis. The loosely textured proliferation of spindled elements resembles cells growing in tissue culture.

ance (6). Nucleoli are small or absent. Although Meister and colleagues reported mild or moderate cellular atypia in up to 70% of their cases (2), the absence of marked cytologic atypia is usually a consistent (and, one might say, prerequisite) finding in nodular fasciitis. The recognition of even occasional bizarre or anaplastic cells should therefore prompt serious reconsideration of the diagnosis (4).

The spindle cells may be randomly oriented, with no consistently recognizable pattern. This feature, combined with a loose myxoid background, produces a characteristic tissue culture–like appearance (Fig. 2) (5). In other areas, however, fusiform cells may form curved bundles or fascicles, producing a whorled appearance (4). Less commonly, a storiform arrangement is appreciated (Fig. 3) (3,6). Areas such as this may occasionally cause confusion with histiocytic tumors, although the storiform arrangement in nodular fasciitis is almost always more subtle than that seen in fibrous histiocytoma.

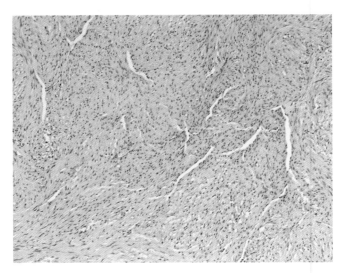

**FIG. 4.** Nodular fasciitis. Clefts often partially divide solid areas of growth.

The background stroma is frequently edematous and myxoid, and is pale or lightly basophilic in hematoxylin and eosin (H&E) stains. It labels positively with Alcian blue, but it is hyaluronidase-sensitive (3,16) and may lie between individual cells or in the cleft-like spaces that further characterize these lesions (Fig. 4). Such clefts, which probably represent a degenerative change, may on occasion enlarge to form microcysts or cysts that are filled with a finely granular basophilic ground substance (Fig. 5) (4,6). These spaces may also contain red blood cells; however, they are not lined with endothelium and therefore do not represent vascular channels (4). Nodular fasciitis is nevertheless a very vascular lesion, containing numerous small, thin-walled vascular channels. This rich vascularity may impart a granulation tissue–like appearance, particularly when there is an associ-

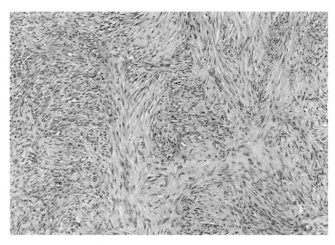

**FIG. 3.** Nodular fasciitis. Areas of more compact proliferation may assume a storiform appearance.

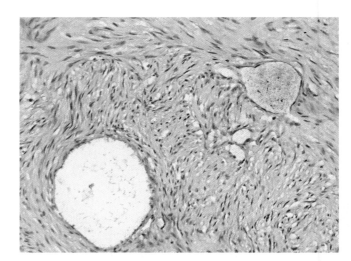

**FIG. 5.** Nodular fasciitis. Expansion of the clefts depicted in Fig. 4 may accumulate ground substance, producing small stromal cysts.

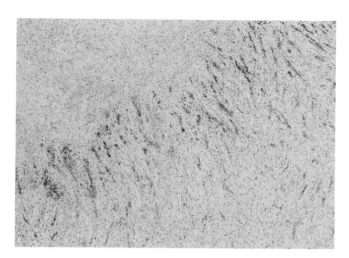

**FIG. 6.** Nodular fasciitis. At the periphery of the lesion, a parallel proliferation of capillaries often forms festoons.

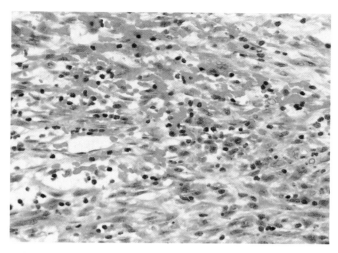

**FIG. 8.** Nodular fasciitis. A chronic inflammatory infiltrate may be seen. In this example, hemosiderin-laden macrophages are also apparent.

ated inflammatory cell infiltrate (2). Supporting vessels are typically lined with plump endothelial cells, some of which appear to obliterate the lumen. Capillaries may also be arranged in parallel, forming vascular festoons, often at the periphery of the lesion (Fig. 6) (5). In some cases of nodular fasciitis, a distinct zonation phenomenon may be appreciated, wherein a vascular palisade encloses a hypocellular, edematous center composed of stellate fibroblast-like cells, and is itself bordered by more cellular areas that are more descriptively typical of nodular fasciitis (4). Allen has emphasized the abrupt transition that may exist between these hypocellular and vascular zones, noting the histologic similarity between this process and tissue repair (4). Bernstein and Lattes have further documented the presence of fibrin in the center of such lesions, arguing that this may represent the remnant of an old hematoma (8). This pattern has been referred to as the repair variant of nodular fasciitis (4).

Red blood cell extravasation is a consistent, if occasion-ally focal, finding in nodular fasciitis, and it may be seen principally in myxoid areas or in the above-mentioned cleft-like spaces (Fig. 7). Somewhat surprisingly, however, hemosiderin is rarely conspicuous in these lesions, although small numbers of siderophages may occasionally be seen (Fig. 8) (2). Notably, erythrocyte extravasation is an uncommon element of fibrohistiocytic tumors and other lesions in the differential diagnosis of nodular fasciitis; hence, this finding carries significant diagnostic weight and should be actively sought.

Vascularity and red blood cell extravasation are less prominent features in more cellular (type 2) or fibrous (type 3) lesions, in which the myxoid ground substance is, to a greater or lesser extent, replaced by a closer apposition of spindle cells or the deposition of delicate, pale-staining collagen (7). Rarely, collagen deposition may be substantial, producing a hyalinized appearance (Fig. 9) (4).

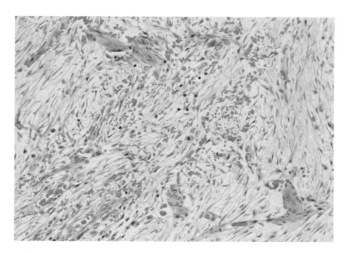

**FIG. 7.** Nodular fasciitis. Extravasation of red blood cells is characteristic of this process.

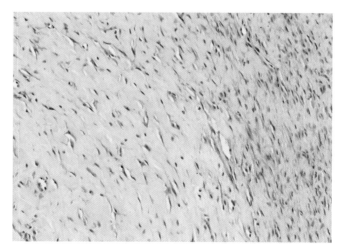

**FIG. 9.** Nodular fasciitis. Stroma may be hyalinized.

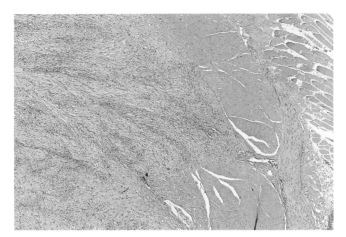

FIG. 10. Nodular fasciitis. In this example, skeletal muscle at the periphery of the lesion is infiltrated by proliferating cells.

The infiltrative capacity of nodular fasciitis is frequently borne out by the presence of finger-like extensions into adjacent tissue that entrap fat, skeletal muscle (Fig. 10), and other elements (7). Perineural extension is occasionally recognized (14). Atrophic or degenerative features in involved muscle may be appreciated but are rarely prominent. Extension into contiguous vascular channels (so-called intravascular fasciitis) is discussed separately in this chapter.

Mitotic figures are such a consistent finding in nodular fasciitis that many investigators have proposed that the diagnosis should not be rendered in their absence (4). Mitotic counts vary from case to case and regionally within a given tumor, but they rarely exceed two or three mitoses per high power ($\times 400$) field (Fig. 11) (3,8). Atypical forms should not be seen (3–7), although Bernstein and Lattes described occasional tripolar mitoses in cases that they otherwise accepted as examples of nodular fasciitis (8).

Meister et al. (2) documented necrosis in 10% of their cases but, in most other series, this was an unusual finding. The difference may be less a discrepancy, in fact, than one of interpretation, since the figures used by Meister and colleagues to illustrate necrosis more closely resemble degenerative changes with microcyst formation rather than tumor necrosis, in our opinion.

As might be anticipated from the name fasciitis, inflammatory cells are usually present. However, they are rarely the predominant feature (see Fig. 8) and, in occasional cases, are not seen at all (2). Hence, it seems unlikely that the inflammatory infiltrate plays a primary pathogenic role. A mixture of cell types is typical, including macrophages and lymphocytes, and, to a lesser extent, plasma cells. Some macrophages have foamy cytoplasm, whereas fewer (as noted previously) contain hemosiderin (2). Polymorphonuclear leukocytes are uncommon (4). The infiltrate may be present in the proliferative areas, at the periphery of the lesions, or in both (8). Giant cells are identified in approximately 50% of cases (2,7,8) and are occasionally a prominent feature (Fig. 11) (4). Some of these have an osteoclast-like appearance, but the precise cell of origin of the giant cell population is uncertain; some authors have suggested a derivation from degenerating muscle fibers, histiocytes, or even fibroblasts (8). A recent immunohistologic study, however, appears to lend support to a histiocytic nature (6). Allen has described the presence of occasional ganglion-like giant cells in otherwise typical examples of nodular fasciitis (4). Such a finding should not lead to significant diagnostic confusion, as it merely emphasizes the considerable histologic overlap that exists between *proliferative fasciitis/myositis* and nodular fasciitis (4).

Rarely, metaplastic foci of osteoid (with or without conspicuous mineralization) or cartilage may be identified in otherwise typical examples of nodular fasciitis. Whereas Bernstein and Lattes describe peripheral maturation of osteoid in their series, most authors have observed a more haphazard arrangement, specifically lacking the zonal qualities that otherwise characterize *myositis ossificans* (1,8,11). The characterization of this process as *fasciitis ossificans* is considered later in this discussion.

The diagnosis of soft tissue tumors by fine needle aspiration is fraught with considerable difficulties, given their cytologic heterogeneity. Recognition of a mesenchymal nature is usually possible, however, and there is usually sufficient evidence on which to base reasonable speculation regarding the biological potential of the lesion. Nevertheless, exact classification within the nosologic spectrum of soft tissue neoplasia is rarely possible (17). Nodular fasciitis typically yields a cellular specimen with collagen fragments and a myxoid background. Spindle cells are usually present, either as small groups or as individual cells. These range from long and slender to plump and ovoid, and exhibit relatively bland nuclear features (18). These findings, when combined with a typical clinical history, should allow the cytologist to render a correct diagnosis. However, in the absence of sufficient history or in the presence of atypical morphologic features or simply a limited specimen, the differential diagnosis broadens to encompass fibrohistiocytic neoplasms, fibromatoses, and peripheral nerve sheath neoplasms (17).

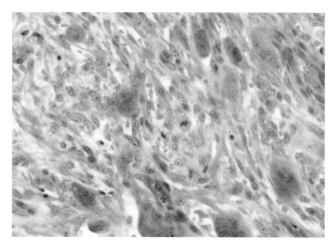

FIG. 11. Nodular fasciitis. Areas with multinucleated giant cells are not an unusual finding. In this example, mitotic activity is evident in the spindle cell population.

Immunohistochemical analysis reveals that the spindle cells of nodular fasciitis are diffusely positive for vimentin and typically display at least focal reactivity for $\alpha$-isoform smooth muscle actin and muscle-specific actin (Fig. 12). The lysosomal marker CD68, which is traditionally used by some as a marker of histiocytic differentiation, labels a small percentage of spindle cells and most giant cells strongly (6).

By electron microscopy, many of the giant cells of nodular fasciitis show features that are consistent with histiocytic differentiation, including irregular cell borders, pinocytotic vesicles, rough endoplasmic reticulum, and secondary lysosomes. The spindle cells contain uniformly shaped elongated nuclei with occasional deep clefts and a solitary, small nucleolus. In addition to abundant rough endoplasmic reticulum, microtubules, and pinocytotic vesicles, these cells may also contain numerous 6- to 7-mm-diameter myofilaments (actin). These typically lie in bundles at the periphery of the cell. (16). As expected from the light microscopic appearance, the stroma shows a varied fine structural appearance. In some areas, the intercellular spaces are relatively featureless, corresponding to myxoid areas by light microscopy. In others, collagen fibers are densely packed and lie in close apposition to cell membranes.

The above-cited combination of histopathologic, immunophenotypic, and electron microscopic features indicates that the predominant cell type in nodular fasciitis is myofibroblastic in nature. This cell population, which exhibits features of both fibroblasts and smooth muscle cells, is a normal constituent of granulation tissue and scars, and it plays a central role in the repair process. It is probably derived from fibroblasts (19,20). Myofibroblasts are an important component of a number of reactive and neoplastic lesions, including fibroinflammatory and repair phenomena, fibromatoses, myofibromatosis, malignant fibrous histiocytomas, and the fibrous stroma associated with selected carcinomas (19). In some instances, atypical single or multinucleated myofibroblasts may be encountered in these

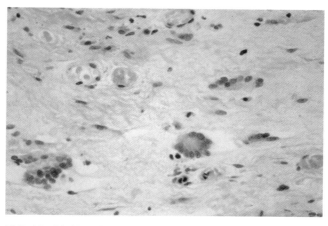

**FIG. 13.** Multinucleated myofibroblasts in the bladder. These cells are immunoreactive for muscle actins. Their presence in reactive inflammatory and neoplastic conditions may account in part for the multinucleated cells seen in nodular fasciitis.

processes (Fig. 13) (21). The latter of these forms may account for some of the osteoclast-like giant cells in nodular fasciitis. Immunophenotypic heterogeneity of myofibroblastic cells has been identified in the spectrum of reactive and neoplastic proliferations. It has been suggested that the expression of actin isoforms by myofibroblasts does not typify the myofibroblasts of normal reparative processes (20), although other studies of phenotypic diversity in myofibroblasts (22), together with our own experience, implies that this observation may be of limited value.

Cytogenetic analysis has been performed in only isolated cases of nodular fasciitis. Both Sawyer et al. (23) and Birdsall et al. (24) reported clonal cytogenetic aberrations in individual examples. However, the former study identified an abnormal karyotype in only 2% of cells examined (23). Hence, the significance of such findings, based as they are on cell culture preparations, remains uncertain. Furthermore, although Birdsall et al. additionally reported a tetraploid cell population in their case report (24), flow cytometric analysis in larger series of nodular fasciitis has repeatedly demonstrated diploid DNA content (13,25). Whether or not cytogenetic and flow cytometric abnormalities are confirmed in future studies, the apparent presence of abnormal karyotypes in benign neoplasms and normal cell populations precludes us from deriving reliable information about the biology of a lesion from adjuvant nonmorphologic data alone (23).

The etiology and nature of this myofibroblastic proliferation therefore remains in doubt, although most authors agree that it is probably a reactive or inflammatory lesion. Given the location of the process in or adjacent to fascial planes, it is possible that various changes in connective tissue, including necrosis, may precipitate nodular fasciitis. In this context, its resemblance to granulation tissue, as already emphasized, suggests that nodular fasciitis might simply represent an abnormal mesenchymal healing response to tissue injury (2,4). This concept is further supported by the recent description of a nodular fasciitis–like stroma in cases of papil-

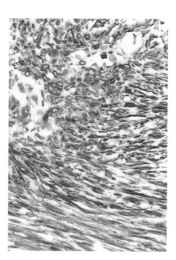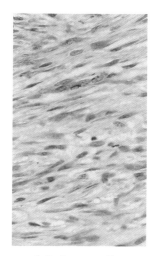

**FIG. 12.** Nodular fasciitis. Immunoreactivity for smooth muscle actin (left) and muscle-specific actin (right) highlights the myofibroblastic nature of nodular fasciitis.

lary thyroid carcinoma where, it was proposed, the tissue injury caused by tumor invasion induced an aberrant myofibroblastic proliferation (26). Unfortunately, as stated above, only a minority of patients give a history of trauma or other tissue damage, and the presumed initiating event in the remainder of cases remains obscure.

Nodular fasciitis is a benign and self-limited process. Resolution following incomplete excision and even after fine needle aspiration is well recognized (2,8,18). There would therefore appear to be no indication for further surgical intervention when grossly or microscopically involved resection margins are encountered. The more aggressive course of two cases reported by Toker (27), one of which resulted in the death of the patient, has not been substantiated by others, and it seems likely that Toker's report in fact describes a different disease process. The fatal case was located initially at the porta hepatis; this location, combined with the clinical course and illustrated histology, suggests to us that this lesion should instead be regarded as an inflammatory myofibroblastic tumor.

Recurrence rates as low as 1–10% are reported in many series, with most occurring within 2 months of initial resection (2–6). In their classic paper, Bernstein and Lattes reviewed the clinical and histologic findings of 18 cases in which recurrence of nodular fasciitis was documented (8). In each example, their review led to a revision of the original diagnosis, with cases being redesignated as fibrous histiocytomas (benign or malignant), fibromatoses, fibrosarcomas, benign peripheral nerve sheath tumors, epithelioid sarcomas, leiomyomas, liposarcomas, or angiosarcomas. They found no recurrences in 116 lesions where careful review confirmed the initial diagnosis of nodular fasciitis. On the basis of these observations, it was proposed (and is now widely held) that nodular fasciitis rarely, if ever, recurs (8). Clinical persistence of the lesion should therefore always prompt a critical review of the initial histology.

The varied histologic appearances of nodular fasciitis require that a wide range of benign and malignant lesions must enter the differential diagnosis. However, by far the most frequent diagnostic consideration is that of *fibrous histiocytoma*. Although benign fibrous histiocytoma is usually a dermal or subcuticular lesion, deeper examples have been increasingly recognized, and the existence of dermal nodular fasciitis makes distinction on the basis of location alone unreliable (15). Similarly, there is a considerable overlap in the histologic and immunohistochemical features of fibrous histiocytomas and nodular fasciitis. Nevertheless, extravasation of red cells remains a useful diagnostic feature in favor of nodular fasciitis, whereas the presence of coarser, blunted nuclear profiles suggests the diagnosis of fibrous histiocytoma (6). The separation of these lesions is still not always possible, and the development of a clinical recurrence may ultimately be required to reach the correct diagnosis in occasional cases.

Distinction of nodular fasciitis from *(myo)fibromatosis* may also be difficult in selected instances. Fibromatosis, in contrast to nodular fasciitis, usually occurs in deep fascia and muscle, sparing the subcutaneous tissue. It is a larger lesion at presentation as well, typically measuring >5 cm in most cases. Slit-like interstitial spaces are not seen, and the prominent myxoid change of nodular fasciitis is unusual. Immunostaining for proliferating cell nuclear antigen (PCNA) may illustrate a different distribution of proliferating cells in these two processes; PCNA staining concentrated at the periphery of the lesion is said to typify nodular fasciitis, whereas evenly distributed proliferative elements are more characteristic of fibromatosis and fibrosarcoma (25). This finding, while of considerable biological interest, has yet to be substantiated and is therefore of unproven diagnostic value.

*Fibrosarcoma*, another frequent misdiagnosis in cases of nodular fasciitis, typically displays a less varied histology, with a prominent herring-bone growth pattern and a more monotonous cell population (4). Other diagnostic considerations, including benign and malignant *peripheral nerve sheath tumors, leiomyoma, leiomyosarcoma,* and *spindle cell angiosarcoma,* are usually readily recognized by a combination of cytologic, histologic, and immunophenotypic features. The occasional demonstration of CD57 immunoreactivity in examples of nodular fasciitis does not, in our experience, complicate this differential diagnosis.

### Intravascular Fasciitis

As noted earlier, the infiltrative nature and rapid growth of nodular fasciitis may result in the involvement of preexisting structures. Perineural extension has been recognized and may account for some of the pain that can be associated with nodular fasciitis (14). Prolapse or invagination into native vascular channels has also been reported, a process that has been designated the intravascular variant of nodular fasciitis by Allen (4). He observed this subtype in 2 of 96 cases of nodular fasciitis. The term "intravascular fasciitis" was more recently applied to histologically identical lesions by Patchefsky and Enzinger (28). In the latter analysis, the lesions exhibited a characteristic multinodular pattern of growth, presumably due to their close association with, or origin from, vascular channels. We consider the latter element a necessary component of lesions diagnosed as intravascular fasciitis, an opinion reflected in the following discussion of this entity.

Intravascular fasciitis is seen in a patient population that is similar to that affected by classical nodular fasciitis. The signs and symptoms of these two lesions are identical. However, in the small number of cases reported by Patchefsky and Enzinger, the duration of complaints in intravascular fasciitis appears to be somewhat longer (28), typically 10–60 months before presentation. Rapid growth is relatively unusual. The anatomic distribution of intravascular lesions is consistent with that of typical nodular fasciitis, although a greater percentage of cases (31%) involves deep soft tissues (28). There is no obvious clinical association with trauma.

Macroscopically, most cases form discrete nodules, but on occasion finger-like projections, which presumably correspond to intravascular growth, may be appreciated. Involvement of specific vessels may be identified by the surgeon at the time of excision (28,29).

Intravascular fasciitis shows the same histologic features as nodular fasciitis, except for the striking angiocentricity that in part defines these lesions (Fig. 14). Involvement of numerous adjacent vascular spaces is responsible for producing a multinodular or plexiform growth pattern (29). These proliferations infiltrate the vascular lumina, occasionally completely filling them. Because of effacement of the native vessels, the nature of these nodular fasciitis-like lesions may only be recognized after careful evaluation of histochemical stains for elastin. Superimposed thrombosis of affected vessels has been documented in one case (28). Both arteries and veins may be affected, and all layers of the vessel wall may be affected. Extensive growth in extravascular soft tissues may occasionally predominate, disguising the vasculocentric pattern. However, smaller nodules of proliferating myofibroblasts can usually be appreciated in small-caliber vessels and perivascular soft tissue remote from the main lesion (15,28), a feature that emphasizes the multifocal origin of this condition.

Recurrence after resection most likely represents growth of either transected intravascular fingers or proliferation of a remote and independent nodule. Such an outcome was described in 2 of the 17 cases reported by Patchefsky and Enzinger (28). However, the admittedly limited literature on this entity supports the contention that intravascular fasciitis is no more aggressive than typical nodular fasciitis, despite its angiocentricity (15,28,29).

The particular differential diagnostic alternative that is most likely to present difficulty in this setting is that of *infantile myofibromatosis (congenital fibromatosis)*. This condition may present as a solitary tumor or as multiple lesions involving bone, viscera, and soft tissues (30). Histologically,

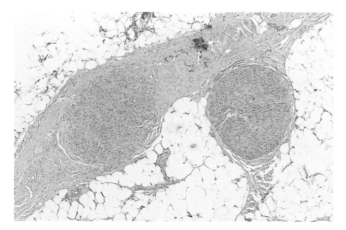

**FIG. 14.** Intravascular fasciitis. At low magnification, the intravascular distribution of proliferating cells results in a multinodular or plexiform appearance.

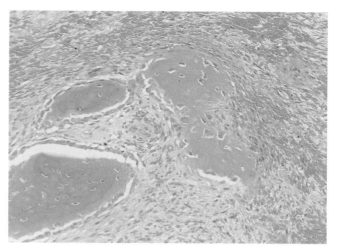

**FIG. 15.** Fasciitis ossificans. Bone trabeculae lined with plump osteoblasts are interspersed with stromal elements (with erythrocyte extravasation) that are otherwise typical of nodular fasciitis.

myofibromatosis consists of interweaving fascicles and nodules of spindle cells (myofibroblasts). Slit-like vascular spaces may produce a hemangiopericytoma-like pattern. With respect to the latter feature, Coffin and Dehner (31), as well as other authors (32;33), have proposed that infantile myofibromatosis is, in fact, part of a histopathologic continuum that is shared with *congenital hemangiopericytoma*. The proliferation of myofibroblastic cells in the intima of vessels, both as an integral part of and remote from the main lesion of intravascular fasciitis, is a diagnostically useful feature, but the myofibroblastic nature of these lesions can clearly cause confusion with the myofibromatoses. However, the latter lesions are typically less myxoid in appearance and do not exhibit the red cell extravasation and inflammatory cell infiltrate of fasciitis (32,33).

### *Fasciitis Ossificans (Ossifying Fasciitis)*

The possible presence of cartilage, osteoid, or woven bone in otherwise typical examples of nodular fasciitis (10,15) has already been cited. Kwittken and Branche (34) have proposed that such lesions be referred to as "fasciitis ossificans." However, because there appears to be no significant clinical or histologic difference between these lesions and other examples of fasciitis (with the obvious exception of focal ossification), the designation "fasciitis with ossification" seems equally appropriate.

The formation of irregular trabeculae of osteoid or woven bone occurs haphazardly throughout the lesion and is typically associated with plump osteoblasts (Fig. 15) (35). The deposition specifically lacks the zonation characteristic of *myositis ossificans,* in which mature bone is formed at the periphery, enveloping an edematous and cellular connective tissue center (see discussion of myositis ossificans). Ossification may occur in either loose cellular areas or in regions with a more dense fibrotic appearance; it is clearly a meta-plastic rather than a dystrophic process (35). The origin of the osteoblastic population in these cases, remote from periosteum as it is, is unknown but presumably derives from an immature mesenchymal precursor.

Ossification in fasciitis is unusual. Only one of the 96 examples of nodular fasciitis reported by Allen displayed this feature (4). Its exact frequency is difficult to gauge, however, because other authors appear to include examples of myositis ossificans among fasciitis-like lesions exhibiting peripheral bone formation (8). Bernstein and Lattes also suggested that overlap lesions exist (8). Given this blurred distinction, the suggestion that the lesions of fasciitis ossificans are usually larger than typical nodular fasciitis must be regarded with some suspicion (8).

### Parosteal Fasciitis (Periosteal Fasciitis, Florid Reactive Periostitis, Fibro-osseous Pseudotumor of the Digit)

Lesions with many of the features of nodular fasciitis occasionally occur in a parosteal location and are associated with prominent osteoid formation. Such lesions have been reported under a number of different names (36–39). Although Spjut and Dorfman (36) correctly indicated that origin from the fascia is not always demonstrable or even likely in these cases, derivation from or involvement of the periosteum is similarly not always recognized; therefore, the designation of parosteal fasciitis (which at least conveys the histologic similarity of the lesion to nodular fasciitis and has historical precedence) should probably be retained (36,37,39).

Parosteal fasciitis may present with either pain or swelling, or both. Some patients complain of tenderness; 11 of the 21 cases reported by Dupree and Enzinger (39) showed redness of the overlying skin. Symptoms are typically present for 2–3 months prior to referral, but the clinical history may occasionally be longer; Spjut and Dorfman reported a case where symptoms had been present for 2 years (36). The condition affects the same age group as nodular fasciitis. Although the initial report (37) described a lesion that occurred exclusively in long bones, the two largest series documented examples in tubular bones of the hands and feet (36,39). Most lesions are 1–4 cm in length and 30–50% of patients give a history of antecedent trauma (36).

Radiologically, most cases of parosteal fasciitis manifest with a soft tissue swelling (Fig. 16). Some show focal calcification, with or without periosteal reaction in the adjacent bone (40). The periosteal reaction is typically smooth or laminated, and may be associated with dense cortical new bone formation. The cortex is typically intact, but cases in which it is eroded and even destroyed have been described (36,37,41). Although most examples of parosteal fasciitis are interpreted by the radiologist as benign, such destructive examples clearly raise the possibility of malignancy. Indeed, Ewing's sarcoma was the favored diagnosis in one case (37).

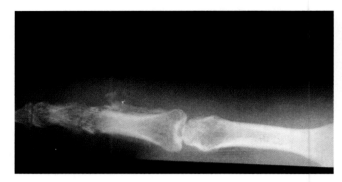

**FIG. 16.** Parosteal fasciitis. Radiographs typically identify a parosteal soft tissue swelling with calcification.

Radiologic progression was documented in one case, with increased density of the periosteal reaction over a period of 1 year (36). Two other examples from the same series appeared as bony protuberances.

Histologically, the lesions are similar to nodular fasciitis (see above), with the familiar loose fascicles of mitotically active spindle cells set in a myxoid or fibrous background (39,40). Small numbers of inflammatory cells are distributed throughout the lesion, and occasional osteoclast-like giant cells may be seen (38). Irregular seams of osteoid, when present, are lined with plump osteoblasts. Small nests of immature cartilage are also a characteristic feature. In some examples, the osteocartilaginous component to a great extent effaces the cellular spindle cell areas, making it difficult to detect the underlying fasciitis pattern (36). These histologic features clearly illustrate the similarity of this lesion to fasciitis ossificans. The description of occasional examples with a more zonal distribution of osteoid additionally highlights an apparent overlap with myositis ossificans, although Hutter et al. (37) and Dupree and Enzinger (39) specifically excluded examples with such peripheral bone deposition from this designation. Furthermore, Hutter et al. emphasized that parosteal fasciitis is essentially a spindle cell proliferation with foci of osteoid production, whereas myositis ossificans, in its maturing form, is a relatively paucicellular lesion dominated by bone.

In addition to fasciitis ossificans and myositis ossificans, other conditions that might be considered in the differential diagnosis include *osteosarcoma, bizarre parosteal osteochondromatous proliferations,* and, less likely, *chronic osteomyelitis.* Osteosarcomas of the parosteal, periosteal, and high-grade surface varieties are, by definition, predominantly or exclusively extramedullary lesions. Although their clinical and radiologic features differ, discrimination between these osteosarcoma subtypes and parosteal fasciitis often rests on histologic criteria. High-grade surface osteosarcoma is readily recognized by its pronounced cytologic atypia, whereas periosteal osteosarcoma is a predominantly chondroblastic tumor that is unlikely to be confused with parosteal fasciitis microscopically. In parosteal osteosarcoma, cytologic atypia is more subtle, and the presence of both cartilage islands and an intervening spindle cell proliferation may complicate the histologic distinction of this lesion from parosteal fasciitis. However, some examples of the former neoplasm contain small foci of a higher-grade sarcoma, and even those that do not have such obvious sarcomatous elements usually exhibit greater cytologic atypia than is permissible in parosteal fasciitis (36).

Bizarre parosteal osteochondromatous proliferation is a reactive condition involving the small bones of the hands and feet (41) that is closely related to parosteal fasciitis. As is described in greater detail later in this chapter, these osteochondromatous lesions are attached to the underlying cortex but show no continuity with the medulla. Histologically, a proliferation of spindle cells lies between islands of occasionally quite atypical (hence, "bizarre") cartilage that matures into bone. These cartilaginous areas possess a characteristic and distinctive blue color that should facilitate the diagnosis.

As relatively few cases of parosteal fasciitis have been reported, the natural history of this lesion is uncertain. However, recurrence, if it is seen at all, appears to be a rare phenomenon. Conservative excision, therefore, is the therapy of choice (36–39).

### Cranial Fasciitis

A lesion that is closely related to parosteal fasciitis and that occurs in the skulls of infants and young children has been described by Lauer and Enzinger (42) under the rubric "cranial fasciitis." This condition typically presents in the first 2 years of life and may even be present at birth (42). Rare cases in later childhood have been documented, and males are more commonly affected than females (43). Most lesions present as a scalp mass, frequently with a short history of rapid growth. Individual examples of this lesion may attain a larger size, but the overwhelming majority are <3 cm, irrespective of the duration of symptoms (42,44). A tenuous history of forceps trauma was recorded in one case, but most lesions have no obvious initiating or precipitating event (42). Although some authors report a predilection for the temporoparietal region, examples of fasciitis have been reported over a wide range of cranial sites; in the largest reported series, no single location was clearly preferred (29,42). Cranial fasciitis is thought to arise from the periosteum, galea, or deep fascia, but an origin from the connective tissue associated with skull sutures has also been suggested. However, in the absence of an obvious predilection for suture lines, this latter possibility seems dubious.

Radiographically, these lesions are soft tissue swellings, frequently (although not invariably) associated with lytic changes in the underlying bone. Erosion of the skull is usually limited to the outer table, producing a saucer-like depression, with or without a sclerotic rim (42,43). Relatively few cases extend through both inner and outer tables of the skull and are attached to the dura mater (42,43).

On both macroscopic and microscopic examination, cranial fasciitis mimics nodular fasciitis. Its gross appearance is varied, with areas of gray–white, rubbery, firm tissue associated with more gelatinous and even frankly cystic regions. Histologically, these lesions consist of a proliferation of spindle to stellate cells that are usually arranged haphazardly but may focally assume a storiform pattern. The background stroma may be myxoid or fibrous. Other features of nodular fasciitis, including a mixed inflammatory cell infiltrate, multinucleated giant cells, red blood cell extravasation, and mitotic figures, are readily appreciated (Fig. 17). As in nodular fasciitis, mitoses are never atypical (42). Occasionally, thickened, acellular fascial or periosteal tissue may be seen at the periphery of the lesion (42).

In two thirds of cases, foci of bone formation are evident (42). This high frequency of osseous metaplasia emphasizes the considerable histologic overlap that exists between cranial fasciitis, parosteal fasciitis, and fasciitis ossificans. Nonetheless, the distinctive clinical setting of cranial fasciitis justifies separation from the other two entities. As might be expected, recurrence is the exception, and conservative excision is the treatment of choice (42–44).

In addition to lesions discussed in relation to other fasciitides, the differential diagnosis of cranial fasciitis includes lesions derived from the underlying bone and meninges. Primary bone tumors and hamartomatous lesions of meningothelial origin (the latter are discussed in Chapter 2) are unlikely to cause diagnostic difficulty. Although cranial fasciitis may penetrate the full thickness of the calvarium and involve the dura, attachment to or origin from the leptomeninges has not been documented. Unless the specimen consists only of a small biopsy, histologic distinction from fibrous variants of *meningioma* is therefore relatively straightforward.

Perhaps more difficult is the separation of cranial fasciitis from *solitary infantile myofibromatosis*, a lesion that fre-

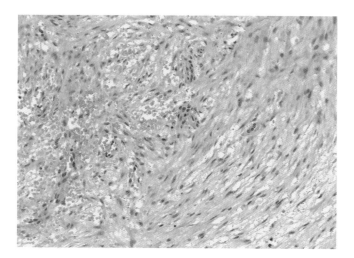

**FIG. 17.** Cranial fasciitis. The histology of this process is indistinguishable from that of nodular fasciitis in other locations.

quently involves cranial bones and presents as a lytic intraosseous lesion. Indeed, some authors believe that the latter condition and cranial fasciitis are one and the same (30).
Histologically, the myofibroblastic elements of solitary infantile myofibromatosis are arranged in interweaving fascicles and nodules in a manner quite reminiscent of fasciitis.
As noted earlier, slit-like vascular spaces may produce a hemangiopericytoma-like pattern in some examples of myofibromatosis. However, as is true of intravascular fasciitis in
extracranial sites, the proliferation of myofibroblastic cells
in the intima of vessels within and remote from the main lesion may help to separate cranial fasciitis from myofibromatosis (30,32). Furthermore, osseous metaplasia, red cell
extravasation, and inflammation are not features of myofibromatosis.

### Proliferative Myositis

In his classic 1958 paper on myositis ossificans, Ackerman described occasional examples in which the characteristic peripheral zone of ossification was absent (45), proposing that these may represent myositis ossificans in evolution.
Similar lesions were first recognized as an entity distinct
from myositis ossificans by Kern in 1960 (46). Proliferative
myositis, as Kern chose to designate this entity, shows considerable clinical and histopathologic overlap with *proliferative fasciitis* (a lesion discussed in somewhat greater detail
later in this chapter), and much of the ensuing text applies
equally to the latter condition.

Proliferative myositis typically presents as a painless soft
tissue swelling. A history of rapid growth is usually volun-
teered, and 68% of patients in the series reported by Enzinger and Dulcey (47) presented to a physician within 2
weeks of onset. Indeed, although occasional cases may exhibit a more sluggish rate of enlargement, rapid growth is
frequently so alarming to patient and clinician alike that
many lesions are surgically resected within a few days of detection (46).

Early reports suggested that proliferative myositis was a
condition that presented in a somewhat older age group than
other fasciitides, with a mean age of 50–55 years (46,47).
However, in their more recent analysis of this entity, Meis
and Enzinger (48) described a series of lesions that developed in children. Clearly, this condition may arise in any
age. Similarly, proliferative myositis may arise in almost any
skeletal muscle group, although most examples occur in
muscles of the chest, upper extremities, and shoulder girdle
region (46,47).

Lesions range in size from 1 to 6 cm and grossly produce
a poorly circumscribed gray–white mass that is typically
centered in the superficial or subepimysial portion of the
muscle, with variable extension into the underlying
parenchyma. In flat muscles, it may involve the entire thickness of the muscle mass (47). Given these macroscopic findings, the histologic appearance is predictable, represented by
a cellular proliferation centered on the connective tissue

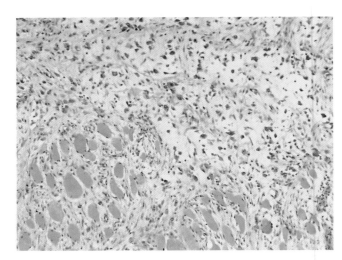

**FIG. 18.** Proliferative myositis. An admixture of myofibroblasts and polygonal and giant cells infiltrate skeletal muscle.

septa of the host skeletal muscle (46–48). The proliferation
expands these normally inconspicuous regions, occasionally
resulting in a thickening that is visible by macroscopic inspection. Two distinct populations constitute the cellular elements of the proliferation. Fibroblast-like spindle cells, arranged haphazardly or in short fascicles, coexist with a
prominent polygonal cell and giant cell population (Fig. 18)
(46,49). The giant cells, which lie singly or in small clusters,
contain abundant basophilic cytoplasm and one or occasionally more vesicular nuclei. Nucleoli are conspicuous, resulting in a ganglion cell–like appearance (Fig. 19). The latter
resemblance is sufficiently convincing to cause the occasional misdiagnosis of proliferative myositis as a *ganglioneuroma*. The giant cells may also exhibit an elongated
appearance, imparting more than a superficial resemblance
to rhabdomyoblasts, a comparison that is heightened by the
presence of intracytoplasmic eosinophilic inclusions, with or
without a demonstrable fibrillary character (47,49).

Mitoses are readily apparent in both the spindle cell and

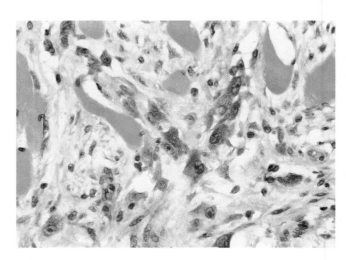

**FIG. 19.** Proliferative myositis. The larger atypical cells in
this process often resemble ganglion cells.

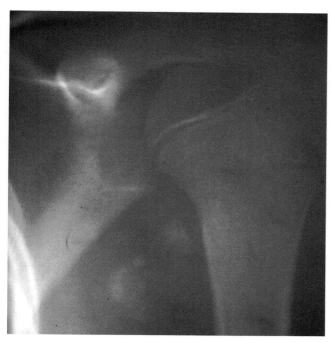

**FIG. 42.** Myositis ossificans. Radiographs taken early in the course of this process show irregular mineralization without distinct zonation.

with the stromal elements (Fig. 46). Mineralization of the osteoid initially occurs in the periphery of the lesion; it is in these areas that ossification first occurs as the lesion matures. In some examples, the matrix in the peripheral zone assumes

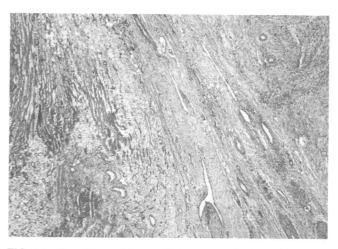

**FIG. 44.** Myositis ossificans. At low magnification, the zonation of the lesion is apparent. The central zone still contains skeletal muscle, whereas intermediate zones are more cellular.

a chondroblastic appearance (Fig. 47), and both immature and mature hyaline cartilage may be seen (106,108).

Beginning 4–6 weeks after the onset of the process, and corresponding to the clinical stage of sharp demarcation and increasing firmness, radiographs reveal increasing mineralization of the peripheral zone (see Fig. 44) (45,106,108). Macroscopically, that portion of the lesion is firm, variegated in appearance, and gritty; bone trabeculae become increasingly conspicuous with time. In the later stage, the central loose fibroblastic zone persists initially, but it is either gradually replaced by paucicellular fibrous tissue or it involutes entirely, resulting in a cystic space. The intermediate zone of osteoblastic differentiation becomes progressively less conspicuous until ossification of the osteoid matrix and cartilaginous elements is complete. In its fully evolved form, the ossified zone resembles mature lamellar bone and may

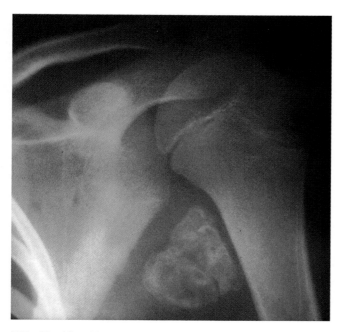

**FIG. 43.** Myositis ossificans. Radiographs of the lesion depicted in Fig. 42 taken 6 weeks later show progressive mineralization, with accentuation of the peripheral zone.

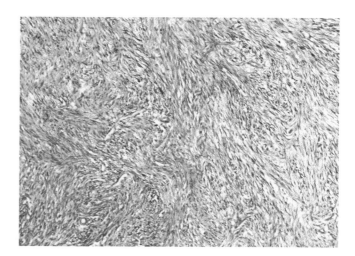

**FIG. 45.** Myositis ossificans. The intermediate zone may be dominated by a fibroblastic proliferation that resembles a fibromatosis or a storiform fibrohistiocytic lesion.

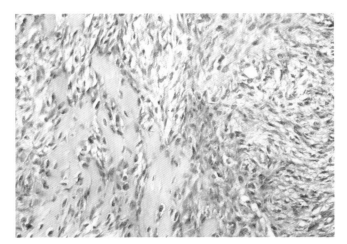

**FIG. 46.** Myositis ossificans. Osteoid is admixed with fibrous elements in the intermediate zone.

envelop adipose tissue (but not marrow elements). Apart from the fact that this lesion resides in soft tissue, the gross and histologic features of fully mature myositis ossificans are virtually indistinguishable from those of a benign *osteoma* (45,108,109).

Throughout the later stages of maturation, the admixture of osseous and cartilaginous elements in the intermediate and peripheral zones may both grossly and radiographically resemble an osteochondromatous proliferation (45,106). However, the absence of a broad base of attachment to underlying cortical bone and the lack of a predilection for the metaphysis of long bones allows for accurate preoperative separation of MO from *osteochondroma*.

Myositis ossificans, when resected, is not generally confused with neoplastic soft tissue–based osteoblastic proliferations or soft tissue metastases of *osteosarcoma* for 3 reasons: (1) the distinct zonation of MO is not recapitulated by

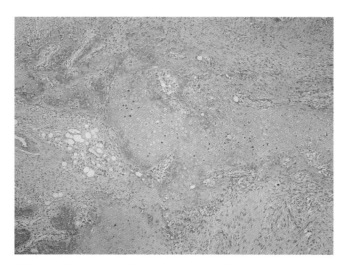

**FIG. 47.** Myositis ossificans. In the peripheral zone, maturing osseous and chondroid elements are admixed.

extraskeletal osteosarcoma; rather, the organization of the ossifying matrix in this latter entity is haphazard, with an admixture or peripheralization of fibroblastic or granulation tissue–like foci; (2) unlike MO, osteosarcoma does not exhibit a sharp demarcation from adjacent reactive nonlesional tissues; aggressive infiltration of soft tissue is more characteristic; and (3) throughout the process of ossification, a single layer of cytologically monotonous but mitotically active osteoblasts rims the developing trabecula in MO. The nuclear pleomorphism and atypical mitotic figures of osteosarcoma effectively exclude the diagnosis of MO (45,108,109). Diagnostic problems generally arise only when immature MO is biopsied; small samples of the intermediate osteoblastic zone, with or without the central proliferative zone, may obviously contain a pleomorphic and variably cellular myofibroblastic proliferation that, particularly in fragment biopsies, may appear to be admixed with immature osteoblastic elements. Careful attention to the cytologic features of the osteoblasts may be helpful, but in limited samples, and without careful evaluation of all available clinical and radiographic information, confident diagnosis of the lesion as a benign reactive process may not be possible, and misdiagnosis is increasingly likely.

Separation of MO from other processes that may occasionally contain foci of ossification rests on attention to the same zonation phenomenon. As discussed briefly in the section on pseudoneoplastic proliferations of (myo) fibroblasts, the lesion known variously as *parosteal fasciitis*, fibro-osseous pseudotumor of digits, or florid reactive periostitis is an inflammatory, occasionally posttraumatic pseudoneoplastic process that often incorporates an active osteoblastic proliferation that results in the formation of lamellar bone (36–39). This lesion, along with osteosarcoma, generally only enters the differential diagnosis of MO when small biopsies are studied in isolation; however, attention to location, a relationship to underlying bone, and a lack of zonation of the osteoblastic elements make the diagnosis of MO unlikely. The immature osteogenic foci of *fracture calluses* may also mimic both MO and osteosarcoma (109); attention to clinical and radiographic details usually resolves this differential diagnosis with certainty.

Although small islands of immature or mature bone may arise in typical cases of *proliferative/nodular fasciitis, proliferative myositis,* and so-called *fasciitis ossificans* (1,2,4,8,11,34,36,47), such areas never dominate the periphery of the lesion and, as such, do not raise a diagnostic problem either radiographically or by gross or histologic examination. In small biopsy samples, the characteristic features of these benign processes (as described earlier in this chapter) are generally well displayed. These include both the loosely textured fibroblastic proliferation with focal erythrocyte extravasation in nodular fasciitis and the ganglion-like cells that are often conspicuous in proliferative myositis. Peripheral zones of ossified tissue may occasionally be encountered in metastases of giant cell tumor of bone, but the characteristic cytohistology of this entity and the unlikely

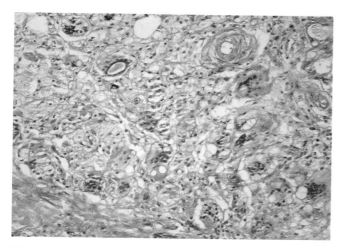

**FIG. 54.** Polyvinylpyrrolidone granuloma. Multinucleated cells and foamy histiocytes predominate.

body reactions, including those seen, for example, in response to extracellular silicone (109). Notably, PVP induces neither tissue necrosis nor significant inflammation, apart from an exuberant foreign body–type histiocytic infiltrate. In cases where systemic infusion has occurred, deposits of PVP in the medulla of both flat and long bones may result in progressively enlarging lytic lesions that may resemble the cystic and fibro-osseous lesions of bone discussed later in this chapter (141,143). In uncommon instances, such lesions may present as pathologic fracture (141). The histologic features of PVP reactions in bone are essentially identical to those seen in soft tissue. Because PVP-saturated matrix may predominate in both soft tissue and bone, the alternative diagnosis of *myxoma* may be contemplated in some cases (109,139). Conversely, the foreign body–laden cells may unusually assume a signet ring configuration and be mistaken for metastases of a *mucin-producing* or *signet ring cell adenocarcinoma* (138,142). In these limited settings, histochemical analyses may be of value because PVP is typically reactive with mucicarmine, Congo red, and colloidal iron preparations, but will not stain with PAS or Alcian blue methods (109,142). Neither myxoma nor adenocarcinoma will exhibit a similar profile, although mistaken diagnoses may potentially result from histochemical analyses that are limited only to mucicarmine stains.

### Infectious Processes Simulating Neoplasms

A variety of infectious organisms have been associated with xanthogranulomatous reactions in soft tissue. Their resemblance to fibrohistiocytic neoplasms may at times be striking, an observation that warrants their inclusion in this discussion.

### Histoid Leprosy

Perhaps the best-characterized infectious pseudoneoplasm is *histoid leprosy* (144,145), a nodular process due to *Mycobacterium leprae* that most often affects the skin and subcutaneous tissues. Often composed of spindled rather than histiocytoid cells, histoid leprosy exhibits considerable histologic overlap with storiform fibrous histiocytomas (see Chapter 14, Figs. 53–55) (109,144). The presence of numerous intracellular acid-fast organisms readily separates this process from a true neoplasm, but without histochemical confirmation of lepromatous organisms and careful attention to a clinical history that typically includes longstanding disease, misdiagnosis is possible. This disease has been discussed in greater detail elsewhere in this text (see Chapter 14).

### "Retroperitoneal Xanthogranuloma"

A variety of gram-positive and gram-negative organisms (especially *Staphylococcus*) may incite a reaction in deep soft tissues, particularly in the retroperitoneum, which is similar to that of histoid leprosy (109). As in the latter entity, the identification of microorganisms is essential to the accurate identification of these lesions. Unlike histoid leprosy, most such lesions contain an abundance of foamy histiocytes (see Fig. 55), and, because of their association with similar visceral (especially renal) xanthogranulomatous infiltrates, they may descriptively be called *retroperitoneal xanthogranulomas* (109,146). Focal abscess formation in these lesions is an important element in their accurate identification as infectious processes. The recognition of an infectious etiology is critical to distinguish this benign condition from the more common xanthogranulomatous lesions in the retroperitoneum that collectively comprise the inflammatory variants of *malignant fibrous histiocytoma* (Fig. 56) and

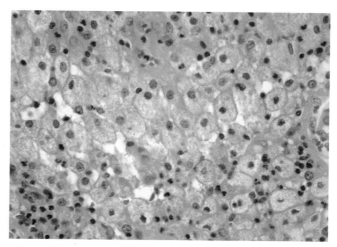

**FIG. 55.** Retroperitoneal xanthogranuloma. The histiocytes have relatively uniform oval nuclei. A background of mononuclear inflammatory cells is also present.

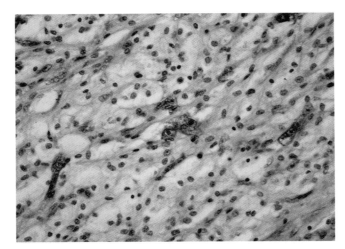

**FIG. 56.** Malignant fibrous histiocytoma. In retroperitoneal malignant fibrous histiocytoma, foam cells may predominate. Separation of the process from retroperitoneal xanthogranuloma depends on recognition of the atypical cell population that composes this neoplastic proliferation.

*leiomyosarcoma* (109,146–149). Notably, the overwhelming majority of reported cases of xanthogranulomatous lesions in the retroperitoneum are ultimately proven to be neoplastic in nature. Nonneoplastic, noninfectious xanthogranulomatous lesions in the retroperitoneum have been only rarely described; many of these are associated with *Erdheim–Chester disease,* a storage disorder presenting in adulthood that generally affects bones, with or without multifocal visceral and soft tissue involvement (150–153). It has been suggested that the term "retroperitoneal xanthogranuloma" be reserved for retroperitoneal involvement by the latter lesions (109).

### Malakoplakia

In genitourinary viscera and in adjacent pelvic or retroperitoneal soft tissues, infection with gram-negative bacteria (especially *Escherichia coli* and *Klebsiella* ssp) and acid-fast organisms may uncommonly provoke a proliferation of granular or vacuolated histiocytes that forms a soft ("malakos") plaque ("plax") in the mucosa or ill-defined masses in the soft tissue (154,155). The latter are more likely to raise the suspicion of neoplasia, although the often exuberant admixture of lymphocytes, plasma cells, and neutrophils seen in these lesions may more closely resemble *inflammatory myofibroblastic tumors* (154).

Histologic examination generally reveals variably cellular aggregates of large histiocytes (van Hansemann's cells) that generally lack cytologic atypia. PAS-positive, diastase-resistant cytoplasmic inclusions are characteristically present. In addition, small targetoid spherules (Michaelis–Guttmann bodies) may be seen both within these cells and resting free in the extracellular stroma (Fig. 57), particularly in older lesions (108,154,155). These bodies contain both organic and inorganic material; the latter are predominantly calcium and phosphate. There is also a variable amount of iron; as a re-

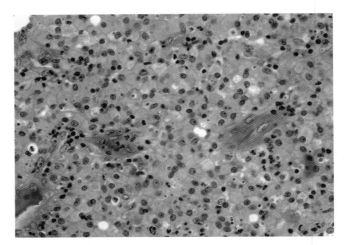

**FIG. 57.** Malakoplakia. A bland histiocytic infiltrate is associated with both intra- and extracellular calcospherules (Michaelis–Guttmann bodies).

sult, histochemical stains for calcium (such as the von Kossa method) are usually positive (Fig. 58), as are stains for elemental iron (155). Gram stains are not usually helpful in these lesions, although some Michaelis–Guttmann bodies may be appropriately gram-negative. Scattered microorganisms may be seen, together with laminated electron-dense Michaelis–Guttmann bodies, within phagolysosomes when representative areas of the lesion are studied ultrastructurally (109,154).

### Mesenchymal Proliferations Due to Infectious Organisms in Immunocompromised Patients

It is interesting that organisms that are often associated with a granulomatous response in immunocompetent individuals may elicit a spindle cell or angiomatous proliferation in immunocompromised patients, particularly those with the

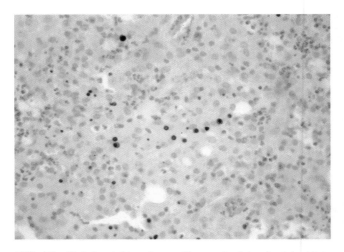

**FIG. 58.** Malakoplakia. A von Kossa (calcium) stain highlights the Michaelis–Guttmann bodies.

acquired immunodeficiency syndrome (AIDS). Because these processes generally do not involve deep soft tissues, they are not discussed in great detail here. Nonetheless, some observations are relevant to pseudoneoplasia in these soft tissue sites.

A variety of infectious species (including *Mycobacterium tuberculosis, kansasii, gordonae,* and *avium-intracellulare,* and *Leishmania infantum)* have been associated with the formation of spindle cell pseudotumors in skin, viscera, bone marrow, and lymph nodes. The most common of these are the atypical mycobacteria (156–161). Although not all patients are immunodeficient, AIDS remains the most common clinical setting in which this process has been recognized. These so-called *mycobacterial spindle cell tumors* are generally solid, often multicentric nodular proliferations of cytologically bland spindled cells that are devoid of vasoformative areas or Kaposiform slit-like spaces (see Chapter 14, Figs. 56–59) (156,157,161). The cells are devoid of atypical nuclear features and generally resemble fibroblasts, although some histiocytic qualities, including numerous lysosomes, are encountered on fine structural analysis (156). The immunophenotype of these lesions is also typical of fibroblasts or myofibroblasts, without evidence of leiomyomatous or neurilemmal differentiation. Nonetheless, macrophage-associated markers such as CD68, lysozyme, and HLA-DR may be positive in most cases (156,158,160). The expected immunoprofile, therefore, is that of a vimentin-reactive spindle cell population, which is variably reactive for desmin (and, in our experience, muscle-specific actin), to the exclusion of $\alpha$-smooth muscle actin, CD57, or CD34. Both Chen (157) and Perrin et al.(158) have described S-100 protein immunoreactivity in series on this unusual process, but most reactivity appeared to be limited to histiocyte-like elements. The critical feature in these lesions is the presence of acid-fast organisms within the spindle cell proliferation. PAS-reactive material is generally indicative of MAI infection, although this is not a specific histochemical reaction (161).

Despite the bland cytology of these cells and absence of vasoformative foci, their pattern of growth and predilection for lymph nodes and viscera often raise the specter of *Kaposi's sarcoma,* a matter of greater concern in some cases because of an abundance of hemosiderin pigment in or adjacent to the lesion. Other spindle cell tumors often mentioned in the differential diagnosis include *spindle cell malignant melanoma, malignant fibrous histiocytoma,* and both benign and malignant *peripheral nerve sheath* and *smooth muscle tumors.* In each case, careful attention to cytologic features and immunohistochemical characteristics will separate infectious spindle cell processes from any of these neoplastic lesions. Less obvious is the separation of mycobacterial spindle cell lesions from intranodal myofibroblastic or smooth muscle proliferations (so-called *intranodal myofibroblastoma),* although even in these cases, as already alluded to, the presence of a myogenic phenotype (with muscle-associated actin or desmin immunoreactivity) is usually sufficient for accurate diagnosis (109). The report of desmin

staining of mycobacterial aggregates in mycobacterial spindle cell tumors by Umlas and colleagues (160) is difficult to defend as anything but spurious, in light of a lack of corroboration in subsequent analyses of this entity.

In contrast to the aforementioned mycobacterial spindle cell tumors, *bacillary angiomatosis* is a vasoformative lesion that results not from mycobacterial infection but rather from infection by *Bartonella henselae* or related species (162–164). Although visceral and superficial soft tissue–based lesions may closely resemble true epithelioid endothelial neoplasms, including *epithelioid* or *histiocytoid hemangiomas* and *epithelioid hemangioendotheliomas,* owing in large part to the presence of large polygonal cells lining ill-defined lobules or clusters of ramifying capillary-like or tubular structures, certain reproducible histologic features separate this cellular response to infection from true neoplastic processes (see Chapter 14, Figs. 48–52). Most important among them is the presence of intralesional, perivascular eosinophilic deposits which, on closer examination, are composed in part of clumps of bacilli that rest in the extracellular matrix or have been engulfed by phagocytic cells (165–167). These structures, in keeping with their known nature, stain with the Warthin–Starry method but are essentially undetectable using other silver impregnation techniques, gram stains, or acid-fast techniques. No such material has been reported in true epithelioid neoplasms of endothelium (109,165,166). Furthermore, the lobular nature of the vascular proliferation in bacillary angiomatosis is distinctive among the lesions in this differential diagnostic group (109,165,167).

It is tempting, based on the similar distribution of bacillary angiomatosis/mycobacterial spindle cell tumors and Kaposi's sarcoma (KS), to lend credence to the hypothesis popularized by Auerbach and Brooks (168) that KS is also an infectious, reactive, nonneoplastic proliferation. The recent identification of a herpes-like virus in lesional tissues from HIV- and non–HIV-infected patients has provided provocative information in this regard (169–171), as have earlier studies reporting the presence of cytomegalovirus-related gene sequences in KS (172,173). Also provocative is the reproducible observation of diploid DNA content by flow cytometry (174) and analyses that identify immunophenotypic and functional attributes of a reactive myofibroblastic or smooth muscle proliferation (109,175). Although the clinical indolence of nonepidemic forms of this disease might support a reactive nature, the propensity for KS to exhibit regional or widespread dissemination or multifocality in immunocompromised patients is difficult to explain in a nonneoplastic paradigm, even if diminished immune surveillance is cited (176). Irrespective of an association with viral genomic sequences or a reactive myofibroblastic phenotype, the atypical cytologic features of KS and aspects of its molecular biologic profile suggest that it should still be regarded as an autonomously proliferating process. This opinion has perhaps its strongest support from results of divergent treatment approaches in KS cases. Undeniable benefit has been derived from antineoplastic interventions, whereas therapies for infectious diseases have generally proven ineffectual.

## Pseudoneoplastic Vascular Proliferations

### *Vegetant Intravascular Papillary Endothelial Hyperplasia*

The lesion attributed eponymically to Masson is nothing more than an organizing vascular (usually venous) thrombus. Because the thrombus may be palpable as a distinct tissue nodule, and because the complexity of endothelial and fibroblastic proliferation with the fibrin matrix of the thrombus often mimics a neoplastic endothelial process, this lesion warrants consideration as a pseudoneoplastic proliferation (see Chapter 14, Figs. 38–40). Its separation from angiosarcoma is generally straightforward, provided that the lesion can be recognized as intravascular, because such a location is almost unknown in malignant endothelial tumors (109). For a more complete description of this process, the reader is referred to Chapter 14.

### *Angiomatoses*

Diffuse vascular proliferations in bone and soft tissue—the so-called angiomatoses and lymphangiomatoses—are mimics of vascular neoplasms, particularly when small incisional biopsies are submitted without reference to the diffuse nature of the mass in question. Diffuse angiomatosis is confused most often with *intramuscular hemangioma*. In general, malignant processes do not enter the differential diagnosis.

Although multifocal soft tissue and visceral vascular proliferations characterize a variety of disorders in childhood, we have confined our description of the angiomatoses to fit the definition of this entity offered by Rao and Weiss (177). They suggested that only those histologically benign vascular proliferations that are confined to large contiguous regions of the body be considered angiomatosis. Most angiomatoses so defined present in childhood or adolescence as diffuse nonhomogeneous expansions of soft tissue compartments, usually with an asymmetric distribution. In their report of 51 examples of this process, Rao and Weiss (177) noted that the lower extremities and buttocks were the most commonly affected sites, followed in order by the chest wall and abdomen, upper extremities, and other sites. Angiomatosis often causes discoloration of the affected region and can be painful, but gigantism of limbs or hemihypertrophy generally do not occur (177–181). The latter manifestation is more likely in localized or regional lymphangiomatosis, wherein lymphatic obstruction results from hamartomatous lymphangiogenesis (182–186). Involvement of bones in angiomatosis and lymphangiomatosis is usually associated with involvement of adjacent soft tissue compartments as well (177,185). Angiomatoses often incorporate a

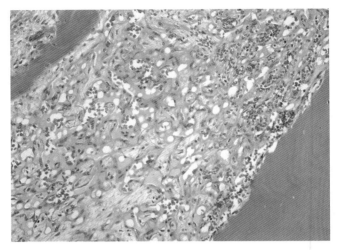

**FIG. 59.** Angiomatosis. A dense capillary proliferation replaces medullary adipose tissue in this example of angiomatosis with osseous involvement.

generous amount of mature adipose tissue, and, for this reason, may be mistaken for *lipomas* on radiographic studies (177). Tumors referred to as infiltrating angiolipomas probably compose a subset of such lesions (178,179,187).

The histology of angiomatosis is quite varied, but all cases are cytologically benign. While some lesions are predominantly or exclusively composed of small capillary spaces in a configuration reminiscent of capillary or intramuscular hemangiomas (Fig. 59), the majority contain an admixture of capillary-sized, venous and cavernous vascular elements (Fig. 60). The venous component often consists of thick-walled vessels with irregular clusters of small capillaries within or adjacent to the vascular wall (Fig. 61). Irregular thinning or attenuation of these vessels is also associated with herniation and tortuous deformity. The latter features are distinctive and may help to separate angiomatosis from circumscribed intramuscular angiomas on histologic

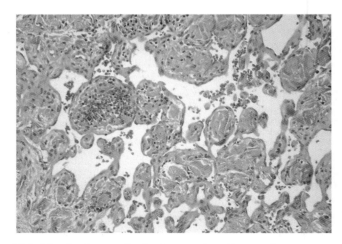

**FIG. 60.** Angiomatosis. A mixture of capillary and cavernous vessels may be seen.

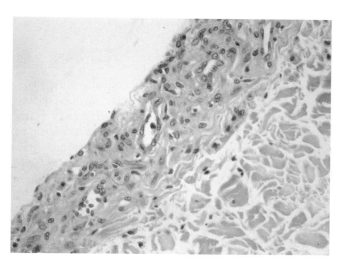

**FIG. 61.** Angiomatosis. The characteristic feature of this case is the proliferation of small capillaries in the wall of larger vessels.

grounds (177,181). In most instances, the diagnosis rests on the clinical examination, wherein a large, diffuse mass should be evident. In the less common lymphangiomatoses occurring in the soft tissues and bones, variously sized anastomosing thin-walled vessels are intimately associated with collections of mature lymphocytes; clustering of small vessels around the walls of veins (typifying angiomatosis) is not observed (183,185).

Surgical extirpation of affected musculature and soft tissue may be offered as treatment in some cases of angiomatosis. However, unlike the more anatomically limited intramuscular angiomas, surgical control is often limited in efficacy, and local recurrence over time is common. Despite locally aggressive recurrent disease, malignant transformation does not occur (177). In contrast to lymphangiomatoses in other soft tissue sites or the viscera, lymphangiomatosis limited to the limbs and bones is not usually an aggressive lesion, although recurrent or persistent disease is seen in most cases (185).

### Spindle Cell Hemangioendothelioma

The discussion of spindle cell hemangioendothelioma (SCH) in a text devoted to pseudoneoplastic disease may be at odds with most accepted classifications of this vasoformative entity (188,189), but there is, in our opinion, suggestive evidence in opposition to traditional interpretations of this condition.

SCH was first described by Weiss and Enzinger (189) as an indolent, nonmetastasizing lesion of the skin that may, despite its lack of systemic spread, exhibit locally destructive growth. SCH presents as an asymptomatic, slowly growing solitary mass, or as a multifocal process involving a limited anatomic region (188–191). The latter attribute likely accounts for regional recurrence up to several centimeters from

previous resection sites (109). Most cases arise in the dermis or subcutis of the distal upper extremity, although anecdotal cases involving deep soft tissue and the spleen have also been reported (109). Lymph node metastases have been documented only once, and because that lesion arose in a radiation field, Enzinger and Weiss believe that it likely underwent radiation-induced malignant transformation and does not reflect the usual natural history of SCH (109).

Gross inspection of resected lesions reveals a nodular, red mass that often contains areas of intralesional thrombosis (188,191). Phleboliths are occasionally encountered. The histologic features of this proliferation are relatively consistent. Although cytologically bland spindle cells dominate some histologic fields, as the name might imply, the lesion is clearly vasoformative, with large cavernous endothelial-lined spaces that often dominate its periphery (Fig. 62) and that also may be interspersed with spindle cell areas. In predominantly spindle cell areas, small clefts are common and may be associated with hemosiderin pigment (Fig. 63). These foci, when viewed in isolation, are reminiscent of *Kaposi's sarcoma*, but in context they are intimately associated with cavernous vascular elements (188–191). SCH differs from Kaposi's sarcoma in four other important respects: (1) spindle cells of SCH are often admixed with rounded or epithelioid cells (188,189,192), some of which may contain intracellular lumina. This is reminiscent of *epithelioid hemangioendothelioma*; (2) the lesion is often partly intravascular—that is, both cavernous and spindled foci may appear to reside partially or completely within large veins that extend into perilesional soft tissue; (3) SCH is not infiltrative of adjacent dermis or soft tissues; and (4) spindle cell elements of SCH do not permeate around small dermal vessels or adnexae (the promontory sign of Kaposi's sarcoma) (109,188,189).

Cells lining cavernous spaces are typically reactive for common endothelial markers, including von Willebrand's

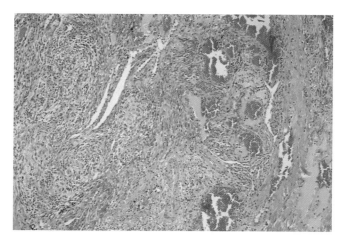

**FIG. 62.** Spindle cell hemangioendothelioma. Cavernous vessels are distributed peripherally around a spindle cell proliferation.

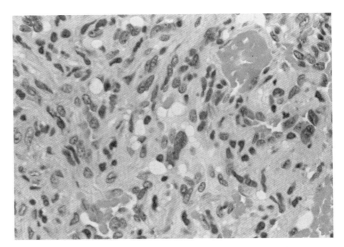

**FIG. 63.** Spindle cell hemangioendothelioma. Cleft-like spaces divide spindle cells. Small oval or epithelioid cells are also present, some of which are vacuolated (intracellular lumens).

factor (factor VIII–related antigen), CD34, and CD31, as are the epithelioid elements in SCH (193). In contrast, the spindle cells, even in areas where vessel-like clefts are present, are nonreactive for these markers. Vimentin immunoreactivity is consistently displayed, and some authors have reported elements of a myofibroblastic or smooth muscle phenotype, including muscle-associated actins (190,193–196). This observation is corroborated by electron microscopic analyses (193,195,196).

Why is this lesion included among the pseudoneoplasms of soft tissue? As already noted, SCH is an indolent process without a natural tendency to metastasize (109). It is cytologically bland and usually devoid of significant mitotic activity. Flow cytometric and cell cycle analyses have demonstrated consistently diploid DNA content and a low proliferative index, with the latter being corroborated by Ki-67 labeling studies (197). This lesion is associated with other vasoformative malformations or pseudoneoplastic proliferations, including the Klippel–Trenaunay syndrome, congenital lymphedema, and early onset varices. SCH may also be a component of the vascular proliferations encountered in Maffucci's syndrome (109,188,191). Finally, the partially intravascular location of SCH, together with ultrastructural evidence of repeated thrombosis of tumoral venous and capillary-like elements (196), suggests that this lesion may result from repeated vascular injury or malformation. It is notable in this context that despite initially proposing a borderline or low-grade malignant nature for SCH (188), Enzinger and Weiss now argue for classifying this entity as a benign neoplasm or vascular malformation (109). As a potential simulator of both Kaposi's sarcoma and epithelioid hemangioendothelioma, SCH thus earns its place in the present discussion.

## Hamartomatous Lesions in Soft Tissue

### Fibrous Hamartoma of Infancy

As a palpable deep dermal or subcuticular mass that is most commonly encountered in the axillae, inguinal regions, or proximal extremities of young children (198,199), fibrous hamartoma of infancy (FHI) often raises clinical concern because of its occasional tendency to be fixed to underlying muscle or fascia. Cut sections reveal a poorly circumscribed, fatty, fibrous mass that only uncommonly exceeds 5 cm in diameter (198).

The histologic features of FHI that most often raise a suspicion of neoplasia pertain to its fibrous elements. Haphazardly arranged, an organoid moderately cellular fibrous trabecula composed of cytologically bland, relatively uniform spindle cells with elongated nuclei that traverse a variably prominent but mature lipomatous element is integral to most examples of FHI (Fig. 64) (109,198,199). However, loosely textured, focally myxoid collections of fusiform cells are also present (Fig. 65) (198). The latter elements, particularly in lesions lacking conspicuous lipomatous components, may be mistaken for *fibromatosis* (Fig. 66) (109). The presence of paucicellular fibrotic zones, particularly with infiltrative peripheral margins, may also result in a histologic impression of *neurofibroma*. Fibromatoses are perhaps the most difficult to reliably separate from FHI, although the particular arrangement of fibrous and immature myxoid elements in FHI is distinctive. However, the occurrence of mature myofibroblastic proliferations in FHI, together with the propensity for FHI to recur as a lesion indistinguishable from fibromatosis, lends credence to speculation that FHI is in fact a variant of *infantile myofibromatosis*.

The immunohistochemical features of FHI are relatively uniform (200–203); the spindle-cell elements, both mature and immature, are intensely reactive for vimentin, and typi-

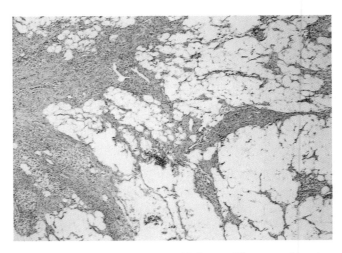

**FIG. 64.** Fibrous hamartoma of infancy. Fibrous trabeculae divide mature adipose tissue.

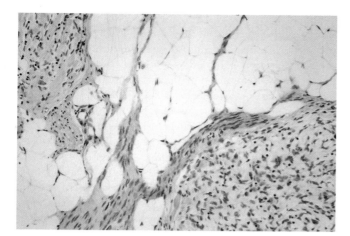

**FIG. 65.** Fibrous hamartoma of infancy. Nodules of spindle cells in a myxoid stroma are admixed with adipose tissue and more hyalinized areas.

cally exhibit generalized reactivity for muscle-specific-and α-smooth muscle actins. Unlike its presence in some other myofibroblastic proliferations, desmin reactivity is, in our experience, uncommon in FHI. S-100 protein is lacking in this lesion, but occasional examples in our experience are CD57 (Leu7)-positive. While the latter finding may complicate the histologic separation of solid examples of FHI from neurofibromas, the absence of generalized myxoid change, and the lack of Meissner corpuscle-like changes in organoid fibrous clusters diminish the likelihood of such confusion.

Ultrastructural analyses of FHI demonstrate that the fibrous trabeculae are populated by elongated cells with varying degrees of fibroblastic or myofibroblastic differentiation (201,202). Dense collagen bundles are often present in infiltrative foci, and loose granular or fibrillar material characterizes the myxoid stroma. Schwann cell and perineural differentiation are lacking.

## Fibrolipomatous Hamartoma

Also known as *lipofibromatous hamartoma*, *neural fibrolipoma*, *neurolipomatosis*, and *macrodystrophia lipomatosa* (with the latter term acknowledging the tendency of this lesion to present with macrodactyly), fibrolipomatous hamartoma (FLH) is usually a congenital nodular or fusiform expansion of large nerves (Fig. 67) in the digits, hands, or distal upper and lower extremities (203–205). Cranial nerve involvement is rare (206). Whereas most lesions are initially asymptomatic, the majority of patients ultimately experience pain, loss of sensation, or paresthesias. The absence of symptoms in some patients, together with a slow growth rate, probably accounts for the fact that most examples present after early childhood. Surgical extirpation, although effective in relieving symptoms, cannot be recommended because marked motor or sensory neural deficits invariably result (205,207).

The histologic features of FLH are distinctive in both biopsy and excisional specimens. Proliferations of perineural and epineural cells result in a concentric cuff of bland spindle cells around large and small nerve branches (Fig. 68). Fibrolipomatous tissue markedly expands the interfascicular stroma and may proliferate in the periphery of the lesion away from the involved nerves (203–205,208,209). Because of the latter feature, occasional misinterpretation of FLH as a *lipoma* is possible. However, misdiagnosis of FLH as an *intraneural lipoma* is less likely because concentric fibrous cuffs of perineural cells are not encountered in isolated intraneural adipose lesions (109). Ossification uncommonly occurs in FLH (210,211), but the presence of metaplastic bone generally does not alter the usual histologic configuration of this hamartomatous process.

Occasionally, a small biopsy of FLH will tangentially or incompletely sample the involved nerve, yielding an asymmetric or eccentric fibrous proliferation that may be mistaken for an *intraneural neurofibroma* or *neuroma*. Immunohistochemistry has some value in the latter instances

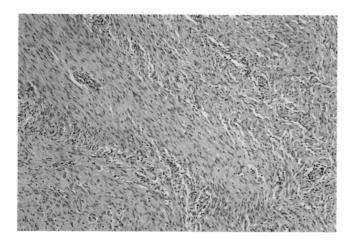

**FIG. 66.** Fibrous hamartoma of infancy. Solid spindle cell areas resemble fibromatosis. Recurrent lesions may be dominated by areas such as this.

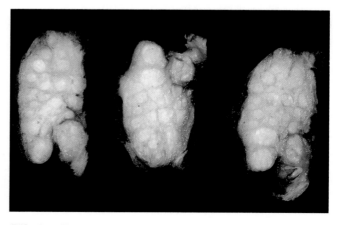

**FIG. 67.** Fibrolipomatous hamartoma. This macroscopic image shows how nerve fascicles appear thickened and separated by an adipose-laden interstitium.

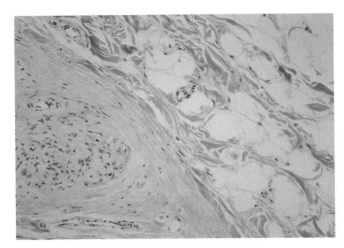

**FIG. 68.** Fibrolipomatous hamartoma. Concentric cuffs of perineural spindle cells surround nerves.

because the concentric perineural elements of FLH are characteristically reactive for epithelial membrane antigen (EMA) (Fig. 69). Sparse EMA-reactive elements (perineural cells) may be admixed with nerve sheath and fibroblastic cells in neurofibroma; in some cases of both neuroma and neurofibroma, a thin rim of EMA reactivity may also be seen around tumor lobules or clusters, but concentric layers of EMA-positive cells are never evident (205). Neuromas and neurofibromas may also be distinguished from FLH in some instances by the presence of neural atrophy in the latter lesion, particularly in longstanding examples (203–205). Electron microscopy confirms the perineural nature of the proliferating cells in FLH, but such an evaluation is not a diagnostic necessity (203,205).

### Neuromuscular Hamartoma (Choristoma)

In relatively few reported instances, mature neural and rhabdomyomatous elements have comprised benign soft tissue masses in young children and, less commonly, in adults. Because these elements do not appear to have proliferative potential, the hamartomatous combination of nerve and skeletal muscle is regarded as a nonneoplastic process distinct from the benign and malignant triton tumors that similarly combine these elements (205,212–222).

The first examples of neuromuscular hamartoma were described by Orlandi in 1895 (221), who regarded them as variants of rhabdomyoma that incorporated mature nerve fibers; more recent studies, however, have stressed their developmental or malformative nature (219). Neuromuscular hamartoma presumably results from the incorporation of skeletal muscle fibers into the developing nerve sheath of large nerve trunks. The sciatic nerve and nerves of the brachial plexus are most commonly affected, although smaller nerves of the head and neck have also been affected. The occurrence of lesions in the central nervous system and in subcutaneous tissue are perhaps most striking (215,220) because in neither site are skeletal muscle elements normally encountered. This has prompted the designation of choristoma that is favored by Mitchell and colleagues (219). Most lesions are well-circumscribed multinodular masses, ranging in size from 2 to 16 cm, that are separated by fibrous bands. Although the majority appear to be intimately associated with nerves, a minority are only superficially infiltrative and can be dissected with little disruption of nerve fibers (219). All examples of neuromuscular hamartoma are composed of variably sized skeletal muscle fibers arranged in bundles or nodules that are inhomogeneously distributed in neural tissue (Fig. 70). Neural elements are also haphazardly arranged, consisting of small fascicles of nerve fibers and Schwann cells that dissect between skeletal muscle elements or are intimately admixed with single-striated muscle fibers. Cellular atypia is never conspicuous in these lesions, and mitotic activity is lacking (219). Dense fibrosis may occasionally dominate portions of the lesion, and it may raise the diagnostic alternative of fi-

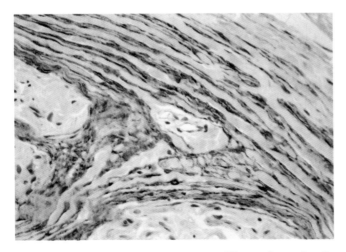

**FIG. 69.** Fibrolipomatous hamartoma. The perineural cells are immunoreactive for epithelial membrane antigen.

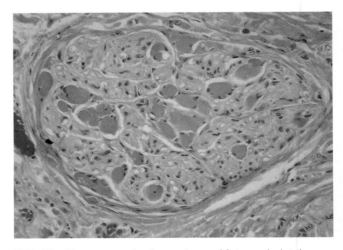

**FIG. 70.** Neuromuscular hamartoma. Mature skeletal muscle cells are interspersed with neural elements within the nerve sheath.

bromatosis infiltrating skeletal muscle and nerve (109). In one example reported by Boman and associates (213), a neuromuscular hamartoma was only identified after amputation for persistently recurrent fibromatosis, suggesting a relationship between those lesions. The recurrence of neuromuscular hamartoma as a lesion indistinguishable from fibromatosis after surgical resection, however, may simply underscore an association between fibromatosis and soft tissue trauma (219).

Differential diagnostic considerations include malignant peripheral nerve sheath tumors with heterologous mesenchymal elements (malignant triton tumors) (205,223,224) and the so-called malignant ectomesenchymoma (225,226). The former of these neoplasms is usually a large, cytologically malignant proliferation of spindle cells or epithelioid elements with immunohistochemical (S-100, CD57, and collagen IV immunoreactivity in the absence of smooth muscle differentiation) and ultrastructural attributes of the peripheral nerve sheath, admixed with collections of heterologous mesenchymal elements that include immature rhabdomyoblastic foci (205,223). The malignant nature of the nerve sheath cells, together with the immaturity of the differentiated skeletal muscle component, clearly distinguishes this entity from neuromuscular hamartoma. Similarly, undifferentiated small round cells having the immunohistochemical features of peripheral neuroectodermal tumor or rhabdomyosarcoma (or both) are admixed with nerve sheath and ganglion cells in *malignant ectomesenchymoma* (225,226). Finally, rare examples of lesions otherwise indistinguishable from benign *peripheral nerve sheath tumor* may contain collections of mature skeletal muscle (227). The latter lesion perhaps more appropriately deserves the appellation benign triton tumor than does neuromuscular hamartoma (205,219).

Surgical resection is usually curative (219). As noted above, secondary fibromatosis–like lesions have been reported in the resection field of at least two examples of neuromuscular hamartoma (109,213), but true lesional recurrence has not been documented. Spontaneous regression after biopsy or subtotal resection has also been reported (219).

### Angiomyolipoma

The juxtaposition of well-vascularized smooth muscle and adipose tissues is a common histologic theme in benign reactive and neoplastic processes (228–235). However, the use of the term "angiomyolipoma" has a very specific connotation, referring to a hamartomatous proliferation of smooth muscle and fatty tissue that most often arises in or subjacent to the renal capsule (109,236,237). Angiomyolipomas often grow to a considerable size and may also primarily involve retroperitoneal soft tissues (109,236). Because the majority of these lesions are asymptomatic, they are often discovered only incidentally. Multicentric and bilateral masses are less common than solitary proliferations;

most of these are encountered in patients with tuberous sclerosis, who collectively constitute roughly one third of all individuals with angiomyolipomas (238–240).

The macroscopic appearance of angiomyolipoma varies considerably, depending on the relative abundance of mature adipose tissue (109). Most cases contain abundant fat, an attribute that is often detected by radiographic imaging (241). In many examples, a broad base of attachment to the renal parenchyma is observed; the adjacent kidney is not replaced by tumor. Loose infiltration of adjacent renal tissue should raise suspicion that the lesion in hand is not in fact an angiomyolipoma. In large examples, areas of hemorrhage may occur; when adipose tissue is not well represented, the firm fibrous appearance of the lesion may resemble either an intrarenal sarcoma or a sarcomatoid carcinoma (109). In general, however, the separation of angiomyolipoma from neoplastic lesions in this site is often more problematic when histologic material is reviewed.

To varying degrees, angiomyolipomas contain histologically mature adipose tissue that is admixed with sheets or bundles of desmin- and muscle-related actin-positive smooth muscle cells (Figs. 71–73)(109,236,237,242). In the latter component, thick muscularized vessels may be conspicuous (Fig. 74). Occasionally, epithelioid smooth muscle cells may be prominent. In some areas, the latter elements may contain prominent cytoplasmic granules and needle-shaped crystals (Fig. 75), imparting a resemblance to cells of the juxtaglomerular apparatus (109,243). Problems in the interpretation of angiomyolipomas arise not so much from any one histologic characteristic of this lesion as from a lack of awareness of the morphologic variations of all of its constituents that may be observed. For example, although the adipose tissue is mature, adipocytes can vary dramatically in size and shape; some may be multivacuolated (Fig. 76). In areas, these changes may closely resemble those of well-differentiated liposarcoma. In smooth muscle elements, considerable nuclear pleomorphism may occasionally raise suspi-

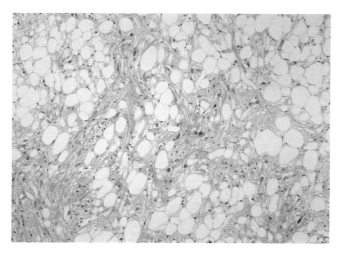

**FIG. 71.** Angiomyolipoma. At low magnification, the admixture of adipose tissue and smooth muscle is apparent.

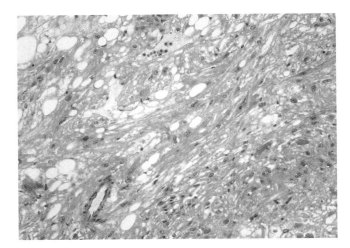

**FIG. 72.** Angiomyolipoma. Some nuclear pleomorphism may be seen in the smooth muscle component, but atypia is usually not pronounced.

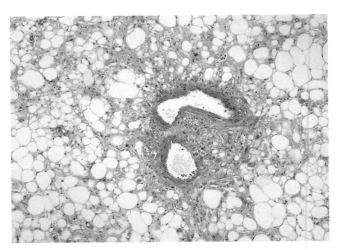

**FIG. 74.** Angiomyolipoma. Thick-walled vessels are characteristic of this condition. Their presence reliably separates angiomyolipomas from the histologically similar benign neoplasm known as myolipoma.

cion of a leiomyosarcoma infiltrating perirenal fat. Cellularity may be quite dense, contributing further to misdiagnosis in some examples (109,236,244,245). Finally, foci of intravascular or lymph nodal growth may rarely occur (Fig. 77) (109,228,240,246,247).

Because of the large size of some angiomyolipomas, the aforementioned atypical histologic features may be deemed sufficient to warrant an interpretation of either *liposarcoma* or *leiomyosarcoma* (109,236). Nevertheless, careful evaluation of the entire lesion will yield two pertinent observations that should confirm its benign nature: (1) the fatty elements are not sclerotic and are not divided by cellular septa containing atypical spindled or multinucleated cells; and (2) despite the presence of small foci of necrosis in the atypical smooth muscle elements of occasional angiomyolipomas, marked nuclear pleomorphism is not accompanied by mitotic activity (109,236,237,244,245). In difficult cases, the

demonstration of HMB-45 immunoreactivity in smooth muscle cells provides reliable evidence in support of this diagnosis (Fig. 78) (237,242,248,249). Among verifiable smooth muscle proliferations (including immunoreactivity for desmin and smooth muscle or muscle-specific actins), staining for HMB-45 is shared only by the proliferative spindle cell elements in *lymphangiomyomatosis* (242). A recent report of HMB-45 reactivity in examples of *renal leiomyoma*, but not *renal leiomyosarcoma* (250), has yet to be corroborated; nevertheless, the potential confusion of spindle cell predominant angiomyolipomas with benign smooth muscle neoplasms in this site may prove problematic in exceptional cases.

The tendency for well-differentiated retroperitoneal liposarcomas to contain variable amounts of mature smooth

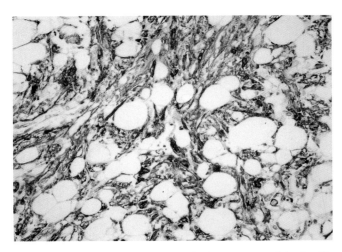

**FIG. 73.** Angiomyolipoma. Desmin immunoreactivity is diffusely displayed in the smooth muscle cells.

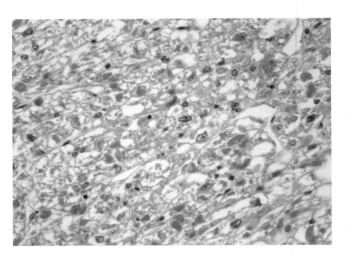

**FIG. 75.** Angiomyolipoma. Eosinophilic cytoplasmic granules and crystalline material are often seen in polygonal or epithelioid smooth muscle cells.

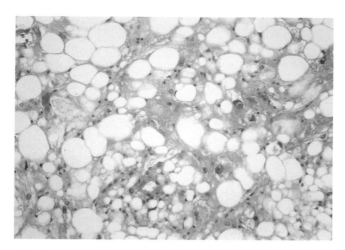

**FIG. 76.** Angiomyolipoma. Atypical nuclei in adipocytes may resemble those of well-differentiated liposarcoma.

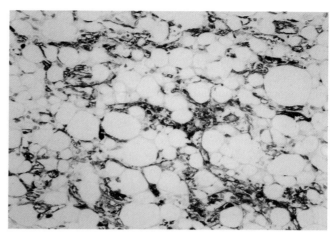

**FIG. 78.** Angiomyolipoma. The smooth muscle cells are typically reactive with HMB-45.

muscle complicates this differential diagnosis (Fig. 119) (229,234,251,252), but, as already emphasized, attention to the cytomorphology of the adipocytic component (with true lipoblasts or floret cells in liposarcomas) and the architectural features of the proliferation are usually sufficient for accurate diagnosis. This peculiar juxtaposition of cellular elements in retroperitoneal sarcomas probably accounts for most examples of lesions thought to represent malignant transformation in angiomyolipomas (109,236). Only two cases have been reported in which features of true malignant transformation have been satisfactorily documented (253,254).

Extrarenal angiomyolipoma-like lesions have been described in several sites, including, but not limited to, the lung (255), spleen (256), liver (257,258), heart (259), mediastinum (109), and spermatic cord (260). Slow growth and indolent clinical behavior may favor a benign diagnosis in

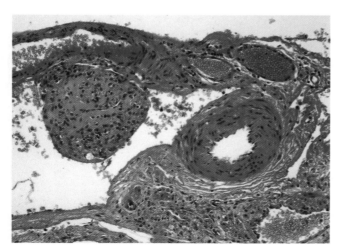

**FIG. 77.** Angiomyolipoma. In this example, intravascular extension of a more solid smooth muscle proliferation is encountered.

these sites, but the presence of mature-appearing adipose tissue and smooth muscle in the last of these locations should be regarded with concern, because well-differentiated liposarcomas also might favor the spermatic cord (109,234). Although the term angiomyolipoma may be applicable to these lesions, HMB-45 staining of smooth muscle elements should now be regarded as an obligate inclusionary criterion for this diagnosis in extrarenal sites. In the absence of such staining, the term *myolipoma* may be more appropriate. Meis and Enzinger (230), Michal (231), and Sonobe and colleagues (233) have used this term in their separate descriptions of partially encapsulated large retroperitoneal myolipomatous tumors that are cytologically bland and not clinically aggressive. Although the processes described in these reports lacked the thickened muscularized vessels or epithelioid smooth muscle elements that are typical of renal angiomyolipomas, there is little else with which to contrast these two entities.

In general, partial nephrectomy or simple excision of soft tissue masses is adequate treatment for angiomyolipoma, although large lesions may require wider resections. Local recurrences generally do not occur (109).

### Stroma-Predominant Fibroproliferative Processes Mimicking Soft Tissue Neoplasms

#### *Elastofibroma*

In many respects, the lesion most commonly referred to as elastofibroma does not represent a pseudoneoplastic process in that its histologic features are distinctive and do not overlap those of well-characterized neoplasms (109,261, 262). Nevertheless, since we have encountered cases wherein elastofibromas were confused with fibromatoses, we felt that the images provided by this unique fibroinflammatory process were worth reviewing here.

Elastofibroma occurs almost exclusively in older adults as

a slowly growing mass between the lower scapular border deep to the rhomboid and latissimus dorsi muscles but superficial to the chest wall. It is often fixed to the ribs and may insinuate into costal periosteum (109,261–264). Similar lesions in other sites are rare (109). Elastofibromas generally are asymptomatic until they assume sufficient size to cause a mass effect, resulting in local tenderness or restriction of scapular movement (109,261,262). As many as 10% of affected individuals present with bilateral subscapular masses (109,261). The latter observation suggests a predisposition for the formation of elastofibromas; the familial distribution of some examples of this entity (261), together with an unusual case of elastofibromatous change associated with a healing gastric ulcer in a patient with bilateral elastofibromas (265), suggests that this predisposition may, in part, be heritable.

On macroscopic examination, elastofibromas are ill-defined, nonencapsulated, firm, fibrous or fibromyxoid masses that are admixed with adipose tissue, especially at the periphery, where the lesion infiltrates adjacent soft tissues. Cystic changes may be conspicuous (109,261,262). Histologically, the mass is paucicellular, with only occasional fibroblasts or myofibroblasts interspersed within haphazardly organized, densely eosinophilic bundles of collagen and elastin fibers (Figs. 79 and 80) (109,261,262,265). The latter are distinctly abnormal, forming thick, beaded structures that when fragmented or cut in cross-section often assume serrated or flower-like configurations (261,262,264,266) that have been given the name "petaloid globules" or "chenille bodies" (109). Histochemical preparations that normally label elastin fibers highlight these elements in dramatic fashion (Fig. 81). The fibers are presumably formed by the sparse (myo)fibroblastic elements that are interspersed throughout the lesion. Ultrastructural examination reveals distinctive, small, non-membrane-bound, granular inclusions in the cy-

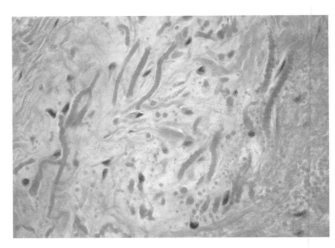

FIG. 80. Elastofibroma. The serrated appearance of elastin fibers is evident at higher magnification.

toplasm of the cells, presumably representing elastin precursors (263,264,266–268). Myofibroblasts in normal or reactive proliferative states do not contain similar structures.

Although the amount and nature of collagens and elastin formed in this process are unusual, the clinical features of elastofibroma suggest that it is likely a variant of the aforementioned *inflammatory myofibroblastic tumors*. The location and slow evolution of the lesion implies a reactive process, and its favored location suggests that the inciting stimulus for this process is traumatic in nature (109,261,262). It is notable in this regard that elastofibroma-like changes have been observed focally in the thoracic fascia in a minority of routine autopsy cases. The latter finding suggests that mechanical trauma, through use and aging, may be an important factor in the development of this lesion (261).

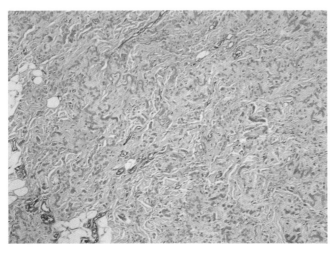

FIG. 79. Elastofibroma. Densely eosinophilic elastic fibers populate a paucicellular fibrous stroma.

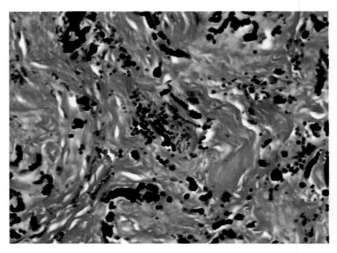

FIG. 81. Elastofibroma. An elastic van Gieson stain highlights the distinctive morphology of elastin fibers.

### Myxoma

The formation of excessive hyalurans and other stromal mucins is generally regarded as a nonspecific characteristic of mesenchymal elements in a variety of reactive and neoplastic processes. Such lesions assume a mucoid or gelatinous consistency because of the tendency of these stromal substances to accumulate water and because of their ability to inhibit polymerization of collagen type I (109). Focal or diffuse stromal myxoid change has been described in virtually all forms of soft tissue sarcoma (but perhaps most importantly in *liposarcoma, leiomyosarcoma, rhabdomyosarcoma,* and *malignant peripheral nerve sheath tumor*), and both osseous and extraskeletal *myxoid chondrosarcomas,* but it also characterizes a group of stroma-predominant, paucicellular, nonneoplastic lesions in bone, skin, and soft tissue that are referred to collectively as *myxomas* (269–277). Because the latter may occasionally mimic myxoid neoplastic lesions in similar anatomic sites, the attributes of these benign reactive tumors should be reviewed.

Although myxomas may arise in a variety of locations (269,270,274,275,277–279), they are most common in the large muscles of the proximal extremities, the gluteal region, and the shoulders. Partly because of their spatial relationship to flat bones and neural plexes in these sites, potential clinical confusion with malignant neoplasms of the soft tissue and bones may be heightened. Children are occasionally afflicted (109,269); however, older adults compose the majority of patients (109,270,277). Most myxomas, apart from a local mass effect, are not symptomatic, and most develop slowly without antecedent trauma. The lesions may occasionally be multifocal, a setting that has in selected cases been associated with monostotic and polyostotic fibrous dysplasia of bone (272,276,280–283). A small number of patients with polyostotic lesions present with Albright's disease (284,285). Miettinen and colleagues (276) have reported that careful skeletal examination may reveal minor abnormalities of the long bones in the majority of patients with intramuscular myxoma.

The macroscopic and microscopic features of intramuscular myxoma are reproducible. Grossly, myxomas are globoid gelatinous masses that either resemble the gray translucence of granulation tissue when poorly collagenized or appear more uniformly pale tan or white in instances where collagen deposition is more pronounced. Cut surfaces are mucoid in consistency; fluid-filled cysts may be conspicuous. Borders appear sharply defined macroscopically, but the lesion is often fixed to adjacent skeletal muscle or fascial planes, bespeaking an infiltrative nature that is corroborated by histologic examination (109,270,277). Because these masses are typically asymptomatic, they tend to reach a relatively large size before presentation, occasionally in excess of 10 cm. Enzinger and Weiss argue in favor of a neoplastic nature (109), but, in general, we feel that inclusion of at least some examples of myxoma as pseudoneoplastic proliferations in bone and soft tissue is more appropriate.

**FIG. 82.** Myxoma. At low magnification, intramuscular myxomas appear to consist of relatively few cells loosely dispersed in a myxoid stroma.

The histologic attributes of myxoma are consistently displayed in noncystic areas throughout any given lesion. The masses are paucicellular, populated by few cytologically bland spindled (Figs. 82 and 83), or, less commonly, stellate cells that are evenly dispersed in a hypovascular, mucicarmine-positive, hyalurinodase-sensitive Alcian blue– and colloidal iron–positive mucoid matrix. Cells have relatively little cytoplasm, and nuclei are small, and often pyknotic, with no mitotic activity. Multinucleated cells are not seen. Loosely arranged reticulin fibers divide the matrix, and variable amounts of mature collagen fibers are present. Scattered macrophages may be seen, some of which may contain intracellular accumulations of lipid, but features of lipoblasts are not apparent. In cells where intracellular lipid is abundant, nuclear profiles are unencumbered (109,269, 270,272,274,277). Although both the macrophages and the

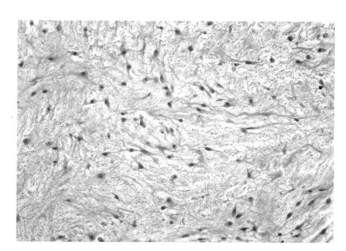

**FIG. 83.** Myxoma. Most cells have sparse eosinophilic cytoplasm and elongated or stellate profiles.

spindle-stellate cells are consistently vimentin-reactive, no immunostaining for S-100 protein is seen in either cell population (109,271). The latter observation further substantiates the lack of lipoblastic differentiation in myxomas. Given the lack of reactivity for CD34, CD57, desmin, and muscle-associated actins, the diagnosis of a myxoid nerve sheath or smooth muscle tumor may also be excluded. This limited immunoprofile suggests a fibroblastic or relatively unspecialized myofibroblastic phenotype, a conclusion that is supported by electron microscopic analyses (271,286).

As suggested earlier, myxomas tend to be infiltrative at their margins, with an intermingling of tumoral and reactive or atrophic muscle or stromal elements. Edema may be pronounced in the periphery of the lesion, and an attenuated condensation of fibrous tissue may form a pseudocapsule around portions of the lesion (109,269,270,277).

Given the characteristic clinical and histologic attributes of myxoma, it is reasonable to expect that careful histopathologic examination will exclude myxoid neoplastic proliferations from consideration in most instances. However, when paucicellular areas are sampled, small biopsies of myxoid soft tissue masses may present difficulties. In such cases, a careful search for nuclear pleomorphism and mitotic activity may provide a rational basis for selecting cases in which histochemical and immunophenotypic analyses will be of value in resolving the differential diagnosis. Needless to say, areas of increased cellularity or vascularity, evidence of true lipoblastic differentiation, association with a large nerve or nerve trunk, or continuity of the lesion with underlying bone should lead one to regard the diagnosis of myxoma with extreme skepticism.

All of the features recounted herein for intramuscular myxoma also apply to myxomas in other sites, particularly those of relevance to this chapter. These include myxomas of the jaws, juxtaarticular myxomas, and cutaneous myxomas (109,269,275,278,279). Although differential diagnosis may vary slightly for each of these myxomatous lesions, the approach to their identification should be the same.

Surgical excision of myxomas is generally curative, although rare recurrences have been reported (109). The nature of these recrudescent lesions is a matter of some conjecture, since Ireland and colleagues (272) described recurring lesions as cellular, a description that is at odds with the characteristic phenotype recounted herein.

## Pseudoneoplastic Processes Affecting Peritoneum and Peritonealized Soft Tissues

Apart from peculiar reactions to foreign materials, pigments, or cellular products as described above, relatively few processes in the peritoneum and peritonealized soft tissues form mass lesions that might be mistaken for a neoplastic process. Mesenchymal, mesothelial, and epithelial proliferations have been implicated, and the more common of these are discussed in greater detail as part of the discussion of pseudoneoplasms of the genital tract and peritoneum (see Chapter 10).

## PSEUDONEOPLASTIC LESIONS OF BONE

The clinically benign nature of most lesions that are ultimately classified as osseous pseudoneoplasms is often established radiographically. Indeed, most of the entities discussed in this section normally present as a radiolucent or heterogeneously mineralized lesion of diaphyseal or metaphyseal bone, with sharply defined, often sclerotic borders. However, in some cases, marked deformity or actual breaching of the cortex by a complex cystic or sclerosing fibro-(chondro-osseous) proliferation might raise the suspicion of an aggressive neoplasm in bone, necessitating careful histopathologic examination to exclude a malignant process from diagnostic consideration. The interpretative problems associated with intraosseous or parosteal pseudoneoplasms are more often histologic because radiographically bland lesions often contain unexpectedly cellular proliferations of fibro- or chondro-osseous tissues (with or without osteoclast-like giant cells) that may be difficult to separate from osteosarcoma, chondrosarcoma, chondroblastoma, and giant cell tumor. The entities that are described in the following discussion are listed in Table 3.

### Fibrous and Fibro-osseous Proliferations of Bone

#### Fibrous Dysplasia

The inclusion of fibrous dysplasia in a discussion of pseudoneoplastic proliferations of bone reflects the bias of the authors, and is likely to have its detractors because neither fibrous dysplasia nor cortical osteofibrous dysplasia (see below) has been granted nonneoplastic status by consensus.

Fibrous dysplasia is a fibroproliferative process in one (monostotic) or several (polyostotic) bones, which manifests a haphazardly distributed osseous component in the form of woven bone (287–295). Patients with polyostotic lesions are almost invariably young children (287,290,294,296,297),

**TABLE 3.** *Pseudoneoplastic lesions in bone*

| |
|---|
| Fibrous and fibro-osseous proliferations in bone |
|   Fibrous dysplasia |
|   Cortical osteofibrous dysplasia |
|   Metaphyseal fibrous defects |
|   Polymorphic Fibro-osseous lesion |
|   Parosteal fasciitis |
| Fibroinflammatory and reactive/reparative lesions |
|   Giant cell reparative granuloma |
|   Bizarre parosteal osteochondromatous proliferation of bone |
|   Synovial chondrometaplasia/chondromatosis |
| Aneurysmal bone cyst |

cal defect arise at or near sites of tendinous insertions, and they initially erode the outer cortical zone. Although trauma is not often an element of the stated clinical history, the location and the early pattern of metaphyseal damage support musculoskeletal injury as an important etiologic factor (342,344,347).

The radiographic appearance of metaphyseal fibrous defects is characteristic, allowing for accurate diagnosis in virtually all cases. Lytic zones have an irregular shape, and are sharply demarcated from adjacent cortical bone by a thin sclerotic rim (Fig. 99). These attributes generally permit confident nonsurgical management of smaller lesions, as well as properly conservative surgical therapy in larger, destabilizing lytic lesions (343,347–349). In this respect, it must be acknowledged that these fibro-osseous lesions may not be pseudoneoplasms in the sense outlined in Chapter 1. However, in cases that present in older children or young adults, the radiographic appearance can be indeterminate. Nonossifying fibroma can, like small fibrous cortical defects, undergo progressive mineralization and remodeling over time, resulting in irregular dense mineralization. This is seen initially in the peripheral zone but ultimately affects the entire

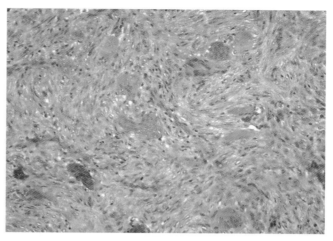

**FIG. 100.** Nonossifying fibroma. Spindled cells arranged in a storiform pattern are admixed with osteoclast-like giant cells.

lesion (347). After pathologic fracture, medullary hemorrhage, periosteal reaction, or early callus formation may further mask the characteristic features of this disease (290).

The gross appearances of nonossifying fibroma and fibrous cortical defect are relatively nondescript. Curetted portions of soft gray–tan or yellow tissue may be accompanied by fragments of reactive bone or callus. In their unusual description of an intact nonossifying fibroma removed as part of an amputation specimen, Mubarek and colleagues (354) emphasized the sharp demarcation of this lesion from cortical bone, a finding that is in keeping with the radiographic features of the entity. Histologic examination reveals a cellular population of well-differentiated fibroblast-like spindle cells arranged haphazardly or in a storiform pattern, with a loose admixture of osteoclast-like multinucleated cells (Fig. 100) and foam cells (xanthoma cells) (Fig. 101). Hemosiderin is often seen within histiocytes but may also be present in spindled and multinucleated cells (Fig. 102). Be-

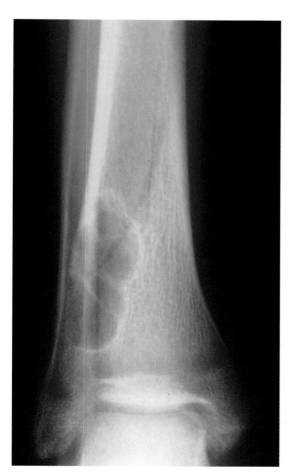

**FIG. 99.** Nonossifying fibroma. A sharply defined lytic lesion of the metaphysis with sclerotic borders typifies nonossifying fibroma.

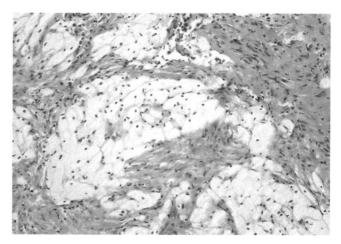

**FIG. 101.** Nonossifying fibroma. Collections of xanthoma (foam) cells are interspersed with spindled elements.

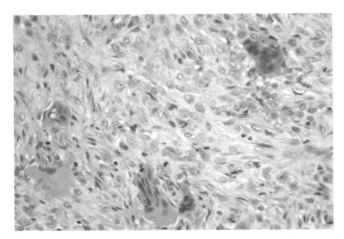

**FIG. 102.** Nonossifying fibroma. Hemosiderin may be seen in spindled cells.

cause foam cells and hemosiderin are more conspicuous in older lesions, these elements are often regarded as regressive in nature. Ossification is not an inherent element of metaphyseal fibrous defects; rather, bony trabeculae are either reactive in nature or represent elements of normal growth and maturation of the cortex at the periphery of the lesion. In either case, bony trabeculae, when present, exhibit an orderly pattern of mineralization with a uniformly distributed population of osteoblasts (290,342,344,355). The latter feature is important to the differential diagnosis of nonossifying fibroma because the presence of bony trabeculae in fibrous stroma might otherwise be mistaken for *fibrous dysplasia* (Fig. 103). The stroma may contain varying amounts of collagen, but dense hyalinization to the exclusion of cellular elements is but a focal phenomenon in a subset of cases. Such areas may also resemble *desmoplastic fibroma*, but the storiform configuration of more typical cellular elements elsewhere in the lesion effectively excludes this diagnostic alternative (290). Malignant transformation probably does not occur, although Kyriakos and Murphy (356) have reported the apparent coincidental occurrence of nonossifying fibroma and osteosarcoma.

Despite numerous immunohistochemical and electron microscopic studies, the character of nonossifying fibroma is unclear (357–362). A recent study by Bejarano and Kyriakos (355) appears to resolve 2 important matters: (1) that the stromal (spindle cells) exhibit a mixed (myo)fibroblastic/histiocytic phenotype, with common reactivity for vimentin, muscle-specific actin, CD68, and HAM-56; and (2) that the stromal cells alone exhibit proliferative potential, and likely serve as the reservoir for maturation into an immunophenotypically similar xanthoma cell population. The mixed phenotype of the spindle cells raises yet another issue because the storiform pattern of spindle cells in nonossifying fibroma, together with the collections of foam cells, often suggests the diagnosis of *benign fibrous histiocytoma*. In fact, it is probably not possible to separate fibrous histiocytoma from nonossifying fibroma on histologic grounds alone (287,363–367). Importantly, fibrous histiocytomas do not show an exclusive predilection for the metaphysis of long bones (involvement is more often diaphyseal, with less common extension to metaphysis or even epiphysis), and they more often arise in axial skeletal sites that are not affected by nonossifying fibromas. Young children may be affected, as is true of nonossifying fibromas, but benign fibrous histiocytomas continue to arise throughout adulthood. In further contrast to nonossifying fibromas, fibrous histiocytomas may be painful lesions even in the absence of fracture. Finally, osseous fibrous histiocytomas may recur after curettage or may behave in a locally aggressive fashion (364), although Bertoni et al. (363) suggest that xanthoma cell–laden examples of such tumors (bearing a striking histologic, if not clinical, resemblance to nonossifying fibroma) are less likely to do so. Some examples of fibrous histiocytoma may breach the cortex and infiltrate into adjacent soft tissue (290). In general, differential diagnosis is only problematic in metaphyseal or diaphyseal lesions in long bones in patients over the age of 25. Given the potential for aggressive clinical behavior of fibrous histiocytoma, erring on the side of surgical management in such cases may be warranted.

### Polymorphic Fibro-osseous Lesion/Liposclerosing Myxofibrous Tumor of Bone

Most pseudoneoplastic lesions of bone exhibit clinical and histologic attributes that allow the surgical pathologist to recognize them as distinct nosologic entities within the heterogeneous spectrum of fibroblastic and chondro-osseous proliferations. Less commonly, fibro-osseous proliferations assume phenotypic configurations that are not easily categorized. Ragsdale has addressed this issue in a discussion of 95 such lesions, in which an admixture of elements that were variously interpreted as nonossifying fibroma, fibrous dys-

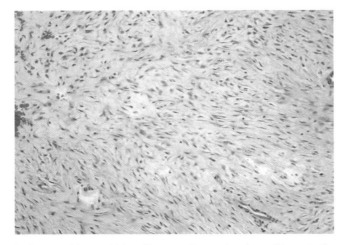

**FIG. 103.** Nonossifying fibroma. Areas dominated by spindle cells may resemble desmoplastic fibroma.

tion), bizarre parosteal osteochondromatous proliferation of bone (BPOP) is a parosteal mass that clinically simulates benign osteochondroma in its presentation but is generally regarded as a benign reactive or reparative process that occasionally is associated with a history of local trauma (41,394). Although BPOP primarily affects bones of the hands and feet (with the exception of the distal phalanges) (41,394–397), these lesions arise in the long bones in 15–20% of cases (41,394,398). A single example of BPOP in the skull has been reported. Its radiographic appearance is relatively nonspecific, but roentgenograms generally illustrate a pattern of benign parosteal heterotopic cortical mineralization in the absence of a periosteal reaction (Fig. 114). There is no obvious cortical flaring, and there is progressive organization of the ossifying elements over time. Despite the latter phenomenon, BPOP lacks the zonation of *myositis ossificans,* and is not generally considered a clinical or radiographic mimic of that lesion (41,394,396). Nevertheless, its parosteal location often raises the diagnostic alternative of the similar inflammatory myofibroblastic and chondro-osseous process known as *parosteal fasciitis* (36–39). Notably, the clinical behavior of this lesion is not predictably indolent; in more than half of the cases reported by Nora et al. (41) and Meneses and colleagues (394), isolated or repeated local recurrences followed surgical resection; in those cases, second recurrences were not uncommon. However, no lesion

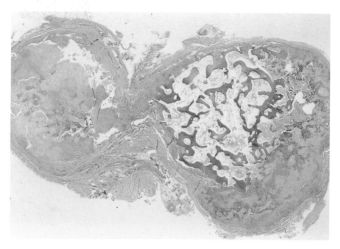

**FIG. 115.** Bizarre parosteal osteochondromatous proliferation (Nora's lesion). At low magnification, a poorly organized osseous proliferation is associated with a distinct cartilaginous cap. (Courtesy of F. Nora, M.D., Medford, OR.)

was infiltrative of soft tissue or adjacent bone, and no patient suffered metastasis.

The histologic features of BPOP are similarly at odds with its radiographic appearances. Although it is primarily a cartilaginous lesion, BPOP invariably contains poorly organized bone and spindled mesenchymal elements (41,290,394). Cartilage often forms a cap at the periphery of the ossifying elements (Fig. 115) but may, in some examples, consist of lobules that undergo an enchondral pattern of ossification separated by septa of cytologically bland spindle cells (Fig. 116). Chondrocytes, as the name of the lesion implies, are often enlarged and cytologically bizarre (Fig. 117); in fact, without careful attention to these lesions at higher magnification, a diagnosis of malignancy may be mistakenly preferred (41). Neither the osseous nor the spindle cell

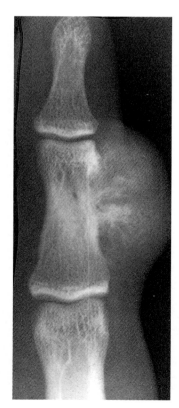

**FIG. 114.** Bizarre parosteal osteochondromatous proliferation (Nora's lesion). In this radiograph, a parosteal-based mass is irregularly mineralized. There is no evidence of a periosteal reaction. (Courtesy of F. Nora, M.D., Medford, OR.)

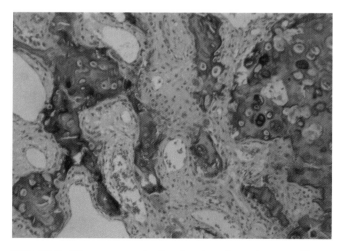

**FIG. 116.** Bizarre parosteal osteochondromatous proliferation (Nora's lesion). Areas of enchondral ossification are separated by a spindle cell stroma. (Courtesy of F. Nora, M.D., Medford, OR.)

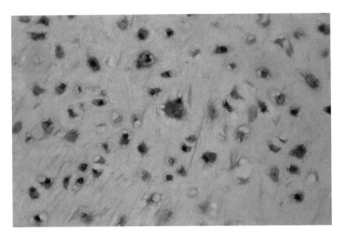

**FIG. 117.** Bizarre parosteal osteochondromatous proliferation (Nora's lesion). Chondrocytes may be quite atypical. (Courtesy of F. Nora, M.D., Medford, OR.)

elements are cytologically atypical, but plump osteoblasts are often associated with mineralizing osteoid matrix (41,290,394).

The histologic differential diagnosis includes many benign and malignant chondro-osseous lesions of bone and soft tissue, including *osteochondroma, subungual exostosis, parosteal fasciitis (florid reactive periositis), parosteal osteosarcoma,* and *chondrosarcoma.* The architecture of BPOP does not fully mimic most examples of osteochondroma in that the fibrous stroma of the former lesion does not include marrow elements, and lacks continuity with the medullary cavity of the affected bone. Furthermore, the osseous elements are not well organized, and occasionally arise directly from spindle cells without the apparent enlistment of osteoblasts. Finally, neither the cellularity nor the cytologic atypia of the cartilaginous elements in BPOP is matched by those of osteochondroma. As Fechner and Mills have suggested, BPOP probably only differs from subungual exostosis in terms of location; the latter lesion occurs on the distal phalanges but is histologically similar to BPOP in most, if not all, respects (290). As mentioned earlier, BPOP does not share radiographic or histologic features with either myositis ossificans or its parosteal imitator, so-called parosteal fasciitis, but its location often suggests the latter diagnostic alternative. Important differences between fasciitis and BPOP include a lack of abundant calcified matrix or cartilaginous elements, and a prominent, often laminated periosteal reaction in the former of these two entities. The bizarre cytologic features of BPOP may mimic those of well-differentiated chondrosarcomas, but the latter lesions are not admixed with fibrous stromal elements, and almost never involve the small bones of the hands and feet (287). Moreover, the doubly nucleated cells with nuclear hyperchromasia that in part define chondrosarcomatous proliferations are lacking in BPOP. Separation of BPOP from parosteal osteosarcoma is also generally possible on clinical grounds because osteosarcoma does not involve the hands and feet with any

great frequency (287). In long bones, the separation of these processes is based on the lack of significant atypia in spindle cell fibro-blastic elements in BPOP (41,394).

### Synovial Chondrometaplasia/Chondromatosis

As a primary chondrometaplasia, this lesion is distinct among pseudoneoplasms in skeletal and articular tissues. Usually monoarticular in nature, synovial chondromatosis arises as a multinodular chondrometaplasia of synovium, bursa, or tendon sheaths in or around the large joints, particularly the knee. The nodules secondarily detach, resting free within the synovial spaces as loose bodies (109,399–404). Extraarticular lesions can also occur (405,406).

The radiographic appearance of chondromatosis in both intra- and extraarticular sites is variable, although most lesions are characteristically radiolucent. Varying degrees of mineralization reflect a tendency for the cartilaginous nodules to calcify or undergo ossification (Fig. 118); heterogeneous patterns of mineralization may be particularly worrisome in extraarticular sites (290,399–402,404).

Histologically, chondromatosis consists principally of mature hyaline cartilage. Nuclei might be hyperchromatic, with large irregular shapes, and multinucleated chondrocytes might be present. Cellular areas might also exhibit varying degrees of mitotic activity, but the overall atypia that typifies

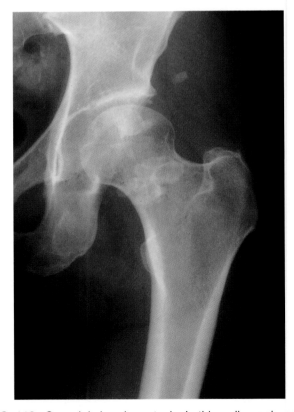

**FIG. 118.** Synovial chondromatosis. In this radiograph, nodules of mineralized tissue are present in synovium.

*chondrosarcoma* is absent. Separation of synovial chondromatosis from enchondroma is never problematic because of the location of the latter tumor, but distinction of metaplastic cartilage from *soft part chondroma* might not be possible in the unusual circumstance when chondromatosis occurs in or near synovial tissues in the hands or feet. This diagnostic separation is complicated in some cases by the increased incidence of true soft tissue cartilaginous neoplasms in patients with synovial chondromatosis (290,400). However, the benign clinical behavior of primary soft tissue chondroma renders this distinction of little practical significance (109).

The pattern of ossification in chondromatosis resembles normal enchondral ossification; osteoblastic atypia is not a feature of that lesion. The nodular pattern of growth likewise precludes the misdiagnosis of *osteochondroma* in both intraarticular and parosteal sites (407). Although malignant transformation to chondrosarcoma has occurred in a few reported instances of synovial chondromatosis (408–411), local recurrence is a far more common complication (290,404).

### Aneurysmal Bone Cyst

Aneurysmal bone cysts are important entities because of their common presence in the metaphysis of long bones or in vertebrae (although virtually any bone in the body may occasionally harbor this entity) (287,391,393), and because of the rapid, painful, and often destructive growth they may exhibit. The large majority of aneurysmal bone cysts occur in young individuals, most often in the second decade of life. Females are only slightly more commonly affected than males. As noted, the lesions are often painful, and they might have been symptomatic for relatively short periods of time before presentation. Pain on palpation is uncommon (287,375,391,393,412–418).

In long bones, the distal femur and proximal tibia are the most common sites of involvement (287,375,391,412, 413,418). In vertebrae, aneurysmal bone cysts often affect the posterior arch and spinous processes (with secondary extension into the vertebral body), and have the peculiar tendency to involve adjacent bones (418). Lesions of small bones of the distal extremities have also been described (287,419). The majority arise in cortical or medullary bone; fewer than 10% primarily affect subperiosteal sites (287,414,420,421).

The radiographic appearance of aneurysmal bone cyst evolves over the life of the lesion (414,420–422). Initially, the lesion is small, is often eccentrically placed in the affected bone, and does not expand the cortex. In this incipient phase, the borders of the lesion are not distinct, and might exhibit a permeative pattern of growth into adjacent cortex or medulla. In the so-called growth phase of the lesion, rapid enlargement is associated with cortical expansion, osteolysis, and cortical destruction. There may be sufficient periosteal injury to evoke changes indistinguishable from the

classic Codman's triangle of *osteosarcoma*, as periosteal new bone growth ensues. In rapidly enlarging lesions, periosteal bone cannot accommodate the lesion, and portions of the cortex may appear to be lost entirely. However, the medullary margins of the lesion are distinct, a feature that may help to distinguish this phase of disease from osteosarcoma or another intraosseous malignancy. Following rapid expansion, aneurysmal bone cyst assumes a more stable course ("stable phase"), wherein the classic radiographic appearance of an expanded, lytic, trabeculated metaphyseal lesion with distinct perilesional sclerosis emerges (Figs. 119 and 120). As the lesion heals, the trabeculae progressively ossify (290).

The gross appearance of aneurysmal bone cyst is not often well displayed in surgical specimens; most are accurately recognized prior to surgery, so that only curetted fragments are submitted for histologic examination (290). In larger pieces of tissue, or when the entire lesion is available for examination, the most conspicuous feature is a catacomb of cavernous or aneurysmal blood-filled spaces (375,391, 392,414,415). The prominence and thickness of more solid trabeculae within the lesion depends on the stage of lesional growth in which the specimen has been obtained. In older lesions, coarse bony trabeculae may be prominent. The lesion, apart from its aneurysmal characteristics, may also be conspicuously cystic with serous and serosanguinous fluid filling irregularly sized spaces. Predominantly or exclusively

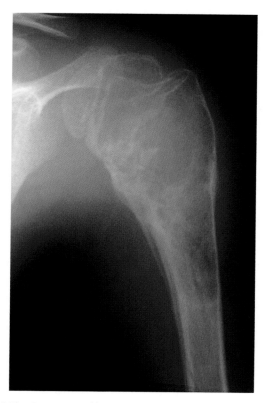

**FIG. 119.** Aneurysmal bone cyst. Medullary expansion is associated with marked thinning of cortical bone.

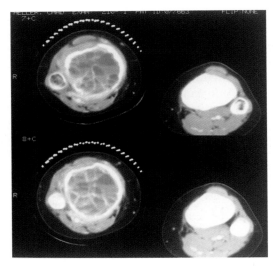

**FIG. 120.** Aneurysmal bone cyst. The heterogeneous appearance of the aneurysmal bone cyst is apparent in this tomographic image. The denser trabeculae correspond to those seen in Fig. 121.

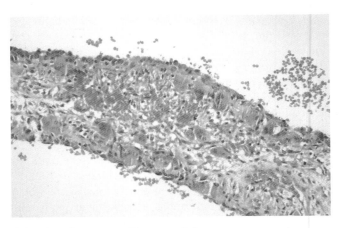

**FIG. 121.** Aneurysmal bone cyst. Large aneurysmal spaces are lined with trabeculae.

solid lesions (so-called solid variants of aneurysmal bone cyst) are uncommon (390,392,423–425).

The histologic features of aneurysmal bone cyst are not uniform from case to case, but they encompass a fairly consistent range of features that allow for unequivocal diagnosis in the majority of cases (287,290,375,391,393,412–418). Cystic or aneurysmal blood-filled spaces, from which the name of the lesion is derived, are characteristic of all but the solid variant lesions. Neither careful histologic, ultrastructural, nor immunohistochemical analyses have identified an endothelial lining on the surface of these spaces (418,425–429), although the presence of arteriovenous malformations within resected aneurysmal bone cysts suggests that vascular trauma may be an important factor in their development (290,412,429). The aneurysmal spaces are separated by fibrous septa of varying thicknesses and configurations (Fig. 121) that are relatively cellular, populated by fibroblasts and an admixture of chondroid or osteoid matrix, multinucleated giant cells, mononuclear histiocytoid cells, and a bland lymphoplasmocytic inflammatory infiltrate. Giant cells may congregate beneath the lining of the blood-filled spaces (Figs. 121 and 122) but do not actually constitute an element of the lining or reside within the space. In many areas, the admixture of cellular elements may resemble those seen in *giant cell reparative granuloma* or *giant cell tumor*, a topic to which we will return.

Ossification within the lesion may be conspicuous in older lesions. Bone formation either arises as a mineralization of osteoid in a manner very similar to that seen in *fibrous dysplasia* or develops together with a rim of primitive chondromyxoid matrix (Fig. 123) (290,392,393,418). The latter, regarded by some as characteristic of aneurysmal bone cyst (392,393), often occupies large areas in the septa that are independent of osteoid and may line the blood-filled spaces.

This characteristic matrix often calcifies in a focal, heterogeneous pattern that clearly distinguishes aneurysmal bone cyst from *chondroblastoma* (287). Osteoid is often conspicuous in calcifying aneurysmal bone cysts, and may assume a linear, trabecular, or lace-like configuration (Fig. 124). The matrix is usually associated with mitotically active but cytologically bland mononuclear cells (Fig. 125). At the periphery of the lesion, aneurysmal spaces may interdigitate with cortical bone; in lesions that have eroded through the cortex, the characteristic histologic components of aneurysmal bone cyst may also be present in extraperiosteal soft tissue (290,418).

In the relatively few reported cases of solid variant aneurysmal bone cyst (390,392,423–425), all of the features evident in the septa of typical examples are represented, including the distinctive chondroid matrix (392). But for lack of aneurysmal spaces, the juxtaposition of these elements bears a strong resemblance to giant cell reparative granuloma. Because most of the solid lesions reported by Sanerkin and colleagues (392) also contained small foci in which

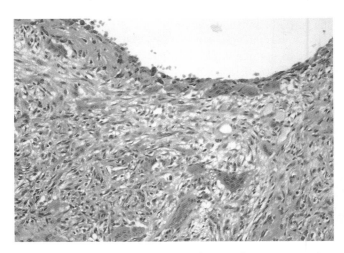

**FIG. 122.** Aneurysmal bone cyst. Giant cells congregate beneath the cyst lining.

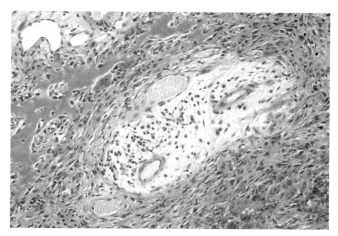

FIG. 123. Aneurysmal bone cyst. Small islands of chondromyxoid tissue are apparent in this example.

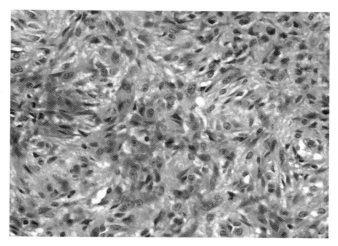

FIG. 125. Aneurysmal bone cyst. The stroma is populated by histiocyte-like mononuclear cells.

ectatic blood-filled spaces were present, the diagnosis of aneurysmal bone cyst may have been justified in that series of cases. However, it is accepted that many lesions histologically characteristic of aneurysmal bone cyst are associated with, or arise as a secondary phenomenon in, several intraosseous lesions (287,375,391,393,412,417,422,430–433). These include giant cell reparative granuloma and giant cell tumor, among others. Although the distributions of aneurysmal bone cyst and giant cell reparative granuloma by definition do not overlap (as already emphasized, in the hands and feet, aneurysmal lesions containing solid foci resembling giant cell reparative granuloma are regarded as examples of the latter), the similarities between these lesions suggest a common histogenesis (290). This relationship also serves to emphasize an important element in diagnostic evaluation; the presence of another recognizable pattern of bone pathology is almost never coincidental, so that the diagnosis of primary aneurysmal bone cyst requires that another disease of bone be excluded first. As many as 50% of metaphyseal le-

sions and nearly 75% of epiphyseal aneurysmal bone cysts are associated with fracture or with another reactive or neoplastic osseous lesion (287,375,391,393,412,417,422, 430–433). Given that the elements of aneurysmal bone cyst may superficially resemble those of *osteosarcoma, osteoblastoma, giant cell tumor, chondroblastoma, chondromyxoid fibroma, fibrous dysplasia,* and *unicameral bone cyst,* careful histologic examination of curetted or resected aneurysmal specimens should never be taken lightly. So common is the association between aneurysmal changes or reparative granuloma–like features and reactive and neoplastic disease of bone that some have suggested that all aneurysmal bone cysts are secondary phenomena and that the inciting pathologic process is overrun or no longer identifiable in those lesions ultimately diagnosed as aneurysmal bone cysts. As noted previously, the radiographic features of cases that are finally interpreted as aneurysmal bone cysts identify a pattern of lesional evolution that does not require the presence of a preexisting or concurrent lesion in bone. However, exclusion of a small inciting lesion that is overrun by aneurysmal changes is not possible in all cases.

Apart from the separation of aneurysmal bone cyst from giant cell reparative granuloma in appendicular sites and the exclusion of a primary underlying lesion associated with aneurysmal bone cyst, the differential diagnosis of this lesion is based on the nature and distribution of its chondro-osseous elements. In this context, the diagnosis of giant cell tumor can be excluded with confidence in most cases. Even though aneurysmal bone cyst exhibits an aggressive nature in some cases, and although blood-filled spaces are admixed with an irregularly mineralizing osteoid and chondroid matrix that contains mitotically active cells, the histologic misinterpretation of this lesion as *telangiectatic osteosarcoma* should be a rare occurrence. However, as Fechner and Mills have reminded us, this may be the biggest diagnostic problem posed by aneurysmal bone cyst (290). In telangiectatic osteosarcoma, compact irregular trabeculae of osteoid are

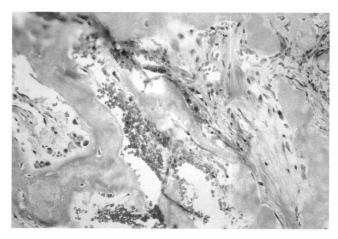

FIG. 124. Aneurysmal bone cyst. Lace-like osteoid may be seen in trabeculae.

associated with cytologically anaplastic osteoblasts that contain atypical mitotic figures, but the presence of a conspicuous giant cell population in septa around large telangiectatic blood-filled spaces may confound the unwary pathologist.

Although large, destructive aneurysmal bone cysts may require surgical resection, curettage or excision with bone grafting is standard therapy (418,419). Unfortunately, recurrence of aneurysmal bone cyst in 6–24 months is relatively common after such treatment (391,418,420,429). Recurrence of aneurysmal changes may also be seen in patients with secondary aneurysmal bone cysts in true neoplasms, although in the majority of such cases, the primary intraosseous process also recurs (375,412,433). Cryotherapy has been reported as a useful adjunct to surgical procedures in some instances (412). In rapidly destructive lesions, particularly those in the vertebrae where neurologic deficits due to cord compression might be unavoidable without aggressive management, low-dose radiotherapy can offer some benefit (290). Malignant transformation in primary aneurysmal bone cyst is usually associated with a prior history of radiation therapy (414,417,418), although Kyriakos and Hardy have reported one case in which no such history was obtained (434).

By definition, aneurysmal bone cyst is an intraosseous lesion, but there are reports of a histologically indistinguishable process occurring primarily in soft tissues. The so-called aneurysmal cyst of soft tissues reported by Rodriguez-Peralto and colleagues is one example of this phenomenon (435). In this lesion, represented by a soft tissue mass in the left shoulder of a 20-year-old woman, aneurysmal blood-filled spaces were separated by trabeculae that were histologically identical to those of typical osseous aneurysmal cysts. In both this case and another reported by Amir and associates (436) in the groin of a 15-year-old boy, the aneurysmal lesion was surrounded by a delicate wall of lamellar bone, imparting a radiographic similarity to myositis ossificans. Neither case exhibited the zonation phenomenon of ossification that is typical of myositis ossificans; rather, each contained trabecular or lace-like osteoid that was associated with woven bone, osteoclast-like giant cells, and an admixture of chondroid elements. A similar but nonossifying aneurysmal giant cell lesion was described in an intravascular site by Petrik and colleagues (437). The common phenotype of these soft tissue lesions and osseous aneurysmal cysts suggests a common histogenesis as well, lending further credence to the concept of aneurysmal bone cyst as a reparative phenomenon in response to injury.

## REFERENCES

1. Dahl I, Angervall L. Pseudosarcomatous proliferative lesions of soft tissue with or without bone formation. *Acta Pathol Microbiol Scand A* 1977;85:577–589.
2. Meister P, Buckmann FW, Konrad E. Nodular fasciitis: (analysis of 100 cases and review of the literature). *Pathol Res Pract* 1978;162: 133–165.
3. Shimizu S, Hashimoto H, Enjoji M. Nodular fasciitis: an analysis of 250 patients. *Pathology* 1984;16:161–166.
4. Allen PW. Nodular fasciitis. *Pathology* 1972;4:9–26.
5. Kleinstiver BJ, Rodrigue HA. Nodular fasciitis: a study of forty-five cases and review of the literature. *J Bone Joint Surg (Am)* 1968;50: 1204–1212.
6. Montgomery EA, Meis JM. Nodular fasciitis: its morphologic spectrum and immunohistochemical profile. *Am J Surg Pathol* 1991;15: 942–948.
7. Price EB, Silliphant WM, Shuman R. Nodular fasciitis: a clinicopathologic analysis of 65 cases. *Am J Clin Pathol* 1961;35:122–136.
8. Bernstein KE, Lattes R. Nodular (pseudosarcomatous) fasciitis, a nonrecurrent lesion: clinicopathologic study of 134 cases. *Cancer* 1982; 49:1668–1678.
9. Allen PW, Allen LJ. Perce, the permissive pathologist: a cautionary tale of one who misdiagnosed a pseudosarcoma, killed the patient and was found out. *Aust N Z J Surg* 1994;64:273–274.
10. Konwaler BE, Keasbey L, Kaplan L. Subcutaneous pseudosarcomatous fibromatosis (fasciitis). *Am J Clin Pathol* 1955;25:241–252
11. Stout AP. Pseudosarcomatous fasciitis in children. *Cancer* 1961;14: 1216–1222.
12. Coffin CM, Reyes A, Furman J, Dehner LP. Nodular fasciitis in children and adolescents. A report of 18 cases (abstract). *Mod Pathol* 1995;8:1P.
13. El-Jabbour JN, Wilson GD, Bennett MH, Burke MM, Davey AT, Eames K. Flow cytometric study of nodular fasciitis, proliferative fasciitis, and proliferative myositis. *Hum Pathol* 1991;22:1146–1149.
14. Hutter RVP, Stewart FW, Foote FW Jr. Fasciitis: a report of 70 cases with follow-up proving the benignity of the lesion. *Cancer* 1962;15: 992–1003.
15. Price SK, Kahn LB, Saxe N. Dermal and intravascular fasciitis: unusual variants of nodular fasciitis. *Am J Dermatopathol* 1993;15: 539–543.
16. Wirman JA. Nodular fasciitis, a lesion of myofibroblasts: an ultrastructural study. *Cancer* 1976;38:2378–2389.
17. Powers CN, Berardo MD, Frable WJ. Fine-needle aspiration biopsy: pitfalls in the diagnosis of spindle-cell lesions. *Diagn Cytopathol* 1994;10:232–241.
18. Stanley MW, Skoog L, Tani EM, Horwitz CA. Nodular fasciitis: spontaneous resolution following diagnosis by fine-needle aspiration. *Diagn Cytopathol* 1993;9:322–324.
19. Hasegawa T, Hirose T, Kudo E, Abe J, Hizawa K. Cytoskeletal characteristics of myofibroblasts in benign, neoplastic and reactive fibroblastic lesions. *Virchows Arch A Path Anat* 1990;416:375–382.
20. Skalli O, Schurch W, Seemayer T, et al. Myofibroblasts from diverse pathologic settings are heterogeneous in their content of actin isoforms and intermediate filament proteins. *Lab Invest* 1989;60: 275–285.
21. Pitt MA, Roberts ISD, Agbamu DA, Eyden BP. The nature of atypical multinucleated stromal cells: a study of 37 cases from different sites. *Histopathology* 1993;23:137–145.
22. Hasegawa T, Hirose T, Kudo E, et al. Cytoskeletal characteristics of myofibroblasts in benign neoplastic and reactive fibroblastic lesions. *Virchows Arch A Path Anat* 1990; 416:375–382.
23. Sawyer JR, Sammartino G, Baker GF, Bell JM. Clonal chromosome aberrations in a case of nodular fasciitis. *Cancer Genet Cytogenet* 1994;76:154–156.
24. Birdsall SH, Shipley JM, Summersgill BM, et al. Cytogenetic findings in a case of nodular fasciitis of the breast. *Cancer Genet Cytogenet* 1995;81:166–168.
25. Oshiro Y, Fukuda T, Tsuneyoshi M. Fibrosarcoma versus fibromatoses and cellular nodular fasciitis: a comparative study of their proliferative activity using proliferating cell nuclear antigen, DNA flow cytometry, and p53. *Am J Surg Pathol* 1994;18:712–719.
26. Chan JKC, Carcangiu ML, Rosai J. Papillary carcinoma of thyroid with exuberant nodular fasciitis-like stroma: report of three cases. *Am J Clin Pathol* 1991;95:309–314.
27. Toker C. Pseudo-sarcomatous fasciitis: further observations indicating the aggressive capabilities of this lesion, and justifying the inclusion of this entity within the category of the fibromatoses. *Ann Surg* 1971;174:994–1001.
28. Patchefsky AS, Enzinger FM. Intravascular fasciitis: a report of 17 cases. *Am J Surg Pathol* 1981;5:29–36.

29. Batsakis JG, El-Naggar AK. Pseudosarcomatous proliferative lesions of soft tissues. *Ann Otol Rhinol Laryngol* 1994;103:578–582.

30. Inwards CY, Unni KK, Beabout JW, Shives TC. Solitary congenital fibromatosis (infantile myofibromatosis) of bone. *Am J Surg Pathol* 1991;15:935–941.

31. Coffin CM, Dehner LP. Fibroblastic-myofibroblastic tumors in children and adolescents: a clinicopathologic study of 108 examples in 103 patients. *Pediatr Pathol* 1991;11:569–588.

32. Coffin CM, Dehner LP. Vascular tumors in children and adolescents: a clinicopathologic study of 228 tumors in 222 patients. *Pathol Annu* 1993;1:97–120.

33. Mentzel T, Calonje E, Nascimento AG, Fletcher CDM. Infantile hemangiopericytoma versus infantile myofibromatosis: study of a series suggesting a continuous spectrum of infantile myofibroblastic lesions. *Am J Surg Pathol* 1994;18:922–930.

34. Kwittken J, Branche M. Fasciitis ossificans. *Am J Clin Pathol* 1969; 51:251–255.

35. Daroca PJ Jr, Pulitzer DR, LoCicero J III. Ossifying fasciitis. *Arch Pathol Lab Med* 1982;106:682–685.

36. Spjut HJ, Dorfman HD. Florid reactive periostitis of the tubular bones of the hands and feet: a benign lesion which may simulate osteosarcoma. *Am J Surg Pathol* 1981;5:423–433.

37. Hutter RVP, Foote FW Jr, Francis KC, Higginbotham NL. Parosteal fasciitis: a self-limited benign process that simulates a malignant neoplasm. *Am J Surg* 1962;104:800–807.

38. Mighell AJ, Stassen LFA. Periosteal fasciitis of the mandible. *Head Neck* 1994;16:282–286.

39. Dupree WB, Enzinger FM. Fibro-osseous pseudotumor of the digits. *Cancer* 1986;58:2103–2109.

40. McCarthy EF, Ireland DCR, Sprague BL, Bonfiglio M. Parosteal (nodular) fasciitis of the hand. *J Bone Joint Surg (Am)* 1976;58: 714–716.

41. Nora FE, Dahlin DC, Beabout JW. Bizarre parosteal osteochondromatous proliferations of the hands and feet. *Am J Surg Pathol* 1983; 7:245–250.

42. Lauer DH, Enzinger FM. Cranial fasciitis of childhood. *Cancer* 1980; 45:401–406.

43. Hunter NS, Bulas DI, Chadduck WM, Chandra R. Cranial fasciitis of childhood. *Pediatr Radiol* 1993;23:398–399.

44. Iqbal K, Saqulain G, Udaipurwala IH, Ashraf J, Aijaz F, Jalisi M. Cranial fasciitis: presentation as a post-auricular mass. *J Laryngol Otol* 1995;109:255–257.

45. Ackerman LV. Extra-osseous localized non-neoplastic bone and cartilage formation (so-called myositis ossificans): clinical and pathological confusion with malignant neoplasms. *J Bone Joint Surg (Am)* 1958;40:279–298.

46. Kern WH. Proliferative myositis, a pseudosarcomatous reaction to injury: a report of seven cases. *Arch Pathol* 1960;69:209–216.

47. Enzinger FM, Dulcey F. Proliferative myositis: report of thirty-three cases. *Cancer* 1967;20:2213–2223.

48. Meis JM, Enzinger FM. Proliferative fasciitis and myositis of childhood. *Am J Surg Pathol* 1992;16:364–372.

49. Lundgren L, Kindblom L, Willems J, Falkmer U, Angervall L. Proliferative myositis and fasciitis: a light and electron microscopic, cytologic, DNA-cytometric and immunohistochemical study. *APMIS* 1992;100:437–448.

50. Brooks JS. Immunohistochemistry of proliferative myositis. *Arch Pathol Lab Med* 1981;105:682.

51. El-Jabbour JN, Bennett MH, Burke MM, Lessells A, O'Halloran A. Proliferative myositis: an immunohistochemical and ultrastructural study. *Am J Surg Pathol* 1991;15:654–659.

52. Ghadially FN, Thomas MJ, Jabi M, Rippstein P. Intracisternal collagen fibrils in proliferative fasciitis and myositis of childhood. *Ultrastruct Pathol* 1993;17:161–168.

53. Chung EB, Enzinger FM. Proliferative fasciitis. *Cancer* 1975;36: 1450–1458.

54. Craver JL, McDivitt RW. Proliferative fasciitis: ultrastructural study of two cases. *Arch Pathol Lab Med* 1981;105:542–545.

55. Dembinski A, Bridge JA, Neff JR, Berger C, Sandberg AA. Trisomy 2 in proliferative fasciitis. *Cancer Genet Cytogenet* 1991;60:27–30.

56. Chow LTC, Chow WH, Lee LCK. Fine needle aspiration (FNA) cytology of proliferative fasciitis: report of a case with immunohistochemical study. *Cytopathology* 1995;6:349–357.

57. Perosio PM, Weiss SW. Ischemic fasciitis: a juxta-skeletal fibroblastic proliferation with a predilection for elderly patients. *Mod Pathol* 1993;6:69–72.

58. Montgomery EA, Meis JM, Mitchell MS, Enzinger FM. Atypical decubital fibroplasia: a distinctive fibroblastic pseudotumor occurring in debilitated patients. *Am J Surg Pathol* 1992;16:708–715.

59. Schepsis AA, Leach RE, Gorzyca J. Plantar fasciitis, etiology, treatment, surgical results, and review of the literature. *Clin Orthop Rel Research* 1991;266:185–196.

60. Chandler TJ, Kibler WB. A biomechanical approach to the prevention, treatment and rehabilitation of plantar fasciitis. *Sports Med* 1993; 15:344–352.

61. DeMaio M, Paine R, Mangine RE, Drez D Jr. Plantar fasciitis. *Orthopedics* 1993;16:1153–1163.

62. Asfar SK, Baraka A, Juma T, Ma Rafie A, Aladeen T, Al Sayer H. Necrotizing fasciitis. *Br J Surg* 1991;78:838–840.

63. Efem SEE. The features and aetiology of Fournier's gangrene. *Postgrad Med J* 1994;70:568–571.

64. Umbert I, Winkelmann RK, Wegener L. Comparison of the pathology of fascia in eosinophilic myalgia syndrome patients and idiopathic eosinophilic fasciitis. *Dermatology* 1993;186:18–22.

65. Champion GD, Saxon JA, Kossard S. The syndrome of palmar fibromatosis (fasciitis) and polyarthritis. *J Rheumatol* 1987;14:1196–1198.

66. Heffner RR Jr, Armbrustmacher VW, Earle KM. Focal myositis. *Cancer* 1977;40:301–306.

67. Colding-Jorgensen E, Laursen H, Lauritzen M. Focal myositis of the thigh: report of two cases. *Acta Neurol Scand* 1993;88:289–292.

68. Heffner RR Jr, Barron SA. Denervating changes in focal myositis, a benign inflammatory pseudotumor. *Arch Pathol Lab Med* 1980;104: 261–264.

69. Isaacson G, Chan KH, Heffner RR Jr. Focal myositis: a new cause for the pediatric neck mass. *Arch Otolaryngol Head Neck Surg* 1991;117: 103–105.

70. Gonzalez-Crussi F, deMello DE, Sotelo-Avila C. Omental-mesenteric myxoid hamartomas. *Am J Surg Pathol* 1983;7:567–578.

71. Coffin CM, Watterson J, Priest JR, Dehner LP. Extrapulmonary inflammatory myofibroblastic tumor (inflammatory pseudotumor): a clinicopathologic and immunohistochemical study of 84 cases. *Am J Surg Pathol* 1995;19:859–872.

72. Tang TT, Segura AD, Oechler HW, et al. Inflammatory myofibrohistiocytic proliferation simulating sarcoma in children. *Cancer* 1990;65: 1626–1634.

73. Meis JM, Enzinger FM. Inflammatory fibrosarcoma of the mesentery and retroperitoneum: a tumor closely simulating inflammatory pseudotumor. *Am J Surg Pathol* 1991;15:1146–1156.

74. Spencer H. The pulmonary plasma cell/histiocytoma complex. *Histopathology* 1984;8:903–916.

75. Pettinato G, Manivel JC, DeRosa N, Dehner LP. Inflammatory myofibroblastic tumor (plasma cell granuloma): clinicopathologic study of 20 cases with immunohistochemical and ultrastructural observations. *Am J Clin Pathol* 1990;94:538–546.

76. Myint MA, Medeiros LJ, Sulaiman RA, Aswad BI, Glantz L. Inflammatory pseudotumor of the ileum. A report of a multifocal, transmural lesion with regional lymph node involvement. *Arch Pathol Lab Med* 1994;118:1138–1142.

77. Day DL, Sane S, Dehner LP. Inflammatory pseudotumor of the mesentery and small intestine. *Pediatr Radiol* 1986;16:210–215.

78. Stringer MD, Ramani P, Yeung CK, Capps SNJ, Kiely EM, Spitz L. Abdominal inflammatory myofibroblastic tumours in children. *Br J Surg* 1992;79:1357–1360.

79. Nam BH, Rha KS, Yoo JY, Park C. Plasma cell granuloma of the temporal bone: a case report. *Head Neck* 1994;16:457–459.

80. Johnston SJ, Beaver BJ, Sun CCJ, Luddy RE, Schwartz AD. Inflammatory pseudotumor of the retroperitoneum. *Maryland Med J* 1991;40:787–790.

81. Chan YF, White J, Brash H. Metachronous pulmonary and cerebral inflammatory pseudotumor in a child. *Pediatr Pathol* 1994;14:805–815.

82. Vujanic GM, Milovanovic D, Aleksandrovic S. Aggressive inflammatory pseudotumor of the abdomen 9 years after therapy for Wilms tumor: a complication, coincidence or association? *Cancer* 1992;70: 2362–2366.

83. Broughan TA, Fischer WL, Tuthill RJ. Vascular invasion by hepatic inflammatory pseudotumor: a clinical study. *Cancer* 1993;71: 2934–2940.

84. Macleod CB, Wakely PE Jr, Frable WJ. Extrapulmonary inflammatory myofibroblastic pseudotumor: a potential cytologic trap in childhood. *Diagn Cytopathol* 1991;7:633–636.

85. Treissman SP, Gillis DA, Lee CLY, Giacomantonio M, Resch L. Omental-mesenteric inflammatory pseudotumor: cytogenetic demonstration of genetic changes and monoclonality in one tumor. *Cancer* 1994;73:1433–1437.

86. Souid AK, Ziemba MC, Dubansky AS, et al. Inflammatory myofibroblastic tumor in children. *Cancer* 1993;72:2042–2048.

87. Arber DA, Kamel OW, van de Rijn M, et al. Frequent presence of the Epstein–Barr virus in inflammatory pseudotumor. *Hum Pathol* 1995; 26:1093–1098.

88. Matsubara O, Tan-Liu NS, Kenny RM, Mark EJ. Inflammatory pseudotumors of the lung: progression from organizing pneumonia to fibrous histiocytoma or to plasma cell granuloma in 32 cases. *Hum Pathol* 1988;19:807–814.

89. Kelly JK, Hwang W-S. Idiopathic retractile (sclerosing) mesenteritis and its differential diagnosis. *Am J Surg Pathol* 1989;13:513–521.

90. Fetsch JF, Montgomery EA, Meis JM. Calcifying fibrous pseudotumor. *Am J Surg Pathol* 1993;17:502–508.

91. Rosenberg NS, Abdul-Karim FW. Childhood fibrous tumor with psammoma bodies. *Arch Pathol Lab Med* 1988;112:798–800.

92. Pinkard NB, Wilson RW, Lawless N, et al. Calcifying fibrous pseudotumor of pleura. A report of three cases of a newly described entity involving the pleura. *Am J Clin Pathol* 1996;105:189–194.

93. Renshaw AA, Pinkus GS, Corson JW. CD34 and AE1/AE3. Diagnostic discriminants in the distinction of solitary fibrous tumor of the pleura from sarcomatoid mesothelioma. *Appl Immunohistochem* 1994;2:94–102.

94. Suster S, Nascimento AG, Miettinen M, Sickel JZ, Moran CA. Solitary fibrous tumors of soft tissue. A clinicopathologic and immunohistochemical study of 12 cases. *Am J Surg Pathol* 1995;19:1257–1266.

95. van de Rijn M, Lombard CM, Rouse RV. Expression of CD34 by solitary fibrous tumor of the pleura, mediastinum, and lung. *Am J Surg Pathol* 1994;18:814–820.

96. Westra WH, Gerald WL, Rosai J. Solitary fibrous tumor. Consistent CD34 immunoreactivity and occurrence in the orbit. *Am J Surg Pathol* 1994;18:992–998.

97. Adelizzi RA, Shockley FK, Peitras JR. Wegener's granulomatosis with ureteric obstruction. *J Rheumatol* 1986;13:448–451.

98. Baker SB, Robinson DR. Unusual renal manifestation of Wegener's granulomatosis: report of two cases. *Am J Med* 1978;64:883–889.

99. Bullen CL, Liesegang TJ, McDonald TJ, De Remee RA. Ocular complications of Wegener's granulomatosis. *Ophthalmology* 1983;90:279–290.

100. Coutu RE, Klein M, Lessel S, Friedman E, Snider GL. Limited form of Wegener's granulomatosis: eye involvement as a major sign. *JAMA* 1975;233:868–871.

101. Gohel VK, Dalinka MK, Israel HL, Libshitz HI. The radiological manifestations of Wegener's granulomatosis. *Br J Radiol* 1973;46:427–432.

102. Goulart RA, Mark EJ, Rosen S. Tumefactions as an extravascular manifestation of Wegener's granulomatosis. *Am J Surg Pathol* 1995;19:145–153.

103. Gutierrez-Rave VM, Ayerza MA. Hilar and mediastinal lymphadenopathy in the limited form of Wegener's granulomatosis. *Thorax* 1991;46:219–220.

104. Hensle TW, Mitchell ME, Crooks KK, Robinson D. Urologic manifestations of Wegener's granulomatosis. *Urology* 1978;12:553–556.

105. Ter Maaten JC, Franssen CS, Niles JL, Raizman AA, Hoorntje SJ. Triple Wegener's granulomatosis involving the urogenital tract. *Nephron* 1993;63:358–359.

106. Nuovo MA, Norman A, Chumas J, Ackerman LV. Myositis ossificans with atypical clinical, radiographic, and pathologic findings: a review of 23 cases. *Skeletal Radiol* 1992;21:87–101.

107. Povysil C, Matejovsky Z. Ultrastructural evidence of myofibroblasts in pseudomalignant myositis ossificans. *Virchows Arch A Path Anat* 1979;381:189–203.

108. Sumiyoshi K, Tsuneyoshi M, Enjoji M. Myositis ossificans. A clinicopathologic study of 21 cases. *Acta Pathol Jpn* 1985;35:1109–1122.

109. Enzinger FM, Weiss SW. *Soft tissue tumors.* 3rd ed. St. Louis: CV Mosby, 1995.

110. Donner LR. Ossifying fibromyxoid tumor of soft parts. Evidence supporting Schwann cell origin. *Hum Pathol* 1992;23:200–202.

111. Enzinger FM, Weiss SW, Liang CY. Ossifying fibromyxoid tumor of soft parts. A clinicopathological analysis of 59 cases. *Am J Surg Pathol* 1989;13:817–827.

112. Kilpatrick SE, Ward WG, Mozes M, et al. Atypical and malignant variants of ossifying fibromyxoid tumor. Clinicopathologic analysis of six cases. *Am J Surg Pathol* 1995;1039–1046.

113. Miettinen M. Ossifying fibromyxoid tumor of soft parts. Additional observations of a distinctive soft tissue tumor. *Am J Clin Pathol* 1991; 95:142–149.

114. Schofield JB, Krausz T, Stamp GW, Fletcher CD, Fisher C, Azzopardi JG. Ossifying fibromyxoid tumor of soft parts. Immunohistochemical and ultrastructural analysis. *Histopathology* 1993; 22:101–112.

115. Yang P, Hirose T, Hasegawa T, Gao Z, Hizawa K. Ossifying fibromyxoid tumor of soft parts. A morphological and immunohistochemical study. *Pathol Int* 1994;44:448–453.

116. Rosai J, Dorfman HD. Sinus histiocytosis with massive lymphadenopathy. A pseudolymphomatous benign disorder. Analysis of 34 cases. *Cancer* 1972;30:1174–1188.

117. Foucar E, Rosai J, Dorfman RF. Sinus histiocytosis with massive lymphadenopathy (Rosai–Dorfman disease). Review of the entity. *Semin Diagn Pathol* 1990;7:19–73.

118. Montgomery EA, Meis JM, Frizzera G. Rosai–Dorfman disease of soft tissue. *Am J Surg Pathol* 1992;16:122–129.

119. Wenig BM, Abbondanzo SL, Childers EL, Kapadia SB, Heffner DR. Extranodal sinus histiocytosis with massive lymphadenopathy (Rosai–Dorfman disease) of the head and neck. *Hum Pathol* 1993;24:483–492.

120. Bonetti F, Chilosi M, Menestrina F, et al. Immunohistological analysis of Rosai–Dorfman histiocytosis. A disease of S100- CD1- histiocytes. *Virchows Arch A Path Anat* 1987;411:129–135.

121. Eisen RN, Buckley PJ, Rosai J. Immunophenotypic characterization of sinus histiocytosis with massive lymphadenopathy (Rosai–Dorfman disease). *Semin Diagn Pathol* 1990;7:74–82.

122. Clement PB. Reactive tumor-like lesions of the peritoneum. *Am J Clin Pathol* 1995;103:673–675.

123. Nascimento AG, Keeney GL, Fletcher CDM. Deciduoid peritoneal mesothelioma. An unusual phenotype affecting young females. *Am J Surg Pathol* 1994;18:439–445.

124. Harada M, Shimada M, Fukuyama M, Kaneko T, Kitazume K, Weiss SW. Crystal-storing histiocytosis associated with lymphoplasmocytic lymphoma mimicking Weber–Christian disease: immunohistochemical, ultrastructural, and gene-rearrangement studies. *Hum Pathol* 1996;27:84–87.

125. Jennette JC, Wilkman AS, Benson JD. IgD myeloma with intracytoplasmic crystalline inclusions. *Am J Clin Pathol* 1980; 75:231–235.

126. Kapadia SB, Enzinger FM, Heffner DK, Hyams VJ, Frizzera G. Crystal-storing histiocytosis associated with lymphoplasmocytic neoplasms. Report of three cases mimicking adult rhabdomyoma. *Am J Surg Pathol* 1993;17:461–467.

127. Mullen B, Chalvardjian A. Crystalline tissue deposits in a case of multiple myeloma. *Arch Pathol Lab Med* 1981;105:94–97.

128. Stavem P, Vandvik B, Skrede S, et al. Needle-like crystals in plasma cells in patients with a plasma cell proliferative disorder. *Scand J Haematol* 1975;14:24–34.

129. Takahashi K, Naito M, Takatsuki K, et al. Multiple myeloma. IgA kappa type, accompanying crystal-storing histiocytosis and amyloidosis. *Acta Pathol Jpn* 1987;37:141–154.

130. Yamamoto T, Hishida A, Honda N, et al. Crystal-storing histiocytosis and crystalline tissue deposition in multiple myeloma. *Arch Pathol Lab Med* 1991;115:351–354.

131. Sobel H, Arvin E, Marquet E, et al. Reactive granular cells in sites of trauma: a cytochemical and ultrastructural study. *Am J Clin Pathol* 1974;61:223–236.

132. Weiss SW, Enzinger FM, Johnson FB. Silica reaction simulating fibrous histiocytoma. *Cancer* 1978;42:2738–2745.

133. Akosa AB, Ali MH, Khoo CT, Evans DM. Angiolymphoid hyperplasia with eosinophilia associated with tetanus toxoid vaccination. *Histopathology* 1990;16:589–593.

134. Lenz TR. Foreign body granuloma caused by jet injection of tetanus toxoid. *Rocky Mt Med J* 1966;63:48.

135. Miliauskas JR, Mukherjee T, Dixon B. Postimmunization (vaccination) injection-site reactions. A report of four cases and review of the literature. *Am J Surg Pathol* 1993;17:516–524.

136. Slater DN, Underwood JC, Durrant TE, Gray T, Hopper IP. Alu-

minum hydroxide granulomas: light and electron microscopic studies and x-ray microanalysis. *Br J Dermatol* 1982;107:103–108.

137. Cabanne F, Chapuis JL, Duperrat B, Putelat R. L infiltration cutanee par la polyvinylpyrrolidone. *Ann Anat Pathol* 1966;11:385–396.

138. Hewan-Lowe K, Hammers Y, Lyons JM, Wilcox CM. Polyvinylpyrrolidone storage disease: a source of error in the diagnosis of signet ring cell gastric adenocarcinoma. *Ultrastruct Pathol* 1994;18:271–278.

139. Hizawa K, Inaba H, Nakanishi S, Otsuka H, Izumi K. Subcutaneous pseudosarcomatous polyvinylpyrrolidone granuloma. *Am J Surg Pathol* 1984;8:393–398.

140. Hueper WC. Bioassay on polyvinylpyrrolidones with limited molecular weight range. *JNCI* 1960;26:229–237.

141. Kepes JJ, Chen WYK, Jim JF. Mucoid dissolution of bones and multiple pathologic fractures in a patient with past history of intravenous administration of polyvinylpyrrolidone (PVP). A case report. *Bone Mineral* 1993;22:33–41.

142. Kuo T-T, Hsueh S. Mucicarminophilic histiocytosis. A polyvinylpyrrolidone (PVP) storage disease simulating signet ring cell carcinoma. *Am J Surg Pathol* 1984;8:419–428.

143. Reske-Nielsen E, Bojsen-Moller M, Vetner M, et al. Polyvinylpyrrolidone-storage disease: light and microscopical, ultrastructural, and chemical verification. *Acta Pathol Microbiol Scand (A)* 1976;84:397–406.

144. Mansfield RE. Histoid leprosy. *Arch Pathol* 1969;87:580–592.

145. Wade HW. Histoid variant of lepromatous leprosy. *Int J Leprosy* 1963;31:129–141.

146. Kahn LB. Retroperitoneal xanthogranuloma and xanthosarcoma (malignant fibrous xanthoma). *Cancer* 1973;31:411–422.

147. Kyriakos M, Kempson RL. Inflammatory fibrous histiocytoma. An aggressive and lethal condition. *Cancer* 1976;37:1584–1606.

148. Merchant W, Calonje E, Fletcher CDM. Inflammatory leiomyosarcoma: a morphological subgroup within the heterogeneous family of so-called inflammatory malignant fibrous histiocytomas. *Histopathology* 1995;27:525–532.

149. Merino MJ, Livolsi VA. Inflammatory malignant fibrous histiocytoma. *Am J Clin Pathol* 1980;73:270–281.

150. Chester W. Regarding lipogranulomas. *Virchows Arch A Path Anat* 1930;279:561–572.

151. Dee P, Westgaard T, Langholm R. Erdheim–Chester disease: case with chronic discharging sinus from bone. *AJR* 1980;134:837–840.

152. Eble JN, Rosenberg AE, Young RH. Retroperitoneal xanthogranuloma in a patient with Erdheim–Chester disease. *Am J Surg Pathol* 1994;18:843–848.

153. Simpson FG, Robinson PJ, Hardy GJ, Losowsky MS. Erdheim–Chester disease associated with retroperitoneal xanthogranuloma. *Br J Radiol* 1979;52:232–235.

154. Damjanov I, Katz SM. Malakoplakia. *Pathol Annu* 1981;16:103–131.

155. Terner JY, Lattes R. Malakoplakia of the colon and retroperitoneum. Report of a case with histochemical study of the Michaelis–Guttmann inclusion bodies. *Am J Clin Pathol* 1965;44:20–31.

156. Branwein M, Choi H-S, Strauchen J, Stoler M, Jagirdir J. Spindle cell reaction to nontuberculous mycobacteriosis in AIDS mimicking a spindle cell neoplasm. Evidence for dual histiocytic and fibroblast-like characteristics of spindle cells. *Virchows Arch A Path Anat* 1990;416:281–286.

157. Chen KTK. Mycobacterial spindle cell pseudotumor of lymph nodes. *Am J Surg Pathol* 1992;16:276–281.

158. Perrin C, Michiels JF, Bernard E, Hofman P, Rosenthal E, Loubiere R. Cutaneous spindle-cell pseudotumors due to *Mycobacterium gordonae* and *Leishmania infantum*. An immunophenotypic study. *Am J Dermatopathol* 1993;15:553–558.

159. Sekosan M, Cleto M, Senseng C, Farolan M, Sekosan J. Spindle cell pseudotumors in the lungs due to *Mycobacterium tuberculosis* in a transplant patient. *Am J Surg Pathol* 1994;18:1065–1068.

160. Umlas J, Federman M. Crawford C, et al. Spindle cell pseudotumor due to *Mycobacterium avium-intracellulare* in patients with acquired immunodeficiency syndrome (AIDS). Positive staining of mycobacteria for cytoskeletal filaments. *Am J Surg Pathol* 1991;15:1181–1187.

161. Wood C, Nickoloff BJ, Todes-Taylor NR. Pseudotumor resulting from atypical mycobacterial infection: a histoid variety of *Mycobacterium avium-intracellulare* complex infection. *Am J Clin Pathol* 1985;83:524–527.

162. Koehler JE, Quinn FD, Berger TG, LeBoit PE, Tappero JW. Isolation of *Rochalimaea* species from cutaneous and osseous lesions of bacillary angiomatosis. *N Engl J Med* 1992;327:1625–1631.

163. Regnery RL, Anderson BE, Clarridge JE III, et al. Characterization of a novel Rochalimaea species, R. henselae sp. nov., isolated from the blood of a febrile human immunodeficiency virus–positive patient. *J Clin Microbiol* 1992;30:265–274.

164. Tompkins DC, Steigbigel RT. Rochalimaea's role in cat scratch disease and bacillary angiomatosis. *Ann Intern Med* 1993;118:388–390.

165. LeBoit PE, Berger TG, Egbert BM, et al. Bacillary angiomatosis. The histopathology and differential diagnosis of a pseudoneoplastic infection in patients with human immunodeficiency virus disease. *Am J Surg Pathol* 1989;13:909–920.

166. Perez-Pitera J, Ariza A, Mate JL, Ojanguren I, Navas-Palacios JJ. Bacillary angiomatosis: a gross mimicker of malignancy. *Histopathology* 1995;26:476–478.

167. Stoler M, Bonfiglio MD, Steigbigel RT, Pereira M. An atypical subcutaneous infection associated with acquired immunodeficiency syndrome. *Am J Clin Pathol* 1983;80:714–718.

168. Auerbach HE, Brooks JJ. Kaposi's sarcoma. Neoplasia or hyperplasia? *Surg Pathol* 1989;2:19–28.

169. Bovenzi P, Mirandola P, Secchiero P, et al. Human herpesvirus 6 (variant A) in Kaposi's sarcoma. *Lancet* 1993;341:1288–1289.

170. Chang Y, Cesarman E, Pessin MS, et al. Human herpesvirus-like DNA sequences in AIDS-associated Kaposi's sarcoma. *Science* 1994;266:1865–1869.

171. Moore PS, Chang Y. Detection of herpesvirus-like DNA sequences in Kaposi's sarcoma in patients with and without HIV infection. *N Engl J Med* 1995;332:1181–1185.

172. Drew WL, Conant MA, Miner RC, et al. Cytomegalovirus and Kaposi's sarcoma in young homosexual men. *Lancet* 1982;2:1255–1257.

173. Ioachim HL, Dorsett B, Melamed J, et al. Cytomegalovirus, angiomatosis, and Kaposi's sarcoma. New observations of a debated relationship. *Mod Pathol* 1992;5:169–178.

174. Fukunaga M, Silverberg SG. Kaposi's sarcoma in patients with acquired immunodeficiency syndrome. A flow cytometric DNA analysis of 26 lesions in 21 patients. *Cancer* 1990;66:758–764.

175. Weich HA, Salahuddin SZ, Gill P, Nakamura S, Gallo RC, Folkmann J. AIDS-associated Kaposi's sarcoma–derived cells in long-term culture express and synthesize smooth muscle actin. *Am J Pathol* 1991;139:1251–1258.

176. Chor PJ, Santa Cruz DJ. Kaposi's sarcoma. A clinicopathologic review and differential diagnosis. *J Cutan Pathol* 1992;19:16–20.

177. Rao VK, Weiss SW. Angiomatosis of soft tissue. An analysis of the histologic features and clinical outcome in 51 cases. *Am J Surg Pathol* 1992;16:764–771.

178. Austin RM, Mack GR, Townsend CM, Lack EE. Infiltrating (intramuscular) lipomas and angiolipomas. *Arch Surg* 1980;115:281–284.

179. Gonzalez-Crussi F, Enneking WF, Arean VM. Infiltrating angiolipoma. *J Bone Joint Surg* 1966;48A:1111–1124.

180. Gutierrez RM, Spjut HJ. Skeletal angiomatosis: report of three cases and review of the literature. *Clin Orthop* 1972;85:82–97.

181. Howat AJ, Campbell PE. Angiomatosis: a vascular malformation of infancy and childhood. *Pathology* 1987;19:377–382.

182. Cohen J, Craig JM. Multiple lymphangiectases of bone. *J Bone Joint Surg (Am)* 1955;37:585–595.

183. Harris R, Prandoni AG. Generalized primary lymphangiomas of bone: report of a case associated with congenital lymphedema of forearm. *Ann Intern Med* 1950;33:1302–1313.

184. Schajowicz F, Aiello CL, Francone MV, Giannini RE. Cystic angiomatosis (hamartomatous haemolymphangiomatosis) of bone. A clinical pathological study of three cases. *J Bone Joint Surg (Br)* 1978;60:100–106.

185. Singh Gomez C, Calonje E, Ferrar DW, Browse NL, Fletcher CDM. Lymphangiomatosis of the limbs. Clinicopathologic analysis of a series with a good prognosis. *Am J Surg Pathol* 1995;19:125–133.

186. Steiner GM, Farman J, Lawson JP. Lymphangiomatosis of bone. *Radiology* 1969;93:1093–1098.

187. Allen PW, Enzinger FM. Hemangiomas of skeletal muscle. An analysis of 89 cases. *Cancer* 1972;29:8–23.

188. Scott GA, Rosai J. Spindle cell hemangioendothelioma. Report of seven additional cases of a recently described vascular neoplasm. *Am J Dermatopathol* 1988;10:281–288.

189. Weiss SW, Enzinger FM. Spindle cell hemangioendothelioma. A low-grade angiosarcoma resembling cavernous hemangioma and Kaposi's sarcoma. *Am J Surg Pathol* 1986;10:521–530.

190. Murakami I, Sarker AB, Teramoto N, Horie Y, Akagi T. Spindle cell

hemangioendothelioma: a report of two cases. *Acta Pathol Jpn* 1993; 43:529–534.

191. Terashi H, Itami S, Kurata S, et al. Spindle cell hemangioendothelioma: report of three cases. *J Dermatol* 1991;18:104–111.

192. Zoltie N, Roberts PF. Spindle cell hemangioendothelioma in association with epithelioid hemangioendothelioma. *Histopathology* 1989; 15:544–546.

193. Fletcher CDM, Beham A, Schmid C. Spindle cell hemangioendothelioma: a clinicopathological and immunohistochemical study indicative of a non-neoplastic lesion. *Histopathology* 1991;18:291–301.

194. Battocchio S, Facchetti F, Brisgotti M. Spindle cell hemangioendothelioma: further evidence against its proposed neoplastic nature. *Histopathology* 1993;22:296–298.

195. Ding J, Hashimoto H, Imayama S, Tsuneyoshi M, Enjoji M. Spindle cell hemangioendothelioma: probably a benign vascular lesion, not a low-grade angiosarcoma. *Virchows Arch A Path Anat* 1992;420: 77–85.

196. Imayama S, Murakamai Y, Hashimoto H, Hori Y. Spindle cell hemangioendothelioma exhibits the ultrastructural features of reactive vascular proliferation, rather than of angiosarcoma. *Am J Clin Pathol* 1992;97:279–287.

197. Hisaoka M, Kuoho H, Aoki T, Hashimoto H. DNA flow cytometric and immunohistochemical analysis of proliferative activity in spindle cell hemangioendothelioma. *Histopathology* 1995;27:451–456.

198. Enzinger FM. Fibrous hamartoma of infancy. *Cancer* 1965;18: 241–248.

199. Maung R, Lindsay R, Trevenen C, Hwang WS. Fibrous hamartoma of infancy. *Hum Pathol* 1987;18:652–653.

200. Fletcher CDM, Powell G, Van Noorden S, McKee PH. Fibrous hamartoma of infancy. A histochemical and immunohistochemical study. *Histopathology* 1988;12:65–74.

201. Groisman G, Lichtig C. Fibrous hamartoma of infancy. An immuno-histochemical and ultrastructural study. *Hum Pathol* 1991;22: 914–918.

202. Michal M, Mukensnabl P, Chlumska A, Kodet R. Fibrous hamartoma of infancy. A study of eight cases with immunohistochemical and electron microscopical findings. *Pathol Res Pract* 1992;188: 1049–1053.

203. Aymard B, Boman-Ferrand F, Vernhes L, et al. Fibrolipomatous hamartoma of peripheral nerves: a clinicopathological analysis of five cases with ultrastructural studies. *Ann Pathol (Paris)* 1987; 7:320–324.

204. Silverman TA, Enzinger FM. Fibrolipomatous hamartoma of nerve. A clinicopathologic analysis of 26 cases. *Am J Surg Pathol* 1985;9:7–14.

205. Swanson PE, Scheithauer BW, Wick MR. Peripheral nerve sheath tumors. Clinicopathologic and immunochemical observations. *Pathol Annu* 1995;2:1–82.

206. Paletta FX, Senay LC Jr. Lipofibromatous hamartoma of median nerve and ulnar nerve. Surgical treatment. *Plast Reconstr Surg* 1981; 68:915–921.

207. Berti E, Roncaroli F. Fibrolipomatous hamartoma of a cranial nerve. *Histopathology* 1994;24:391–392.

208. Amadio PC, Reiman HM, Dobyns JH. Lipofibromatous hamartoma of nerve. *J Hand Surg (Am)* 1988;13:67–75.

209. Johnson RJ, Bonfiglio M. Lipofibromatous hamartoma of the median nerve. *J Bone Joint Surg (Am)* 1969;51:984–990.

210. Drut R. Ossifying fibrolipomatous hamartoma of the ulnar nerve. *Pediatr Pathol* 1988;8:179–184.

211. Louis DS, Dick HM. Ossifying fibrolipoma of the median nerve. *J Bone Joint Surg (Am)* 1973;55:1082–1084.

212. Awasthi D, Kline DG, Bechman EN. Neuromuscular hamartoma (benign Triton tumor) of the brachial plexus. *J Neurosurg* 1991;75: 795–797.

213. Boman F, Palan C, Floquet A, Floquet J, Lascombes P. Neuromuscular hamartoma. *Ann Pathol* 1991;11:36–41.

214. Bonneau R, Brochu P. Neuromuscular choristoma: a clinicopathologic study of two cases. *Am J Surg Pathol* 1983;7:521–528.

215. Chapon F, Hubert P, Mandard JC, Rivrain Y, Lechevalier B. Spinal lipoma associated with a neuromuscular hamartoma. Report of one case. *Ann Pathol* 1991;11:345–348.

216. Chen KTK. Neuromuscular hamartoma. *J Surg Oncol* 1984;26: 258–260.

217. Louhimo I, Rapola J. Intraneural muscular hamartoma: a report of two cases in small children. *J Pediatr Surg* 1972;7:696–699.

218. Markel SF, Enzinger FM. Neuromuscular hamartoma: a benign Triton

219. Mitchell A, Scheithauer BW, Ostertag H, Sephernia A, Sav A. Neuromuscular choristoma. *Am J Clin Pathol* 1995;103:460–465.

220. O'Connell JX, Rosenberg AE. Multiple cutaneous neuromuscular choristomas: report of a case and review of the literature. *Am J Surg Pathol* 1990;14:93–96.

221. Orlandi E. A case of rhabdomyoma of the sciatic nerve. *Archivio per la Scienze Mediche* 1985;19:113–117.

222. Zwick DL, Livingston K, Clapp L, Kosnik E, Yates A. Intracranial trigeminal nerve rhabdomyoma/choristoma in a child: a case report and discussion of possible histogenesis. *Hum Pathol* 1989;20: 390–392.

223. Ducatman BS, Scheithauer BW. Malignant peripheral nerve sheath tumors with divergent differentiation. *Cancer* 1984;54:1049–1057.

224. Woodruff JM, Chernik NL, Smith MC, et al. Peripheral nerve tumors with rhabdomyosarcomatous differentiation (malignant Triton tumors). *Cancer* 1973;32:426–439.

225. Karcioglu Z, Someren A, Mathes SJ. Ectomesenchymoma. A malignant tumor of migratory neural crest (ectomesenchyme) remnants showing ganglionic, schwannian, melanocytic and rhabdomyoblastic differentiation. *Cancer* 1977;39:2486–2496.

226. Kawamoto EH, Weidner N, Agostino RM Jr, Jaffe R. Malignant ectomesenchymoma of soft tissue. Report of two cases and review of the literature. *Cancer* 1987;59:1791–1802.

227. Azzopardi JG, Eusebi V, Tison V, Betts BM. Neurofibroma with rhabdomyomatous differentiation. Benign Triton tumor of the vagina. *Histopathology* 1983;7:561–572.

228. Brescia RJ, Tazelaar HD, Hobbs J, Miller AW. Intravascular lipoleiomyomatosis. A report of two cases. *Hum Pathol* 1989;20: 252–256.

229. Evans HL. Smooth muscle in atypical lipomatous tumors. A report of three cases. *Am J Surg Pathol* 1990;14:714–718.

230. Meis JM, Enzinger FM. Myolipoma of soft tissue. *Am J Surg Pathol* 1991;15:121–125.

231. Michal M. Retroperitoneal myolipoma. A tumour mimicking retroperitoneal angiomyolipoma and liposarcoma with myosarcomatous differentiation. *Histopathology* 1994;25:86–88.

232. Scurry JP, Carey MP, Targett CS, Dowling JP. Soft tissue lipoleiomyoma. *Pathology* 1991;23:360–362.

233. Sonobe H, Ohtsuki Y, Iwata J, Furihata M, Ido E, Hamada I. Myolipoma of the round ligament: report of a case with a review of the English literature. *Virchows Arch A Path Anat* 1995;427:455–458.

234. Suster S, Wong T-Y, Moran CA. Sarcomas with combined features of liposarcoma and leiomyosarcoma. Study of two cases with an unusual soft-tissue tumor showing dual lineage differentiation. *Am J Surg Pathol* 1993;17:905–911.

235. Tallini G, Erlandson RA, Brennan WF, Woodruff JM. Divergent myosarcomatous differentiation in retroperitoneal liposarcoma. *Am J Surg Pathol* 1993;17:546–556.

236. Hruban RH, Bhagavan BS, Epstein JI. Massive retroperitoneal angiomyolipoma. A lesion that may be confused with well-differentiated liposarcoma. *Am J Clin Pathol* 1989;92:8005–8008.

237. Kaiserling E, Kroeber S, Xiao J-C, Schaumberg-Lever G. Angiomyolipoma of the kidney. Immunoreactivity with HMB-45. Light and electron-microscopic findings. *Histopathology* 1994;25:41–48.

238. Monteforte WJ Jr, Kohnen PW. Angiomyolipomas in a case of lymphangiomyomatosis syndrome: relationship to tuberous sclerosis. *Cancer* 1974;34:317–321.

239. Price EB, Mostofi FK. Symptomatic angiomyolipoma of the kidney. *Cancer* 1965;18:761–774.

240. Taylor RS, Joseph DB, Kohaut EC, et al. Renal angiomyolipoma associated with lymph node involvement and renal cell carcinoma in patients with tuberous sclerosis. *J Urol* 1989;141:930–935.

241. Sherman JL, Hartman DS, Friedman AC, et al. Angiomyolipoma: computed tomograhic-pathologic correlation of 17 cases. *AJR* 1981; 137:1221–1226.

242. Chan JKC, Tsang WYW, Pau MY, et al. Lymphangiomyomatosis and angiomyolipoma: closely related entities characterized by hamartomatous proliferation of HMB–45 positive smooth muscle. *Histopathology* 1993;22:445–455.

243. Mukai M, Torikata C, Iri H, et al. Crystalloids in angiomyolipoma: a previously unnoticed phenomenon of renal angiomyolipoma occurring at high frequency. *Am J Surg Pathol* 1992;16:1–10.

244. Berg JW. Angiomyoliposarcoma of kidney (malignant hamartoma-

tous angiomyolipoma) in a case with solitary metastases from bronchogenic carcinoma. *Cancer* 1955;8:759–771.

245. Umeyama T, Saito Y, Tomaru Y, et al. Bilateral renal angiomyolipoma associated with bilateral renal vein and inferior vena caval thrombi. *J Urol* 1992;148:1885–1892.

246. Ansari SJ, Stephenson RA, Mackay B. Angiomyolipoma of the kidney with lymph node involvement. *Ultrastruct Pathol* 1991;15:531–538.

247. Brecher ME, Gill WB, Straus FH. Angiomyolipoma with regional lymph node involvement and long-term follow-up study. *Hum Pathol* 1986;17:962–963.

248. Pea M, Bonetti F, Zamboni G, et al. Melanocyte marker HMB-45 is regularly expressed in angiomyolipoma of the kidney. *Pathology* 1991;23:185–188.

249. Sturtz CL, Dabbs DJ. Angiomyolipomas: the nature and expression of the HMB-45 antigen. *Mod Pathol* 1994;7:842–845.

250. Bonsib SM. HMB-45 reactivity in renal smooth muscle neoplasms (abstract). *Mod Pathol* 1996;9:71A.

251. McCormick D, Mentzel T, Beham A, Fletcher CDM. Dedifferentiated liposarcoma. Clinicopathologic analysis of 32 cases suggesting a better prognostic subgroup among pleomorphic sarcomas. *Am J Surg Pathol* 1994;18:1213–1223.

252. Weiss SW, Rao VK. Well differentiated liposarcoma (atypical lipoma) of deep soft tissue of the extremities, retroperitoneum, and miscellaneous sites: a follow-up study of 92 cases with analysis of the incidence of dedifferentiation. *Am J Surg Pathol* 1992;16:1051–1058.

253. Ferry JA, Malt RA, Young RH. Renal angiomyolipoma with sarcomatous transformation and pulmonary metastases. *Am J Surg Pathol* 1991;15:1083–1088.

254. Lowe BA, Brewer J, Houghton DC, et al. Malignant transformation of angiomyolipoma. *J Urol* 1992;147:1356–1360.

255. Guinee DG Jr, Thornberry DS, Azumi N, Przygodzky RM, Koss MN, Travis WD. Unique pulmonary presentation of an angiomyolipoma. Analysis of the clinical, radiographic, and histopathologic features. *Am J Surg Pathol* 1995;19:476–480.

256. Hulbert JC, Graf R. Involvement of the spleen by renal angiomyolipoma: metastasis or multicentricity. *J Urol* 1983;130:328–331.

257. Terris B, Flejou J-F, Picot R, Belghiti J, Henin D. Hepatic angiomyolipoma. A report of four cases with immunohistochemical and DNA-flow cytometric studies. *Arch Pathol Lab Med* 1996;120:68–72.

258. Weeks DA, Malott RL, Arensen M, Zuppan C, Aitken D, Mierau G. Hepatic angiomyolipoma with striated granules and positivity with melanoma specific antibody (HMB-45); report of two cases. *Ultrastruct Pathol* 1991;15:563–571.

259. Shimuzu M, Manabe T, Tazelaar HD, et al. Intramyocardial angiomyolipoma. *Am J Surg Pathol* 1994;18:1164–1169.

260. Castillenti TA, Bertin AP. Angiomyolipoma of the spermatic cord: case report and review of the literature. *J Urol* 1989;142:1308–1313.

261. Nagamine N, Nohara Y, Ito E. Elastofibroma in Okinawa. A clinicopathologic study of 170 cases. *Cancer* 1982;50:1794–1805.

262. Stemmerman GN, Stout AP. Elastofibroma dorsi. *Am J Clin Pathol* 1963;37:490–506.

263. Banfield WG, Lee CK. Elastofibroma. An electron microscopic study. *JNCI* 1968;40:1067–1077.

264. Kindblom L-G, Spicer SS. Elastofibroma. A correlated light and electron microscopic study. *Virchows Arch A Path Anat* 1982;396:127–140.

265. Enjoji M, Sumiyoshi K, Sueyuski K. Elastofibromatous lesion of the stomach in a patient with elastofibroma dorsi. *Am J Surg Pathol* 1985;9:233–237.

266. Kahn HJ, Hanna WM. Aberrant elastic in elastofibroma. An immunohistochemical and ultrastructural study. *Ultrastruct Pathol* 1995;19:45–50.

267. Dixon AY, Lee SH. An ultrastructural study of elastofibromas. *Hum Pathol* 1980;11:257–262.

268. Govoni E, Severi B, Laschi R, Lorenzini P, Ronchetti IP, Baccarani M. Elastofibroma. An in vivo model of abnormal neoelastogenesis. *Ultrastruct Pathol* 1988;12:327–339.

269. Dutz W, Stout AP. The myxoma in childhood. *Cancer* 1961;14:629–634.

270. Enzinger FM. Intramuscular myxoma. A review and follow-up study of 34 cases. *Am J Clin Pathol* 1965;43:104–113.

271. Hashimoto H, Tsuneyoshi M, Daimaru Y, Enjoji M, Shinohara N. Intramuscular myxoma. A clinicopathologic, immunohistochemical, and electron microscopic study. *Cancer* 1986;58:740–747.

272. Ireland DCR, Soule EH, Ivins JC. Myxoma of somatic soft tissues. A report of 58 patients, 3 with multiple tumors and fibrous dysplasia of bone. *Mayo Clin Proc* 1973;48:401–410.

273. Kindblom L, Steiner B, Angervall L. Intramuscular myxoma. *Cancer* 1974;34:1737–1744.

274. Mackenzie DH. The myxoid tumors of somatic soft tissues. *Am J Surg Pathol* 1981;5:443–458.

275. Meis JM, Enzinger FM. Juxta-articular myxoma. A clinical and pathologic study of 65 cases. *Hum Pathol* 1992;23:639–646.

276. Miettinen M, Hockerstedt K, Reitamo J, Totterman S. Intramuscular myxoma. A clinicopathological study of twenty three cases. *Am J Clin Pathol* 1985;84:265–272.

277. Stout AP. Myxoma, the tumor of primitive mesenchyme. *Ann Surg* 1948;127:706–719.

278. Allen PW, Dymoock RB, MacCormack LB. Superficial angiomyxomas with and without epithelial components. Report of 30 tumors in 28 patients. *Am J Surg Pathol* 1988;12:519–530.

279. Carney JA, Gordon H, Carpenter PC, Shenoy BV, Go VLW. The complex of myxomas, spotty pigmentation and endocrine overactivity. *Medicine* 1985;64:270–283.

280. Aoki T, Kuoho H, Hisaoka M, Hashimoto H, Nakata H, Sakai A. Intramuscular myxoma with fibrous dysplasia. A report of two cases with a review of the literature. *Pathol Int* 1995;45:165–171.

281. Blasier RD, Ryan JR, Schaldenbrand MF. Multiple myxomata of soft tissue associated with polyostotic fibrous dysplasia: a case report. *Clin Orthop* 1986;206:211–215.

282. Sedmak DD, Hart WR, Belhobek GH, et al. Massive intramuscular myxoma associated with fibrous dysplasia of bone. *Cleve Clin Q* 1983;50:469–472.

283. Wirth WA, Leavitt D, Enzinger FM. Multiple intramuscular myxomas: another extraskeletal manifestation of fibrous dysplasia. *Cancer* 1971;27:1167–1173.

284. Lever EG, Pettingale KW. Albright's syndrome associated with a soft-tissue myxoma and hypophosphataemic osteomalacia: report of a case and review of the literature. *J Bone Joint Surg (Br)* 1983;65:621–624.

285. Logel RJ. Recurrent intramuscular myxoma associated with Albright's syndrome. Case report and review of the literature. *J Bone Joint Surg (Am)* 1976;58:565–561.

286. Feldman PS. A comparative study including ultrastructure of intramuscular myxoma and myxoid liposarcoma. *Cancer* 1979;43:512–525.

287. Unni KK. *Dahlin's bone tumors: general aspects and data on 11,087 cases.* 5th ed. Philadelphia: Lippincott-Raven, 1996.

288. Drolshagen LF, Reynolds WA, Marcus NW. Fibrocartilaginous dysplasia of bone. *Radiology* 1985;156:32.

289. Fechner RE. Problematic lesions of the craniofacial bones. *Am J Surg Pathol* 1989;13(Suppl 1):17–30.

290. Fechner RE, Mills SE. *Tumors of the bones and joints. Atlas of tumor pathology.* Series 3. Fascicle 6. Washington, DC: Armed Forces Institute of Pathology, 1993.

291. Harris WH, Dudley HR Jr, Barry RJ. The natural history of fibrous dysplasia. *J Bone Joint Surg (Am)* 1962;44:207–233.

292. Henry A. Monostotic fibrous dysplasia. *J Bone Joint Surg (Br)* 1969;51:300–306.

293. Lichtenstein L. Polyostotic fibrous dysplasia. *Arch Surg* 1938;36:874–898.

294. Lichtenstein L, Jaffe HL. Fibrous dysplasia: a condition affecting one, several or many bones, the graver case of which may present with abnormal pigmentation of skin, premature sexual development, hyperthyroidism or still other extraskeletal abnormalities. *Arch Pathol* 1942;33:777–816.

295. Reed RJ. Fibrous dysplasia of bone. A review of 25 cases. *Arch Pathol* 1963;75:480–495.

296. Albright F, Butler AM, Hampton AO, Smith P. Syndrome characterized by osteitis fibrosa disseminata, areas of pigmentation and endocrine dysfunction with precocious puberty in females. *N Engl J Med* 1937;216:727–746.

297. Pelzmann KS, Nagel DZ, Salyer WR. Case report 114 (polyostotic fibrous dysplasia and fibrochondrodysplasia). *Skeletal Radiol* 1980;5:116–118.

298. Dorfman HD, Ishida T, Tsuneyoshi M. Exophytic variant of fibrous dysplasia (fibrous dysplasia protuberans). *Hum Pathol* 1994;25:1234–1237.

299. Ishida T, Dorfman HD. Massive chondroid differentiation in fibrous dysplasia of bone (fibrocartilaginous dysplasia). *Am J Surg Pathol* 1993;17:924–930.

300. Bulychova IV, Unni KK, Bertoni F, Beabout JW. Fibrocartilagenous mesenchymoma of bone. *Am J Surg Pathol* 1993;17:830–836.

301. Greco MA, Steiner GC. Ultrastructure of fibrous dysplasia of bone. A study of its fibrous, osseous, and cartilaginous components. *Ultrastruct Pathol* 1986;10:55–66.

302. Povysil C, Matejovsky Z. Fibro-osseous lesion with calcified spherules (cementifying fibromalike lesion) of the tibia. *Ultrastruct Pathol* 1993;17:25–34.

303. Sissons HA, Steiner GC, Dorfman HD. Calcified spherules in fibroosseous lesions of bone. *Arch Pathol Lab Med* 1993;117:284–290.

304. Voytek TM, Ro JY, Edeiken J, Ayala AG. Fibrous dysplasia and cemento-ossifying fibroma. A histologic spectrum. *Am J Surg Pathol* 1995;19:775–781.

305. Dabska M, Buraczewski J. On malignant transformation in fibrous dysplasia of bone. *Oncology* 1972;26:369–383.

306. DeSmet AA, Travers H, Neff JR. Chondrosarcoma occurring in a patient with polyostotic fibrous dysplasia. *Skeletal Radiol* 1981;7:197–201.

307. Feintuch TA. Chondrosarcoma arising in a cartilaginous area of previously irradiated fibrous dysplasia. *Cancer* 1973;31:877–881.

308. Halawa M, Aziz AA. Chondrosarcoma in fibrous dysplasia of the pelvis. A case report and review of the literature. *J Bone Joint Surg (Br)* 1984;66:760–764.

309. Huvos AG, Higginbotham NL, Miller TR. Bone sarcomas arising in fibrous dysplasia. *J Bone Joint Surg (Am)* 1972;54:1047–1056.

310. Ishida T, Machinami R, Kojima T, Kikuchi F. Malignant fibrous histiocytoma and osteosarcoma in association with fibrous dysplasia of bone. Report of three cases. *Pathol Res Pract* 1992;188:757–763.

311. Ruggieri P, Sim FH, Bond JR, Unni KK. Malignancies in fibrous dysplasia. *Cancer* 1994;73:1411–1424.

312. Taconis WK. Osteosarcoma in fibrous dysplasia. *Skeletal Radiol* 1988;17:163–170.

313. Yabut SM Jr, Kenan S, Sissons HA, Lewis MM. Malignant transformation of fibrous dysplasia. A case report and review of the literature. *Clin Orthop* 1988;228:281–289.

314. Campanacci M. Osteofibrous dysplasia of the long bones—a new clinical entity. *Ital J Orthop Traumatol* 1976;2:221–237.

315. Campanacci M, Laus M. Osteofibrous dysplasia of the tibia and fibula. *J Bone Joint Surg (Am)* 1981;63:367–375.

316. Campbell CJ, Hawk T. A variant of fibrous dysplasia (osteofibrous dysplasia). *J Bone Joint Surg (Am)* 1982;64:231–236.

317. Castellote A, Garcia-Pena P, Lucaya J, Lorenzo J. Osteofibrous dysplasia. A report of two cases. *Skeletal Radiol* 1988;17:483–486.

318. Kempson RL. Ossifying fibroma of the long bones. *Arch Pathol* 1966;82:218–233.

319. Nakashima Y, Yamamuro T, Fujiwara Y, et al. Osteofibrous dysplasia (ossifying fibroma of long bones). *Cancer* 1983;52:909–914.

320. Park Y-K, Unni KK, McLeod RA, Pritchard DJ. Osteofibrous dysplasia: clinicopathologic study of 80 cases. *Hum Pathol* 1993;24:1339–1347.

321. Markel SF. Ossifying fibroma of long bone. Its distinction from fibrous dysplasia and its association with adamantinoma of long bone. *Am J Clin Pathol* 1978;69:91–97.

322. Resnick CS, Young JW, Levine AM, Aisner SC. Case report 604. Osteofibrous dysplasia (ossifying fibroma) of the tibia. *Skeletal Radiol* 1990;19:217–219.

323. Benassi MS, Campanacci L, Gamberi G, et al. Cytokeratin expression and distribution in adamantinoma of the long bones and osteofibrous dysplasia of tibia and fibula. An immunohistochemical study correlated to histogenesis. *Histopathology* 1994;25:71–76.

324. Ishida T, Iijima T, Kikuchi F, et al. A clinicopathological and immunohistochemical study of osteofibrous dysplasia, differentiated adamantinoma and adamantinoma of long bones. *Skeletal Radiol* 1992;21:493–502.

325. Sweet DE, Vihn TN, Devaney K. Cortical osteofibrous dysplasia of long bone and its relationship to adamantinoma. *Am J Surg Pathol* 1992;16:282–290.

326. Baker PL, Dockerty MB, Coventry MB. Adamantinoma (so-called) of the long bones. Review of the literature and a report of three new cases. *J Bone Joint Surg (Am)* 1954;36:704–720.

327. Campanacci M, Laus M, Guinti A, Gitalis S, Bertoni F. Adamantinoma of the long bones. The experience of the Instituto Ortopedico Rizzolo. *Am J Surg Pathol* 1981;5:533–542.

328. Czerniak B, Rojas-Corona RR, Dorfman HD. Morphologic diversity of long bone adamantinoma. The concept of differentiated (regress-ing) adamantinoma and its relationship to osteofibrous dysplasia. *Cancer* 1989;64:2319–2334.

329. Keeney GL, Unni KK, Beabout JW, Pritchard DJ. Adamantinoma of long bones. A clinicopathologic study of 85 cases. *Cancer* 1989;64:730–737.

330. Knapp RH, Wick MR, Scheithauer BW, Unni KK. Adamantinoma of bone. An electron microscopic and immunohistochemical study. *Virchows Arch A Path Anat* 1982;398:75–86.

331. Mills SE, Rosai J. Adamantinoma of the pretibial soft tissue. Clinicopathologic features, differential diagnosis, and possible relationship to intraosseous disease. *Am J Clin Pathol* 1985;83:108–114.

332. Mori H, Yamamoto S, Hiramatsu K, Miura T, Moon NF. Adamantinoma of the tibia: ultrastructural and immunohistochemical study with reference to histogenesis. *Clin Orthop* 1984;190:299–311.

333. Perez-Atayde AR, Kozakewich HPW, Gordon FV. Adamantinoma of tibia: an ultrastructural and immunohistochemical study. *Cancer* 1985;55:1015–1023.

334. Pieterse AS, Smith PS, McClure J. Adamantinoma of long bones: clinical, pathological, and ultrastructural features. *J Clin Pathol* 1982;35:780–786.

335. Weiss SW, Dorfman HD. Adamantinoma of long bone. An analysis of nine new cases with emphasis on metastasizing lesions and fibrous dysplasia-like changes. *Hum Pathol* 1977;8:141–153.

336. Rosai J, Pinkus GS. Immunohistochemical demonstration of epithelial differentiation in adamantinoma of the tibia. *Am J Surg Pathol* 1982;6:427–434.

337. Johnson LC. Congenital pseudoarthrosis, adamantinoma of long bone and intracortical fibrous dysplasia of the tibia. *J Bone Joint Surg (Am)* 1972;54:1355–1358.

338. Levack B, Revell PA, Roper BA. Adamantinoma associated with fibrous dysplasia. *Int Orthop* 1986;10:253–259.

339. Schajowicz F, Santini-Araujo E. Adamantinoma of the tibia masked by fibrous dysplasia. Report of three cases. *Clin Orthop Res* 1989;238:294–301.

340. Ueda Y, Roessner A, Bosse A, Edel G, Bocker W. Juvenile intracortical adamantinoma of the tibia with predominantly osteofibrous dysplasia-like features. *Pathol Res Pract* 1991;187:1039–1043.

341. Bridge JA, Dembinski A, De Boer J, Travis J, Neff JR. Clonal chromosomal abnormalities in osteofibrous dysplasia. Implications for histopathogenesis and its relationship with adamantinoma. *Cancer* 1994;73:1746–1752.

342. Caffey J. On fibrous defects in cortical walls of growing tubular bones: their radiologic appearance, structure, prevalence, natural course, and diagnostic significance. *Adv Pediatr* 1955;7:13–51.

343. Cunningham JB, Ackerman LV. Metaphyseal fibrous defects. *J Bone Joint Surg (Am)* 1956;38:797–808.

344. Hatcher CH. The pathogenesis of localized fibrous lesions in the metaphysis of long bones. *Ann Surg* 1945;122:1016–1030.

345. Jaffe HL, Lichtenstein L. Non-osteogenic fibroma of bone. *Am J Pathol* 1942;18:205–221.

346. Lazarus SS, Trombetta LD. Nonossifying fibroma or benign lipoblastoma of bone—an electron microscopic and histochemical study. *Histopathology* 1982;6:793–805.

347. Ritschl P, Karmel F, Hajek P. Fibrous metaphyseal defects—determination of their origin and natural history using a radiomorphological study. *Skeletal Radiol* 1988;17:8–15.

348. Young JW, Levine AM, Dorfman HD. Case report 293. Nonossifying fibroma (NOF) of the upper tibial diametaphysis, with considerable increase in size over a three-year period. *Skeletal Radiol* 1984;12:294–297.

349. Moser RP Jr, Sweet DR, Hanseman DB, Madewell JE. Multiple skeletal fibroxanthomas: radiologic-pathologic correlation of 72 cases. *Skeletal Radiol* 1987;16:353–359.

350. Campanacci M, Laus M, Boriani S. Multiple nonossifying fibromata with extraskeletal anomalies: a new syndrome? *J Bone Joint Surg (Br)* 1983;65:627–632.

351. Mirra JM, Gold RH, Rand F. Disseminated nonossifying fibromas in association with cafe-au-lait spots (Jaffe-Campanacci syndrome). *Clin Orthop* 1982;168:192–205.

352. Arata MA, Peterson HA, Dahlin DC. Pathologic fracture through nonossifying fibroma. Review of the Mayo Clinic experience. *J Bone Joint Surg (Am)* 1981;63:980–988.

353. Drennan DB, Maylahn DJ, Fahey JJ. Fractures through large nonossifying fibromas. *Clin Orthop* 1974;103:82–88.

354. Mubarak S, Saltzstein SL, Daniel DM. Nonossifying fibroma. Report of an intact lesion. *Am J Clin Pathol* 1974;6:697–701.

*Pathology of Pseudoneoplastic Lesions,*
edited by M. R. Wick, P. A. Humphrey, and J. H. Ritter.
Lippincott-Raven Publishers, Philadelphia © 1997.

# CHAPTER 13

# Pseudoneoplastic Lesions of the Hematolymphoid System

Stefano Rosati and Glauco Frizzera

The hematolymphoid system, which, for the purposes of this chapter, includes lymph nodes, spleen, and bone marrow, is home to many different cell types. Each type might be the origin of a true neoplasm, and each might be involved—usually with other cell types—in a response to a stimulus. Although the two sets of processes are usually distinguishable, there are florid reactive lesions in which the high degree of cellularity and the extensive disturbance of the normal architecture closely simulate a malignancy. Some of them may

actually be precursor lesions to a true neoplasm, or "preneoplastic." Awareness of these extremes is essential because—in any equivocal case—it suggests caution in relying on morphology only and dictates recourse to additional studies before a diagnosis of malignancy is rendered.

## LYMPH NODES

In the following discussion, these florid reactions will be categorized first by the main cell type involved (lymphoid, histiocytic/dendritic, and stromal/endothelial) and second by the tissue compartment primarily affected.

S. Rosati and G. Frizzera: Department of Pathology, New York University Medical Center, New York, New York 10016.

# LYMPHOID HYPERPLASIAS SIMULATING NEOPLASMS

According to the functional compartment in which they mainly occur, and thus the histologic pattern of growth produced in the lymph node (LN), these reactions can be recognized as follicular, paracortical, or diffuse, when the limits of the original compartment are transgressed and the proliferation obscures the recognition of other topographic landmarks of the LN.

Reactions with a nodular (follicular) pattern include atypical follicular (germinal center) hyperplasia, progressive transformation of germinal centers, Castleman's disease of the hyaline-vascular type, and Kimura's disease. A predominant involvement of the paracortical areas is characteristic of the immunoblastic reactions observed in viral infections or hypersensitivity to drugs. A diffuse, quasiobliterative pattern is observed in what, for lack of a more specific term, can be called "atypical lymphoproliferative disorders."

## Atypical Follicular (Germinal Center) Hyperplasia

In the usual immune response the secondary follicles feature two sharply defined structures: a germinal center (GC) and its surrounding mantle zone (MZ). The former is the site of clonal expansion of antigen-primed B cells and formation of memory cells (1). In the process the immunoglobulins (Ig) undergo class switching (from IgMD to IgG or IgA) and variable region somatic hypermutation (which gives rise to antibodies of higher affinity for the antigen) (2,3). The lymphoid cells with no or low affinity for the antigens present on the follicular dendritic cells (FDCs) undergo apoptosis (programmed cell death), whereas those expressing high-affinity antibodies become either effector plasma cells that will home in on the bone marrow or memory cells to home in on the MZ or the marginal zone (4). There are several morphologic expressions of these physiologic processes: the polarization of the GC into two main areas, the dark proliferative zone and the light zone, richer in FDCs; the abundance of large cells and mitotic figures, especially in the dark zone; the presence of single-cell necrosis and the associated tingible body macrophages; the complex cellular composition, which includes GC cells (small cleaved and large noncleaved cells), as well as FDCs and small T cells (1). The MZ contains only small lymphoid cells, largely composed of long-lived recirculating memory cells, and rare dendritic cells.

An abnormality in the formation of the GC is not uncommon and finds its explanation in a defect of the complex immunoregulatory mechanisms that underlie it (5,6). Thus it is found in a variety of disorders associated with proven abnormal function(s) and, by analogy, if such are not evident, a more subtle derangement of immune function can reasonably be suspected. Similar changes in the GCs, in fact, are also seen as part of the complex picture of atypical lymphoproliferative disorders, in association with striking abnor-

malities in the paracortex. "Atypical" germinal cell hyperplasia (GCH), as we use it here, is a generic term for any process in which GCs predominate, to the point of largely obscuring the other compartments of the LN, but do not conform to the usual morphology of reactive secondary follicles. These lesions go beyond the "florid follicular hyperplasia" of HIV-infected individuals, in which, in spite of their large size, the GCs are still clearly recognizable as such and alternate with recognizable paracortical areas and with sinuses, often showing monocytoid B-cell hyperplasia (7).

### Clinical Features

Atypical GCH is a manifestation of many diseases; thus, no consistent clinical picture is associated with it. In our experience, most patients manifest one or more symptoms and signs of an autoimmune disorder, especially Sjögren's syndrome or rheumatoid arthritis (8,9), or those of a hypersensitivity syndrome related to the intake of drugs (10). However, we have seen similar findings in patients with genetically determined immunodeficiencies (11) and, rarely, with HIV infection. A request to the clinician for additional clinical information and laboratory tests that may help rule out or confirm these four possible situations is reasonable in any case of atypical GCH.

### Histologic Findings

Of the many morphologies that atypical GCH can take, two are most frequent and characteristic. In one form, the GCs are tightly crowded, serpiginous in shape, and interconnected, so that it is difficult to distinguish each individual one from the other (Fig. 1A, B). They are "naked" in that no MZ separates them from the reduced intervening areas of paracortex, and they feature a prominent "starry-sky" pattern. The predominant GC cells are noncleaved cells of intermediate or large size. In the second form, obvious nodular areas are seen continuous with one another, with lack of a clear distinction between GC and MZ (Fig. 2A). Large cells of the noncleaved type seem to predominate in the central areas of the nodule, without forming a cohesive aggregate. They are also numerous at its periphery, so that there is no clear demarcation between GC and MZ, or between MZ and paracortex, where large cells are also seen (Fig. 2B). This second set of features may be summarized under the term "dissolution of GC" (12). The cell composition of the GCs is unusual; intermingled with the transformed cells is a predominance of small round lymphocytes, and the typical small cleaved cells of the GCs are difficult to find.

### Differential Diagnosis

Criteria that help in the histopathologic distinction of follicular hyperplasia from *follicular lymphoma (FL)* were first

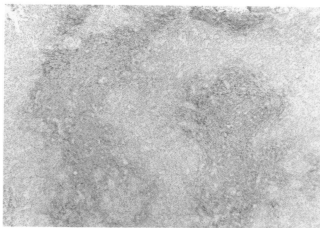

**FIG. 1.** Atypical germinal center (GC) hyperplasia with ill-defined, serpiginous, and confluent GCs (bluish, darker areas) **(A)**. Often these can be only identified with certainty by bringing out the follicular dendritic cell network **(B)** (immunoperoxidase with 1F8/CD21).

proposed by Rappaport (13) and are still largely valid. These, reviewed and expanded by Nathwani et al. (14), can be summarized as follows. Contrary to the findings in GCH, the follicles of FLs are crowded together, with few intervening nonfollicular structures. They are often seen in the capsule and pericapsular tissues, are relatively uniform in size and shape where they have not become confluent, have ill-defined borders due to the infiltration of the neoplastic cells in the paracortex, and do not show polarization. While a mixed small and large cell composition is of no help in the differential diagnosis, a uniform large cell or small cleaved cell population is an abnormal finding, observed only in FLs. It cannot be stressed enough that no single criterion is by itself sufficient to discriminate between the two processes, and that all must be factored into the decision. Additional criteria may be used more specifically for the distinction of

the two forms of atypical GCH described above from FL. The first, with naked GCs, may be misinterpreted as an FL of large cell type; it differs from FL in the serpiginous and interconnected configuration of the GCs and in their sharp borders. The morphology of the "dissolution of GCs" is quite reminiscent of that produced by FL of mixed cell type; however, these abnormal reactive GCs lack both the cohesion and the striking component of small cleaved cells usually seen in the nodules of FL.

Most of the uncertainties in the differential diagnosis can be solved by immunophenotypic studies. The most relevant of these is the demonstration of light chain restriction in frozen sections; this is, however, often frustrated by technical problems and, moreover, up to 9% of FLs do not express Igs (15). In these cases, the breakdown or the disappearance of the reticular polyclonal Ig staining on the surface of the

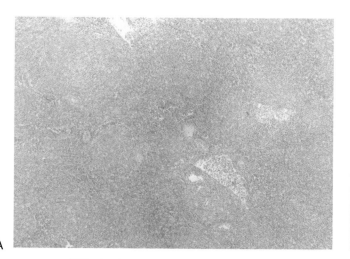
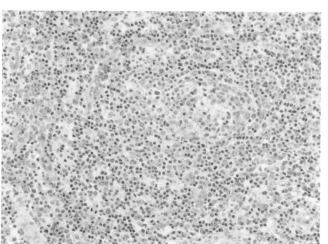

**FIG. 2.** Atypical germinal center (GC) hyperplasia with "dissolution" of the GCs. **A:** The GCs are roundish and ill defined. **B:** The lack of cohesion of the GC cells and the abundance of large transformed cells in the mantle zone and paracortex make the recognition of these different compartments difficult.

FDCs distinctly favors FL (15). Other criteria have been suggested. Neoplastic GCs, but not hyperplastic ones, react with the monoclonal antibody (Moab) 41H (15), and the Moab MT2, which decorates the mantle zone and paracortical lymphocytes, reacts with a proportion of FLs variable from 45% (16) up to 97% (17,18), but not hyperplastic GCs. Anti-bcl-2 Moabs have reactivity similar to that of MT2 and have demonstrated expression of bcl-2 in the nodules of FLs in a consistent proportion (85–90%) of cases, whether studied in frozen or paraffin sections (19–21). In a head-to-head comparison, these antibodies appear to be superior to MT2 in both sensitivity and ease of interpretation (22). It should be remembered that the reactivity with both Moabs, in order to be attributed to the neoplastic GC cells, should always be evaluated against a stain that brings out the T cells (which also are MT2 and bcl-2-positive) in the same areas.

The evaluation of the network of FDCs with a number of Moabs, reactive in frozen sections (R4/23, Ki-M4), paraffin sections (Ki-M4P, Ki-DRC1), or both (1F8/CD21, CD35), in order to distinguish reactive from neoplastic follicles, is of uncertain use. Both the intensity and the configuration of this network have been found to be very similar in the two situations (23). Although we have consistently observed a breakdown and irregularity of the FDC network in atypical GCH, indistinguishable changes can also be seen in FL, especially in areas where they tend to become diffuse in pattern (23). However, more detailed studies of other surface characteristics of the FDCs have revealed differences that should be evaluated for their practical use in this differential diagnosis. In fact, FDCs harvested from FLs demonstrate a loss of several adhesion molecules (CD11b, CD29, CD49b, CD49c) normally present on these cells, a loss that is possibly indicative of a reduced capacity for cohesion among the FDCs that is associated with malignant follicles (24).

In difficult cases in which the diagnostic dilemma between atypical GCH and FL has not been solved by immunophenotyping, genomic analysis may be the last resort but does not necessarily provide a definitive answer. Rearrangement of the Ig heavy and/or light chain is found in all FLs (25–27); however, it was also observed in 18% of histologically typical florid reactive follicular hyperplasia in patients with HIV infection (28). Thus the detection of a rearrangement band, while indicative of a clonal population in the tissue, does not by itself portend the clinical behavior of a lymphoma. Similarly, a rearrangement of the bcl-2 oncogene, the molecular counterpart of the t(14;18), is detected in FL with an incidence varying from 65% to 86%, depending on the technique used (29); however, it was also found by modifications of the polymerase chain reaction (PCR) in a large proportion (10–54%) of hyperplastic lymphoid tissues (30–32), suggesting that it may not be sufficient either in lymphomagenesis or, as a corollary, in the diagnosis of FL (33).

It is apparent that in some cases a definitive diagnosis may not be forthcoming by any of the analyses described above. At times, history, clinical or laboratory findings, or the short-term evolution of the lymphadenopathy (such as a regression without therapy) may still provide an answer. It is, however, entirely appropriate, in all unresolved cases, to propose a diagnosis of atypical follicular proliferation and adopt a "wait-and-see" attitude because if the process is neoplastic, the behavior in most cases is that of a low-grade lymphoma. It is essential in these cases that if the lymphadenopathy persists or progresses, another biopsy should be obtained, which should also be studied by immunophenotypic and immunogenotypic techniques, in order to compare the results with those already accrued. The detection of the same rearranged band of the Ig genes or bcl-2 oncogene would define the process as neoplastic.

### Evolution, Treatment, and Prognosis

These are, of course, as varied as the many different diseases that can manifest as atypical GCH in the LNs. There are no longitudinal studies of such lymphoid lesions, evaluated so completely that their diagnosis, and thus the interpretation of their evolution, is beyond doubt. In three studies, proliferations characterized by "atypical" follicular hyperplasia had very diverse evolutions, testifying to the variability of the criteria leading to such diagnosis: no patient, in one study (34), and only one of two in another (35), developed lymphoma on follow-up. In contrast, all had clonal rearrangement of the Ig genes and developed lymphoma in a median time of 3.5 months, in a third series (9). Data about the development of lymphoma in patients with rheumatoid arthritis are conflicting, but it appears that those with reactive follicular hyperplasia are not at increased risk (36). None of the patients with Sjögren's syndrome who manifested in their nodes reactive follicular hyperplasia developed lymphoma, but one of two showing an "atypical" lymphoproliferation did so (37). These data may appear to contrast with those reported for cases of myoepithelial sialoadenitis with or without Sjögren's syndrome: 58% (38) to 74% (39) of these glands also contain lymphoma. This contrast, however, is explained by the recent concept that lymphomas arising in salivary glands with myoepithelial sialoadenitis are "marginal cell lymphomas" of the mucosa-associated lymphoid tissue (MALT) type, not FLs (39), and thus are unrelated to GCs. The reactive GCH observed in the LNs of these patients is probably only an expression of their general B-cell hyperreactivity, and this does not seem to be prone to progress to an FL. This last observation also might well apply to the atypical GCHs in patients with immunodeficiency, either congenitally determined or acquired (AIDS). In fact, while lymphomas are known to develop in both situations with an incidence higher than in the normal population, only exceptionally are they of the follicular type (40,41) and thus suspected to arise in the original GCH.

It is, however, theoretically possible that in reactive GCs, which are in fact oligoclonal (2), a GC neoplasm might develop. This might be the case—and would be a worthwhile area of inquiry—in those atypical GCHs that cannot be attributed to any of the above discussed etiologies, and may thus represent forms of atypical lymphoproliferative disorders, specifically manifesting an abnormality in the regulatory mechanisms of GC formation. In some such atypical GCHs we have, in fact, observed monoclonal plasma cell proliferations limited to one or few GCs (42).

## Progressive Transformation of Germinal Centers

Progressive transformation of germinal centers (PTGC), described two decades ago by Lennert and Müller-Hermelink (43), is relatively uncommon. It has been reported in 3.5% of chronic nonspecific lymphadenitis (44) or approximately 10% of lymph nodes with reactive follicular hyperplasia (45). Although much is known today about its histopathologic and immunophenotypic characteristics, it is still unclear what it represents. It is considered by some to be a physiologic form of GC response (46) or an early transient stage in the normal development of the follicle within the so-called composite nodule (47). Others regard it as a form of abnormal development of the follicle, based on an undetermined immunoregulatory defect (48). The interest in this process is largely due to its proposed relationship to Hodgkin's disease (HD) of the nodular lymphocyte predominance type (nodular paragranuloma), with which it shares uncanny histopathologic and immunophenotypic similarities. A relationship with HD—which precedes, coexists with, or follows a lymph node biopsy with PTGC—is obtained in approximately 30% of cases. We discuss first PTGC in its uncomplicated form, as seen in the majority of cases.

### Clinical Features

Reactive lymph nodes showing PTGC are observed over a wide age range, but most commonly occur in the second and third decades, the median age being 27.5 years in one series (49). The majority (77%) of patients are male, and present with large, solitary, and asymptomatic lymphadenopathy of recent onset, most often in the cervical or axillary region (44,49,50). In occasional cases, the lymphadenopathy has been present for several years (50), or may involve unusual areas (paragastric, mesenteric) (44) or multiple LN groups (50). PTGC has also been observed in extranodal sites, such as the skin or the oral cavity (44).

### Histologic Findings (44,48–50)

PTGC is seen in greatly enlarged LNs and in the background of usual reactive follicular hyperplasia and preserved LN architecture (Fig. 3A). A few or many follicles appear much larger than normal reactive follicles and are characterized by a prominent mantle zone and ill-defined GCs (Fig. 3B). These are actually infiltrated by the small lymphocytes, and the GC cell component is spread apart and difficult to recognize as such. Sparse epithelioid histiocytes are commonly seen in the mantle zone (44,50).

### Immunophenotyping

The follicular nature of these nodules is well brought about by stains for FDCs, which show an enlarged and broken down network (Fig. 4A); interestingly, these FDCs do not bear Igs (44). The predominant cells in the progressively transformed GCs are small and large B cells, but numerous T cells are also present, which are predominantly of the CD4 subset and which express the natural killer (NK) marker CD57 (Leu7) (48) (Fig. 4B).

### Differential Diagnosis

At times, it may be difficult to distinguish PTGC from the process of *follicle lysis*, which may also be found in the same LN (50). Follicle lysis was originally described in patients

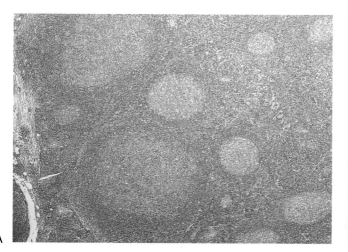
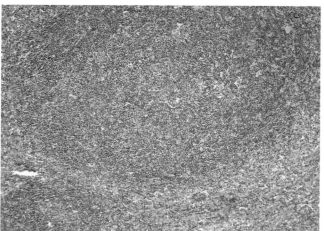

A          B

**FIG. 3.** Progressive transformation of germinal center (GC). **A:** The two transformed GCs are much larger than the surrounding hyperplastic GCs. **B:** This follicle shows a predominance of small lymphoid cells and no clear distinction between GC and mantle zone.

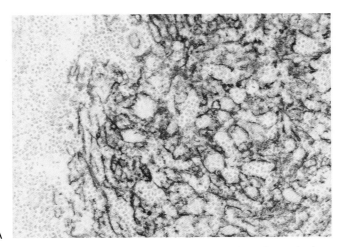
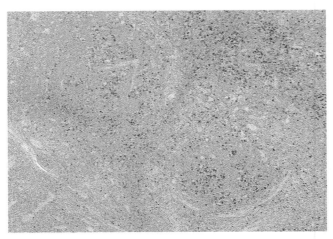

A                                                                                                         B

**FIG. 4.** Progressive transformation of germinal center (GC). **A:** A stain with 1F8/CD21 demonstrates the open network of follicular dendritic cells. **B:** Abundant Leu7/CD57-positive small cells are seen within the progressively transformed GCs.

with HIV infection (51) but may also be observed in usual reactive LNs (52,53). Like PTGC, it also features enlarged follicles and GC breakdown by small lymphocytes, but differs from PTGC in several regards: there is no expanded MZ; the GC cell component is collected in irregular but compact clusters; and these are sharply separated, rather than infiltrated, by collections of small lymphocytes and by red blood cells.

The most difficult differential diagnosis is with *nodular paragranuloma,* with which PTGC may be associated in the same LN; at times the distinction may, in fact, be arbitrary. At low power, nodular paragranuloma is to be suspected when nodules with features of PTGC become crowded and confluent, producing a distortion, if not complete obliteration, of the nodal architecture, and when clusters of epithelioid, rather than single and separated, histiocytes are seen (44), often encircling the nodules (54). The hallmark of nodular paragranuloma is the presence of the classic atypical large cells, with abundant cytoplasm and multilobulated nuclei, the so-called lymphocytic and histiocytic (L&H) cells (55) or "popcorn" cells. There may also be binucleated cells closely reminiscent of diagnostic Reed–Sternberg cells.

The immunophenotypic characteristics of nodular paragranuloma are indistinguishable from those of PTGC: the nodules are supported by an irregular network of FDCs, and are predominantly composed of small and large B cells, including the L&H cells, associated with abundant CD4-positive T cells, which also express CD57 (48,56). The large B cells in some cases express detectable surface and/or cytoplasmic Igs, but no light chain restriction is detected in these cells in the vast majority of the studies reported (56–59). However, in a recent study, where stainings for kappa and lambda Ig light chains were compared in each nodule in serial paraffin sections, almost all cases of nodular paragranuloma were said to express monoclonal Igs (60). This finding would certainly favor nodular paragranuloma over PTGC in a contentious case, as would the presence of chromosomal abnormalities, which are, at least in rare cases, present in

nodular paragranuloma (61). Genomic studies for Ig gene rearrangement have mostly been negative in nodular paragranuloma (62–64) and would, therefore, be of little help in the distinction. Thus, the distinction of PTGC from nodular paragranuloma generally rests on histopathology.

*Evolution, Treatment, and Prognosis*

One characteristic feature of patients with PTGC is that the lymphadenopathy may be persistent (50) and often recurs, in which case it again shows evidence of PTGC. Recurrent lymphadenopathy was reported to occur in 32% of patients with PTGC unassociated with HD, at intervals variable from a few months to 15 years (median 3 years) from the first biopsy (45). This is seen most often—but not necessarily—in the same LN group that was originally involved. In this series of patients, followed for up to 20 years (median 4) and in a smaller one, composed of five young men with shorter follow-up (1–10 years; median 2) (50), none developed HD, and all are alive and well, with the exception of one subject, who developed an apparently unrelated seminoma.

There is, however, some relationship between PTGC and HD, which is now discussed. Collating the experience of three large series in the literature (44,45,49), totaling 138 patients with lymphadenopathy featuring PTGC, an association with HD was found in 27% of them: PTGC was preceded by HD in 17%, coexisted with HD in 7% and was followed by HD in only 3%. All cases of HD that coexisted with PTGC in the same or in different LN groups, or followed an LN biopsy with PTGC, were of the nodular paragranuloma type. The presence of the two lesions in the same LN, with aspects of transition from one to the other, and the fact that the peak of incidence for nodular paragranuloma is 20 years later than that of PTGC (44), as well as the histoimmunophenotypic similarities already mentioned, have led to the concept that PTGC is a precursor lesion of nodular paragranuloma. The risk of this evolution is apparently very small (3%), even though it remains possible, as suggested by Hansmann et al. (44), that there are additional cases in which this possible transformation has been prevented by the excision of the LN containing PTGC. Thus, while it is important for the pathologist to thoroughly examine any biopsy with PTGC for the presence of nodular paragranuloma, and a request for a careful follow-up and a biopsy of any future lymphadenopathy is reasonable, no undue alarm should be created in the patient.

One is left with the problem of what causes PTGC. If it represents a physiologic form of GC development (47), one would expect its incidence in LN biopsies to be higher than 3–10%. The abnormality of both the FDCs and of the cellular composition, especially the abundance of CD57-positive T cells, strongly suggest the existence of some form of altered immunoregulation in the formation of the GC (48). HD that precedes 17% of the lymphadenopathies with PTGC and is in these cases equally of nodular paragranuloma or of the classic types may be responsible for the changes of PTGC, via the altered immunity that is characteristic of the disease. Delineation of the causes of dysimmunity in the larger (70%) proportion of cases of PTGC that are not associated with HD remains a challenge for future research.

## Castleman's Disease of Hyaline-Vascular Type

In contrast with the preceding LN lesions, this one represents a distinct clinicopathologic entity. It is also the only one, we believe, that fits the original description by Castleman et al. (65) and as such truly deserves this eponym. It should be clearly distinguished from the so-called plasma cell (66) and systemic (67,68) or multicentric (69) variants of Castleman's disease, which despite some morphologic similarities and perhaps some overlapping with the hyaline-vascular type are distinctly different biological entities. Hyaline-vascular Castleman's disease (HV CD) is composed of a lymphoid and a stromovascular component, either or both of which, in some cases, may simulate neoplasms. Both sets of differential diagnoses are discussed at this point for practical reasons, even though the stromal proliferation in HV CD would be more correctly included in a later section (stromovascular proliferations).

### Clinical Features

These have already been reviewed in detail (70) and are only briefly summarized here. The lesion presents in a wide range of ages, from 12 to 69 years (median, 33 years), with no gender predilection. It is most often an incidental finding in an asymptomatic patient or is discovered because of resulting compression phenomena. In several cases, in a retrospective review of radiographic studies, it was shown to have been present for many years, as long as 24 (66). Constitutional symptoms or laboratory abnormalities [low hemoglobin values, elevated erythrocyte sedimentation rate (ESR), or hypergammaglobulinemia] are present only in a minority (10%) of patients. Single case reports have described a whole host of unusual associations, such as with retarded growth, myasthenia gravis, nephrotic syndrome, peripheral neuropathy, erythema nodosum, temporal arteritis, or a familial pattern (70).

The lesions are found in a variety of locations. This process presents most commonly in the mediastinum, abdomen, and cervical LNs and less frequently in other LN groups or extranodal sites, such as the larynx, vulva, pericardium, cranium, subcutis, or skeletal muscle (70). The distribution among the three most common sites varies somewhat between a series of well-proven but otherwise unselected cases collected from the literature (70), and the series we reviewed at the AFIP (71). This was, respectively, 52%, 26%, and 15% in the former, but 28%, 16%, and 38% in the latter. These differences, we believe, can be accounted for by the frequent case reporting of mediastinal and abdominal lesions in the surgical literature, as opposed to the overall representation of these lesions in the practice of pathology laboratories. In cases in which angiography was performed, hypertrophic arterial supply and abundant intralesional vascularity were documented, and profuse bleeding is often reported at surgery (70). The lesion size varied from 3 to 25 cm in major dimensions, with most being between 7 and 10 cm.

Patients with the stroma-rich variant, which we identified recently (see below), were somewhat distinct: a very high proportion of them (80%) were women, all were adults (18 or older), and patients presented most often with an abdominal mass (rather than cervical and mediastinal, as in the other forms of HV CD) (71).

### Histologic Findings

HV CD is characterized by a combination of abnormal follicles, hypervascular interfollicular tissue containing clusters of plasmacytoid monocytes, and lack of sinuses (65,71,72) (Fig. 5A). The *follicles* are abnormal in several regards: they often show complex, "geographic" configuration (73); there is a marked predominance of the MZ over the GC, and an increased vascularity in both; and the GCs, frequently multiple in the same follicle, are mostly of the classic HV type (65) (Fig. 5B). The HV morphology corresponds to a decrease in the lymphoid component and a predominance of FDCs and blood vessels, often with sclerosis, resulting in a hypocellular, more eosinophilic look to the GC. Abnormal dystrophic FDCs, with multiple nuclei, clumped chromatin, and little recognizable cytoplasm (74) are quite common, both in the GC and in the MZ. In the latter, the much-stressed "onion-skin" arrangement of the small lymphocytes may or may not be present.

The *interfollicular areas* show marked vascularity, due to both small arteries and high-endothelial venules, and are populated by small lymphoid cells, various types of stromal cells (histiocytes, histiocytic dendritic cells, fibroblastic reticulum cells) (71), and, more distinctly, by an abundant component of plasmacytoid monocytes (71,75,76), a re-

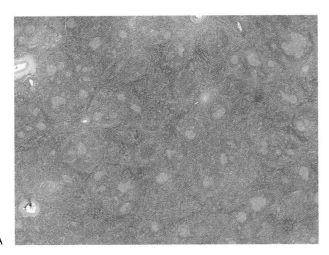
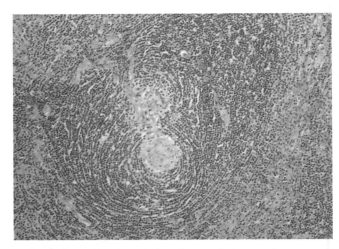

**FIG. 5.** Hyaline-vascular (HV) Castleman's disease. **A:** Typical combination of abundance of abnormal follicles, hypervascular interfollicular tissue, and lack of sinuses. **B:** HV germinal center surrounded by small lymphoid cells in "onion-skin" arrangement.

cently described cell type with possible antigen presenting and secretory properties (77,78). These cells, characterized by a medium size, round to oval nuclei with very fine chromatin, and pale eosinophilic, eccentric cytoplasm (79), are more easily recognizable when they form clusters or large sheets associated with the characteristic single-cell necrosis, but they are also found scattered singly. Only a minority (<5%) of the 102 cases in our series showed a relevant "inflammatory" cell component in the interfollicular areas (plasma cells, immunoblasts, eosinophils, or epithelioid macrophages), as commonly observed in usual reactive LNs.

One of the most characteristic features of HV CD is the *absence of sinuses* within the lesional tissue (65,71,72). These, however, may be observed at the periphery of the lesion, where residual, more or less compressed uninvolved portions of LN may be found. *Additional changes,* commonly but not consistently seen in HV CD, include the presence of a fibrotic capsule, often with abnormally large and dilated blood vessels; bands of fibrosis; and areas of calcification or bone formation. Rarely, a lipomatous component has been reported (80), which, added to abnormal blood vessels, produced a hamartomatous appearance. Deposits of amyloid have been described in rare cases of CD, classified as HV or "mixed" type [reviewed in Ordi et al. (81)], but their consistent localization in the abdomen or multicentric presentation (both typical features of CD of the plasma cell type) and the association with evidence of systemic amyloidosis suggest that these cases may in fact represent CD of the plasma cell type instead.

*Variants*

In our study we have observed striking differences in the proportion of follicular (lymphoid) to intrafollicular (stromovascular) components from lesion to lesion. In addition to cases showing the "classic" mixture of the two in approxi-

mately equal proportions, there were cases with a predominant follicular component (over 50% of the lesional area) (Fig. 6), and others with a predominant stromovascular component (over 75% of the lesional area) (71). It is these two histopathologic extremes that may simulate and be misdiagnosed as neoplasms. While the former has already been described as the "lymphoid variant" by Keller et al. (66), the latter, which we have only recently identified, needs to be stressed here.

In this form, which we refer to as the "stroma-rich variant," a diffuse stroma predominates, populated by small lymphocytes, abundant and often spindly stromal cells, and sparse plasmacytoid monocytes. This stroma is traversed by abundant small blood vessels. The follicles are widely dispersed and often minute, and show GCs with HV morphology, and MZs infiltrated by blood vessels. Within the

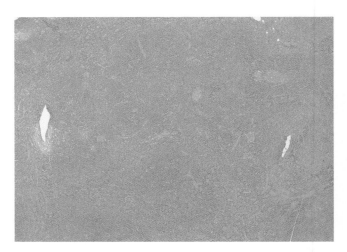

**FIG. 6.** Hyaline-vascular (HV) Castleman's disease, follicular (lymphoid) variant. Crowded follicles are separated by increased blood vessels. Only rare HV germinal centers are seen.

stroma, in a fifth of the cases, one may observe focal, ill-defined, or nodular proliferations, which due to their distinct morphology and immunophenotype we described as angiomyoid, angiohistiocytic reticulum cell, and/or follicular dendritic cell (FDC) types. The angiomyoid growths have a storiform pattern with crowded, much ramified blood vessels associated with abundant spindle cells and a reduced lymphoid component (Fig. 7A, B). The angiohistiocytic reticulum cell type also features an increased, complex network of blood vessels, but contains abundant lymphocytes and stromal cells with no prominent spindling or storiform pattern. Finally, the FDC foci show a loose, storiform pattern due to spindle cells, intermixed with abundant lymphocytes and spread-out, thinned blood vessels; the cytologic appearances vary from very sparse, thin elongated cells (hyperplasia?) to more crowded, plumper and more atypical spindle to polygonal cells (neoplasm?).

### Immunophenotyping

Immunohistochemical studies are not of great help in the diagnosis of CD HV but have provided important clues to an understanding of its pathogenesis (70). The follicles are supported by a dense network of FDCs in the MZ and an even denser one in the GC, as shown by reagents such as DRC 1 (R4/23), 1F8 (CD21), or Ki-M4, and contain B cells, varying numbers of T cells and sparse Leu7 (CD57)-positive cells. The prominent vascularity is best seen with Q-BEND10 (CD34) in the follicles and with anti–factor VIII antibodies in the interfollicular areas; in the latter, the majority of the blood vessels show strong reactivity with two antibodies, HECA-452 and MECA-79, that characterize the high endothelial venules of the LNs (82,83). In the interfollicular areas there are abundant T lymphocytes, and staining with CD68 reagents, such as KP-1, highlights the abundant plasmacytoid monocytes (which are also HECA-452-positive,

but MECA-79 negative). In addition, there are stromal cells of different type, also seen in reactive LNs. These include cells with dendritic or spindle morphology, decorated with KP-1, or histiocytic dendritic cells (46); and cells with similar morphology, but reactive with anti-smooth muscle actin and antivimentin antibodies, corresponding to the fibroblastic reticulum cells of Müller-Hermelink et al. (84) and the myoid cells of Pinkus et al. (85,86). It is through the distinct immunohistochemical reactivities of the predominant cell component that the histopathologically different growths found in the stroma-rich variant can be recognized as of angiomyoid, histiocytic dendritic cell or FDC type.

### Pathogenesis

The very distinct histoimmunophenotypic characteristics outlined above are so different from those of CD of the plasma cell type that they cannot be given the same pathogenetic explanation accepted today for the latter disease. The combination of features of CD of the plasma cell type (preservation of the nodal architecture, including sinuses; hyperplasia of the GCs; and abundance of plasma cells) has long been interpreted as an expression of an abnormal immune response (66,87). It is believed that the key cells in this response are an abnormal mantle cell population of CD5-positive B cells (88,89) and that their proliferation and differentiation to plasma cells is due to excessive production of interleukin-6 (IL-6) by the hyperplastic GCs (90–92).

This, however, cannot explain the combination of abnormalities of the follicles (poor development of the GCs and preponderance of the MZ), lack of sinuses, increase in plasmacytoid monocytes, and hypervascularity that characterizes HV CD. In the past, pathogenetic theories for it have included hyperplasia (65,66,87) or hamartoma (73,93,94). And more recent studies have proposed a role for an acquired T-cell immunodeficiency (95) or for a dysplasia of FDCs

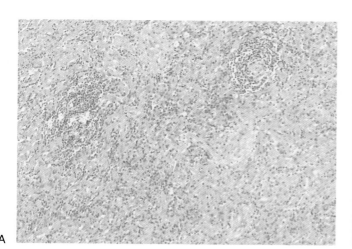
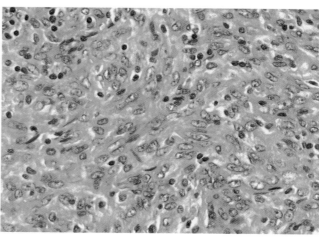

**FIG. 7.** Hyaline-vascular (HV) Castleman's disease with focal angiomyoid growth. **A:** Only two small follicles are recognizable within a hypervascular and storiform growth. **B:** This is composed of plump endothelial and spindle cells.

(74) in the pathogenesis of GC abnormalities. We tend to agree with the suggestion that the classic HV GC represents a primary defect in the development of the GC rather than a regressive phenomenon ["regressive transformation" (46)] occurring after its formation and, like others (74,96), suspect that these changes reflect an abnormality of the FDCs rather than of the lymphoid cells.

Based on our findings and the working hypothesis that plasmacytoid monocytes are the precursors of both FDCs and sinus-lining cells (Parwaresch et al., personal communication), we have further proposed a possible explanation that would link the abnormalities of the follicles to the abundance of plasmacytoid monocytes and the lack of sinuses (71). In this scenario, HV CD would originate wherever an antigenic stimulus involves an LN containing abnormal plasmacytoid monocytes that are unable to develop into sinus-lining cells and FDCs. The ensuing response would be abnormal in that stimulated but functionally blocked plasmacytoid monocytes would accumulate locally, but no sinuses or functional GCs would form. The lack of sinuses would lead to decreased influx of antigens and explain the poor reactivity of this lymphoid tissue. However, the presence of normal high endothelial venules would allow recirculating lymphocytes to enter the tissue and to accumulate in, and thus expand, the MZ, resulting in slow but progressive formation of a mass. We are at a loss to explain the marked vascularity of this tissue and the variety of stromovascular responses that we and others (97–99) have observed in it, as well as the continuum from a predominantly lymphoid to a predominantly stromal growth (successive phases of the same response or diverse and unrelated tissue responses?). As the B-cell hyperreactivity that characterizes CD of the plasma cell type has been attributed to overproduction of cytokines, i.e., specific B-cell growth factors, so it is likely that other factors are at play in HV CD, acting this time on the stromal component, and stimulating angiogenesis and stromal cell outgrowth.

*Differential Diagnosis*

HV CD of both the classic and the follicular types may suggest a lymphoma with a follicular pattern of growth. When the follicles are small and somewhat regular in shape and the GCs small and ill defined, a *follicular lymphoma* may be considered in view of the lack of recognizable normal architecture. However, we have seen only two cases of follicular lymphoma in which the nodules had central structures of HV type, and the round nuclei of the small cells, the absence of large noncleaved cells (centroblasts), and the very rich interfollicular vascularity all mitigate against a diagnosis of follicular lymphoma. When, on the contrary, the follicles are large and confluent, a similarity with a *nodular mantle cell lymphoma* [mantle zone lymphoma (100)] may be seen. In such a case, one could not rely on the cytologic characteristics of the mantle cells, but the presence of HV changes in the GCs would be unusual for mantle zone lym-

phoma, as would be the prominent interfollicular vascularity and the abundance of plasmacytoid monocytes. In cases of persisting doubt, an FDC reagent would show in HV CD a tight network, much different from the loose and open one seen in mantle cell lymphoma (101), and T-cell staining would bring out the almost exclusive T-cell composition of the interfollicular areas and their sharp delimitation from the negative nodules, both unexpected in the expanding nodules of a lymphoma.

Much more difficult could be the distinction of focal stromal cell growths arising in HV CD from a neoplasm. The crowded, ramified blood vessels of the angiohistiocytic dendritic cell foci and, even more, of the angiomyoid growths, with their spindling, plump endothelia, and storiform pattern, can easily be misinterpreted as *vascular neoplasms*. These, in fact, have been reported to arise in the context of CD (98) and, in at least two cases, have been proven to be such by the development of distant metastases. However, the regularity of the vascular pattern throughout the lesion, the absence of cellular atypia and mitoses, and, in difficult cases, the demonstration of high-endothelial venule differentiation in the blood vessels (reactivity with HECA-452 and MECA-79) and the distinct cell population (histiocytic dendritic cells or myoid cells) associated with them would help to identify these vascular proliferations as nonneoplastic.

The *foci of FDC type* that we (71,106) and others (99) have observed in HV CD raise the issue of distinguishing between non-neoplastic proliferations, and true neoplasm, akin to the FDC sarcoma of the LN, to which the more cellular of these foci bear an uncanny similarity by virtue of their nodular pattern, spindling, abundance of intermingled lymphocytes, and FDC reactivity of the spindle cells (102–104). As experience with these lesions is still very limited, this distinction would need to rely for now on the absence or presence of standard criteria for malignancy, such as evidence of invasion of adjacent soft tissue, rich cellularity, numerous mitoses, nuclear atypia and necrosis.

The common presence of giant, multinucleated, dystrophic FDCs in HV CD should be kept in mind and not interpreted as evidence of malignancy. Described first by Ruco et al. (74), they are characterized by the clumped chromatin pattern, suggestive of a degenerating cell. The nuclei may be very large and multiple, and the cytoplasm either abundant, possibly with phagocytosed cells or material, or so inconspicuous that the cells are difficult to recognize. They are present either in the follicles, where they arise, or appear in the interfollicular areas, a memory, so to speak, of a GC that has been wiped away by the stromal outgrowth. A few of these cells can be found, after careful search, in almost all cases of HV CD. However, in rare cases they may be so abundant and bizarre and are associated with such a florid stromal cell proliferation as to suggest a *malignant fibrous histiocytoma* (MFH). HV CD, however, differs from MFH by the dystrophic characteristic of the nuclei and the lack of mitoses. The even distribution of the proliferative process between HV GCs, without mass formation or infiltrative characteristics, is an additional feature to help exclude a neoplastic diagnosis.

### Evolution, Treatment, and Prognosis

HV CD is a benign disorder that is best treated by surgical excision. Cases that include symptoms and laboratory abnormalities show resolution of these associated features following excision. Radiation therapy has been used in cases not amenable to surgery but has been less effective than excision (66). Some lesions are said to have recurred (71), and in rare patients HV CD was histologically documented in successive biopsies (see ref. 70). However, most of these "secondary lesions" were at the same site as the primary lesion, suggesting persistence of the disease in adjacent nodes not included in the surgical procedure rather than recurrence. The term recurrence might not be applicable to cases occurring at different sites either, given the possibility that HV CD may in rare cases be multicentric.

The possibility of a neoplasm developing in HV CD is exceedingly small. The case of FDC neoplasms has already been mentioned: these have shown the potential for recurrences and distant metastases at variable intervals (18 months to 11 years) (106). As we said before, only two cases of vascular neoplasms in which metastases have occurred have been reported (98). Other cases of "vascular neoplasia," particularly those with uneventful follow-up (98,105), probably represent examples of the angiomyoid growths, as described above. In the patients of our original series (71), and in those of a more recent series (106), follow-up from 14 months to 16 years provided no evidence of recurrence or dissemination of the angiomyoid growths, supporting their hyperplastic rather than neoplastic nature. The same applies to the cases we have seen with abundant bizarre giant cells, simulating MFH.

There are rare reported cases of HV CD associated with, or said to have "progressed to," lymphoma. In two reports the non-Hodgkin's lymphoma was of the follicular type. One is said to have developed at the same site as an HV CD excised 8 years before (107). However, the illustrations of the neoplastic nodules said to be focally observed in the original HV CD are unconvincing, as are those of another case said to contain follicular lymphoma and HV CD at the same inguinal nodal site (105). A third case is a diffuse large cell lymphoma of the stomach in a patient in whom an incisional biopsy of an adjacent retroperitoneal mass was interpreted as showing HV CD (108). These cases clearly demonstrate that an association of HV CD with a non-Hodgkin's lymphoma, if it exists at all, is probably coincidental. Lesions consistent with HV CD have also predated Hodgkin's disease, in one case only (109), or been found in association with Hodgkin's disease, in several cases (110–113). The former situation may be a coincidental occurrence of two separate diseases; however, it is generally agreed (110–112,114) that changes in CD of HV, plasma cell (111,113,114), or mixed (110) type in association with HD simply represent a morphologic manifestation of the abnormal immune status found in this disorder rather than CD proper. Similar changes are, in fact, also observed in other situations of immunodeficiency, particularly in HIV infection (115,116).

In conclusion, it can be said that only rarely do neoplasms arise in HV CD. The reported associations of HV CD with lymphoma are probably coincidental, whereas other (vascular neoplasms and FDC tumors) might be thought of as a progression of the stromovascular proliferation that characterizes the disease. This is, of course, in contrast with the not uncommon occurrence of neoplasms in CD of the plasma cell type, especially multicentric or systemic (70). In keeping with the clear histogenetic distinction we have drawn between these two forms of disease, these are neoplasms of lymphoid origin (plasmacytoma, lymphoma) or immunodeficiency-related (Kaposi's sarcoma).

## Kimura's Disease

Kimura's disease (KiD) is a chronic inflammatory condition of unknown cause that was first described, and is particularly common, among Asians (117–121). However, it also occurs in Caucasians (122). In the Western literature KiD has long been—and still is—confused with histiocytoid (123) or *epithelioid hemangioma (EH)* (124). One of the reasons for this confusion is the erratic use of the term "angiolymphoid hyperplasia with eosinophilia" (ALHE) for both: this term describes well the main histologic features of KiD and thus, in our opinion, could be an acceptable synonym for it (125–128); however, it is also often applied to EH (129–133), and inappropriately so because EH may be a neoplastic process that can lack the lymphoid and eosinophilic component (121). The distinctiveness of KiD vis-à-ris EH is well supported by several recent series (120–122, 133–136); these findings are summarized here, with emphasis on the nodal manifestations of the disease.

### Clinical Findings

KiD affects any age, with means ranging between 26 and 40 years, and predominantly men (M/F = 5:1) (121). It manifests with subcutaneous or deep soft tissue nodules and/or salivary gland swelling (137). While centered most frequently in the head and neck region, especially around the ears, it may rarely involve other areas, such as the trunk, axilla, groin, and extremities. The subcutaneous nodules are usually sizable (2–10 cm), may be solitary or multiple, and have often been present for years (median 4) (121,133). For the purposes of our discussion, it is to be noted that clinical lymphadenopathy is present in up to two thirds of the patients. Elevated serum IgE levels and peripheral eosinophilia are very common laboratory findings (133,137); the latter has been attributed to production of IL-5 in the lesion (128,138) or by peripheral blood lymphocytes (139). Proteinuria or other evidence of renal disease was found in about 12% of patients in the literature (140–142).

### Histopathologic Findings

The lesions in the subcutis, soft tissue, and salivary glands are characterized by lymphoid hyperplasia, an abundance of nondescript and usually thin-walled blood vessels, and intense infiltration with eosinophils. The follicles often show prominent GCs; these may be hypervascularized, infiltrated, and/or destroyed by eosinophils ("eosinophilic folliculolysis") (133), and they contain deposits of eosinophilic material and occasionally polykaryocytes of the Warthin–Finkeldey type. Sclerosis is common in the lesions. The combination of numerous eosinophils, polykaryocytes, vascular proliferation, and sclerosis help diagnose KiD in fine needle aspirates (133).

All of the above findings are also observed in the adjacent LNs (Fig. 8A). In addition to vascularization, proteinaceous deposits, and eosinophilia, the GCs can show necrosis (120). Characteristically, the blood vessels are largely represented by high-endothelial venules, as in the usual reactive LN (Fig. 8B). Eosinophils vary from few to very numerous, may form eosinophilic abscesses (Fig. 8C), and may also infiltrate the

perinodal tissue (133). The distribution of B and T cells is as expected in a reactive LN (133); the T cells are predominantly activated CD4+ cells (143). In some cases, reticular deposits of IgE can be demonstrated in the GCs and IgE-bearing mast cells in the paracortex (120).

It has been stressed (120,133) that none of the above features is specific, including the reticular staining pattern of IgE in the GCs (144), but it is their combination that is highly characteristic of KiD, in the presence of an appropriate clinical presentation. These features and the association with atopic dermatitis (143,145), nephrotic syndrome (140–142), and ulcerative colitis (125) point to an immunologically mediated reaction. IL-5 mRNA has been detected in the LN of one case of KiD; the overproduction of this cytokine by activated T cells may account for both the hypereosinophilia and, via enhancement of the ability of IL-4 to induce IgE synthesis in cultured B cells, the elevated IgE levels found in this disease (138). The trapping of IgE–antigen complexes on the FDCs would produce the characteristic pattern of deposition in the GCs, and degranulation of eosinophils might explain the sclerosis seen in most cases of KiD (120).

While these observations make up a good histogenetic scenario, it is unclear what the initial antigenic stimulus or stimuli might be. However, in at least three recent contribu-

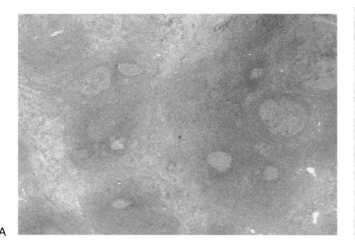

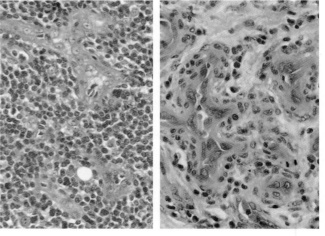

**FIG. 8.** Kimura's disease (KiD). **A:** Characteristic combination of hyperplastic germinal centers (GCs), fibrosis, and eosinophilic abscess (right upper field). **B:** The typical high-endothelial venules of KiD, on the left, are compared with the abnormal vessels of an epithelioid hemangioendothelioma, on the right. **C:** An eosinophilic abscess is seen, as well as eosinophilic infiltration in a GC ("eosinophilic folliculolysis").

tions, histologically identical lesions in the soft tissue (reported under the term ALHE) were clearly etiologically related to recent vaccination in the same area (126,127,146). *Candida albicans* could be another causative agent, as stimulation with *Candida* antigens resulted in local production of IL-5 (128) and the serum IgEs in one patient were specific for this organism (142).

### Differential Diagnosis

Histologic features similar to KiD can be seen in EH, as was stated before, in spindle and epithelioid hemangioendothelioma, and possibly in Hodgkin's disease. *EH* and *KiD* share several histopathologic and clinical features. Histopathologically, ALHE is observed in both; clinically, both affect young adults, involve mainly the head and neck region, and might recur. However, whatever the nature of EH, neoplastic or, at least in a proportion of cases, reactive (129), this disorder is mainly characterized by an angiomatous proliferation, with well-formed vascular lumina surrounded by a fibromyxoid matrix and lined with tall, plump endothelial cells, with folded nuclei and eosinophilic cytoplasm, at times containing vacuoles (123,124) (Fig. 8B). It is part of the spectrum of epithelioid vascular tumors, which also includes epithelioid hemangioendothelioma and its variants spindle and epithelioid, and polymorphous hemangioendothelioma (147). In EH the lymphoid and eosinophilic component may be inconspicuous or be absent (121); reactive GCs, proteinaceous deposits, polykaryocytes, and fibrosis are much less common, and folliculolysis is not seen (121,133). EH can develop in almost any tissue in the body, and in the skin it forms small papules or superficial nodules, which tend to be multiple and to bleed easily and have a much shorter duration than KiD. Peripheral eosinophilia and elevated serum IgE levels are less common. More importantly, as it relates to this chapter, clinical lymphadenopathy is uncommon (<20%) and, when enlarged, the LNs only show reactive changes (121). Primary EH of the LN is a very rare occurrence (130,148) and thus would be the least likely choice in the differential diagnosis with KiD.

We have seen a case of primary nodal *spindle and epithelioid hemangioendothelioma* in which a small area of spindle and epithelioid cell proliferation and sparse isolated clusters of eosinophilic polygonal cells with vacuoles were associated with florid GCs with proteinaceous deposits, increased vascularity, marked infiltration of eosinophils, and sclerosis, totally consistent with KiD. This lesion recurred several times in the cervical LNs of a young man. As pointed out in another case, the abundance of eosinophils, the association with fibrosis, and the occasional polykaryocytes seen in KiD might also suggest *Hodgkin's disease,* of interfollicular or nodular sclerosis type (130); however, the polykaryocytes never have the prominent nucleoli of Reed–Sternberg cells and are often found, unlike any Reed–Sternberg cell, within hyperplastic GCs.

### Evolution, Treatment, and Prognosis

The lesions of KiD persist for years and, after excision, may be followed by new lesions at other sites or, in 15–40% of cases (121), by one or more recurrences at the same site. Prednisolone produces only transient resolution of the lesions (141); pentoxifylline has also resulted in responses (149). No neoplastic evolution has ever been reported.

## Paracortical Immunoblastic Hyperplasias

The general term paracortical immunoblastic hyperplasia (PIH) includes any lesion that mainly expresses itself with an expansion of the paracortex due to a proliferation of large transformed lymphoid cells and an increase in high-endothelial venules (HEVs). These features are regular manifestations of the nodal response to a great many stimuli, but are particularly florid in the following clinical situations: infectious mononucleosis and other viral infections, postvaccinial lymphadenitis, and hypersensitivity reactions to medicaments. In all of these, the degree of immunoblastic proliferation and of associated mitotic activity might be so pronounced as to imitate a large cell non-Hodgkin's lymphoma, and the not uncommon occurrence of Reed–Sternberg–like atypical immunoblasts may evoke the possibility of HD.

Because all of these processes share both some basic histologic features and require the same differential diagnosis, they are treated together in this section. Even though their specific characteristics are mentioned when appropriate, no comprehensive account of each of these numerous clinicopathologic entities can be offered within the limits of this chapter.

### Clinical Findings

Symptomatic *infectious mononucleosis (IM)* is an uncommon disease in developing countries, where EBV infection occurs early in life. It is instead more prevalent in the West, where exposure to EBV is delayed by better hygienic conditions. Here it usually affects adolescents and young adults, but may develop at any age (150). The classic presentation, after an incubation of 3–7 weeks, includes the triad of fever, pharyngitis, and lymphadenopathy, usually localized to the neck, often with flu-like symptoms and with (52%) or without splenomegaly (151). The diagnosis is supported by the laboratory findings of absolute lymphocytosis, with more than 10% atypical cells, heterophile antibody titers over 1:56 in the Paul–Bunnell–Davidson test or positive Mono-Latex test, and virus-specific serologic tests (anti-VCA-IgM and IgG, anti-EA of the diffuse type, and no anti-EBNA antibodies) (152).

In these classic cases, it has been said that an LN biopsy would be "a complication of IM" (153)! However, this could be performed in the rare patient in whom the diagnosis of IM is not considered due to atypical clinical presentations, such as one or more of the following: very young age or older age than usual; generalized lymphadenopathy; predominant manifestations of complications (hepatitis, severe autoimmune hemolysis, hemophagocytic syndrome, etc.) (150); early observation, before lymphocytosis develops (1 week after the onset of IM); negative heterophile antibody test (154).

*Herpes simplex virus (HSV)* in the immunocompetent patient typically causes skin or mucosal lesions, such as oral or genital ulcers or keratoconjunctivitis, and only rarely acute encephalitis in the adult or hepatoadrenal necrosis in infants (155,156). In contrast, in the immunocompromised patient it may produce visceral infections, most often in the esophagus and lower respiratory tract, which may become disseminated. Lymphadenopathy caused by HSV is a rare event but has been the subject of many recent reports.

In one group of cases, it was an accompaniment of the classic mucocutaneous lesions in immunocompetent patients and was self-limited. Some of these patients had localized, mostly inguinal, LN enlargement, synchronous with or following the detection of genital herpes (157–159); others presented with fever, flu-like symptoms, and generalized lymphadenopathy associated with widespread erythematous or macular skin rash (156,160,161). Another group of cases includes patients with subtle or overt immunodeficiencies. In some of these, the lymphadenopathy was part of a disseminated visceral HSV infection with grave prognosis (162–165); in a few others, who had hematopoietic malignancies, it was a localized manifestation mostly associated with genital herpes (166,167). Two of the latter, however, died rapidly with disseminated infection and malignancy (166,167).

Primary *cytomegalovirus infection* might be congenital and involve the lymph nodes as part of a disseminated infection, or it might develop in the adult. At the later age, in the immunocompetent host, it manifests itself as a mild and self-limited disease, most frequently in the form of an IM syndrome that is completely similar to that caused by EBV, except for the lack of the characteristic pharyngitis. In the immunodeficient host, it is a more virulent disease in the form of IM syndrome, pneumonia, or hepatitis (168). In *measles* lymphadenopathy usually appears simultaneously or slightly after the classic mucocutaneous rash, but it may also occur during the prodromal stage and be cause for concern, leading to an LN biopsy. Similarly, the lymphadenopathy of *varicella-zoster infection* is associated with localized skin lesions or is part of the disseminated disease of patients with cancer or otherwise immunodepressed. However, an LN biopsy might be done unusually, if the lymphadenopathy precedes the appearance of the vesicular skin lesions. In that case, the etiology could be determined by the detection of intranuclear viral particles by EM and of viral antigens by fluorescence immunohistochemistry (169).

*Postvaccinial lymphadenopathy* was described initially in response to smallpox (vaccinia) vaccination, but similar responses may also follow other immunizations (170), such as to measles (171), rubella (170,172), and typhoid (173). In the classic series of Hartsock (174), the lymphadenopathy developed over a wide time range following vaccination (7–190 days), with a median of 14, and was mostly localized to the left supraclavicular region. Very importantly, the history of vaccination—which may have helped avoid a biopsy—had been overlooked during the preoperative evaluation in 14 of the 20 (70%) patients!

Localized or generalized lymphadenopathy is a common manifestation of untoward *reactions to medicaments*. In the long list of offenders (36), which include *para*-aminosalicylic acid, phenylmetazone, indomethacin, sulfonamides, penicillins, tetracyclines, and many other (175–178), the most commonly reported are anticonvulsants, such as various derivatives of phenytoin and carbamazepine (179). From our review of "Dilantin-associated" lymphadenopathy, it is clear that many different benign and malignant lymphoid lesions can be observed in patients taking this medication but that only a small minority of these can be attributed to the drug with any degree of certainty (10), all of the others representing either "late effects" or pure coincidence. The lesions that most likely represent actual hypersensitivity reactions to phenytoins are characterized by (a) PIH *and* GC reactions (see below), (b) a relatively short lag time from (re)exposure to the drug (from a few weeks to a few months), and (c) associations with one or more of the classic manifestations of a hypersensitivity syndrome (10), i.e., fever, skin rash, arthralgias, eosinophilia, and, less commonly, evidence of hepatic or bone marrow dysfunction (10,179,180). Similar lesions, characterized by PIH with atrophic GCs, developed at much longer intervals and were not associated with hypersensitivity syndrome. Even though the causal connection is more tenuous, they may represent "late effects." In fact, adverse reactions to drugs may clinically mimic a variety of acute infectious diseases and lymphoproliferative disorders (177,178).

### Histopathologic Findings

The morphologic manifestations of IM in LNs are variable and run the gamut from (a) predominantly immunoblastic proliferation to (b) prominent necrosis and (c) hemophagocytic histiocytic hyperplasia (181). As any combination of these findings may be observed in a single case, this general categorization is useful only insofar as it alerts the pathologist to consider EBV infection in the differential diagnosis of very different histopathologies. Only the first two situations are discussed at this point, as the third is best included in a later section.

The classic immunoblastic proliferative form of IM has been exhaustively described several times (153,154, 182–185). This manifests as an activated node with expansion of the paracortex, filling of the sinuses with transformed lymphoid cells, and GC hyperplasia or atrophy may be present in various proportions (182,185). This produces a blurring, but not an obliteration, of the LN architecture (Fig. 9A). The involvement of the LN may be nonuniform (185). At

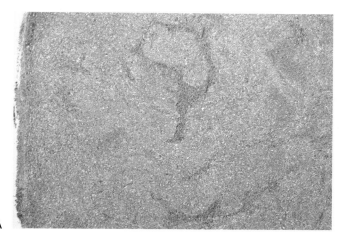 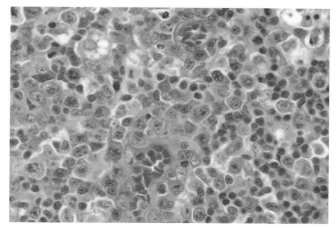

**FIG. 9.** Infectious mononucleosis (IM) lymphadenopathy. **A:** The diffuse expansion of the paracortex spares only small compressed follicles. **B:** Spectrum of lymphocyte transformation, with many immunoblasts and plasma cells. Several necrotic cells are seen *(right upper field)*.

low power, the paracortex may show a mottled appearance due to sparse immunoblasts in the background of small lymphocytes or, more often, a polymorphous sheet of transformed lymphoid cells studded with mitoses and single-cell necrosis (Fig. 9B). This characteristic polymorphous cellularity includes lymphocytes of various size, with open chromatin, visible nucleolus, and increasingly greater amounts of cytoplasm, up to large immunoblasts with pale amphophilic or plasmacytoid cytoplasm. Smaller plasmacytoid cells and plasma cells are numerous. In addition, sparse histiocytes, with or without necrotic debris, or ill-defined small granulomas can be seen, but very rarely eosinophils. The immunoblasts may show even marked nuclear atypia, leading to bi- or multinucleated cells that simulate Reed–Sternberg cells (183). There are abundant HEVs. The sinuses are often distended by transformed lymphocytes, or monocytoid B cells, and by intensely stained lymph nodes. The GCs may appear hyperplastic (182,183,185) or small and inconspicuous.

Necrosis is a consistent feature of IM. Most common is single cell necrosis, in the form of contracted eosinophilic apoptotic cells or clusters of karyorrhectic debris. Larger necrotic foci can also be seen in usual IM, but very extensive necrosis, leading to destruction of most or all of the LN, is characteristic of fatal cases (153,186). These manifest clinically with an aggressive course complicated by superimposed opportunistic infections, and multiple organ failure or hemorrhages. They are most often associated with the X-linked lymphoproliferative (Duncan's) syndrome, which is due to an ill-defined genetic immunoregulatory defect that renders the male affected individuals uniquely vulnerable to EBV infection (187). In addition, sporadic fatal cases, not genetically determined, have been reported (188–190).

The histologic manifestations of *HSV lymphadenitis* are very similar to those of IM in any of the four clinical situations described above (Fig. 10A): they include PIH, with increased vascularity, sinuses filled with immunoblasts or

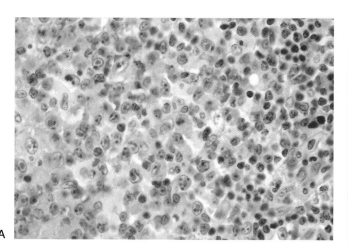 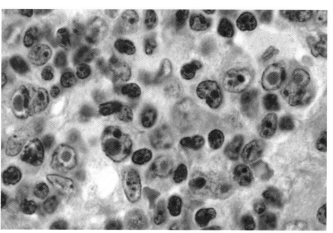

**FIG. 10.** HSV lymphadenopathy. **A:** Very marked proliferation of immunoblasts, many of which show eosinophilic nuclear inclusions. **B:** These are seen at higher power, surrounded by a clear halo.

monocytoid B cells, hyperplastic or atrophic GCs, and necrosis, the last feature apparently being more extensive in immunodeficient patients (166,167). Some unusual findings are reported in the appearance of HSV lymphadenitis. The foci of necrosis are either of the suppurative or ischemic type, and they are interpreted as "early" or "late," respectively (158,166). The necrotic areas may be surrounded by mononucleated or multinucleated cells with viral inclusions (157,160,167), by a rim of macrophages (158,160), or granulation tissue in the case of infarcts (167); or by histiocytes with erythrophagocytosis (159). Eosinophils are occasionally present (156), and lymphoma can be found in the same node (166,167). The inclusions are mostly nuclear in location (Fig. 10B) and take the form of either pale ground glass nuclei or Cowdry type A eosinophilic globules with a surrounding halo (156,157); rarely, they may be seen in the cytoplasm (158).

*Cytomegalovirus (CMV) lymphadenitis* has no specific features, except for the presence of the characteristic cytomegalic cells, with prominent intranuclear Cowdry type A inclusions and/or granular cytoplasmic inclusions (191,192). Predominant paracortical involvement, germinal center hyperplasia, or a mixture of the two is reported (193,194), which—by extrapolating serial studies of CMV lymphadenopathy in guinea pigs—probably reflects an early, late, or intermediate stage of the development of the disease (195). Multinucleated giant cells can be seen in *varicellazoster infection* (94) and both in *measles* and in *measles vaccination* (Warthin–Finkeldey cells) (171,196); in measles they have been shown to be the result of the fusion of noninfected B cells caused by the F-surface protein of virions released by infected cells (197). Similar cells seen in other reactive conditions have a T-cell phenotype (CD3+ CD43+ OPD4+) (198).

The nodal response to *medicaments* is very variable: atypical follicular hyperplasia (199), vasculitis (107,200), granulomatous reactions, and others have been reported, but the most common pattern is that of a PIH, indistinguishable from IM, including the presence of immunoblasts in the sinuses (10), necrosis, and Reed–Sternberg–like cells (36). Several cases with features of classic AILD have also been reported in response to Dilantin (36,201–206) and to carbamazepine (205, 207) and these seem to have a better prognosis than AILD in general (204–206). In our study of lymphadenopathies arising in patients treated with Dilantin, we found such a vast array of morphologies as to suggest that most represented a coincidental finding. The pattern associated with hypersensitivity featured both prominent PIH and reactions of the GCs, in the form of either common hyperplasia or "dissolution," as described earlier. Eosinophilia, a common finding in other series (179), was uncommon in our cases.

*Special Studies*

The proliferating cells in the tissues of IM represent a mixture of B and T immunoblasts, in various proportions (208–212). T cells usually predominate and are mainly CD8+ cells (209,213,214). Both CD4+ and CD8+ cells are activated and include a large population of UCHL-1/ CD45RO+ memory cells (213). The immunoblasts all express LCA/CD45 and most also express CD30 (215). In contrast, the large, atypical, Reed–Sternberg–like cells, 50–75% of which are L26/CD20+ and also express CD30, are LCA−; thus, they closely imitate the phenotype of the Reed–Sternberg cells in Hodgkin's disease, from which they are distinguished by being CD15− (215,216). EBV is present in all EM lesions (152) and can be detected with various approaches (217). For detecting EBV-DNA, Southern blotting, PCR, and *in situ* hybridization (ISH) have been used. The first of these methods, by determining the composition of the terminal repeats of the episomal and linear forms of the virus, is also useful in recognizing the poly- versus monoclonal nature and the latent versus lytic form of the EBV present in a given tissue. In addition, by evaluating the variations in the EBNA2 and EBNA3A, 3B, and 3C genes, it allows the distinction of two viral biotypes or strains, type 1 (A) or 2 (B). More commonly, viral products are assayed by ISH, northern blotting, or reverse transcriptase PCR. The detection of the EBV, encoded small RNAs (EBER1, 2) by ISH is especially useful, given the great abundance of these transcripts. Finally, immunohistochemical detection of virus-associated proteins (mainly EBNA2 and LMP1) has been used in the study of EBV-associated disorders. In IM, ISH for internal DNA repeats of the EBV genome (209–211,218) or EBER1 (219) and immunohistochemistry for LMP1 (215,216,220) demonstrate reactivity in many cells throughout the node or the interfollicular areas of the tonsil. The expression of EBNA2 through −6 and LMP1, in addition to EBNA1, produces the phenotype of EBV-immortalized lymphoblastoid cell lines (221). A combination of *in situ* and immunohistochemical techniques, in a study of tonsils of patients with IM, has demonstrated that EBER1 and 2 are present mainly in B cells, of immunoblastic, plasmacytoid, and small lymphocytic morphology, and in sparse T cells, but never in the epithelium, suggesting that, contrary to established opinion, it is the B cells, rather than the epithelium, that are the reservoir of the virus in the oral cavity (222). In another study as well (218), small lymphocytes in the GCs, endothelia, and sinus-lining cells have rarely been found to contain EBV-DNA by ISH.

In most of the cases of *HSV lymphadenitis,* the etiology was proven by the reactivity in the nucleus, cytoplasm, or both with antibodies to viral proteins (156,166), by ISH with anti-DNA probes (166,167), or by the detection of viral particles on electron microscopy (156,159). In the few immunophenotypic studies done, the immunoblasts and the cells containing the inclusions were shown to be T cells (156,159), in agreement with experimental data of replication of HSV in mitogen-stimulated T cells, as well as in B cells and macrophages (223). The infected cells bore neither B or T cell markers in another study (167).

In immunophenotypic studies of *CMV lymphadenitis,* al-

*Differential Diagnosis*

AIL-like lesions need to be differentiated both from other lymph node immune responses and from lymphomas. The line between AIL proper and *other benign lymph node reactions,* such as some hypersensitivity responses or autoimmune-associated lymphadenopathies (237) that may closely imitate it, is not, in fact, a definite one. The presence of GCs has been taken to exclude AIL in favor of "hyperimmune reactions" (238,281); we would agree with this only if the GCs have the usual hyperplastic morphology, because abnormal forms of GC reactivity are not uncommon in AIL (11). Hypocellularity and proteinaceous interstitial material (250) are helpful features, not seen in other immune responses. AIL differs from *other ALPDs,* such as systemic Castleman's disease and systemic polyclonal immunoblastic proliferations, because of its diffuse, rather than nodular, growth pattern, very marked vascularity, and the lack of massive plasmacytosis. The distinction of AIL proper from *AIL lymphoma* is even more difficult and subjective. There seems to be a general agreement (11), however, that the presence of clusters of "clear cells" favors a lymphoma (Fig. 12B), particularly, in our opinion, if these are mainly large cells. Immunophenotypic abnormalities of the proliferating T cells would also suggest a lymphoma. Whether the detection of clonal rearrangement bands of TCR and/or Ig heavy chain genes or single-cell changes on cytogenetics by itself qualifies the proliferation as lymphoma is debatable, since—as already said—both have been shown to disappear with time in some cases (244,261,264). As we suggested (282), only in the presence of a complete concordance of morphologic, immunophenotypic, and genotypic findings would we feel completely confident in diagnosing an AIL-like lesion as AIL proper or AILL. In all cases, judgment of the clinical situation and tempo of the disease has great importance and might override pathologic considerations in the management of the single patient. The possibility of misdiagnosing AIL as *Hodgkin's disease,* suggested in one of the original papers (202), seems to be more remote, despite the occurrence of eosinophils, epithelioid histiocytes, and occasional giant multinucleated cells in AIL. HD, in fact, would be ruled out in the presence of the very prominent vascularity, the spectrum of lymphoid transformation, and the numerous mitoses that characterize AIL.

*Evolution, Treatment, and Prognosis*

The clinical course of AIL is aggressive in most cases, but may vary from one or more episodes controlled by therapy to rapid progression refractory to therapy. Evolution to malignant lymphoma diagnosed histologically (usually of high grade, and of both B- and T-cell phenotype) (269) has been reported with an incidence variable from 0 to 35%, or in a total of 11% of the evaluable patients (11). Intercurrent infections are the most common cause of death (62%). In different series the overall mortality rate varied from 48% to 72%

and the median survival from 11 to 30 months (244). There is no consensus as to the best treatment for AIL: steroids alone have produced complete remission (mostly not durable, however) in approximately half of patients; the efficacy of single-agent chemotherapy is controversial; and multiple-agent chemotherapy has obtained complete remissions in 58% of patients overall (243). In recent trials, an aggressive 10-drug regimen, with or without initial prednisone (283), or doxorubicin-containing regimens (257), have not fared better; and experimental approaches with IFN$\alpha$ (284) or CSA (285) have had some success in a small number of cases.

A plethora of prognostic factors have been proposed, both clinical and pathologic (249,255,278,279,286,287). Among the former, the most consistently favorable one is achievement of complete, versus partial or no, remission; and negative factors include rashes, drug-related onset of disease, allergic history, and elevated serum lactic dehydrogenase and other laboratory abnormalities. Among the latter, the occurrence of immunoblastic clusters predicted poor outcome in both patients treated with steroids and those who received chemotherapy (249), as did a high proliferative index (>25% Ki-67+ cells) (255,256,287) and the presence of clonal rearrangements of the TCR$\beta$ gene (256); in contrast, abundance of eosinophils might be associated with a better outcome (201,287).

### Multicentric Castleman's Disease

Multicentric Castleman's disease (MCD) has been reported independently by several groups under different terms: multicentric angiofollicular lymphoid hyperplasia (69), angiofollicular and plasmocytic polyadenopathy (288), systemic lymphoproliferative disorder with morphologic features of CD (67,68), idiopathic plasmocytic lymphadenopathy with polyclonal hypergammaglobulinemia (289), plasma cell dyscrasia (290,291), and lymphogranulomatosis X with excessive plasmacytosis (238). The common features in these reports were a characteristic morphology, similar to that of CD of the plasma cell type (PC CD), and a characteristic clinical picture. It has become clear, however, that neither is specific. On the one hand, identical histologic nodal changes can be found in several other situations: autoimmune diseases, especially rheumatoid arthritis (292) and Sjögren's syndrome, HIV-related lymphadenopathy (115, 293), nodal or disseminated Kaposi's sarcoma (294,295), reactions to coexistent or adjacent malignancies or to skin diseases, vaccination, etc. On the other hand, the clinical presentation may suggest an autoimmune or collagen vascular disease, an infection, or a malignancy. Thus, the definition of MCD is by necessity a composite one and, in our opinion, requires four criteria:

1. The histopathology of PC CD.
2. The presentation as a predominantly lymphadenopathic disease, which consistently involves multiple and peripheral nodal groups.

3. Manifestations of involvement of multiple systems, including bone marrow, liver, kidney, and nervous system.
4. Exclusion of all other obvious causes for the above histology.

So defined, the process is of unknown etiology. Whether it represents a unique entity or just the expression of a common pathogenetic pathway is still unclear.

*Clinical Findings*

These have been recently reviewed (296) and are only summarized here. The median age of the patients is 64 years (age range 19–85); only rare cases have been reported in children and adolescents (297–300). About 66% of the cases occur in women. The onset of disease may be abrupt and dramatic or vague and indolent. Almost all patients present with symptoms, often severe. These include, in order of frequency, malaise, fever, night sweats, and weight loss. Lymphadenopathy is constant and involves multiple peripheral node groups; abdominal and mediastinal nodes are enlarged at presentation only in 10–15% of patients, but more frequently as the disease progresses. Hepatosplenomegaly is also observed in the majority of patients, up to more than 75% over the course of the disease. Less constant are edema tations (29%), and rheumatologic signs and symptoms. The skin changes are mostly localized or generalized maculopapular rashes; however, there are rare reports of distinctive "glomeruloid hemangiomas" (301), violaceous nodules composed of plasma cell infiltrates in the Japanese literature (302,303), or vitiligo (304). Not uncommon is severe sensory-motor peripheral neuropathy, which overlaps the picture of the so-called POEMS syndrome (see below), but there may be other neurologic manifestations, such as seizures, aphasia, dysarthria, coma, or pseudotumor cerebri cerebrospinal fluid (305,306). In some patients direct cerebrospinal fluid (CNS) or cerebrospinal fluid (CSF) involvement has been proven microscopically (307–309). A variety of rheumatologic manifestations have been reported, such as arthralgias, joint effusions, myalgias, keratoconjunctivitis sicca, Raynaud's phenomenon, as well as serologic findings (68), but none of sufficient degree as to permit a definitive diagnosis of a rheumatic disease.

Laboratory abnormalities are constant and greatly variable. Very common are anemia (89%), often of moderate to severe degree (<10 g/dl) and of chronic disease type, and thrombocytopenia (61%), at times proven to be immune in type (298,304). Most patients also have an elevated erythrocyte sedimentation rate (95%) and hypergammaglobulinemia (85%). Serum monoclonal spikes have been detected in rare cases, in association, as discussed below, with clonal plasma cell populations in the LNs (310–313). Renal dysfunction is quite frequent; it may be manifested by proteinuria (83%), hematuria, and renal insufficiency, and may contribute to hypoalbuminemia (100%). A nephrotic syndrome has been occasionally reported (68,314–317). Finally, liver function tests are quite frequently abnormal (69%).

There is often an overlap, and resulting confusion, between MCD and a clinicopathologic constellation that has been variably referred to as Takatsuki's (318) or Crow-Fukase's (319) or POEMS (320,321) syndrome. This last acronym summarizes the principal features as Polyneuropathy, Organomegaly (lymphadenopathy, splenomegaly), Endocrinopathy (diabetes mellitus, gynecomastia, amenorrhea), M proteins in the serum, and Skin lesions (pigmentation, hypertrichosis, sclerosis, hemangiomas) (291, 322–325). This complex has been reported in association with osteosclerotic myeloma and, in the lymph nodes, with the histopathology of PC CD. It appears to us and to others (322) that the two disorders, MCD and POEMS syndrome, although possibly related, are not identical and that their similarities may be due to some shared mechanisms, such as the antitissue effects of Igs produced by the plasma cells (321), and to a shared nodal histology, which—as we discuss below—is nonspecific, or common laboratory findings, such as serum monoclonal gammopathy. Thus, to deal with these "overlap" cases, we would start by recognizing that the POEMS syndrome may be associated, on the one hand, with MCD and, on the other hand, with osteosclerotic or, rarely, osteolytic (318,319) myeloma. We would then diagnose cases of the former type as true MCD manifesting with POEMS syndrome (306,322), and cases of the latter type as myelomas associated with *PC CD-like* lesions and POEMS syndrome (324,326,327).

*Histopathologic Findings*

The nodal architecture is blurred but recognizable. The low-power examination shows an expansion of the GCs, resulting in a vaguely nodular pattern, highly vascularized interfollicular areas, and often dilated sinuses filled with hyperchromatic lymph (Fig. 13A). The GCs may be hyperplastic, but most often manifest the classic abnormalities of ALPDs: ill-defined borders, with large cells spreading out in the mantle zone; increased vascularity; loose cellularity; abundance of pale eosinophilic cells (FDCs and epithelioid histiocytes); proteinaceous deposits; or the characteristic hyaline-vascular appearance. We have not found in the GCs the dysplastic dendritic cells characteristic of the localized HV variant of CD (74). The interfollicular tissue is rich in ramified HEVs, immunoblasts, plasma cells, and intermediate and immature plasmacytoid elements (Fig. 13B); there is frequently single-cell necrosis and a starry-sky appearance, with macrophages containing miniature, contracted plasma cells; and mitoses are numerous. This is the pattern that we referred to as "proliferative" (67) (Fig. 14A), and that requires differentiation from a lymphoma. In our study, where we examined multiple biopsies in the same patients, other patterns were also found at one time or another in the course of the disease: an "accumulative" pattern, in which mature

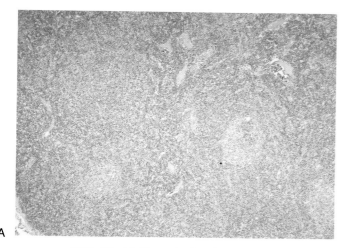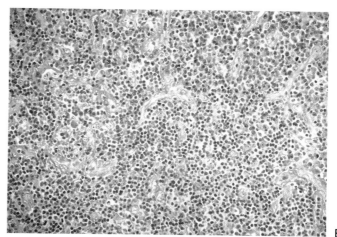

**FIG. 13.** Multicentric Castleman's disease. **A:** Abnormal follicles with intervening plasmacytosis. **B:** Rich vascularity and abundant plasma cells.

plasma cells predominated and were not associated with any increase in vascularity, immunoblastic proliferation, or mitoses (Fig. 14B); a burned-out stage, with predominantly hyaline-vascular GCs, sclerotic blood vessels, and sparse plasma cells; and completely nonspecific reactive hyperplasia of the node (67). This histopathologic variability during the evolution of the disease, on the one hand, justifies the need, in some cases, for additional biopsies in order to correctly diagnose this disorder. On the other hand, it may explain the reports of multicentric CD "of hyaline-vascular type" (these being, in our opinion, cases of the plasma cell type caught at a burned-out stage).

*Special Studies*

Only few immunophenotypic studies of MCD have been reported (92,95,328), and their findings are similar to those in the localized PC variant of CD. The follicles are characterized by a rich, often expanded and disrupted, network of FDCs, detected with the DRC-1 (92) or R4/23 (88,95) antibody, and by an abundant vascular component highlighted with factor VIII, *Ulex europaeus*, and laminin stains (88). The MZs are mainly composed of small cells that, in addition to B-cell-associated antigens and polyclonal IgM+D+, also express the pan-T antigen CD5 (88), which is not expressed by normal mantle cells. The follicles also contain T cells of both the CD4+ and CD8+ subsets and a variable number of Leu7/CD57+ cells (88,328). The interfollicular areas contain many T cells, predominantly of the CD4+ subset (88,92), admixed with an abundant population of polyclonal plasma cells (69,88,328–330). There are numerous reports in the literature that describe in MCD, as in localized CD, the development of a monoclonal plasma cell component, either diffusely replacing the interfollicular areas or

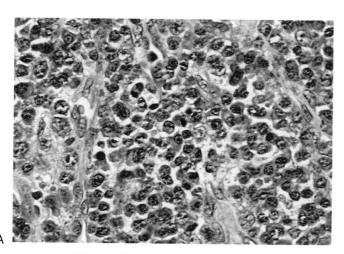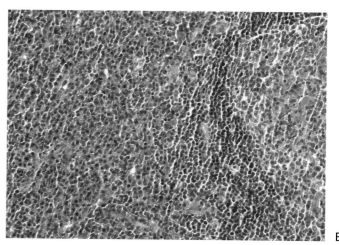

**FIG. 14.** Multicentric Castleman's disease. **A:** In the "proliferative" pattern, in addition to plasma cells, numerous large transformed cells are seen. **B:** In the "accumulative" pattern, mature plasma cells predominate, and blood vessels are sparse.

forming definite nodules (88,291,310,322,328,331). These focal proliferations were mostly of IgG or IgA type and were often associated with a monoclonal serum spike. The clinical implications of this component, which has been compared to a lymph node–based type of benign monoclonal gammopathy (328), are unclear; there was, in fact, no progression to a generalized disease in two reports (328,332), but the follow-up was short. The phenomenon of a clonal plasma cell population arising in lymph node lesions with the histopathology of PC CD is particularly common (29%) in cases associated with the POEMS syndrome (291).

Recently, several groups have studied the production of interleukins in the tissues of CD by identifying the protein products by immunohistochemical methods or the appropriate mRNA by *in situ* hybridization techniques (90–92, 280,333), and their findings are distinctly discordant. IL-6 has been detected in the GCs of MCD by some (92), but not by others (90,333), in the GCs of localized PC CD (280), or only in those of localized PC CD associated with systemic symptoms (91); the reactive cells have been identified as GC B cells by some (92,280) and as FDCs by others (91). Scattered IL-6-producing cells were found in the interfollicular areas by most (90,91,280,333), and were identified as macrophages, interdigitating cells, endothelia, lymphocytes, or immunoblasts. Sparse IL-1α- and IL-1β-producing cells were detected in the interfollicular areas with the same (280) or different (91) distribution seen in normal controls, but IL-1β+ cells were abundant and predominant over the IL-6+ cells in cases of MCD with POEMS (90). In some patients with PC CD (90,92,334), but not all (331), increased levels of IL-6 in the serum have been reported and correlate with the presence of hypergammaglobulinemia, and acute phase reactants, and symptoms (92); and IL-6 was produced in culture by peripheral blood mononuclear cells, identified as monocytes (333). Levels of IL-1β were also found to be elevated in some patients with MCD and the POEMS syndrome (90), but not in others (331).

There are few molecular studies (88,97,331,335,336), and only one (331) cytogenetic analysis of MCD. A rearrangement of antigen receptor genes was detected in 8 of 11 cases evaluated (73%); this involved the Ig heavy chain region in most cases, with or without rearrangement of the Ig light chain or TCRβ region. In two cases, a discordance was noted between immunophenotypic and immunogenotypic clonality findings (polyclonal immunostaining and Igl chain rearrangement; monoclonal immunostain and germ line Ig genes) (331). In this last study, a poorly defined karyotypic abnormality was found in two metaphases from one case, i.e., ins(1)(1pter—1cen::?::1cen—1qter) (331).

*Pathogenesis*

It is clear from clinical and pathologic data that despite some overlapping with autoimmune diseases, lymphoproliferation rather than tissue/cell injury is the essential feature of MCD (68). This disorder can be characterized histopatho-logically as a systemic unregulated B-cell proliferation, resulting in sustained production and accumulation of plasma cells. As in all ALPDs, there is a built-in risk that such a proliferation may give rise to clonal growths. These run the gamut from small clones, only recognizable by molecular genetic analysis, to immunohistochemically detectable monoclonal plasma cell components of indolent nature (328), to plasma cell dyscrasias and bona fide lymphoma.

Recent studies have identified some of the factors involved in MCD and provided the outlines of a convincing pathogenetic scenario, but the etiology(ies) and other questions remain open. The finding that the mantle zone lymphocytes in MCD, but not in reactive follicles, express CD5 (88), and the frequent occurrence of autoimmune manifestations have suggested that MCD might be *another disease of the CD5 + subset of B cells,* characteristically associated with autoantibody production (89). The excessive proliferation and plasma cell differentiation of this subset, as well as many signs and symptoms of MCD (fever, fatigue, myalgias, anemia, etc.), may be accounted for by an *abnormal production of specific cytokines,* known to have similar effects (296). Cultured LN cells from patients with CD have been shown to produce high levels of B-cell differentiation factor without any mitogenic stimulation (337). Both IL-6 and IL-1β, as discussed above, are produced by LN cells (and IL-6 also by peripheral blood mononuclear cells), and are found in high levels in the serum. And, finally, genetic manipulation of mice with coding sequences of IL-6 has reproduced a CD-like syndrome (338). A third, but less well-studied, factor is an *underlying defect of immunoregulation,* suggested by several lines of evidence: the occurrence of the disorder in older age groups, with senescent immune system; the striking histopathologic similarities of the nodal lesions of MCD and those observed in patients with immunodeficiencies (genetically determined or acquired); the association with Kaposi's sarcoma, a known "opportunistic" neoplasm; the frequent occurrence of infectious complications; and, finally, the actual demonstration of altered T- and NK-cell function in some of the patients so evaluated (95,311,339, 340). The initial stimulus for the lymphoproliferation in MCD is not known: the EBV genome has been detected in some cases in our study (336), but not in others (331); other viruses, infectious agents, or exposure to drugs, as in AIL, might be other possible initiating events. The reported association of Kaposi's sarcoma-associated herpesvirus [human herpesvirus (HHV)-8] with MCD in some patients (340A, 340b) is largely based, we believe, on a loose definition of MCD, on PCR-positive and Southern blot-negative findings, and on the concurrence of KS and homosexuality as risk factors in these patients (340b).

The relationship of MCD to the localized form of CD is a moot point (68). Although they share many histopathologic and clinical similarities, there are some subtle pathologic and striking clinical differences between them. In our experience, the disruption of the architecture and the abnormalities of the GCs are more prominent in the systemic form, as is the dilatation of the sinuses in one study (328). Clinically, MCD occurs in older patients, presents consistently with mainly peripheral rather than central adenopathy, has a more aggressive clinical course and a higher fatality rate, and is more frequently associated with infections and the development of malignancies (67,341). It is not clear whether these differences are due to a "more profound immunologic deficit" in the multicentric versus the localized disease (69) or rather indicate "different immune mechanisms" (91) or other pathogenetic differences, such as in etiologic agents or routes of involvement. Whatever the answer to these issues, it is clear from experience that the management of these two disorders is distinctly different: the localized form is surgically treatable, whereas MCD in most cases requires systemic therapy (68).

### Differential Diagnosis

In its "proliferative" form MCD requires differentiation, on the one hand, from other ALPDs and, on the other hand, from lymphomas showing marked plasmacytoid differentiation. The distinction from AIL has already been mentioned. In comparison with *systemic polyclonal immunoblastic proliferations* (see below), with which it shares striking immunoblastic and plasmacytoid differentiation, MCD shows less distortion of the architecture, greater prominence of the GCs, and rich vascularization. In MC, in addition, autoimmune hemolytic anemia is less common and less severe, and marked plasmacytosis of the peripheral blood is not a feature. The distinction from *lymphoplasmacytoid and immunoblastic lymphomas* is based on the recognition of persisting topographic markings throughout the LN, the abnormal reactive features of the GCs, the prominent vascularization, and the lack of nuclear atypia, as well as, in most cases, a polyclonal pattern on immunohistochemistry. In the occasional cases showing a striking preponderance of a population expressing one light chain, one would rely on an intermixed or adjacent background of cells bearing the other light chain to favor MCD versus lymphoma. Only histochemical evidence of monoclonality throughout the lesional tissue and/or rearrangement of both heavy and light Ig chains, rather than of the heavy chain alone, would strongly support a lymphoma in borderline cases.

The distinction of the "accumulative" pattern of MCD from *nodal plasmacytoma* is usually easy, based on the preservation of GCs and sinuses throughout the LN, the wide spectrum of plasmacytoid forms, and the lack of nuclear atypia. In cases of MCD with clonal excess, the same approach as discussed above for plasmacytoid lymphoma would apply.

### Evolution, Treatment, and Prognosis

Three different patterns of evolution can be discerned in the largest reported series of MCD. In some patients, the disease has a protracted, but relatively indolent, stable course; in others its evolution is punctuated by episodic exacerba-

tions and remissions; and in a small minority the course is aggressive and rapidly fatal (67,68). In our review of the literature (11), the mortality rate is high (50%), with a median survival of only 27 months; however, in our own series, this median was 30 months for the patients who died, but 97+ for those who survived (11). The most common cause of death is intercurrent infections, followed by renal failure, progressive lymphoproliferation, and malignancies.

The magnitude of the risk of malignancies is difficult to evaluate with certainty, due to the bias involved in the overreporting of cases with this specific complication. In a collation of 88 literature patients with MCD (series and single case reports), we found 11 cases of synchronous or metachronous Kaposi's sarcoma (12.5%), 8 of non-Hodgkin's lymphoma (9%), mostly of the immunoblastic plasmacytoid type, and 8 of plasma cell dyscrasia (9%) (11). In fact, however, in only rare instances has the diagnosis of lymphoma been documented immunophenotypically (342–345). In addition, some of the cases reported as nodal plasmacytoma, with short or no follow-up (335,346), may represent examples of the indolent clonal plasma cell growths discussed above rather than a clinical malignancy. The association of "Castleman's disease" with HD has been reported only in cases of localized CD and, with the exception of one metachronous case (109), obviously represents a CD-like reaction superimposed on, or adjacent to, HD (110,113,114), possibly resulting from the production of IL-6 by Reed–Sternberg cells and macrophages (347).

The information on treatment of MCD is limited, and an evaluation of the efficacy of the different approaches is difficult. The use of high doses of corticosteroids has produced long remissions in some patients (68,317). With chemotherapy, either as single agent or combination, good responses have also been obtained, but usually incomplete and nondurable. Rarely, either radiation therapy of the involved field (307) or removal of an involved large spleen (68) has led to sustained abatement of the clinical manifestations. In practice, based on our experience and the data available, the following strategy seems appropriate. If therapy is required, in the absence of a spontaneous remission, corticosteroids (which are less toxic in this patient population than are cytotoxic chemotherapy) are the first choice. They may be followed by chemotherapy in resistant cases, or by surgery or radiation therapy in cases with a more localized bulk of disease (296).

Statistical evaluation of survivals in our series (68) indicates that the three clinical features that together best predicted a fatal outcome were male gender, mediastinal enlargement, and an episodic pattern of disease ($p = 0.002$), but only one histologic feature was significantly associated with fatal outcome, i.e., the finding of only the proliferative pattern in multiple biopsies ($p = 0.005$).

### Posttransplant Lymphoproliferations

Posttransplant lymphoproliferations (PT-LPDs) are uncommon processes in the practice of pathology, but their study has provided precious insights into the pathogenesis of lymphoproliferative disorders. With the uncommon exceptions of cases of T-cell neoplasms and Hodgkin's disease, the PT-LPDs are B-cell proliferations and include a wide histologic spectrum of lesions. Almost all are causally related to EBV and result from its immortalizing effects on infected cells and from abnormalities of the immune response to it.

### Clinical Features

The incidence of PT-LPDs varies somewhat in different series, a function of both the type of graft and the regimen used for immunosuppression. It is around 1% for recipients of renal transplants and 2% for liver transplant recipients, and it varies from 1.8% to 11.4% for heart, from 4.6% to 9.4% for heart/lung, and from 0.6% to 7.4% for bone marrow transplants (BMT) (11,348,349). The highest of these figures is mostly obtained from the initial reports on patients treated with cyclosporine A (CSA) or triple therapy [CSA, azathioprine (AZT), and prednisone] or from a series in which high doses (>75 mg) of OKT3 were used (350). Dose reduction and monitoring of serum levels of the drug sharply reduced the incidence of PT-LPDs associated with the use of CSA from 9–13% to 0–1.5% (11). In recent series, the incidence of post-BMT LPDs is 0.6–0.7% (351,352). There might also be a relationship with the interval from transplant: in a recent large multicenter study, the overall incidence of LPDs in recipients of kidney and heart transplant was greater in the first year after transplantation (0.2% and 1.2%, respectively) than in later years (0.04% and 0.3% per year) (353).

There has also been a change in the clinical presentation of these disorders with the evolution from conventional immunosuppression (antilymphocyte globulin, AZT, and steroids) to more modern regimens used in solid organ transplantation (354). In patients treated with CSA, the LPDs tend to develop at a shorter interval from transplantation (median 4.5 months versus mean 9 months with conventional immunosuppression). Those patients treated with CSA also tend to have more often lesions in the lymph nodes and in the oropharyngeal tissue, and less often in the CNS and other unusual extranodal sites. Usual types of presentation today include: involvement of the head and neck lymph nodes with an IM-like illness; a localized tumor mass in the tonsil, gastrointestinal tract, or lung; or organ dysfunction (355–357). Disseminated LPD at presentation is instead uncommon (10–14%) (11), as is the involvement of some type of allograft: cardiac graft LPDs were reported in 18% of heart transplant recipients with LPDs, and renal allograft involvement in 14% of those with kidney transplant (353). In contrast, 60% of heart/lung transplant patients with LPDs showed lesions of the grafted lung (358). The clinical pattern of LPDs arising in BMT recipients is unique in that they develop at very short intervals from transplantation (median

2.5 months), are often disseminated at presentation, and have a rapid course and high mortality rate (232,351,352). With few exceptions, in most of the patients with PT-LPDs there is evidence of primary EBV infection or reactivation, as documented by serology and by an increased oropharyngeal shedding of the virus (359–361). The rare cases of *plasma cell neoplasia* present either as extramedullary plasmacytoma or classic multiple myeloma (357,362,363). The former were often multiple, developed at short intervals from transplantation (median 7 months) and could be treated with reduced immunosuppression, with or without radiotherapy for localized lesions; the latter occurred at much longer intervals (median 3.5 years) and required chemotherapy, as there appears to be no response to reduction of immunosuppression (357,362,363).

The clinical presentation of *T-cell LPDs*, of which a recent review has collected 25 examples to date (364), is similar to that of their B-cell counterpart. These have developed mostly after renal transplantation, again at a shorter interval in patients treated with CSA (median 1.5 years) than in patients treated with conventional immunosuppression (median 10 years) (364). Among those of the peripheral T-cell type the large majority were localized extranodal lesions, and a few were disseminated at presentation; the survival in the latter group was mostly a matter of a few days, while the median survival in the former group was 7 months. The very rare reported cases of posttransplant *Hodgkin's disease* (reviewed in ref. 365) were nodal in presentation and occurred at a 2- to 7-year interval from transplantation (365,366).

### Histopathologic Findings

The morphologic features of LPDs developing in transplant recipients are very variable and may even differ in different sites in the same patient.

1. One group of lesions is *not different from tissue reactions seen in immunocompetent patients*. In LNs or tonsils, classic IM can be seen, as a clinical pattern of "uncomplicated IM" has been reported in some PT patients (367). In tonsils or other sites, there can be bland inflammatory infiltrates rich in plasma cells, with only sparse large transformed cells, which have been referred to as "minimally polymorphic" (355) and, by us, as "plasma cell hyperplasia" (357).

2. The *"polymorphic" lesions* that we have described are the most common in our experience and others' (355, 357) and include a spectrum of lymphoproliferations that in both degree and cellular composition differ from those of the general patient population. They are characterized by extensive disturbance of the organ architecture (in the LNs, residual GCs are rarely observed, and there is extensive infiltration of the capsule) (Fig. 15A) and invasion of soft tissues, blood vessels, and nerves. The infiltrate is composed of a mixture of small and large cells of different types, from lymphoplasmacytoid

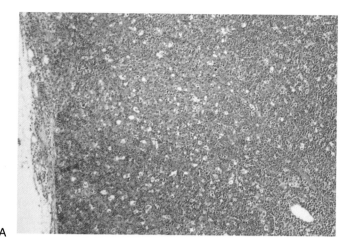
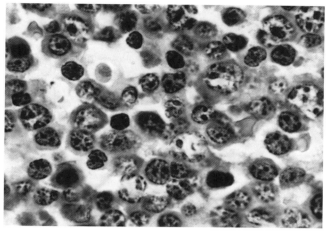

**FIG. 15.** Posttransplant polymorphic B-cell hyperplasia. **A:** Diffuse proliferation in the node and capsule, with prominent single-cell necrosis. **B:** Note the marked plasma cell differentiation, the lack of atypia, and the single-cell necrosis.

forms, plasma cells, and immunoblasts to cells resembling small cleaved and large noncleaved cells (368). When first attempting to correlate histologic patterns with clinical features and outcomes, we distinguished polymorphic B-cell hyperplasia (PBH) from polymorphic B-cell lymphoma (PBL). The former (Fig. 15B) shows very prominent plasmacytoid differentiation, lack of or minimal nuclear atypia, and minimal necrosis (limited to single cells or small groups of cells); the latter (Fig. 16A, B), in contrast, shows less plasmacytoid differentiation, rather marked nuclear atypia (with some of the cells being multinucleated and even Reed–Sternberg–like), and extensive areas of necrosis, often with ramified borders, producing a "geographic pattern." While these two forms are usually quite distinct, we have also occasionally seen intermediate patterns between the two, such as PBH with sparse atypical cells or more necrosis than expected (232).

3. Another large category includes tumors that, by way of contrast with the previous lesions, have been referred to as "*monomorphic*" and are similar to those encountered in the general immunocompetent population (355). While appropriate to neoplasms diagnosable as large or small noncleaved cell type, the term is not always appropriate for those of the immunoblastic lymphoma type, many of which have a distinct component of lymphoplasmacytoid forms associated with the immunoblasts. In our use of the term (357,369), the immunoblastic type differs from PBL in the prominence of homogeneous, intensely stained cytoplasm and large central nucleoli of the immunoblasts and the absence of cells with small cleaved cell morphology.

4. The rare cases of *plasma cell neoplasia,* as said already, include extramedullary plasmacytomas and multiple myeloma (357,362).

5. There are, finally, uncommon cases of *T-cell lymphoma*

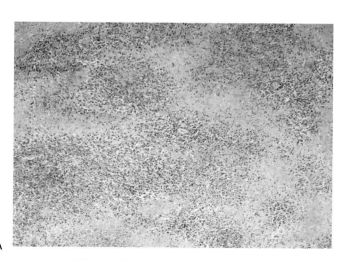
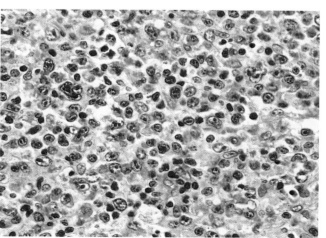

**FIG. 16.** Posttransplant polymorphic B-cell lymphoma. **A:** Abundance of necrosis with a geographic pattern. **B:** The proliferation shows limited plasma cell differentiation and striking atypia.

[reviewed by van Gorp et al. (364)] and even more rare cases of *HD* [reviewed by Doyle et al. (365)]. Most of the former fell into the categories of pleomorphic cell (medium or large); most of the latter included lymphoblastic, cutaneous T-cell, immunoblastic, and anaplastic large cell lymphomas. In most reports of HD, the diagnosis was based only on morphology (any type, except lymphocyte predominance). Only in one recent case were the Reed–Sternberg cells shown to have the classic null, CD15+, CD30+ immunophenotype; they also contained EBER by *in situ* hybridization (366).

*Special Studies*

In the B-cell LPDs, which are the overwhelming majority, the pattern of cytoplasmic or surface immunoglobulin expression varies. In a collation of cases from the literature, most cases (36%) were polyclonal, others (29%) were monoclonal, and 20% were Ig− but expressed HLA-Dr and B-cell antigens; in the remaining cases (15%), specimens from different sites in the same patients yielded diverse patterns of Ig expression (370) This heterogeneity is confirmed in recent series (361,371). In addition to B-cell antigens (CD19, CD20, CD22, and, less often, CD21), the proliferating cells were found to express CD23 in most cases and, consistently, adhesion molecules such as LFA/CD11a, ICAM-1/CD54 and LFA-3/CD58 (361). In two cases, the large cells, which had the morphology of anaplastic large cells and a B-cell phenotype, were CD30+ and EMA+ (372). A more or less abundant component of small reactive T cells is present, of both CD4+ and CD8+ subsets (361). In almost all of the B-cell LPDs of transplant recipients, there is evidence for the presence of EBV gene products of the latent cycle, represented by the immunohistochemical detection of EBNA2, LMP1 (361,373), and EBNA3 (361). Products of the lytic cycle (VCA, MA, and EA) are not expressed, but in one study the immediately early lytic protein ZTA (BZLF1) was detected in a small number of cells (374). In *T-cell neoplasms,* the phenotype was as expected by their histologic type, except for a higher incidence of the CD8+ or CD4−8− phenotype among the peripheral cell lymphomas (364).

Molecular genetic studies of PT-LPDs have provided further evidence both of the heterogeneity of the Ig expression and of the presence of EBV (375). In most of the B-cell lesions, whatever their histologic type and their pattern of Ig expression, monoclonal rearrangement bands are identified (355,376,377). However, in a small number of cases (372,376,378), no Ig gene rearrangements were found. In patients in whom multiple specimens are obtained, one of three possible rearrangement patterns may be detected: identical bands at different sites, suggesting the metastatic dissemination of one clone (377–379); different clonal bands, indicating multiple clonal proliferations (377); or, less commonly, multiple faint rearrangement bands, which are interpreted as oligoclonal proliferations (380). Another marker of clonality is based on the consistency, within the progeny of an infected cell, in the number of EBV terminal repeats that each

infecting virus expresses in its episomal (circular) form, a consistency that is reflected in a single band in Southern blot hybridization. By this method it has again been proven that most PT-LPDs are monoclonal or oligoclonal proliferations (372,377,381,382). The molecular techniques already discussed for IM (Southern, PCR, *in situ* hybridization) have been employed to document, in almost all cases of PT-LPDs, with rare exceptions (363,383), the presence of the EBV genome (371,372,384–388) or the products of its gene expression, especially EBERs by *in situ* hybridization (362,389,390). With this last technique, the PT-LPDs demonstrate localization of EBV in the majority of the proliferating cells (211), but not with uniform intensity (384). As a result of all of these studies, both immunohistochemical and molecular, it was concluded that the pattern of EBV latency gene expression in PT-LPDs is like that of lymphoblastoid cell lines, i.e., unrestricted or of type III (EBNA1+, 2+, 3+, LMP+ and EBER+) (361,373,391). However, more recently, it has been shown that the pool of EBV-infected B cells in PT-LPDs is more heterogeneous, also containing a HD-like restricted latent, or type II population (EBNA1+, EBNA2−, LMP1+/−, LMP2+ and EBER+), as well as cells in the lytic cycle. The selective growth of one or another would depend on the degree of immunosuppression, with a good residual T-cell response leading to the expansion of the type II population and a poor T-cell response being reflected in an expansion of the type III population (392). The etiologic role of EBV is less strong among the T-cell PT-LPDs: in only 4 of 14 cases analyzed was EBV demonstrated in the lymphoid lesion by Southern blot analysis and ISH (393–395). Finally, molecular techniques have recently revealed that PT-LPDs may be associated with oncogene activation and/or abnormalities of tumor suppressor genes. Rearrangements of c-myc were detected only in monomorphic lymphomas and one with "dysplastic plasmacytoid differentiation" in one study (376), and in the immunoblastic plasmacytoid/multiple myeloma group of our study (357). In addition, in this morphologic group we found alterations of N-ras and the p53 tumor suppressor genes. The lesions with these genomic changes did not respond to discontinuation of immunosuppression and required systemic chemotherapy (357,376).

There are only sparse reports of cytogenetic analysis of PT-LPDs, and they do not show any specific karyotypic pattern (232,368,394,396,397). The most frequent lesions (that appear in more than five cases) are in chromosomes 6 and 11. The former is mainly involved in translocations (with different chromosomes and at different breakpoints) or is lost. The latter shows trisomy or duplication, changes that have also been described in secondary (post-therapy) lymphomas (398). The classic translocation of Burkitt's lymphoma, another EBV-associated lymphoproliferation, has been detected in only one case (399). As in AIL-like lesions, unrelated clones (232,397) or nonclonal abnormalities (394,396, 397) have been reported, again suggesting a multiclonal origin for PT-LPDs.

## Pathogenesis

The information acquired in the studies cited above has revealed the main outlines of a pathogenetic scenario for PT-LPDs, although many issues remain unresolved. Clearly there are three main factors at play: the infection with EBV, abnormalities of the immune response to it, and cytogenetic/genomic changes. The *essential role of EBV* is supported by many lines of evidence, which have been recently reviewed (11): increased oropharyngeal shedding of the virus, serologic evidence of infection (primary or reactivation), detection of the EBV genome or its products, and the experimental reproduction of these lymphoproliferations in animals (233,400,401). Several of the EBV gene products have immortalizing effects on the infected lymphoid cells: EBNA1, by increasing c-myc expression; EBNA2, by up-regulating expression of LMP1, which, in turn, increases bcl-2 expression (402); and BHRF1 and EBNA5, by adding to the anti-apoptotic effect of bcl-2 (403). This excessive EBV-driven proliferation is not held in check due to *abnormalities of the cytotoxic T-cell and NK-cell response to EBV-related proteins,* especially EBNA2 and LMP1, that result from the immunosuppressive regimens used in transplant recipients (404–410). Some of these effects are mediated by increased production of IL-6 by B and T cells and macrophages; IL-6, in fact, reduces the NK-cell and T-cell cytotoxic activity (411) and functions as an autocrine mechanism in B-cell proliferation (412,413). The *chronic antigenic stimulation* produced by the graft could be another source for an excessive production of IL-6, as chronic inflammation is in other situations (414). The role of *genetic changes* mentioned above in the pathogenesis of PT-LPDs is still unclear. However, correlation of histopathologic, genomic, and clinical patterns in our recent study has not only confirmed the progression from polyclonal to monoclonal proliferations but has also suggested a further step in the development of these lesions. This occurs with the intervention of genomic mechanisms (c-myc, N-ras, p53), which render the lymphoproliferation unresponsive to a reduction of the immunosuppression and the restoration of the host immune system. A double, and not necessarily contradictory, role for c-myc has recently been suggested: in the presence of an anti-apoptotic effect, due to viral products, such as BHRF1, or to bcl-2 or p53, c-myc may push the cells toward malignant transformation; but, in the absence of such an effect, c-myc activation can push the cells toward programmed cell death (403).

A recent observation that it is time that we "discern a more sophisticated underlying mechanism than the crude concepts of immunosuppression or immunostimulation that would explain the markedly different lymphoma risks seen in various groups with marked immune abnormalities" (415) applies especially well to PT-LPDs. Because EBV infection and immune abnormalities are factors operative in all transplant recipients, but only a small minority of them develop LPDs, additional more subtle explanations are being investigated today: the role of primary EBV infection after, versus before,

transplantation (416,417), of deletions in the LMP1 gene (418), of the low-level expression of LFA-1 (361) and down-regulation of EBNA2 and LMP1 (392) in escaping immunosurveillance, of reduced production of antibodies to EBNA1, EBNA2, and EBNA-LP (392,419), or of T-cell depletion of the donor marrow (420). Other factors may be relevant and need to be investigated, such as the donor versus recipient origin of the infected B cells (351,361), the increased susceptibility to and interaction of EBV with other viruses (232,351), and the role of other cytokines (TNFα, TNFβ, IL-10) (421).

## Differential Diagnosis

In the transplant recipient the polymorphic lesions (PBCH and PBCL) are usually easily recognizable. They are characterized by hypercellularity, the characteristic mixture of lymphoplasmacytoid and immunoblastic elements with small angulated cells and nonimmunoblastic large cells, the abundance of mitoses, the presence of necrosis (single cell or minimal in PBCH or extensive and ramified in PBCL), and the infiltration of normal structures. However, the clear-cut histopathologic differences between PBCH and PBCL do not appear at this point to correspond to differences by other criteria available today. Thus the distinction between PBCH and PBCL is less important than their separation, as a group, from usual tissue reactions in the immunocompetent host, on one side, and from immunoblastic lymphoma, on the other side. This distinction has important treatment implications that are discussed below. PBCH differs from *"plasma cell hyperplasia"* and *"uncomplicated"* IM in the greater complexity of the cellular composition, greater degree of cellularity, and features of invasiveness; in both of the latter disorders the involvement of the nodal architecture is uneven, and residual normal structures persist. PBCH differs from *immunoblastic lymphoma* in the presence of a nonimmunoblastic component of small and large cells and the lack of nuclear atypia, and PBCL differs from it in the scarce plasmacytoid differentiation. EBV studies can be of help in these differential diagnoses. In one study (384), EBV DNA was found by ISH in all tissues involved by PT-LPD, but not in "inflammatory mononuclear infiltrates . . . without histopathologic evidence of PT-LPD." And, in another study, in cases of "uncomplicated" IM, only 10–20% of the cells showed EBV nucleic acid by ISH, versus the majority of the neoplastic cells in PBCL; one case of PBCH "showed only weak and focal cellular localization of grains over background" (211).

## Evolution, Treatment, and Prognosis

The heterogeneity of PT-LPDs makes it difficult to provide a meaningful categorization of these disorders for the purposes of management and prognosis. In the absence of such a system, management has been largely empirical, adding to the complexity of evaluating and comparing clinical course and outcome in different studies: antiviral therapy (359,360), high-dose chemotherapy or radiation therapy (377,422–424), anti-B-cell monoclonal antibody therapy (234), high-dose gammaglobulin and IFNα (425), and reduction or discontinuation of immunosuppression (349) have been used with mixed success in different settings. The last approach is based on the rationale that the expression of EBV-associated proteins, which are targets of T-cell responses, and of adhesion molecules, which facilitate their interaction with normal B and T cells, makes PT-LPDs susceptible to destruction by the host immune system, when restored by reduction of iatrogenic immune suppression or stimulated by cytokines (373).

The LPDs in recipients of BMTs appear to be more severe and more frequently fatal than those of solid organ transplant recipients (232,351); risk factors in these patients are HLA mismatch, T-cell depletion of the donor bone marrow (which may impart an inability to reconstitute normal immune function), the occurrence of graft-versus-host disease, and anti-CD3 therapy (232,351,352). In recipients of solid organ transplants donor-derived, but not host-derived, PT-LPDs are mostly limited to the allograft and have not been fatal (426). The load of EBV must be very relevant to evolution and prognosis: increased intensity of signal in biopsy material studied by ISH (388,389), on the one side, and the number of peripheral blood EBV-infected lymphocytes (which was greater in patients who developed primary EBV infection after their transplant) (416,419), on the other side, were good predictors of the development of LPDs in transplant recipients. Late occurrence of the LPDs (one year after transplantation) was associated with more frequent dissemination, poorer response to decreased immunosuppression, and higher mortality rate than early occurrence in one series (422), but such correlation did not hold in our study (356). The type of immunosuppressive regimen used and the resulting degree of immunosuppression are clearly important risk factors, as illustrated by high-incidence figures quoted above for OKT-3 and triple therapy, and the relatively low incidence of PT-LPDs in old regimens using ALG, which might have a cytotoxic effect on activated B and T cells (427). Lesions in the gastrointestinal tract and lung responded better to reduction in immunosuppression and were associated with a better survival than those at other extranodal sites in our series (356). Increased levels of serum IL-6 were detected in transplant recipients who developed LPDs (428), and decreased levels of anti-EBNA1, -EBNA2, and -EBNA-LP antibodies (which correlated with increased numbers of EBV-infected blood lymphocytes) might be useful prognostic markers to monitor and/or predict the development of PT-LPDs (419).

Histologic distinctions (PBCH, PBCL, and monomorphic lesions) and clonality have shown inconsistent correlations with clinical course and outcome (232,355,356). However, the presence of strong clonal Ig gene rearrangement bands, with or without rearrangements of c-myc, correlated with

poor response to reduction of immunosuppression in the Pittsburgh series (355,376). In a recent analysis of the PT-LPDs at Columbia University, good correlations emerged among histopathologic classification, molecular genetic characteristics, and clinical evolution (357), suggesting the existence of three distinct clinicopathologic categories: (a) plasmocytic hyperplasias were most often diagnosed in the oropharynx or the lymph nodes, had polyclonal patterns of Ig genes and EBV-fused termini, and lacked oncogene and tumor suppressor gene alterations; (b) polymorphic lesions (PBCH and PBCL) arose in lymph nodes or extranodal organs, had monoclonal patterns, and similarly lacked the above genomic alterations; (c) immunoblastic lymphoma and multiple myeloma presented with disseminated disease, were monoclonal according to both criteria, and contained alterations of one or more oncogene or tumor suppressor genes (N-ras, c-myc, p53). Whereas the first two categories of LPDs tended to regress with discontinuation of immune suppression or resolved with more aggressive intervention, the third did not respond to reduced immune suppression and progressed rapidly (429). These data, although they need to be confirmed by other studies, seem to offer an accurate system for approaching the management of PT-LPDs based on pathologic criteria: reduction of immunosuppression and antiviral therapy can be used initially in every case, while molecular data are being obtained on the biopsy; these or other nonaggressive approaches may be continued if no genomic abnormalities are detected, but aggressive chemotherapy (423,424) is probably required when such are found.

### Systemic Polyclonal Immunoblastic Proliferations

The term "systemic polyclonal immunoblastic proliferation" (SPIP) has been used recently to describe the clinicopathologic presentation of a group of patients (430–432) with a process that fits well into the category of ALPDs. The combination of clinical and histopathologic features seen in these patients has been previously reported in the literature. The earliest report might be that of Forster and Moeschlin (433) on a patient interpreted as manifesting "extramedullary leukemic plasmacytoma with dysproteinemia and acquired hemolytic anemia," but similar cases were described later under the term "diffuse sarcomatosis with plasmocytic differentiation" (434). With the addition of two patients whom we have seen and are reporting on (A. Marcelli and G. Frizzera, unpublished observations), 15 such cases represent what we believe to be, by a unique combination of clinical, laboratory, and pathologic findings, a distinct new member of the ALPDs.

### Clinical Findings

With the exception of one patient (430), whose LPD might be an expression of his acquired immunodeficiency syndrome (AIDS)—and thus is not considered further in this discussion—all patients were older adults, 53–78 years of age (median 60), and mostly men (9 men, 6 women). They presented with severe systemic symptoms, often of acute onset, generalized lymphadenopathy (79%), and hepatosplenomegaly. Fifty-seven percent had skin rashes and 29% had jaundice. The most consistent laboratory abnormality was the presence of numerous immunocytes, ranging from plasma cells to large immunoblasts, both in the peripheral blood (100% of cases) and the bone marrow (86% of cases). Other common laboratory findings included positive Coombs' test, polyclonal gammopathy, elevated ESR, and anemia. Thrombocytopenia (<100,000/L) was observed in 65% and leukocytosis (>1500/L) in 60%.

### Histopathologic Findings

The characteristic changes in the peripheral blood and bone marrow are discussed later in this chapter. A description of the LN pathology is given in two of the reports (430,434) and matches our experience with our two patients. The LN architecture is largely obliterated by a diffuse lymphoid proliferation (Fig. 17A) that also involves the capsule. Portions of the sinuses and rare GCs, mostly atrophic, can occasionally be seen. The infiltrate is composed of a spectrum of plasmacytoid elements, mature and immature, and large immunoblasts, without nuclear atypia (Fig. 17B). Mitotic activity is brisk. There is only moderate vascularity. The same spectrum of plasmacytoid differentiation was observed in the portal triads and, focally, in the sinusoids in one case (432).

### Other Pathologic Findings

Immunostains for cytoplasmic Igs have shown a polyclonal pattern (430,432). Both B and T cells can be identified. In contrast with the evidence in the hepatic infiltrate (432), where the large cells were B in type and the small cells were T, we found in one of our nodes a surprisingly great population of large T cells and these were shown—by double staining with CD3 polyclonal antiserum and with MIB (Ki-67)—to be actively proliferating. Molecular analysis of one of our cases demonstrated oligoclonal B-cell populations but germ line configuration of the TCR genes. Cytogenetic studies, done in two reported cases (430) and in both of our own, showed clonal abnormalities in all. In three of them, there were chromosomal translocations producing a break at 14q32, including one with the classic t(14;18) of follicular lymphoma; in the remaining case, there was a t(5;9)(p14;q32). This last abnormality is not a recurrent change in neoplasia, but breaks at 9q32 have been found to recur in multiple myeloma and plasma cell leukemia (435).

These findings obviously have relevance in the pathogenesis of these lesions, suggesting that, as in B-cell LPDs, a clonal proliferation might arise in them when an unknown oncogene is joined to the Ig heavy chain gene. The initial stimulus for the proliferation is at this point unknown, even though this might have been related in one patient to *Pseudomonas aeruginosa* septicemia (432) and several other patients had evidence of autoimmune phenomena (430,434). As in PC CD, it is possible that IL-6 might have a role (436,437) not only as a factor in the B-cell proliferation and plasmacytoid differentiation but also in producing some of the characteristic laboratory and clinical findings in these patients. Some of these findings, in fact, closely mimic those observed in rheumatoid arthritis, in which a role for IL-6 is well recognized (438). Finally, as many characteristics of SPIP were seen in a patient with AIDS (430), a form of more subtle deficiency in the other patients might also underlie, and partially account for, the excessive B-cell proliferation that characterizes this disorder.

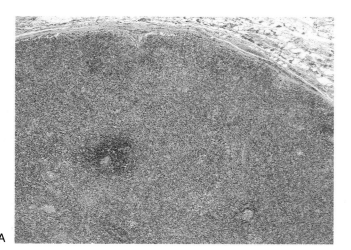
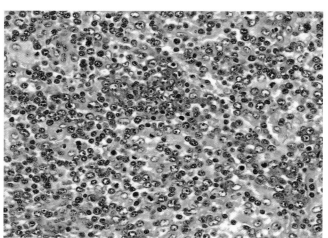

**FIG. 17.** Systemic polyclonal immunoblastic proliferation. **A:** Diffuse expansion of the paracortex, with recognizable small germinal centers and peripheral sinuses. **B:** Massive proliferation of immunoblasts and plasmacytoid cells.

*Differential Diagnosis*

Although SPIP shares many of the histologic features of other ALPDs, it has some distinctive characteristics. This disorder is different from *AIL* in that it is hypercellular, the plasmacytoid differentiation is very prominent, and the vascular component is moderate at best. From a clinical point of view, patients with SPIP have a higher incidence of Coombs' test positivity, peripheral plasmacytosis, and thrombocytopenia than those with AIL. SPIP is also different from *MCD*, despite the abundant plasmacytoid differentiation, because it lacks the follicular pattern, the abundance of abnormal hyperplastic GCs, and the rich vascularity typical of *MCD*. In addition, the incidence of Coombs' test positivity and peripheral plasmacytosis is much higher than in patients with PC CD. The most difficult differential diagnosis is with a *lymphoplasmacytoid or immunoblastic lymphoma*. The preservation of some topographic markings of the LN and the lack of nuclear atypia are suggestive criteria, and the polyclonal pattern of Ig staining provides definitive evidence in favor of SPIP.

*Evolution, Treatment, and Prognosis*

The treatment of these patients was variable and consisted of multiple drug chemotherapy in seven of them, steroids and cyclophosphamide or vincristine in five, and steroids alone in two. All patients improved initially, and half of them can be considered to be free of disease by clinical and laboratory parameters. The demise in the others was due to superimposed infections. Recognition of this entity is thus important, as it identifies a particularly acute and severe, but curable, form of ALPD.

## HISTIOCYTIC/DENDRITIC CELL PROLIFERATIONS SIMULATING NEOPLASMS

### Hemophagocytic Syndromes

The finding of histiocytic hyperplasia with erythrophagocytosis is not uncommon in lymph nodes. It may be a purely histologic feature of no clinical relevance in such different situations as after recent blood transfusions (439), in mediastinal nodes of cystic fibrosis (440), or in axillary LNs of patients who underwent breast biopsy (441). However, it may also be one expression of a severe clinicopathologic hemophagocytic syndrome (HPS), which can be fatal. Thus, on the one hand, this finding should always prompt a request for clinical and laboratory evidence of a systemic disorder; on the other hand, "one is wiser to record the presence of hemophagocytosis as a descriptor, and not embellish it as a syndrome" if such evidence is not forthcoming (440).

HPSs may develop in very diverse contexts, accounting for some clinical and pathologic differences:

1. *Immunodeficiencies:* (a) genetically determined, such as the familial hemophagocytic lymphohistiocytosis (FHL) (442) or the Chediak–Higashi syndrome (443); (b) iatrogenic, such as in transplant recipients (444) or secondary to steroid therapy (445); and (c) ill-defined disorders of immunoregulation, such as seen in abnormal responses to EBV ("fatal infectious mononucleosis") (446–448) or other infectious agents: viruses, such as CMV (449), varicella-zoster (445), adenovirus (444), influenza A (450), HIV (451), which prompted the original designation of "virus-associated hemophagocytic syndrome" (444); bacteria (452,453); chlamydia (454); protozoa (455); and others. This last set of "primary" infectious HPS and the familial form, FHL, which are often clinically indistinguishable in young children, have been recently unified under the term "hemophagocytic lymphohistiocytosis" (HLH) (440,456).
2. *T-cell or NK-cell lymphomas/leukemias* (449,457–462) and, more rarely, B-cell neoplasms (463–466).
3. *Drug reactions,* for example to phenytoins (467) or *lipid-rich parenteral alimentation* (468).
4. *Systemic lupus erythematosus* (SLE) (469).

*Clinical Findings*

The clinical presentation of HPS is pleomorphic and may mimic infectious mononucleosis, septicemia, hematologic malignancies, encephalitis, and systemic autoimmune disorders. Thus the diagnosis is difficult and is often obtained, in fact, only postmortem (456). Although the presentation may vary according to the clinical context in which the HPS develops (470), the complete syndrome, as seen in HLH, includes the following: persistent fever (for a week or longer) and other severe systemic symptoms; splenomegaly, mostly with hepatomegaly; pulmonary infiltrates (471); skin rash; lymphadenopathy and laboratory abnormalities (cytopenias, especially thrombocytopenia, hypertriglyceridemia, and/or hypofibrinogenemia; abnormal LFTs; abnormal coagulation parameters; and CSF pleocytosis) (440,442,456). An increased serum level of multiple cytokines or cytokine-associated factors (IL-1, IL-2 receptor, IL-6, IFN$\gamma$, macrophage colony-stimulating factor, TNF$\alpha$) is a characteristic finding of the active phase of the disease (472–478) and obviously has an important pathogenetic role discussed below. Immunologic defects in these patients are often subtle (446–448, 479).

The cases of familial type are distinguished by a family history (the pattern of inheritance being autosomal recessive) or parental consanguinity, the very early age of onset (<2 years in 80–90% of cases), and a poor prognosis (440, 442,470). Evidence of viral infection, especially EBV, has been obtained in some cases, and there are multiple immune defects (440,442).

*Histologic Findings*

The HPSs are histologically characterized by histiocytic proliferation with hemophagocytosis, most easily found in

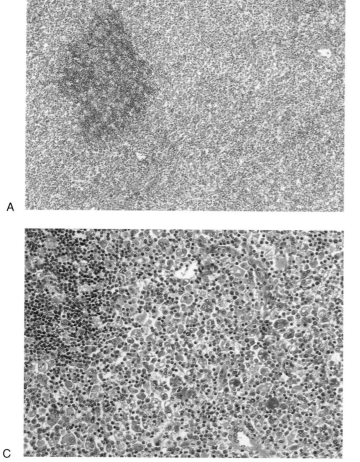

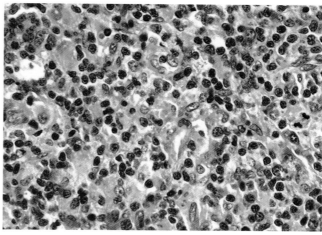

**FIG. 18.** Hemophagocytic syndrome. **A:** Paracortical distribution of the process, with a residual follicle. **B:** Sparsity of hemophagocytic cells in the context of lymphoid activation. **C:** Very abundant component of hemophagocytic cells.

the LNs, in the spleen (red pulp), in the liver (portal triads and, less prominently, the hepatic lobules), but not as often in the bone marrow (456). The nodal involvement is predominantly paracortical (Fig. 18A) but also extends to the sinuses. It may vary from sparse hemophagocytic histiocytes, difficult to recognize in the context of a lymphoid proliferation (Fig. 18B), to a massive infiltration of histiocytes throughout the node, recognizable at low power (Fig. 18C) (479). The histiocytes may contain one or many rare red blood cells, as well as other blood cells, and may show no nuclear atypicality and few or no mitoses.

In an HPS not associated with a neoplasm, there may be a rich lymphoid background composed of many small lymphocytes, as well as activated lymphoid cells, due to an underlying infection, especially viral; however, lymphoid depletion develops in later stages (444,456,480). Burned-out GCs may be seen, as well as foci of nonsuppurative necrosis (447,481). Fibrinoid necrosis of the blood vessels and hematoxylinophilic bodies were features of the acute lupus HPS in one study (469). In the HPS arising on a T- or NK-cell neoplasm, the lymphoid component shows cytologic atypicalities and abundant mitoses, and there are other features typi-

cal of the tumor (panniculitic pattern, angiocentricity and angiodestruction, etc.). Therefore, the presence of histiocytic hyperplasia with hemophagocytosis requires not only a search for clinical and laboratory signs of an HPS, but also a thorough evaluation of the lymphoid component in order to recognize the presence of an underlying malignancy.

*Special Studies*

The immunophenotype of the histiocytes is usually that of mature macrophages, but in one well-studied case it was a "hybrid" between that of macrophages and that of Langerhans cells (CD1α+ and S-100β+) (482). In HPSs non-associated with neoplasm, the lymphoid infiltrate is composed predominantly of T cells (483–486), which are of CD8+ type (483,484), and rare B cells (483). In addition, a considerable number of CD56+ CD57− NK cells have been reported, which, by double labeling with CD3, were shown to be distinct from T cells (483). In several of these studies, the proliferating cells, of either T- or NK-cell type, have been shown to be mono- or biclonal by hybridization analysis of the T-cell receptor genes or the EBV-fused termini (483–485,487). There are, on the other hand, reported cases of T-cell proliferations, one presenting as EBV-associated HPS (488) or developing in two siblings with FHL (489), that were interpreted as T-cell lymphomas based on the very same molecular criteria. Cases like these raise the issue of whether the presence of T-cell clones in patients with aggressive IM or HPS is synonymous with lymphoma and puts them in the category of EBV-associated T-cell lymphomas with HPS (461) or whether, as in EBV-related posttransplant LPDs and other B-cell ALPDs, a multistep process needs to be considered that requires additional genomic changes for a clone to become a bona fide neoplasm.

Among the infectious agents detected in HPS, EBV appears to be the most common in the USA [58% (490)] and in Asia (461,481,485–487,491,492). It can present as fulminant IM, most frequently in very young children (484–487,492), or in association with an NK-cell proliferation (459,483) or T-cell lymphomas (461,490,493); in the last instance, EBV-related HPS can be the initial clinical manifestation ("malignant histiocytosis–like peripheral T-cell lymphoma") or develop at relapse or even in clinical remission of the lymphoma (493). The evidence for the etiologic role of EBV comes from serology (448,486,487,492), Southern blot analysis (478,483–485,487,494), PCR (481,487), or in situ hybridization (484,486,490) techniques. By double labeling methods EBV has been detected in T cells (485,486,490), NK cells (483), and B cells (490).

### Pathogenesis

It has recently become clear that the array of cytokines and other factors, which are found in excessive levels in the serum of patients during the active phase of HPS but decrease during a remission (459,473,475–478), may account for many of the clinical and pathologic manifestations of the disease (440,442). From this notion and the recognition of an association with specific clinical situations, mentioned at the beginning of this section, a plausible pathogenetic scenario has emerged for the HPSs.

In non-neoplasia-associated HPS, it is probable that varied states of immunodeficiency account for an abnormal immune response to infectious agents; this would result in the CD8+ T cells producing an excess of lymphokines, such as GM-CSF and IFNγ, which leads to histiocytic hyperplasia and activation, with increased hemophagocytosis (456,459, 476,477). The activated histiocytes, in turn, by producing excessive monokines, such as prostaglandins (495), IL-6, and TNFα (456,475,477), would be responsible for many of the manifestations of the disease, including fever, lipid abnormalities, cytopenias, and coagulopathy (440,442,456).

In HPS associated with neoplasia, it is probably the lymphokines produced by the neoplastic T cells that stimulate the histiocytes with the same consequences. This notion is supported by the detection of such a factor in cell culture supernatants from angiocentric immunoproliferative lesions (457). Finally, the histiocytic hyperplasia and increased hemophagocytosis occurring in HPS associated with drugs or SLE are thought to be due to a stimulation by antihematopoietic antibodies or immune complexes (469).

### Differential Diagnosis

The essential distinction is between HPSs associated and not associated with a *T-cell or NK-cell neoplasm*. In the former, beyond the histiocytic hyperplasia and hemophagocytosis, one should look for the disruption of the nodal architecture and other characteristic pathologic features that allow the identification of the underlying neoplasm: the immature chromatin pattern and high mitotic activity of acute lymphoblastic leukemia (449); the cytologic atypia and numerous mitoses described in the peripheral T-cell lymphomas (458,461); the subcutaneous location, panniculitic pattern of infiltration, cellular atypia, and karyorrhectic debris of the neoplasms reported by Gonzalez et al. (460); or the extranodal location and angiocentric and angioinvasive features, with or without necrosis, of "angiocentric" T-cell/NK-cell lymphomas (496). HPS, especially if associated with a background lymphoid activation, can be confused with the *lymphohistiocytic T-cell lymphoma,* which is also characterized by an abundance of histiocytes intermingled with small and large lymphoid cells (497); however, in this neoplasm, in contrast to HPS, the nodal architecture is effaced, the histiocytes only occasionally contain erythrocytes, and the large lymphoid cells are atypical and all express CD30.

### Evolution, Treatment, and Prognosis

Although the course of HPS can be atypical and insidious (456), in most cases it is aggressive and rapidly fatal, due to complications specifically related to HPS, such as sepsis, bleeding, CNS involvement or CNS failure (440,442,498), and/or complications of the neoplasm, when this is the underlying disease (466). Mortality was high in patients given only supportive therapy or specific therapy for the underlying disease: in one series including neoplasia-associated and non-neoplasia-associated cases, it was 45% (466); in another, with similar patients and also familial cases, 92% of subjects died, mostly in a matter of days (490). FHL (442,456,470), EBV-related HPS in children (492), and HPS in EBV-associated peripheral T-cell lymphoma (493) were almost uniformly fatal. The first successful treatment of HPS was with etoposide (VP-16) and intrathecal methotrexate (442), but despite initially good response to these regimens, most patients relapsed and died within 2 years from onset of disease (442,487). However, HLA-matched BMT in remission (499) or anti-T-cell activation approaches (steroids, antithymocyte globulin, and CSA) (500,501) seem to hold some promise for continuous remission.

Several factors seem to have prognostic value. In a large

pediatric series, age under 2 years at presentation, but not familiality, was a significant predictor of mortality (470). Increased serum levels of IFNγ (>4.5 U/ml), independently from the association or not with EBV, predicted poor survival (475,478), as did the presence of DIC (466), and serum levels of IL-6 (>300 ng/L) and IL-2 receptor (>10,000 U/ml) (475).

## Mycobacterial Spindle Cell Pseudotumor

The unusual tissue reaction known as mycobacterial spindle cell tumor (MSP), similar to that described in the "histoid" variant of lepromatous leprosy (502), is produced by mycobacteria, most often atypical (*M. avium-intracellulare* and *M. kansasii*), in immunosuppressed patients, especially those with AIDS. It has been reported in the skin (503,504), spleen (505), bone marrow (506), and lung (507), but most frequently in the LNs. There are, in fact, nine reports of nodal MSP (503,506,508,509), and we have seen four other such cases (unpublished observations).

### Clinical Findings

All patients, except one, were men, ranging in age from 25 to 59 years (median 33). All had AIDS, and most belonged to the gay risk group. One of our patients was a 5-year-old girl born to an HIV-infected mother. No specific clinical pattern emerges from the few reports that provide enough information. In most cases, infectious systemic symptoms and lymphadenopathy, localized or generalized, were the presenting manifestations (506,508). In three patients, the MSP was an incidental finding: in an enlarged mesenteric LN obtained during surgery for a bleeding duodenal ulcer, in one reported case (508), and in a splenic hilar node obtained during splenectomy for pancytopenia and in mesenteric nodes adjacent to an ileal large cell lymphoma, in two of our cases.

### Histopathologic Findings

All cases demonstrated a spindle cell proliferation producing a total or subtotal obliteration of the nodal architecture. The proliferation is usually diffuse, but a nodular growth, with coalescent or rather sharply defined separated nodules, has also been observed by us and by others (508). The spindle cells form intersecting cohesive fascicles, which focally produce a storiform pattern (Fig. 19A), and are separated by aggregates of lymphocytes and plasma cells and by sparse thin blood vessels. On a tangential cut, the cells may assume an epithelioid polygonal shape. The spindle cells have oval, thin or plump nuclei, and eosinophilic cytoplasm but in some areas may have a bluish hue. Foamy cells and multinucleated histiocytic cells, typical of mycobacterial infections (509), are uncommon, as are prominent nucleoli, atypical cells, and mitoses (503,508).

This basic pattern may be modified by thin trabecular or coarse scar-like fibrosis, loose areas of necrosis containing free and phagocytosed karyorrhectic debris, and microabscesses (506).

### Special Studies

The spindle cells contain very abundant acid-fast bacilli, often in parallel arrangement (Fig. 19B). The bacilli are also periodic acid–Schiff (PAS)–positive (508), and we and others (508) have observed a strong reaction with Grocott silver methenamine. Immunophenotypic studies of MSP are somewhat contradictory. In one study, antibodies to various intermediate filaments, such as desmin, actin, keratin, and tubulin, have been found to react with the bacilli within the spindle cells, This reactivity, shared by atypical mycobacteria *M. tuberculosis*, and *M. leprae* (506), may be due to the presence of intermediate filament-like material in the bacilli or to cross-reactivity with bacillary antigenic determinants (506). Others have not found reactivity for actin (505,508) or

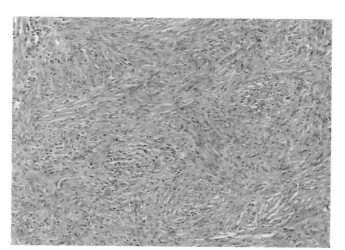
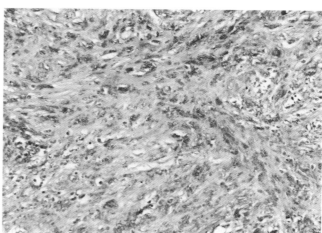

A                                                                                          B

**FIG. 19.** Mycobacterial spindle cell tumor. **A:** Intersecting fascicles of spindle cells. **B:** Large number of bacilli are seen in the spindle cells with an AFB stain.

desmin (508) and the spindle cells are said to be vimentin-positive (508) or negative (505). It is agreed, however, that they express histiocyte-associated markers, such as MAC387, HAM56, $\alpha_1$-antichymotrypsin, and lysozyme (503,505,508), and, in cryostat sections, LCA/CD45, HLA-Dr, and CD14 (503). On electron microscopy, the cells have features of fibroblasts (503), as they contain abundant dilated rough endoplasmic reticulum (ER) and are invested with collagen (503). They also show features of histiocytes, as they contain lysosomes and phagocytosed bacilli (503,506); these may contain the lipid vacuoles pathognomonic of *M. avium-intracellulare* (506). The cells lack filaments and any other features that would suggest a smooth muscle cell origin (506).

In culture, the bacilli producing MSP have been identified as *M. avium-intracellulare* in most nodal and nonnodal cases. *M. kansasii* was grown in our pediatric LN lesion and in one MSP of the skin (503), and *M. tuberculosis* was grown in one lung MSP (507). There are no clear explanations why these bacilli produce a spindle cell reaction in some cases, rather than the usual epithelioid or foamy appearance that is common in these infections (510). HIV might not be a relevant factor because it is missing in transplant recipients and in histoid leprosis, which is histologically so similar to MSP (503). Abnormal immune regulation probably has a role, as it is common to both HIV-infected patients and transplant recipients, and has been implicated in the formation of the granulomas of lepromatous leprosis (511). However, given the rarity of MSP in both of the above situations, other factors are obviously necessary, such as, perhaps, a special individual (genetic) immunologic makeup (507).

*Differential Diagnosis*

The relevance of this infectious response lies in the possibility of misinterpreting it as one of the various other benign or malignant spindle cell lesions of the LN, not only on histologic grounds, but also on immunohistochemistry, in view of the reactivity of its cells for actin and desmin (506). *Bacillary angiomatosis* (BA) may be a consideration in the uncommon cases with a nodular growth pattern; however, MSP shows no conspicuous blood vessel component, no thick foamy endothelia, nor the edematous background with amphophilic interstitial material typical of BA (512). In *inflammatory pseudotumor* the spindle cells do not form cohesive fascicles and are associated with a rich vascular and inflammatory reactive component and with vasculopathy (513). *Kaposi's sarcoma,* a serious consideration in immunosuppressed patients such as those with MSP, shows a richer vascular component and greater atypia and hyaline globules, and lacks a prominent storiform pattern. Similarly, *spindle and epithelioid cell hemangioendothelioma* will show vascular formation and tall, eosinophilic cells, often with large cytoplasmic vacuoles (124). The spindle cells of *follicular dendritic cell sarcoma* form looser fascicles, diffusely sprin-

kled with small lymphocytes, rather than solid cohesive fascicles as in MSP, and show cellular atypia of variable degree (103). The *palisaded myofibroblastoma* is distinguished by the amianthoid fibers and the frequent hemorrhages (514, 515). The cells of *metastatic spindle cell melanoma* and *intranodal leiomyosarcoma* (516) show various degrees of nuclear atypia and numerous mitoses, which are not found in MSP. The very rare *intranodal leiomyoma* (517) is possibly the most difficult differential diagnosis.

In this and all other doubtful cases, any evidence of more conventional mycobacterial infection should be sought to support a diagnosis of MSP, such as hints of pale blue cytoplasm (510), foamy cells, or necrosis, and stains for acid-fast bacilli should be promptly obtained.

*Evolution, Treatment, and Prognosis*

The course and prognosis of MSP depend on the degree of dissemination of the infection and the associated pathology in these fragile patients. Those in whom MSP, in the LNs or any other organ, was but one expression of disseminated mycobacterial infection had an aggressive and fatal course (506–508). Those patients in whom the disease was localized recovered with appropriate antimycobacterial therapy (isoniazid, rifampin, etc.) (506,508), or even without therapy (504,506).

## Kikuchi's Disease (KD) or Histiocytic Necrotizing Lymphadenitis

Kikuchi's disease (KD) features a complex cytologic composition including both cells of histiocytic/monocytic type and transformed T lymphocytes; it is due to the latter component that it may closely imitate a large cell lymphoma. However, it is discussed at this point because the pivotal cell in this process is, in fact, a cell type, the so-called plasmacytoid monocyte (PcM) (518–522), that is thought today to be of monocytic origin. KD was originally described by Kikuchi (523) and, independently, in the Japanese literature, by Fujimoto et al. (524).

*Clinical Features*

KD has been reported first, and is more frequent, among Asians (525–527), but it is not uncommon in the West, where several sizable series have been reported (522, 528–532). It affects predominantly women, and the mean age of onset is between 25 and 30 years (519,528,531). However, the male-to-female ratio varies from 1:3 (519,528) to 1:9 in an American series (531) and patients' ages range from 9 to 75 (519,530). Patients may be asymptomatic or present with fever or flu-like symptoms. The lymphadenopathy is most often localized and cervical. Concurrent or isolated axillary or inguinal lymphadenopathy and generalized lymph node involvement are unusual (525,528). So is hepato- or splenomegaly (528). Erythematous or papular skin rashes are common in some series from Asia, and these have been shown to be identical to the LN lesions (533,534) both histologically and immunophenotypically. Whether KD could present, and be diagnosed, as an isolated skin lesion in the absence of lymph node involvement is unclear (533,535). Hepatic lesions simulating metastases are unique (536). Elevated ESR and leukopenia are the most frequent laboratory abnormalities; hypergammaglobulinemia and abnormal LFTs have also been reported (519,526,530). Cultures for microorganisms have been consistently negative. Bone marrow involvement has been described in one case report only (537). In one case, persistence of disease was associated with an increase in B cells, activated CD30 lymphoid cells, and NK cells in the bone marrow and peripheral blood (538).

### Histologic Findings

The process involves focally or, most often, extensively the LN and may occasionally extend into the capsule and the perinodal tissue (519). It is characterized by pale cellular and/or necrotic foci localized in the paracortex (Fig. 20A, B) and separated by hyperplastic germinal centers and areas of paracortical hyperplasia with a starry-sky pattern (519,529).

The paracortical foci display variable features from case to case and in the same case. The early lesions are very cellular, are composed predominantly of PcMs (Fig. 21A) and activated lymphoid cells, and contain only scattered nuclear debris. The PcMs have oval or round eccentric nuclei, with fine chromatin and inconspicuous nucleoli, and pale cytoplasm. The transformed lymphoid cells are recognizable on the basis of a thicker nuclear membrane, coarser chromatin pattern, more prominent nucleoli, and more basophilic cytoplasm (Fig. 21B). This cellular proliferation is associated

with sparse mitoses. In later foci the nuclear debris is more abundant, and with it one sees an increase in histiocytes of diverse morphology (Fig. 21C). Characteristic are large cells with cellular debris and a nucleus compressed at the periphery ("crescentic histiocytes"); less frequent are "signet ring" histiocytes, with similar nuclei, but homogeneous basophilic, eosinophilic, or clear cytoplasm, and foamy cells with central round nuclei (519). In more advanced foci there is predominant coagulative necrosis and less cellularity, which in some cases may be seen as a peripheral rim to these foci. Finally, foci of granulation tissue, with hypocellularity, marked vascularity, and delicate sclerosis, have been described in rare cases and may be a reparative phase of the necrotic process. Lack of neutrophils is a consistent characteristic of KD at all stages (519,528–530), and it allows its distinction from the lymphadenopathy of systemic lupus erythematosus and bacterial lymphadenitides (528). The combination of karyorrhectic debris, crescentic histiocytes, and PcMs permits the diagnosis of KD by fine needle aspiration (539,540).

The paracortical areas between the cellular/necrotic foci often feature a scattering of histiocytes and immunoblasts, producing a starry-sky pattern, and—more importantly—small collections of PcMs with single-cell necrosis, which are an important clue in this characteristic type of necrotic process. The GCs are hyperplastic or, rarely, necrotic.

### Other Pathologic Features

Immunophenotypic studies confirm the complex cytologic composition of the paracortical foci. CD68 antibodies, such as KP-1 or Ki-M1p (521), highlight both the abundant, coarsely granular cytoplasm of the macrophages and the sharp rim or dot-like polar reactivity of the cytoplasm of the PcMs (518,521). In frozen tissue, the macrophages, but not the PcMs, were reported to also express CD11b and CD11c

A

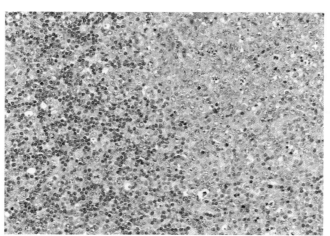

B

**FIG. 20.** Kikuchi's disease. **A:** Ill-defined pale focus of abnormal cell infiltration with necrosis. **B:** The focus is composed of large cells interspersed with necrotic debris. Immunoblasts and histiocytes in the adjacent area account for a starry-sky pattern at low power.

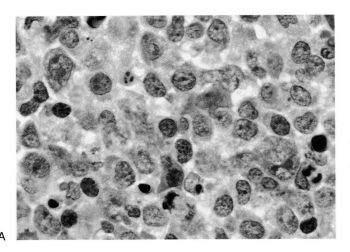

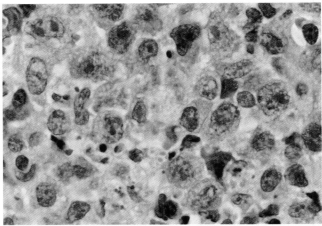

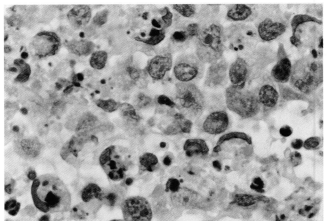

**FIG. 21.** Kikuchi's disease, heterogeneous cell composition. **A:** Area with predominant plasmacytoid monocytes and rare immunoblasts. **B:** Another area with predominant immunoblasts. **C:** An area with predominant histiocytes, some showing the characteristic crescentic nucleus.

(522) and CD15 (541). Characteristically, the PcMs coexpress LN2/CD74 and MT1/CD43 in paraffin tissue (79), and, in frozen sections, CD45, CD4, and CD10 (522), but not CD2 (520). The lymphoid elements in the lesion are almost exclusively T cells, predominantly of the CD8+ cytotoxic/ suppressor subset (522,527,541,542). By double staining with the cell proliferation marker Ki-67, it has been shown that the proliferating cells in the lesion are largely CD8+ (541). By double staining it also appears that the majority of the CD4+ cells were not T cells but rather PcMs because they lacked other T-cell markers but expressed Ki-M1p (542).

All of these findings are in keeping with the proposal by Facchetti et al. that KD represents an abortive granulomatous response (518). Contrary to the usual granulomatous reaction in which histiocytes are associated with a predominant CD4+ T-cell population and mature into large epithelioid cells, it is suggested that KD includes PcMs that do not develop into epithelioid cells and are accompanied predominantly by CD8+ cytotoxic T cells; these last cells are responsible for the necrotic evolution of the lesion. There are, however, no clues at present as to the etiology of the process. *Toxoplasma* (543), *Brucella* (544), and *Yersinia enterocolitica* (520,545) have been considered as possible agents, and some findings, such as the presence of tubu-

loreticular structures (546) and the abundance of IFNα-producing cells (547), have pointed to the possible role of viruses. However, by Southern blot analysis, no genome of human herpesvirus-6 (HHV-6) (548), EBV, CMV, herpes simplex virus, or varicella-zoster virus (549) was found; by PCR, the HHV-6 genome was detected in almost all cases in one series (548), but in no case in another (550); and, by PCR or *in situ* hybridization, the EBV genome was detected in no greater proportion of cases than in other reactive LNs and in a low number of cells, suggesting a latent infection rather than direct causal relation (549,550). Others have proposed that at least some cases of KD might be a forme fruste of systemic lupus erythematosus (SLE) (530,551). Some reports of coexisting KD and SLE (552,553) only stress the histologic similarity of the two diseases. It is, finally, possible that multiple etiologies underlie the disease; in one reported case, for instance, an LN with the histology of KD was found in the area of drainage of a malignant fibrous histiocytoma (554). Rare familial cases have been reported (527).

*Differential Diagnosis*

The most common misdiagnosis of KD is *malignant lymphoma of large cell type (MLCL)* (530). This is particularly true, of course, in the early, hypercellular phases of the disease. The following features are most important to avoid such misinterpretation (519,529,530). Multiple, distinct paracortical foci of involvement, separated by normal paracortex, follicles, and sinuses, are uncommon in DLCL, in which a continuous infiltrate focally obliterating all architectural structures would be expected most often. The polymorphous composition (transformed lymphocytes, as well as PcMs and histiocytes of different types) and relative paucity of mitoses of KD contrast with the uniformity of the large cell population and abundant mitoses seen in DLCL; crescentic histiocytes, in particular, seem to be unique to KD (519). The mottling and the aggregates of PcMs in the adjacent paracortical areas are common in KD but would be rare coincidental findings in DLCL. If doubts still persist, the immunophenotypic findings of abundant CD68+ PcMs admixed with large T cells would help rule out a DLCL.

*Evolution, Treatment, and Prognosis*

The disease is self-limited. The symptoms and signs usually disappear in <2 months (525), with or without therapy. Antibiotics have not been effective (555), but simple antipyretic or steroid treatment has obtained good responses (525,530,537). In a few cases recurrence of the disease has been reported (519,527,530,556), as has later development of SLE (528,530). There is only one reported fatal case; this patient died of heart failure, and at autopsy showed extensive LN involvement by KD, and cardiomyopathy, which was attributed to either large amounts of cytokines produced by the histiocytes or to a stress response (557).

## STROMOVASCULAR PROLIFERATIONS SIMULATING NEOPLASMS

### Inflammatory Pseudotumor

Inflammatory pseudotumor (IPT), first described by us in 1988 (513), may represent a difficult diagnostic problem, in part because of its rarity and in part because it might closely mimic other reactive conditions and lymphomas. Rather than a disease due to a specific etiologic agent, we consider it a distinctive pattern of nodal reaction, probably initiated by different stimuli. In addition to our original 10 cases (513, 558), only one other large series (559) and two case reports have been published (560,561), for a total of 26. However, we have since seen numerous other cases in consultation, suggesting that the lesion is not beyond the everyday experience of pathologists.

*Clinical Findings*

IPT of the LN affects either gender equally, at any age; the age range is 9 to 82 years, with a median of 30, but almost half of the patients affected were in the third and fourth decades. There are no repetitive findings in the past history,

but three patients had associated malignancies (513,558), and in one patient the lesion was preceded by a trauma in the region (513). Seventy-two percent of patients presented with fever, with or without other symptoms, such as night sweats, loss of weight, fatigue, and malaise. The duration of symptoms varied from a few days to 5 years, but in most cases several months. Not unusually the fever recurred periodically, from daily to monthly or at longer intervals. Lymphadenopathy was a constant finding and was mostly localized to one (42%) or more (46%) nodal regions on the same side of the diaphragm; in only 12% of cases was it disseminated. Most frequently involved were the peripheral (50%) or abdominal (23%) LN groups rather than the mediastinal ones (8%). Splenomegaly was recorded in 42% of patients and hepatomegaly in 18%. Laboratory abnormalities, detected in slightly more than half of patients, included elevated ESR (70%), hypergammaglobulinemia (50%), and anemia (45%), as well as a host of other uncommon findings.

*Histologic Findings*

The distinctive feature of this process is the predominant involvement of the connective tissue framework of the LN, i.e., the hilum, the capsule, and the trabeculae, with expansion of these areas and extension into the paracortical region, on the one hand, and into the perinodal soft tissues, on the other. Thus, at low power, one often sees a pale nodule at the center of the LN and/or prominent thickening of the capsule and trabeculae (Fig. 22A, B). These might appear as ramified anastomosing branches or, when cut transversally, as isolated nodules within the LN substance. In rare cases there may only partial involvement of the LN by the process (559).

At higher power, constant features are marked vascularity with vasculopathy; an abundance of spindle cells of various types, best identified immunohistochemically (558,559); and a polymorphous reactive cellular infiltrate. The combination of these features produces variable patterns and cell composition from case to case and in the same case. Edema, rich granulation tissue–like vascularity, and neutrophilic and lymphoplasmacellular infiltrate may predominate; or chronic inflammatory infiltrate and spindle cell proliferation, or fibrosis with abundant spindle cells and less florid reactive cell components may do so (Fig. 23A). A storiform pattern is frequently obtained in parallel with the number of spindle cells and the increase in fibrosis (Fig. 23B). Vascular changes are present in most, but not all (559), cases of IPT. The most common are a subendothelial lymphoid infiltrate and obliteration of the vascular wall and lumen by a florid inflammatory tissue with spindle cells and capillaries (Fig. 23C). Both lesions are often appreciated fully only when highlighting the remnants of the muscular wall with antidesmin or anti–smooth muscle actin antibodies (513,558). Less commonly, thrombosis of small capillaries (513) or fibrinoid necrosis of larger vessels (559,561) may be found. The nodal tissue adjacent to the areas with IPT manifests, in most cases, only nonspecific mild reactive fea-

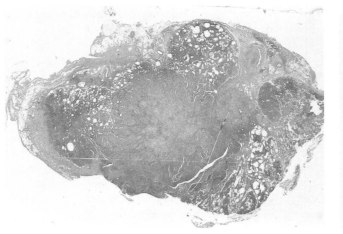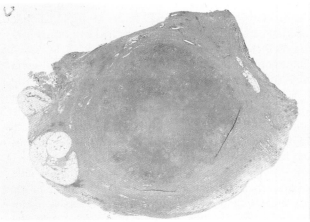

A

B

**FIG. 22.** Inflammatory pseudotumor. **A:** Characteristic thickening of the hilum and, focally, of the capsule and the trabeculae. **B:** Predominant involvement of the capsule, with intranodal sclerosis.

tures or, occasionally (559), paracortical hyperplasia with necrosis, suggesting a viral reaction.

Of equal importance for the diagnosis of IPT as the presence of the classic findings described above are the lack of cellular atypia and the sparseness of mitoses; the highest mitotic count in our series was 6 per 10 hpf (10× eyepieces and 40× objective). In addition, although we cannot exclude necrosis which might be rarely observed (559), lack of necrosis has been a consistent feature of our original cases and the many others we have seen since.

*Special Studies*

Immunohistochemical analyses of IPT have shown that the lymphoid cells present are predominantly of T-cell type (558,559), equally of the CD4+ and CD8+ subsets (558), and that the plasma cell population is polyclonal. The spindle cell component is heterogeneous and includes (558) smaller spindle cells corresponding to activated histiocytes, which coexpress vimentin and macrophage-associated markers (KP-1/CD68, CD14, lysozyme, $\alpha_1$-antichymotrypsin); larger vimentin-positive fibroblasts; and spindle cells expressing muscle-specific actin, i.e., myofibroblasts. The proportion of these cell types obviously varies in different cases and even in different areas of the same case (559), thus perhaps explaining the predominance of fibroblasts and histiocytic spindle cells in our series versus the abundance of myofibroblasts in another study (559). In our interpretation of our data, in contrast with IPT of other organs where the myofibroblasts predominate (562), the spindle histiocytic cells may be the pivotal cell type in nodal IPT, analogous to the "fibrohistiocytoid cells" found in granulation tissue and sundry chronic inflammatory conditions (563).

This cell type is a likely candidate for the production and release of cytokines, which may account for both local histopathologic aspects of IPT and systemic manifestation of the disease. Both IL-1 and TNFα, which has similar effects, induce microthrombosis, endothelial cell and fibroblast pro-

liferation, and possibly B-cell stimulation and differentiation through secretion of IL-6 by these cells, all features characteristically observed in IPT. In addition, IL-1 produces systemic effects, such as fever, weight loss, and production of acute phase reactants, which are also characteristic of IPT. This hypothesis of ours (513,558) has been recently confirmed by the detection of both IL-1β and IL-6 in RNA transcripts in spindle cells and lymphocytes of IPT of LN (563a). There are, however, other aspects of IPT, such as the preferential involvement of the connective tissue framework and the vascular lesions, that are not clearly explained by cytokine production and require the postulation of additional unknown pathogenetic factors (513).

*Differential Diagnosis*

A whole host of *other reactive LN lesions* have been discussed in the differential diagnosis with IPT (513,559). However, in our experience it is CD, vasculitides, and certain infectious processes that may present difficult problems. CD often shows bands of early or advanced fibrosis, reactive GCs, and plasmacytosis that may suggest IPT, especially on a small biopsy; it does not, however, show the complex cytologic composition, especially the spindle cells, storiform pattern, and vasculopathy of IPT. Due to the vasculitis and the associated inflammatory reaction in the adjacent connective tissue, SLE may mimic IPT, but it is distinguished from it by the vascular fibrinoid necrosis—which is rare in IPT, the frequent necrotic areas in the node, the associated activation of the paracortex, and the hematoxylinophilic clumps of material in the sinuses. Syphilis and other infectious processes associated with extensive chronic inflammatory cell infiltrate, fibrosis, and possible vasculitis might be difficult differential considerations. They are recognized by virtue of a granulomatous component and necrosis, which is very rarely—if ever—observed in IPT, and by the lack of the characteristic spindle cell component and storiform pattern of IPT. The differential diagnosis with the mycobacterial spindle cell pseudotumor has already been discussed.

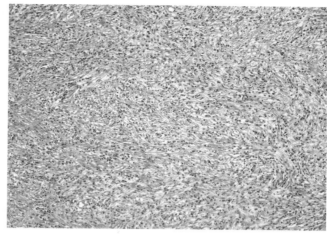

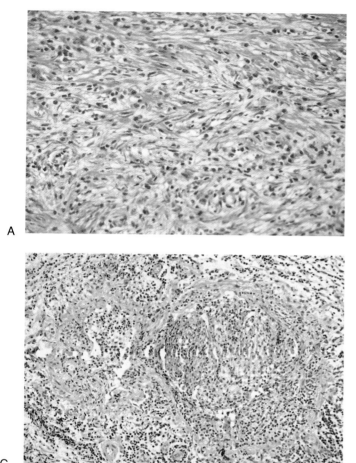

**FIG. 23.** Inflammatory pseudotumor. **A:** Predominance of spindle cells, with sparse lymphocytes and plasma cells. **B:** Vague storiform pattern of the spindle cell proliferation. **C:** Intravascular obliterative growth of the proliferation, with barely recognizable residual muscular coat.

IPT requires differentiation from *any neoplasm that features spindle cells and a storiform pattern and involves the LN:* inflammatory malignant fibrous histiocytoma (564), palisaded myofibroblastoma (514), spindle and epithelioid cell hemangioendothelioma (565,566), and intranodal leiomyoma (517) or leiomyosarcoma (516). Contrary to all of these, however, IPT is obviously localized to preexisting nodal structures, is associated with a complex and variable cell composition, and shows evidence of vasculopathy. In addition, it lacks cellular atypia and numerous mitoses, as well as other characteristics specific to each of these neoplasms, such as the hemorrhage and amianthoid fibers of myofibroblastoma; the irregular vascular spaces lined with epithelioid endothelia of hemangioendothelioma; or the cohesiveness and uniform cytology of the fascicles of muscle cell tumors.

Some features of IPT may also imitate the very rare *dendritic* or *interdigitating cell sarcomas* of the LN (103) or, more importantly, HD. The former, however, are more monomorphic and atypical in cytology, and lack the inflammatory infiltrate so characteristic of IPT (559). IPT shares with *Hodgkin's disease* a mixed cellular infiltrate, capsular and intranodal fibrosis, and, in some cases [a "fibroblastic"

type of nodular sclerosis (567) or lymphoid depletion], a prominent fibroblastic proliferation, but is distinguished from it by the absence of atypical Reed–Sternberg cells and their variants. In cases in which the differential diagnosis of IPT from all of these neoplasms is not solved by morphologic examination, the immunophenotypic characteristics of the component cells are so different that they can be relied on for a definitive diagnosis.

*Evolution, Treatment, and Prognosis*

The evolution of the disease seems to be largely correlated with the type of clinical presentation (513,558,559). A group of patients, the largest (76%), presented with symptoms, often severe and of long duration, had mostly extensive ("stage II") or disseminated lymphadenopathy, with frequent involvement of central LN stations, and often manifested laboratory abnormalities. In this group, the disease tended to be more persistent if not progressive, to be resistant to various treatments (antibiotics, steroids, indomethacin, AZT) used before or after LN excision, and to recur at other nodal sites. The remaining patients had asymptomatic disease, with localized LN involvement, mostly at peripheral sites, and with minimal or no laboratory abnormalities. This group was cured with the excision of the IPT and had no known recurrences.

The management of patients with IPT is so varied that no preferable treatment seems to emerge from the published reports. Indomethacin and steroids, the most commonly used agents, appear to control the disease, but inconsistently. Amelioration of symptoms or cure was obtained with splenectomy in two patients. Chemotherapy (CHOP or CVP), used because of a misdiagnosis of lymphoma in one patient, and as a last resort to control the disease in another, was curative in both. With a follow-up of 7–40 months (median 26), all patients reported are alive and well. Three of them, however, still require treatment with indomethacin or steroids, and one still has lymphadenopathy when off treatment. Thus, although IPT is obviously a reactive process, it may be a persistent, even severe one to bear for some patients and a difficult one to control for the clinician.

## Bacillary Angiomatosis

Bacillary angiomatosis (BA) is a pseudoneoplastic angiogenic infectious disease caused by microorganisms of the *Bartonella* (formerly *Rochalimaea*) species, *B. henselae*

and, less frequently, *B. quintana* and *B. elizabethae*, which also cause bacillary peliosis of the liver and spleen, septicemia, endocarditis, and cat-scratch disease (CSD) (568). The first reports are those of Stoler et al. (569) and Waldo et al. (570), who described cutaneous vascular lesions in patients with HIV infection; in the former, bacteria were identified with silver stain and by electron microscopy, and in the latter the lesion was thought to be a form of "histiocytoid hemangioma." It was a group at New York University (571), however, that gave the first complete description of a vascular proliferative process, "epithelioid angiomatosis," that involved skin, mucosae, and multiple visceral organs of a series of HIV-positive patients. This process was soon recognized as infectious in etiology, hence the term BA (512), and was initially attributed to the CSD bacillus (572–574). While additional expressions of the disorder were being reported [bacillary peliosis of liver and spleen (575), lymph node involvement (576), septicemia (577)], the causative agent became better identified, first as a previously uncharacterized rickettsia-like organism, most closely related to *Rochalimaea quintana* (578), then as a new species, *R. henselae* (579) or *Bartonella henselae*. This and other members of the species are unrelated to *Afipia felis* (577,580), the then-presumed agent of CSD. Several good reviews of BA are now available (581–586).

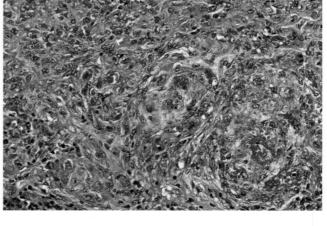

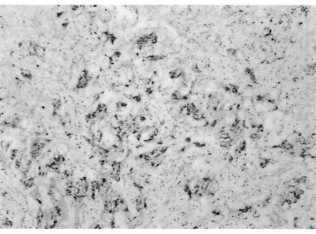

**FIG. 24.** Bacillary angiomatosis. **A:** The pale cellular nodules stand out in the dark lymphoid tissue. **B:** Whorls of plump endothelial cells, with clumps of eosinophilic material. **C:** Numerous clusters of argyrophilic bacteria are seen in this Warthin–Starry stain.

## Clinical Findings

BA is a typical opportunistic infection, which occurs in immunocompromised patients, especially in those infected with HIV, but also in those with hematopoietic malignancies (587) or recipients of transplants (576,588). However, rarely it may occur also in immunocompetent individuals (589–592). It presents with general febrile symptoms (593) and signs of involvement of a variety of organs: skin (512,571,594), mucosae (571,595), liver and spleen (575,596), lymph nodes (576), bone marrow (593), bones [with symptomatic osteolytic lesions (597)], lung [with polypoid endobronchial lesions (598,599)], and CNS (600). There may be wide visceral dissemination (571,601) or septicemia (577,588), as well as association with other opportunistic infections and Kaposi's sarcoma (602,603).

## Histologic Findings

In the classical form of nodal involvement (576), similar to that described in the skin (512), discrete or confluent nodules are seen, composed of blood vessels, with plump endothelia (Fig. 24A, B). The vessels may have well-recognizable, even ectatic, lumina or may form solid areas, with lumina barely visible. The endothelia have oval, vesicular nuclei, at times with moderate atypia, and pale vacuolated cytoplasm. Between the blood vessels there is an edematous background, containing an interstitial eosinophilic material, which corresponds to large clumps of bacteria (Fig. 24C); in addition, there can be foamy histiocytes, abundant polymorphonuclears, or extravasated red blood cells. It is clear, however, that this *classic nodulovascular form* is only one in a rather wide spectrum of lesions due to *B. henselae*, which includes other angioformative and nonangioformative morphologies, in addition to the suppurative-granulomatous reaction typical of CSD. *Peliotic changes* have been described in abdominal lymph nodes, in association with bacillary pe-

liosis of the liver and spleen (604); the characteristic peliotic cavities, without lining cells, were separated by fibromyxoid areas with eosinophilic material and by classic vascular nodules. In our series (605), we also observed *diffuse angiomatous* proliferation and a *vasculonecrotic* response. The former simulated either capillary hemangioma (with lobules of small congested vessels lined with thin endothelia) (Fig. 25A) or endothelioid hemangioma (with irregular lumina lined with large eosinophilic cuboidal endothelia); the latter featured ill-defined patches containing small blood vessels with flat endothelium, intermingled with collections of small histiocytes (immature granulomas) and often centered by non-suppurative necrosis (karyorrhectic debris) (Fig. 25B). Clumps of eosinophilic material between the vessels were seen in all of these forms but were more difficult to find in the vasculonecrotic lesions. Finally, Slater et al. (606) have described an unusual *nonangiogenic lesion,* composed of nodules of lymphocytes and nonepithelioid macrophages.

## Special Studies

Immunohistochemical studies of BA have documented the endothelial markings (CD34, *Ulex europaeus,* factor VIII) of both the cells lining the lumina and intervascular spindle cells and the presence of a component of histiocytes (KP-1/CD68+, factor XIII+) in the intervascular area (512,571,605,607). The definitive diagnosis of BA is based on the identification of the bacilli within what appears to be, on hematoxylin and eosin (H&E) staining, an amorphous amphophilic material. These present as haphazard clusters of gram-negative rods revealed by silver impregnation with the Warthin–Starry method and by Giemsa stain (608). "Optimally performed Warthin–Starry stains will deposit a thin rim of silver on nuclear membranes and punctate dots on nucleoli" of adjacent cells (609). The bacilli are said to always be interstitial (512), but have also been found within the cytoplasm of macrophages (576) and of sinusoidal cells in a

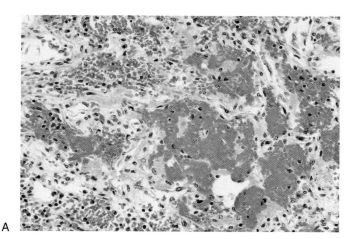
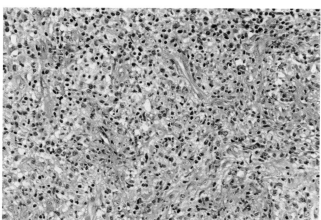

A     B

**FIG. 25.** Bacillary angiomatosis. **A:** Lesion with open and focally dilated vascular lumina. Note the clumps of amphophilic material. **B:** Abundance of small blood vessels in an infiltrate of lymphoid cells and histiocytes, with focal initial necrosis.

peliotic liver (604). *B. henselae* and *B. quintana* may be specifically identified in tissue sections with the use of polyclonal antisera that are today available (606,610,611) and in fresh or paraffin-embedded material by PCR techniques (578,583,590,612). On electron microscopy the bacilli have characteristic trilaminar cell walls (575,576,588,607). Isolation of the bacilli by culture is difficult because they are both fastidious and slow growing (568).

It is agreed today that most of the cases of BA are caused by *B. henselae* or, less commonly, *B. quintana* (568,609, 612) and that there is often an association with scratch or bite by a cat (612). It is unclear, however, why *B. henselae* would usually cause CSD (613) and at other times BA or septicemia, or why *B. quintana* would usually cause trench fever but at other times BA (609). The patient's immune response might be relevant, as might factors produced by the bacilli. In our study there was a rough correlation between histology of the nodal lesions and the amount of bacilli, the histiocytic patterns being associated with less and the angiogenic patterns with more bacilli, suggesting a better immune response in the former than in the latter (605). In agreement with these findings, infection with *B. henselae* in immunocompetent individuals usually manifests with the clinical and histologic features typical of CSD (613) and only rarely with those typical of BA. In patients with slight or no immune deficiency, BA may be limited to the site of inoculation (587,589,591,592), whereas in those with severe immunocompromise it is usually disseminated (609). Microbial factors, however, are also operative. The similarities in the histologic lesions due to *B. henselae* and those due to *B. bacilliformis* (so-called verruga peruana) (614), as well as the DNA relatedness of the two microorganisms (577), have suggested that *B. henselae*, like *B. bacilliformis* (615), may produce an angiogenic factor that accounts for BA and peliosis of the liver and spleen (575,576,609). Thus, clinical and histopathologic manifestations may reflect the balance between the pathogenic characteristics of the causal agent and the immune response of the host (605).

*Differential Diagnosis*

Both the classic nodulovascular (576) and the diffuse angiomatous (605) forms of BA require differentiation from other vascular neoformations, such as capillary hemangioma, epithelioid hemangioma/hemangioendothelioma, Kaposi's sarcoma, and vascular transformation of the sinuses. In both, the essential element for a correct diagnosis is the recognition of the characteristic amorphous, fibrillary, amphophilic interstitial material that requires the demonstration of bacteria with the appropriate stains. Also characteristically (if not consistently) seen in BA, but not in *(epithelioid) angiomas* and KS, are edema and neutrophils in the intervascular stroma (576). In addition, the pale-staining, finely vacuolated character of the endothelial cytoplasm in BA differs from the intensely pink cytoplasm and the sharply defined vacuoles of epithelioid tumors. In comparison to *KS,*

the blood vessels of BA are better formed, do not show jagged contours or hyaline globules, and are not associated with fascicles of, but rather only sparse, spindle cells (609, 616). As opposed to *vascular transformation of sinuses,* BA is not centered on the sinuses, its blood vessels have a tall rather than flattened endothelium, and clumps of eosinophilic material are prominent (616).

*Evolution, Treatment, and Prognosis*

The clinical course of BA is variable, and depends on the severity of the immunocompromise, the dissemination of the disease, the presence of other complications, and the organs involved. Thus the disease may be limited to the skin in immunocompetent or mildly immunodeficient hosts or may be disseminated in patients with AIDS. Fatalities, due to liver failure (604), laryngeal obstruction, or disseminated intravascular coagulation (571), occurred only before the recognition of the infectious nature of the process. BA is, in fact, exquisitely sensitive to various antibiotics, especially erythromycin (583,601,603), doxycycline (583), and azithromycin (617), and the prompt response to these drugs has helped differentiate simultaneous skin lesions of BA and KS occurring in the same patients (602,603). It is also possible that prophylaxis for mycobacteria with clarithromycin might be responsible for decreasing the incidence of BA in HIV-infected patients (609). However, there is the possibility of relapses, which might require lifelong suppressive therapy (581).

**Vascular Transformation of Sinuses**

Vascular transformation of sinuses (VTS) is a reactive vasoproliferative lesion developing in the LNs in response to lymphatic or venous obstruction. It has little or no clinical importance, except for the risk of being misdiagnosed as Kaposi's sarcoma and, as we will discuss below, for alerting the pathologist to the possibility of a tumor in the vicinity. Since the original description of Haferkamp and Lennert (618), only a few cases have been reported (619–623). To these, one may add the rare cases of "nodal angiomatosis" (624), which most probably represent a variant of VTS (616). In addition, a large series of 76 cases has been recently reported from the Stanford group, which has revealed a much larger spectrum of clinical associations and histopathologic patterns (616).

*Clinical Findings*

The reported cases are distributed equally between male and female individuals and fairly evenly among any age group from 3 to 82 years (median 44) (616). Most cases were an incidental finding in LNs excised in varied clinical contexts, such as with an adjacent tumor mass (34%); at staging laparotomy for lymphoma (14%) or at LN dissection in can-

*Pathologic Findings*

The reported spleen weights vary widely, from 60 to 1790 g (median 380 g) in the largest series (661). The hamartomas vary in size from 1.5 to 15 cm (median 5 cm) and are usually single (661); in fact, multiple lesions were observed in only three patients in this surgical series (15%) (661), and in rare others (695,702). However, in the small group of patients that manifested hematologic symptoms, the gross findings appear to be distinctly different: the spleen weighed from 300 to 4560 g (median 957 g), and the lesions were larger (<1–19 cm, median 7 cm) and much more frequently (47%) multiple (694). As already said, these differences are in part due to the inclusion of cases of hemangioma/hemangiomatosis. Hamartomas are roundish, well-circumscribed, often bulging nodules, usually darker than the surrounding compressed parenchyma, and often contain yellowish areas of fibrosis (661).

On histologic examination they are poorly demarcated from the surrounding parenchyma, and are composed of a tangle of irregular, tortuous sinuses lined with endothelium (Fig. 33A, B); their lumina may be thinned by surrounding fibrosis or dilated. Between them, there are no regular cords but only lymphocytes, macrophages, and numerous mast cells; and with silver stains and PAS one sees a disorderly arrangement of the reticulin fibers and often a lack of ring fibers (661). In the context of the lesion there are no trabeculae, arterioles, or large veins and, importantly, no follicles or periarteriolar lymphoid sheaths. Considerable morphologic variations have been described in this basic pattern, including the presence of trilineage extramedullary hematopoiesis (15/20 cases); marked plasmacytosis (12/20); and, more rarely, foamy histiocytes with prominent phagocytosis of erythrocytes and platelets, and association with lymphoma or other splenic pathology (661,667). In fact, in the vast majority of cases, the adjacent parenchyma is normal (693).

*Special Studies*

Only a few immunohistochemical studies have been dedicated to splenic hamartomas. The endothelia have been shown to have all of the characteristics of the sinus-lining cells, as they are vimentin-positive, factor VIII–related antigen–positive, $\alpha_1$-antitrypsin-positive, and $\alpha_1$-antichymotrypsin-positive, and, on cryostat sections, nonspecific esterase–positive, alkaline phosphatase-negative (661). Like the normal sinus lining cells of the spleen, they express CD8 (697) and characteristically lack CD34 (698). The macrophages between the blood vessels express the expected markers (lysozyme, Ki-M7, and Ki-M8); B and T cells are very sparse (661)

These findings confirm that these lesions are composed exclusively of red pulp components, and support the notion that they are hamartomas in the classic sense. This concept may also receive support from reports of splenic hamartomas associated with hamartomas in other organs in the context of tuberous sclerosis (703,704). The fact that the spleen weight and the size of the hamartoma were greater in female than in male patients has suggested a possible role of hormonal factors in its development (694).

*Differential Diagnosis*

It is difficult at times to distinguish, on the basis of histology alone, the red pulp hamartoma from *small vessel hemangioma* (as opposed to the usual cavernous hemangioma). In our experience, the former has a uniform pattern throughout: the lumina of the blood vessels are more crowded, elongated, and tortuous, and are separated by disorganized lymphoid cells and macrophages. The hemangioma, in contrast, has a striking lobular pattern (Fig. 34A, B): the lobules, separated by fibrosis, are composed of a loose tangle of stromal cells and ill-defined vascular channels, and contain abundant

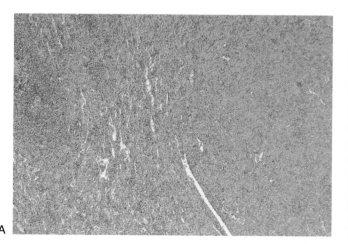

A                                                                                                    B

**FIG. 33.** Red pulp hamartoma. In each photograph, an ill-defined solid nodule, of uniform composition and with poorly recognizable sinuses (**B**) is contrasted with normal splenic tissue (**A**).

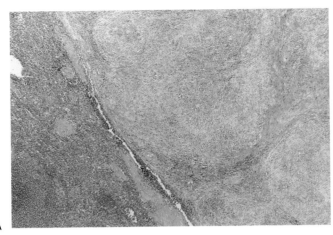
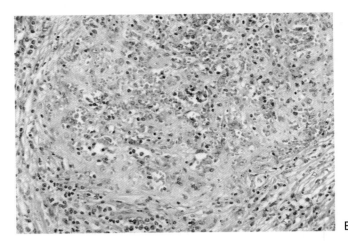

**FIG. 34.** Cord capillary hemangioma. **A:** A mass with a clear nodular pattern and fibrosis compresses residual normal splenic tissue *(left lower field).* **B:** The nodules are composed of clusters of small blood vessels.

extravasated cells and fibrin; on the basis of the reactivity of their endothelial cells (CD34+, but factor VIII–related antigen−), we have identified them as cord capillary hemangiomas (698). In contrast, the endothelia of hamartoma express the staining pattern of sinus lining cells (CD34−, factor VIII–related antigen+). In addition, the endothelial cells of hamartomas, but not those of hemangiomas, express CD8 (697) and are alkaline phosphatase− (661).

Only the rare cases of hamartomas with marked lymphoid cell and plasma cell infiltration (661) might suggest a *lymphoplasmacytoid lymphoma;* these, however, should be correctly identified by their roundish, relatively defined borders with the adjacent parenchyma and by the underlying rich vascularity.

*Evolution, Treatment, and Prognosis*

The hamartoma is a self-contained process, despite the fact that it may reach large dimensions, and only requires surgical treatment. The course after splenectomy has been uneventful in all cases.

**BONE MARROW**

The following discussion of the most common pseudoneoplastic bone marrow processes reviews them based primarily on the main cell lineage involved (erythroid, granulocytic, lymphoid/plasmacellular, and histiocytic).

**ERYTHROID HYPERPLASIAS SIMULATING NEOPLASMS**

**Megaloblastic Anemias and Related Conditions**

Megaloblastic anemias (MA) comprise a group of nonneoplastic disorders of different etiology, whose common denominator is represented by retarded DNA synthesis and altered cell growth. Considering the wide spectrum of disease processes that can be associated with similar hematologic abnormalities, one may choose the terms "megaloblastosis" or "megaloblastic state" when referring to what can be regarded as a hematologic syndrome rather than a specific entity on its own. Megaloblastosis may be secondary to deficiencies of vitamin B$_{12}$ and/or folic acid as well as to inherited or acquired disorders of the DNA synthesis, the latter being related to the administration of drugs (e.g., antineoplastic) or to the exposure to other chemical toxic compounds (705). Regardless of its origin, the impaired DNA synthesis typical of the megaloblastic states alters the mechanisms regulating cell growth. Both vitamin B$_{12}$ and folic acid play essential roles in the biosynthesis of the cellular DNA, and the lack of these cofactors impairs the mitotic process, particularly in the tissues characterized by a rapid cell turnover. RNA synthesis, however, is not affected, allowing cytoplasmic components (such as hemoglobin) to be synthesized in excess. The ultimate result is an increase in cell size; hence the term used to designate these diseases. Retarded DNA synthesis as part of a metabolic defect is common to all of the megaloblastic anemias, which differ only in the mechanisms responsible for their occurrences.

*Clinical Features*

An extremely broad spectrum of disease states can give rise to MA (705); the features of only some of them are briefly recapitulated here. Pernicious anemia (PA) is the prototype of the megaloblastic states. In its classical clinical picture, PA is characterized by symptoms of anemia, sore tongue, gastrointestinal complaints, and neurologic abnormalities typically consequent to the degeneration of the white matter of the dorsolateral columns of the spinal cord. The clinical manifestations of the disease are related to a deficient absorption of vitamin B$_{12}$ in the terminal ileum owing to the lack of Castle's "intrinsic factor" (a vitamin $B_{12}$-binding protein) in the gastric juice. In the adult type, the disease is associated with gastric atrophy and achylia, whereas in the congenital form only the secretion of the intrinsic factor is impaired. The clinical and hematologic features of folate deficiency resemble those of the lack of vitamin $B_{12}$, except for the absence of signs of neurologic involvement; when these are present in a patient with inadequate folate stores, they are generally indicative of a coexistent $B_{12}$ deficiency or of other processes. A megaloblastic state of variable severity can also be seen in the setting of HIV infection, frequently as a result of the administration of drugs of known myelotoxic potential. High doses of trimethoprim (which, in combination with sulfamethoxazole, is used in the treatment of *Pneumocystis carinii* pneumonia) can interfere with the activity of the human dihydrofolate reductase, resulting in acute megaloblastic anemia, reversible with folinic acid (706,707). In addition, it has been suggested that the HIV/AIDS-related ineffective hematopoiesis, which is often associated with dysmyelopoietic changes involving multiple cell lineages, might be due to virus-induced alteration(s) of the bone marrow stromal environment rather than to direct viral infection of the human hematopoietic progenitors (708).

*Morphologic Findings*

The following description is primarily centered on the morphologic changes observed in the peripheral blood and bone marrow of patients who are deficient in vitamin $B_{12}$ and/or folic acid.

**Peripheral blood.** The red cell series shows normochromic, macrocytic anemia that is often severe and characterized by the presence of large oval erythrocytes ("macrocytes") and reticulocytopenia. Red cell macrocytosis precedes the development of anemia and may be a clue for an early diagnosis. When anemia is severe, considerable erythrocyte anisopoikilocytosis and red cell fragmentation can be seen, along with circulating erythroid precursors. The leukocyte count may be normal or there may be neutropenia. Notably, hypersegmented neutrophils (mature granulocytes with six or more nuclear lobes) are present and are one of the earliest signs of megaloblastosis (Fig. 35). Platelet counts may be normal or, in severe cases, reduced. The morphologic changes are attended by abnormalities in numerous hematologic indices, including an increase in the red cell mean corpuscular volume (MCV) due to the presence of oval macrocytes and in the red cell volume distribution width (RDW) secondary to erythrocyte anisopoikilocytosis.

**Bone marrow.** In the core biopsy sections, the marrow is generally hypercellular and may exhibit a "packed" appearance. The most prominent finding is a marked erythroid hyperplasia with a considerable shift toward immaturity. Large, early erythroid precursors are particularly evident, and stand out because of their arrangement in sizable clusters. They are recognizable by virtue of their large, round-to-oval nuclei with finely dispersed chromatin and characteris-

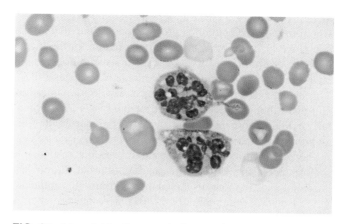

**FIG. 35.** Megaloblastic anemia in a peripheral blood smear. Hypersegmented neutrophils with cytoplasmic vacuoles, marked red cell abnormalities, and thrombocytopenia are recognizable.

tically prominent, often comma-shaped nucleoli frequently abutting on the nuclear membrane (Fig. 36). Another characteristic of these erythroid precursors is the presence of a discernible rim of amphophilic to basophilic cytoplasm. A paranuclear clear zone corresponding to the Golgi apparatus can also be seen, and is sometimes large enough to produce an indentation of the nuclear profile. There is usually an increased number of mitoses, and some of these can be seen within the erythroid colonies. The granulocytic series is usually hyperplastic too, although this is often difficult to appreciate because of the hypercellular erythroid background. Although maturation to the neutrophil stage is present, large metamyelocytes and band forms as well as neutrophils with bizarrely shaped nuclei are frequent, and constitute another typical finding. Megakaryocytes may be normal or decreased in number, depending on the severity of the process.

The cytologic features of the megaloblastic hematopoiesis are best appreciated in the marrow smears. As in the marrow core sections, the early erythroid megaloblasts are recog-

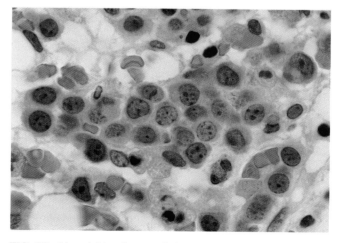

**FIG. 36.** Megaloblastic anemia in the bone marrow biopsy. A typical colony of early erythroid megaloblasts.

nized by virtue of their large size and abundant cytoplasm, which in the Wright-stained preparations is blue and agranular (Fig. 37A). Another characteristic feature of the megaloblastic erythroid precursors is their unusually delicate nuclear chromatin, described as "particulate" or "sieve-like." This change affects all of the stages of erythroid maturation, and even though early erythroid megaloblasts are particularly evident, more mature but abnormal polychromatophilic and orthochromatic ("late") megaloblasts are present as well. In these cells, progressive hemoglobinization is responsible for the increasing cytoplasmic acidophilia, but the nuclear chromatin is still more dispersed than appropriate for the degree of cytoplasmic maturation (709). This phenomenon is referred to as "nuclear-cytoplasmic dissociation," and is typically part of the morphologic spectrum of changes associated with MA. Premature karyorrhexis of the erythroid precursors may also be seen. The neutrophil series often shows a mild shift toward immaturity. As noted, "giant" metamyelocytes and band forms are present (Fig. 37B). These are larger than their normal counterparts, and their nuclei are

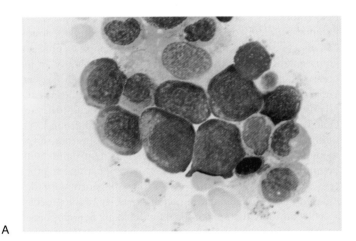

A

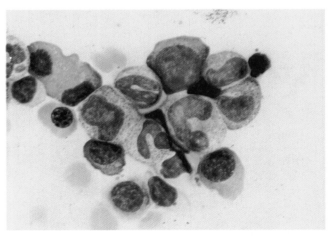

B

**FIG. 37.** Megaloblastic anemia in the marrow smears. **A:** Early erythroid megaloblasts with finely dispersed chromatin and blue, agranular cytoplasm. **B:** A cluster of granulocytes with a giant neutrophilic band *(center)*.

often markedly abnormal. The identification of giant metamyelocytes and giant band forms becomes diagnostically important when the megaloblastic features of the erythroid series are masked by a coexisting iron deficiency (709). The changes involving the megakaryocytic component are usually less pronounced than those affecting the erythroid or granulocytic series, but in severe megaloblastic states megakaryocytes might be reduced and display hyperlobated nuclei with abnormally fine chromatin. Iron stains show erythroid precursors containing abnormally prominent cytoplasmic iron granules, and some ringed sideroblasts (erythroblasts in which the iron granules are arranged in a collar around the nuclear membrane) may also be observed. The storage iron deposited in histiocytes is increased.

*Differential Diagnosis*

A common differential diagnostic problem is the distinction of megaloblastic states from *myelodysplastic syndromes (MDSs)*. MDSs comprise a group of clonal, often preleukemic bone marrow disorders characterized by ineffective hematopoiesis, resulting in peripheral blood cytopenias despite a hypercellular or normocellular bone marrow frequently exhibiting an increase in immature precursors (710). One of the defining features of the MDSs is the morphologic evidence of dysplasia (711). This may involve one or more hematopoietic cell lineages, and the erythroid series is frequently and severely affected (Fig. 38A). Clonal cytogenetic abnormalities and an increase in peripheral blood and/or bone marrow myeloblasts can be seen as well, particularly in the more severe forms. The differential diagnosis between nonclonal megaloblastic states and true myelodysplastic processes can be difficult based on morphology alone because several of the abnormalities observed in the former (e.g., peripheral blood cytopenias with oval macrocytosis, reticulocytopenia and neutrophil hypersegmentation, or prominent bone marrow megaloblastic-like changes) are seen in numerous MDSs as well. Indeed, despite the profound biological difference existing between these two classes of hematopoietic disorders, in both of them hematopoiesis is inadequate and ineffective.

The investigation of the body levels of vitamin $B_{12}$ and folic acid is obviously essential in the distinction of MA from MDS with megaloblastic-like changes. In addition, certain features of granulocytic and megakaryocytic dyspoiesis such as a definite increase in myeloblasts, nuclear hypolobation ("pseudo–Pelger–Huet" change), or cytoplasmic hypogranularity of the mature neutrophils (Fig. 38B) and the presence of small megakaryocytes with hypolobated or widely separated nuclei and fully mature cytoplasm (Fig. 38C, D) are not features of megaloblastosis but rather suggest a true MDS. In addition, if a deficiency in vitamin $B_{12}$ and/or folate is present, the appropriate treatment will result in a predictable sequence of quantitative and qualitative changes in both the peripheral blood and the bone marrow

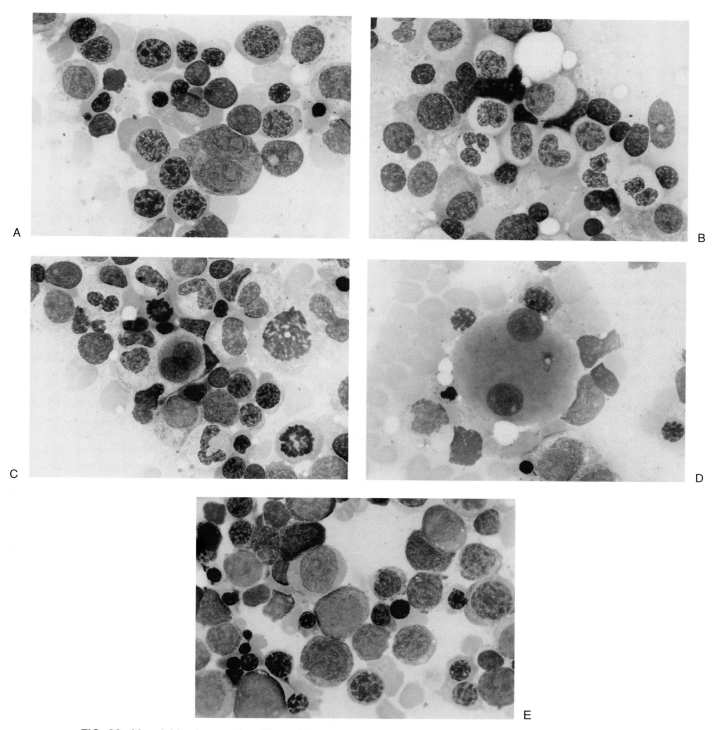

**FIG. 38.** Megaloblastic anemia, differential diagnosis in the marrow smears. **A:** Myelodysplastic syndrome (MDS): abnormal erythroid precursors showing binuclearity, marked megaloblastoid change, and nuclear–cytoplasmic dissociation. **B:** MDS: dysplastic granulocytes with hypogranular cytoplasm and abnormally hypolobated nuclei. **C:** MDS: a micromegakaryocyte *(center)*. Note cell size. **D:** MDS: this megakaryocyte is of normal size, but the two nuclei are abnormally spaced. **E:** Acute erythroleukemia. Marked erythroid hyperplasia is present; some erythroid maturation is still observed. In this case, erythroblasts accounted for 71% of all nucleated marrow elements; myeloblasts were 10.5%.

(705). Recognition of these changes is of considerable help in the differential diagnosis, and may avoid recourse to additional procedures. In the peripheral blood, the earliest sign of hematologic response to vitamin therapy is an increase in reticulocytes, whose extent is proportionate to the severity of the preexisting anemia. Reticulocytosis begins after 2–3 days of optimal therapy, peaks on day 5–8, and gradually returns to normal levels thereafter. Hemoglobin levels return to normal in 4–8 weeks, whereas the MCV decreases progressively after a transient increase due to the appearance of numerous reticulocytes. Neutrophil and platelet counts usually normalize within a week, and hypersegmented neutrophils disappear after 2 weeks. During the hematologic recovery, some circulating granulocytic and erythroid precursors may be seen in the peripheral blood smear. In the bone marrow, the megaloblastic erythropoiesis is rapidly reversed as early as 24–48 hours after initiation of therapy, whereas the abnormal metamyelocytes and bands tend to persist for at least a week. On the other side, the abnormal hematopoiesis of true MDS will show no sign of recovery following vitamin administration, due to its preneoplastic rather than dysmetabolic nature.

Lastly, approximately 40–70% of MDSs are characterized by persistent clonal cytogenetic abnormalities, frequently consisting of loss of genetic material (712). Although these karyotypic abnormalities do not generally relate to specific morphologic subtypes of MDS, they consistently tend to affect some chromosomes (e.g., chromosomes 5, 7, 8, 20) more often than others. In contrast, chromosome studies in megaloblastic anemias have identified a variety of nonspecific karyotypic abnormalities that disappear with therapy (713).

According to the recommendations of the French–American–British (FAB) cooperative group, the diagnosis of *acute myelogenous leukemia (AML)* requires that immature myeloid cells with the features of myeloblasts (as best evaluated in smear preparations) account for 30% or more of the peripheral blood or bone marrow nucleated cells (714). Because in MA the bone marrow is often markedly hypercellular, and, the early megaloblasts may resemble leukemic cells due to their immature appearance, a diagnosis of acute leukemia may be entertained, particularly when the findings observed in the histological sections are not (or cannot be) correlated with the results of the appropriate laboratory studies and with the morphologic findings of the peripheral blood and bone marrow smears. As previously noted, the examination of the marrow aspirate is most helpful in the recognition of the features indicative of a megaloblastic state.

If the bone marrow smears are not available or the marrow aspiration has been unsuccessful, recognition of the histologic findings typical of the megaloblastic anemias is necessary. It is helpful to consider that in the bone marrow biopsy sections the normal erythroid precursors tend to occur in cohesive "colonies," and that this architectural feature is still somewhat maintained in megaloblastic states, even though clusters of large, immature megaloblasts may be of unusual size and poorly defined, so as to create the impression that the cells tend to form sheets or are irregularly distributed in the marrow spaces. In addition, in well-prepared sections early erythroid megaloblasts are recognizable by virtue of their previously mentioned cytologic features, and the identification of giant metamyelocytes and giant bands is usually possible as well. All of these findings may at least suggest the possibility of a pseudoleukemic process and may prompt further investigation or laboratory studies. There are, however, occasional cases of megaloblastic anemias presenting with "atypical" clinicomorphologic features, most often due to the coexistence of infectious processes (715). In these instances, peripheral blood leukemoid reactions or pancytopenias associated with a bone marrow maturational arrest involving the granulocytic lineage may occur. A misdiagnosis of leukemia can be avoided by the evaluation of the serum levels of vitamin B$_{12}$ and folate. However unusual, these cases indicate that the clinicomorphologic picture of MA may occasionally be more heterogeneous than expected.

An uncommon form of AML that MA may morphologically resemble is the *M6 (acute erythroleukemia) subtype* of the FAB classification. In M6 AML the neoplastic clone exhibits prominent evidence of erythroid and myeloid differentiation. The FAB criteria for the diagnosis of AML M6 require that bone marrow erythroid precursors account for 50% or more of all marrow nucleated cells, and that myeloblasts represent 30% or more of the remaining nonerythroid elements (714). Based on these criteria, a diagnosis of AML M6 can therefore be made even in the presence of relatively low myeloblast counts. The clinical, morphologic, and cytogenetic features of erythroleukemia have been recently reviewed (716). The blood and bone marrow findings can be extremely heterogeneous, depending on the extent and degree of proliferation and differentiation of the erythroid component. In particular, the bone marrow picture may be fairly uniform or markedly pleomorphic. The marrow is usually hypercellular with marked erythroid hyperplasia. Varying from case to case, the erythroid component may be primarily composed of immature elements or may display evidence of more advanced, although abnormal, maturation (Fig. 38E). Dyserythropoiesis is often severe, and may take the form of marked megaloblastic-like change, nuclear lobulation, multinuclearity, karyorrhexis, and ringed sideroblasts. Cytoplasmic vacuolization and PAS positivity of the erythroid precursors are also common. Of importance are the frequent findings of granulocytic and megakaryocytic dysplasia and impaired maturation. Myeloblasts can vary in number, but by definition they should account for 30% or more of the nonerythroid marrow elements. Erythroleukemia is distinguished from the megaloblastic anemias by virtue of its lack of evidence of B$_{12}$ or folate deficiency, the severe dysplastic changes involving multiple cell lineages, and the high incidence of cytogenetic abnormalities.

The histologic features of MA may rarely resemble bone marrow involvement by *lymphoma* or *metastatic carcinoma*. Knowledge of the clinical history, the appropriate laboratory data and, if necessary, immunohistochemical stains using antibodies raised against various B- and T-lymphocyte-associated antigens, cytoplasmic intermediate filaments expressed by epithelial cells (cytokeratins), and erythroid-associated markers such as hemoglobin A (717) will help to establish the correct diagnosis.

### Evolution, Treatment, and Prognosis

In most cases of MA the appropriate vitamin therapy results in the normalization of the hematologic abnormalities. If there have been signs or symptoms indicative of neurologic lesions, the extent of their improvement depends on the duration of the disease; manifestations that have been present for short periods of time are likely to be reversible, whereas those of longstanding duration may, to a certain degree, persist. Attention should also be paid to the correction of underlying disorders responsible for the megaloblastic state, such as small bowel bacterial overgrowth, fish tapeworm infection, discontinuation of drugs interfering with DNA synthesis, and so forth. Notably, some inherited disorders affecting the biosynthesis of the purine or pyrimidine nucleotides will not respond to $B_{12}$ or folate treatment: in these cases replacement therapy with the appropriate compounds (e.g., uridine in orotic aciduria) is necessary (705).

## GRANULOCYTIC HYPERPLASIAS SIMULATING NEOPLASMS

### Leukemoid Reactions

Leukemoid reactions (LRs) comprise a heterogeneous group of nonneoplastic hematologic responses characterized by an increase in the peripheral blood leukocyte counts due to a variety of underlying disease states. The granulocytic, monocytic, and lymphoid lineages may be variously affected. The magnitude of the leukocytosis and the possible presence of "atypical" morphologic features may raise differential diagnostic problems between reactive LR and leukemic processes. The most common type of LR involves the neutrophil lineage, and is discussed in detail.

#### Neutrophilic Leukemoid Reactions

##### Clinical and Pathogenetic Features

Neutrophilic LRs are common hematologic responses to a variety of stimuli. Underlying causes include infectious processes, autoimmune disorders, concurrent hematologic and nonhematologic neoplasia, nonneoplastic hematologic disorders, endocrinopathies, and other conditions such as burns, tissue necrosis, acute hemorrhage or hemolysis, chemical poisoning, or drug administration (718). Clinically, patients with neutrophilic LRs are often acutely ill with overt evidence of infection, trauma, inflammatory disorders, or other systemic diseases. Exceptions to this rule, however, may be encountered.

The peripheral blood and bone marrow changes of neutrophilic LRs are due to an increased release of hematopoietic cytokines such as granulocyte- and granulocyte/macrophage colony-stimulating factor (G-CSF/GM-CSF). Production of these growth factors is controlled by a complex regulatory network involving several cell types. For instance, in inflammation- or infection-associated LRs, antigen-activated macrophages secrete TNF$\alpha$ and IL-1, which in turn stimulate the bone marrow stromal cells (e.g., fibroblasts, endothelial cells) to produce growth factors specific for the granulocytic/monocytic series (719–722). Inappropriate production of hematopoietic growth factors responsible for LR may be seen in some patients affected by malignant tumors (723, 724).

##### Morphologic Findings

**Peripheral blood.** Leukocytosis with neutrophilia, increased band forms, and possible appearance of more immature granulocyte precursors are the hallmarks of neutrophilic LRs (Fig. 39A). The extent of the leukocytosis is variable; some authors consider LRs to be present when the leukocyte count exceeds 25,000–30,000/µL (725). Mature neutrophils typically show features of "activation" such as increased azurophilic ("toxic") granulation, cytoplasmic vacuolization, and Dohle bodies. These are sky-blue round or oval inclusions seen in the peripheral areas of the neutrophil cytoplasm, and consist of lamellar aggregates of rough endoplasmic reticulum (726). Anemia and thrombocytopenia are also common, although the platelet count may sometimes be increased; some circulating erythroid precursors can be noted. In some cases, neutrophilic leukocytosis of variable degree may be associated with a more pronounced shift toward immaturity. This occurrence has been described in patients with tuberculosis or malignant tumors, often metastatic to the bone (718). An important laboratory finding associated with LRs is the increased neutrophil alkaline phosphatase (NAP) score.

**Bone marrow.** The core biopsy sections (Fig. 39B) are hypercellular due to hyperplasia and shift toward immaturity of the granulocytic series, which gives rise to an increase in the M/E ratio. Erythropoiesis may be normal or reduced but is qualitatively normal. Megakaryocytes are often prominent (727), particularly if peripheral thrombocytosis is present. Their morphology is normal, although "naked" nuclei may be numerous. The features observed in the bone marrow aspirate recapitulate those observed in the peripheral blood smears and bone marrow biopsy.

##### Differential Diagnosis

The main differential diagnostic problem is the distinction of neutrophilic LRs from the chronic phase of *chronic myelogenous leukemia (CML)*. CML is the prototype of the chronic myeloproliferative disorders and was the first human neoplasm discovered to be associated with a specific cytoge-

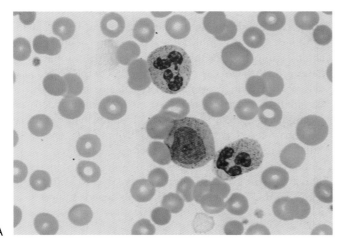 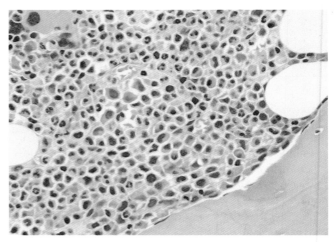

**FIG. 39.** Leukemoid reaction. **A:** The peripheral blood smear shows mature neutrophils with toxic granules and a leftward shift. (Courtesy of the Laboratory of Hematology of the New York University Medical Center.) **B:** The marrow biopsy demonstrates hypercellularity and granulocytic hyperplasia.

netic abnormality, i.e., the presence of a minute, abnormal chromosome (the "Philadelphia" chromosome) (728). It was subsequently recognized that CML is characterized by a reciprocal translocation involving the long arms of chromosomes 9 and 22, and that the originally described "minute" chromosome is a shortened chromosome 22 generated by the translocation (729). The Philadelphia chromosome is detected by karyotypic analysis in 90–95% of cases of CML (730), and its identification is essential for the diagnosis. The t(9;22) leads to the relocation of the protooncogene ABL (the normal cellular counterpart of the Abelson murine leukemia virus) from its normal site on chromosome 9 to chromosome 22, where it joins the sequences of a 5.8-kilobase pair region, the "breakpoint cluster region" (bcr), which is in turn part of the larger BCR gene (731). The chimeric

BCR-ABL gene is actively transcribed into mRNA, leading to the appearance of an abnormal 210-kDa protein having enhanced tyrosine kinase activity as compared to the normal ABL protein. It is generally assumed that these events play important but incompletely understood roles in the pathogenesis of CML.

The peripheral blood findings of CML (Fig. 40A) consist of neutrophilic leukocytosis (usually in excess of 50,000 per $\mu$l) associated with basophilia, anemia, and, frequently, thrombocytosis and eosinophilia (732). The blood smear shows a whole spectrum of immature and mature granulocytes, and the frequency of each granulocyte type increases with increasing cell maturation, with the exception of a myelocyte "bulge." Notably, peripheral blood basophilia is a constant feature of CML. Indeed, basophilia is often ob-

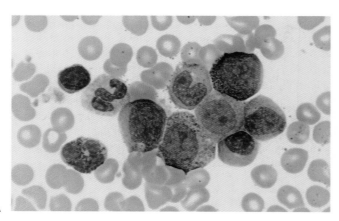 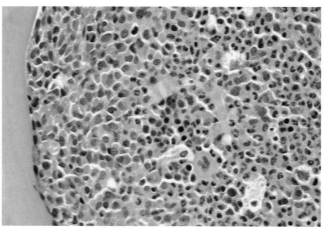

**FIG. 40.** Philadelphia-positive chronic myelogenous leukemia. **A:** The peripheral blood smear shows a whole spectrum of immature and mature granulocytes. A basophil is present *(left)*. **B:** The bone marrow biopsy is markedly hypercellular due to granulocytic hyperplasia. Expanded paratrabecular cuffs of immature granulocytes are visible; mature neutrophils are numerous in the central areas of the marrow spaces.

served in the setting of clonal hematopoietic disorders, and only rarely may it be seen in association with renal diseases, hypothyroidism, some viral infections, and ulcerative colitis (718). In addition, in CML the NAP score is usually decreased. The bone marrow (Fig. 40B) is markedly hypercellular with considerable granulocytic hyperplasia; expanded paratrabecular and perivascular cuffs of immature granulocytes, primarily consisting of promyelocytes and myelocytes, are prominent. Erythropoiesis is variably represented, but the M/E ratio is usually markedly increased. Megakaryocytes can vary in number, but are more frequently normal or increased, and are typically smaller than normal. Some reticulin fibrosis is generally present, and is at times marked, particularly during the evolution of the disease. In distinguishing neutrophilic LRs from CML, the examination of the peripheral blood smear and the evaluation of the above-mentioned laboratory findings are essential because the histopathologic changes observed in the core biopsy may sometimes be deceptively similar. LRs differ from CML in that the increase in the circulating immature granulocytes is not as marked as in the latter, basophilia is not observed, and the NAP score is increased. Most importantly, the Philadelphia chromosome (or its molecular counterpart, the BCR/ABL chimeric gene) is never observed.

Although these findings and the clinical history usually allow the differential diagnosis, difficulties may arise in some CML patients who present with slightly elevated leukocyte counts and minimal hematologic abnormalities ("early" CML). In these cases, a thorough laboratory workup as well as cytogenetic and/or molecular studies are necessary. It needs to be emphasized that basophilia, thrombocytosis, and a decrease in the NAP score are the earliest manifestations of CML, and may precede the typical clinical picture of the disease by several years (733).

Another chronic myeloproliferative disorder to be considered in the differential diagnosis with reactive LRs is *chronic neutrophilic leukemia (CNL)*. CNL is a very rare disorder that usually affects adult or elderly patients who present with anemia, splenomegaly, and peripheral blood leukocyte counts in excess of $30,000/\mu l$, with a predominance of mature neutrophils and band forms (734). The neutrophils may show toxic granulation and Dohle bodies. Laboratory findings include an increase in the NAP score as well as elevated serum levels of vitamin $B_{12}$ and uric acid. The bone marrow is hypercellular with granulocytic or, sometimes, trilineage hyperplasia with normal maturation and no significant increase in myeloblasts. Chromosome abnormalities have rarely been detected, but no specific aberration has been described. An association between CNL and polycythemia vera (another chronic myeloproliferative disorder) has been described (735,736). Survival in CNL has been reported to range from a few months to several years. During the course of the disease, evolution to a blastic phase may supervene. CNL must be distinguished from other myeloproliferative disorders as well as from reactive neutrophilia. Unlike CML, and similarly to LRs, in CNL peripheral blood basophilia is

absent, the NAP score is increased, and cytogenetic studies show no evidence of the Philadelphia chromosome. The diagnosis of CNL is one of exclusion, and should be considered only after other, more common clonal hematopoietic disorders have been excluded and all of the possible etiologies of reactive neutrophilia (including occult malignancies producing granulocytopoietic growth factors) have been eliminated.

### Evolution, Treatment, and Prognosis

These are determined by the cause of the LR. It has to be emphasized that an LR of unexplained origin may be the telltale sign of a serious underlying disorder.

## Peripheral Blood and Bone Marrow Changes Following Growth Factor (G-CSF/GM-CSF) Treatment

As previously alluded to, granulocyte colony-stimulating factor (G-CSF) and granulocyte/macrophage colony-stimulating factor (GM-CSF) are hematopoietic cytokines capable of influencing the proliferation, differentiation, and functional state of the myeloid cells, and are nowadays widely used in the treatment of neutropenias. G-CSF is selective for the neutrophil lineage, whereas GM-CSF has been shown to act on monocytes and eosinophils, in addition to neutrophils (737).

Neutropenia is a common occurrence in patients with malignancies, particularly when high-dose myelotoxic drugs are administered in the setting of cytoreductive treatment or in preparation for a bone marrow transplant. After administration of G-CSF or GM-CSF many patients will respond with a pronounced proliferation of granulocytic elements. If the original disease is a myelogenous leukemia, it may be difficult to decide on morphologic grounds alone whether or not residual disease is still present. The following paragraphs briefly describe the main morphologic and quantitative changes that can be sequentially observed in the peripheral blood and bone marrow following administration of G-CSF or GM-CSF, and outline some differential diagnostic criteria.

### Morphologic Findings

These have been recently reviewed in detail (738,739) and are not summarized here.

**Peripheral blood.** The changes resemble those seen in LRs, and consist of a neutrophilic leukocytosis occurring within 7–10 days after initiation of the treatment. The extent of the leukocytosis is variable. Bone marrow transplant recipients often have a blunted response to the growth factor treatment, and some do not respond at all. In the typical cases, left shift and toxic changes in the mature neutrophils are present; of note, some abnormal hypo- or hypersegmented forms as well as hypogranular neutrophils may be seen. Among the immature granulocytes, myelocytes predominate and are present in most cases, but some promyelocytes and even occasional myeloblasts (not exceeding 2–3% of the differential count) can be identified during the period of maximum response, which tends to occur after 10–15 days of therapy. Transient monocytosis, eosinophilia, and lymphocytosis (particularly of the large granular lymphocyte type) have also been reported, although these changes are not as consistently present as those involving the neutrophil lineage. Neutrophilia is accompanied by an increase in neutrophil alkaline phosphatase levels. Following discontinuation of the growth factors, the leukocyte count decreases progressively and rapidly, usually returning to the baseline levels within a week.

**Bone marrow.** The bone marrow changes tend to be more prominent immediately before or after the first appearance of the neutrophils in the blood, and have been arbitrarily categorized as "early" and "late." Early changes are those occurring within the 3 days preceding or following a peripheral blood absolute neutrophil count of 500 or more neutrophils per microliter. In the core biopsy, they typically consist of sparse clusters of immature granulocytes scattered in a hypocellular bone marrow (Fig. 41). These clusters can be seen away from the normal paratrabecular and/or perivascular sites of early granulocytopoiesis. The marrow aspirate smears show relative granulocytic hyperplasia with a predominance of promyelocytes and myelocytes (Fig. 42). These often display cytologic features suggestive of regeneration, such as large size, increased but evenly distributed azurophilic cytoplasmic granules, and prominent areas of perinuclear cytoplasmic clearing corresponding to the Golgi zone (740). The myelocytes often have increased cytoplasmic basophilia and inconspicuous secondary (specific) granules. Mitoses can be frequent, whereas mature neutrophils

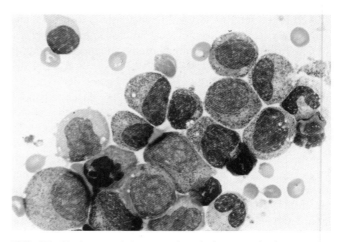

**FIG. 42.** Early growth factor–related changes. In the marrow smears, promyelocytes, and myelocytes with prominent cytoplasmic azurophilic granules predominate. Cytoplasmic vacuolization is present. (Courtesy of Dr. R. McKenna, University of Texas Southwestern Medical Center.)

are few, and those seen show toxic granulation. There should be no significant increase in myeloblasts, although blast counts in excess of 5% have been reported by some (740). There may be an increase in eosinophils.

The late bone marrow changes have been defined as those observed from the time of the maximum peripheral blood WBC response through the week following cessation of the therapy. In general, they are less distinctive than those observed early on. The marrow may be hypo- or hypercellular with a normal or increased M/E ratio due to granulocytic hyperplasia. The neutrophil series shows a progressive decrease in the most immature granulocytic precursors (myeloblasts and promyelocytes) and a predominance of myelocytes, metamyelocytes, and segmented neutrophils exhibiting toxic granulation of variable intensity. After discontinuation of the treatment, the marrow cellularity decreases progressively in the following 4–8 weeks.

*Differential Diagnosis*

The effects of G-CSF/GM-CSF treatment can be regarded as the iatrogenic counterpart of the florid granulocytic hyperplasias due to an exuberant release of *endogenous* hematopoietic growth factors that may follow toxic marrow injury, infection, or inflammation. The features of cellular immaturity observed during the early response to the treatment may simulate a *de novo* acute myelogenous leukemia (AML) or, more frequently, *persistent AML after chemotherapy*. As a rule, this diagnostic problem requires a thorough knowledge of the clinical history and the review of the original diagnostic material. Furthermore, the core biopsy morphology should always be interpreted in the light of the quantitative and qualitative findings observed in the peripheral blood and bone marrow aspirate smears. In particular, the identification of "toxic" changes in the peripheral blood

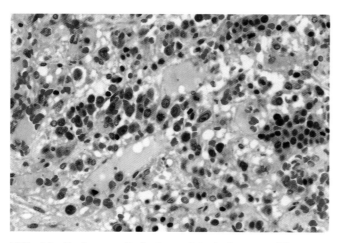

**FIG. 41.** Early growth factor–related changes. The core biopsy shows a hypocellular marrow with acute post-chemotherapy effects. A cluster of immature granulocytes *(left)* and an erythroid colony *(right)* are seen. (Courtesy of Dr. R. McKenna, University of Texas Southwestern Medical Center.)

granulocytes is suggestive of a regenerative process. It has to be considered that rare circulating myeloblasts can be seen in the peripheral smear of patients receiving growth factors, but they usually do not exceed 3% of the differential count and are primarily seen during the period of maximum leukocytosis. Their presence, therefore, does not necessarily imply persistent leukemia, especially if other features suggestive of regeneration are present. On the other side, peripheral blood myeloblast in excess of 3% of the differential count or prolonged persistence of myeloblasts and lack of recovery of the other hematologic indices are worrisome, and suggest that further evaluation is necessary. The presence of Auer rods is considered evidence of persistent leukemia.

In the bone marrow, both the cytologic features of the immature granulocytes (as best seen in the aspirate smears) and the overall cellular composition of the hematopoietic population must be evaluated. As previously mentioned, the early changes of G-CSF/GM-CSF treatment are marked by a predominance of large, reactive-appearing promyelocytes and myelocytes with no significant increase in myeloblasts. On the other side, severe dysplasia (particularly if involving multiple cell lineages) is suspicious for residual disease, and Auer rods are diagnostic of it. Patients treated for acute promyelocytic leukemia (APL) and receiving growth factors may be difficult to evaluate because regenerating promyelocytes may resemble APL cells. In addition, the treatment may be responsible for a prolonged survival of residual leukemic cells (741). In each case, careful evaluation of the cytologic details is essential; however, additional cytogenetic, molecular, and/or immunophenotypic studies are often necessary too. In some cases, the distinction between growth factor effects and residual leukemia requires discontinuation of the treatment and subsequent bone marrow reexamination after 1 or 2 weeks.

### Evolution, Treatment, and Prognosis

G-CSF and GM-CSF are extensively used in the treatment of neutropenia, but several reports suggest that some caution should be exercised because they may stimulate the growth of both normal and neoplastic myelogenous precursors (741–743). Evolution to myelodysplastic syndromes and/or leukemias after treatment with G-CSF for aplastic anemia has been described (744).

## LYMPHOID/PLASMACELLULAR HYPERPLASIAS SIMULATING NEOPLASMS

### Reactive Lymphoid Lesions

Reactive lymphoid lesions (RLLs) can be identified in a considerable proportion (18–47%) of all bone marrow specimens (745). Their characteristics are best appreciated in the histologic sections. In some cases the distinction between benign and malignant bone marrow lymphoid infiltrates is

straightforward, and can be accomplished on a purely histologic basis, but recourse to additional techniques is often necessary to solve differential diagnostic problems. Flow cytometry immunophenotyping, immunofluorescence microscopy, cytogenetics, and gene rearrangement analysis are often very helpful in the evaluation of the clonality of marrow lymphoid lesions, even though these studies generally necessitate that fresh samples of bone marrow aspirate or peripheral blood be sent to fully equipped laboratories. In addition, the recent generation of polyclonal or monoclonal antibodies raised against cytoplasmic or surface antigens resistant to the process of paraffin embedding has made it possible to perform the *in situ* immunophenotypic characterization of the hematopoietic cells in conventionally processed bone marrow specimens (746). Paraffin immunohistochemistry is of considerable importance when marrow fibrosis hampers a successful aspiration.

Lastly, the importance of a careful examination of the peripheral blood has to be emphasized. Lymphoma cells can be identified in the blood smears of approximately 50% of patients with bone marrow involvement by non-Hodgkin's lymphomas, and are most frequently observed in low-grade, small cell disorders (747). The actual incidence, however, is likely higher because small populations of morphologically undetectable circulating neoplastic cells can be identified by flow cytometry or gene rearrangement studies (748,749). Blood involvement without bone marrow disease is rare, and positive peripheral blood results can help in the interpretation of bone marrow specimens with "atypical" or "borderline" morphologic features.

### Clinical Features

Marrow RLLs are not associated with any specific clinical setting, and may be seen in clinically healthy individuals as well as in patients affected by a number of disease processes. They are more common in adult or elderly subjects and in females, in whom they are usually not associated with any particular disease. In younger individuals, RLLs often coexist with inflammatory or immune-mediated disorders including HIV infection.

### Morphologic Findings

**Peripheral blood.** There are no specific peripheral blood changes or abnormal laboratory data. If abnormalities are found, they are generally secondary to an associated disorder.

**Bone marrow.** Three main morphologic types of reactive focal infiltrates are recognized: lymphoid aggregates, polymorphous lymphohistiocytic lesions, and germinal centers.

*Reactive lymphoid aggregates* (RLAs) (Fig. 43A, B) range in size from 50 to 1000 μm, may be solitary or multiple, and are in general randomly scattered in the marrow spaces, away from the osseous trabeculae. They are usually well circumscribed and primarily composed of loosely arranged small, mature lymphocytes often admixed with some histiocytes and plasma cells. A few eosinophils and mast cells may be observed as well. RLAs are frequently centered or traversed by small blood vessels, and exhibit a distinct network of reticulin fibers.

*Reactive polymorphous lymphohistiocytic lesions* (RPLLs) (Fig. 43C, D) are less common and are often associated with diseases characterized by an abnormal functioning of the immune system such as connective tissue disorders, immune-mediated cytopenias, or HIV infection. In these instances, the lesions may be single or multiple, large and poorly defined, and exhibit a polycellular composition including small lymphocytes, scattered larger "transformed" lymphoid cells, epithelioid histiocytes, plasma cells, eosinophils, and mast cells. Blood vessels are often present. Both the small and the larger lymphoid cells may display some nuclear irregulari-

ties, and mitoses may be seen. Reticulin fibers are generally prominent.

*Germinal centers* (GCs) (Fig. 43E, F) are the rarest type of bone marrow RLL. Their frequency has been estimated at about 0.8% of all bone marrow specimens (750). They are more often seen in young individuals and in female patients, frequently in the context of an inflammatory or autoimmune disorder. Bone marrow GCs are usually single and randomly scattered in the marrow spaces. They consist of a central area featuring a mixed population of large noncleaved cells, small cleaved cells, and scattered tingible body histiocytes, surrounded by a peripheral cuff of small round lymphocytes forming a mantle zone.

### Differential Diagnosis

Reactive bone marrow lymphoid lesions need to be distinguished from both *Hodgkin's disease (HD)* and *non-*

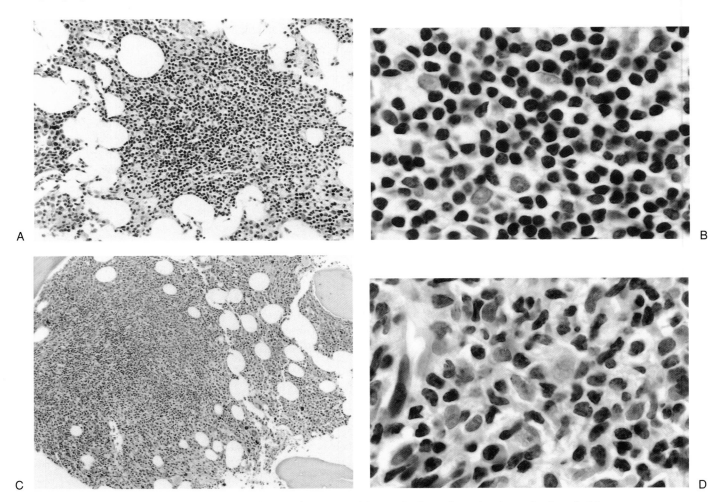

**FIG. 43.** Reactive lymphoid lesions in the marrow biopsy. **A:** A medium-sized reactive lymphoid aggregate with well-circumscribed borders. **B:** At a higher power, most of the cells are small lymphocytes without nuclear atypia, admixed with a few histiocytes and plasma cells. **C:** A large polymorphous lymphohistiocytic lesion in a patient with HIV infection. **D:** At a higher power, small lymphocytes with irregular nuclear contours are admixed with numerous histiocytes. In these lesions, epithelioid macrophages and scattered large transformed lymphocytes may also be seen. *(continued)*

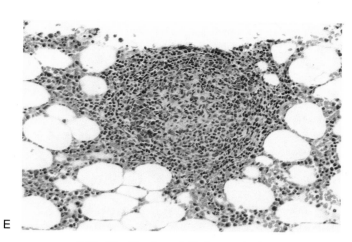 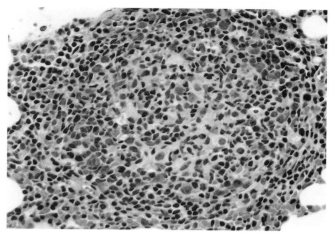

**FIG. 43.** *Continued* **E:** A germinal center. **F:** At a higher power, well-defined borders and a mixed cell population of large noncleaved and small cleaved cells are evident.

*Hodgkin's lymphoma (NHL)*. Before discussing the differential diagnostic criteria, it may be useful to outline some general considerations pertinent to the bone marrow involvement during the course of these hematopoietic malignancies.

Marrow involvement occurs in about 10–15% of cases of *HD*, and is more frequent in the lymphocyte depletion and mixed cellularity categories (751). Patients are typically adult or elderly men with clinically advanced disease. The criteria for the diagnosis of HD in the bone marrow differ depending on whether or not a previous diagnosis of HD has been established. In the first instance, the following recommendations should be followed (751,752):

1. HD can be diagnosed when typical Reed–Sternberg (R-S) cells or their mononuclear variants are seen in one of the cellular environments appropriate for HD.
2. The presence of "atypical histiocytes" lacking the features of diagnostic cells in one of the cellular environments appropriate for HD or in focal or diffuse areas of fibrosis is strongly suggestive of involvement.
3. Fibrosis or necrosis alone is to be regarded as suspicious.

When there is no previous history of HD, it is required that typical R-S cells be identified in a cellular background that is appropriate for HD. Examination of serial sections and paraffin immunohistochemistry are often necessary to support the initial morphologic impression. If uncertainties persist, a repeat biopsy is recommended, unless other evidence of stage IV disease is found. Marrow lesions of HD may be focal (20–30% of cases) or diffuse (70–80%); in the latter, entire marrow spaces between the bony trabeculae are replaced by Hodgkin's tissue. All of the morphologic patterns observed in the lymph nodes involved by HD can be recapitulated in the bone marrow. The R-S cells or their variants

(Fig. 44A, B) are always found in a stromal reaction typical of HD and not in areas of otherwise unremarkable marrow. In general, the infiltrates are cytologically polymorphous: the "appropriate cellular environment" of HD typically consists of a mixed population of benign-looking small lymphocytes, histiocytes, plasma cells, eosinophils, and neutrophils, in which rare or numerous R-S cells and/or mononuclear variants are interspersed. A marked epithelioid reaction may be observed (Fig. 44C). Reticulin and/or collagen fibrosis is constantly present, and at times collagen fibrosis is so intense as to obscure the florid, polymorphous appearance characteristic of Hodgkin's tissue. Paraffin immunostains help to highlight the diagnostic cells when these are sparse and to recognize their distinctive immunophenotypic profile. In fact, in most cases of HD of the nonlymphocyte predominance type, the R-S cells and their variants are reactive for CD15 (Leu-M1), CD30 (Ber-H2), and CD74 (LN-2) but do not express CD45 (leukocyte common antigen) or EMA (epithelial membrane antigen), and only infrequently are B- or T-cell-associated antigens detected (753). Classification of HD based on the bone marrow biopsy alone is not recommended: the marrow biopsy may be too small to fully evaluate architecture and cytology, and the histologic subtype of HD may appear different in the lymph node and bone marrow obtained from the same patient.

The overall frequency of marrow involvement by *NHL* ranges from approximately 30% to 50% (751), but the actual incidence varies according to the B- or T-cell lineage and histopathologic category. As a rule, the NHLs that more often involve the bone marrow are the low-grade, small cell lymphomas (the majority of which are of B-cell origin), the various histotypes of peripheral T-cell lymphomas, and the high-grade lymphomas of lymphoblastic and small noncleaved cell types. Neoplastic lymphoid infiltrates may exhibit a focal, interstitial, or diffuse distribution, and more than one pattern might be seen in an individual case. Focal

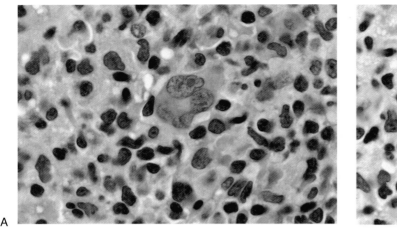

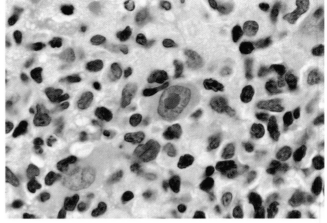

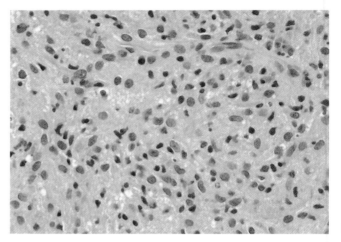

**FIG. 44.** Hodgkin's disease in the marrow biopsy. **A:** A Reed–Sternberg cell. **B:** A mononuclear variant. **C:** Intense epithelioid cell reaction with sparse eosinophils.

lesions are more frequent, and can be paratrabecular or randomly distributed within the marrow spaces (Fig. 45 A, B). Lymphoid infiltrates distinctly streaming along the bony surfaces are always atypical and suspicious for malignancy, whereas the random, nonparatrabecular pattern lacks diagnostic specificity by itself, and other criteria need to be considered in the differential diagnosis (see below). Interstitial involvement is often associated with significant sparing of the normal hematopoietic elements, and might be difficult to identify, whereas diffuse lesions replace entire areas of hematopoietic tissue between the bony trabeculae. Some histotypes of NHL may show a preferential pattern of bone marrow involvement. For instance, paratrabecular lymphoid infiltrates primarily composed of small cleaved cells are typical of the lymphomas of follicular center cell origin, whereas the lesions of other small B-cell malignancies are often randomly scattered, and more rarely interstitial or paratrabecular.

A description of the clinical, morphologic, and immunophenotypic characteristics of the various histotypes of NHL is beyond the limits of this discussion. However, the features of *peripheral T-cell lymphomas (PTCLs)* are rele-

vant enough to the purposes of this chapter to deserve a brief mention. PTCLs comprise a heterogeneous group of post-thymic (i.e., nonlymphoblastic) lymphoproliferations other than mycosis fungoides and the chronic lymphoid leukemias of T-cell origin. Based on their growth pattern and cytology, the majority of PTCLs are classified as "diffuse mixed (small and large) cell" lymphomas according to the Working Formulation proposals for the classification of the NHL (754). Other, less common cases may be predominantly composed of large or small T cells. Rare in the Western countries, PTCLs usually affect adults, often disseminated at the time of diagnosis, and tend to pursue an aggressive clinical course. Immunophenotypically, most PTCL express a CD4+ helper-inducer phenotype (755), but abnormal antigenic profiles (eg, loss of one or more pan-T-cell markers; CD4/CD8 double-positive or double-negative phenotypes) are not uncommon (15). Several antibodies are currently available for the immunologic characterization of PTCLs in paraffin sections, and the use of polyclonal anti-CD3 in combination with monoclonal antibodies recognizing the T-cell associated-CD45R0 isoform of the leukocyte common antigen (e.g., UCHL-1) is recommended for the diagnosis of

PTCL in routinely processed specimens (756). Bone marrow involvement occurs in about 70% of cases (757,758). The lesions are focal or diffuse, and are characterized by a pleomorphic lymphoid infiltrate often admixed with an abundant polycellular reactive population including plasma cells, eosinophils, neutrophils, and epithelioid histiocytes (Fig. 45C, D). Increased vascularity and reticulin fibrosis are common, and large cells resembling R-S cells may be encountered. It has been emphasized that the histopathology of PTCL in the bone marrow is not pathognomonic, and that PTCL may closely resemble other processes such as Hodgkin's disease, some B-cell lymphomas, mast cell disease, and the reactive polymorphous lymphohistiocytic lesions commonly associated with immunologic disorders (757). Whenever possible, the diagnosis of PTCL in the bone marrow should be supported by the clinical history, immunophenotypic and/or immunogenotypic studies, and review of any previous diagnostic material. Paraffin immuno-stains demonstrate the T-cell lineage of the *atypical* lymphoid cells in most cases.

Each of the previously discussed main categories of marrow RLL presents its own differential diagnostic problems. RLAs must be distinguished from the focal, nonparatrabecular lesions often seen in low-grade, small cell, non-Hodgkin's lymphomas. In general, morphologic features suggestive of a reactive nature are unifocality or sparsity of the lymphoid aggregates, lack of a distinct association with the osseous trabeculae, small size, well-circumscribed margins, and predominance of a population of loosely-arranged small lymphocytes admixed with a minor component of histiocytes, mature plasma cells, eosinophils and mast cells, absence of significant nuclear atypia and mitotic figures, and presence of small blood vessels. In contrast, suggestive of malignancy are pronounced multifocality of the lesions, paratrabecular streaming, large size, poorly-delimited margins, unusually compact and/or monomorphic cellularity and significant nuclear atypia or mitotic activity. Exceptions, however, are common. To overcome the limitations of conventional morphology, some recent studies have attempted to identify possible differences between reactive and neo-

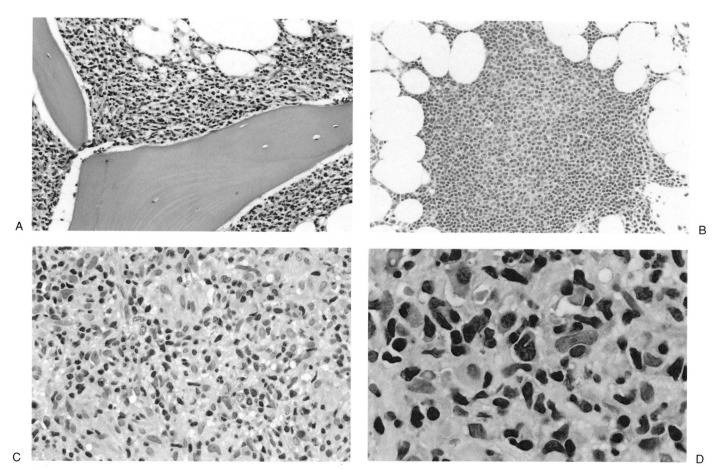

**FIG. 45.** Non-Hodgkin's lymphomas in the marrow biopsy. **A:** A focal paratrabecular lesion. **B:** A focal nonparatrabecular lesion of well-differentiated lymphocytic lymphoma. The pale central area is a "proliferation center." **C:** A peripheral T-cell lymphoma. Bone marrow lesions are typically characterized by a polymorphous cellularity and numerous epithelioid histiocytes. **D:** At a higher power, small and large atypical lymphoid cells are admixed with histiocytes, plasma cells, and eosinophils.

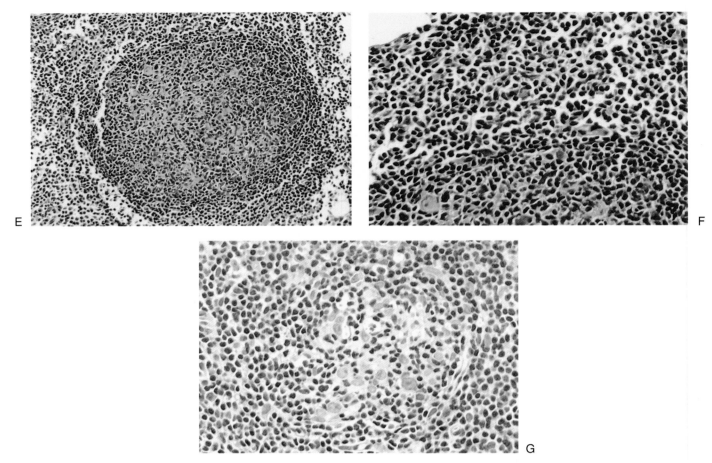

**FIG. 45.** *Continued* **E:** A nodular lesion of follicular lymphoma. Compare with Fig. 43E. **F:** At a higher power, small lymphoid cells are seen streaming outside the main nodule. **G:** Mantle cell lymphoma. Residual larger germinal center cells surrounded by the smaller neoplastic lymphocytes.

plastic marrow B-cell lymphoid aggregates by means of paraffin immunohistochemistry. For instance, it has been described that RLAs are often compartmentalized in a central area consisting primarily of B cells and in a peripheral zone rich in T cells. Focal B-cell neoplastic infiltrates may also contain a component of reactive T lymphocytes, but the zonal arrangement observed in reactive aggregates may be lost (759). Other authors have reported that the staining pattern of marrow lymphoid aggregates for the B-cell associated marker recognized by the antibody L26 (CD20) may discriminate between reactive and neoplastic small B-cell lesions. The former are reported to show a "mixed" pattern of positivity (even distribution of CD20-positive and CD20-negative cells) or a "focally homogeneous" staining (collections of CD20-positive cells surrounded by or surrounding CD20-negative cells), while the latter tend to show "homogeneous" L26 positivity (uniform staining of the majority of the cells throughout the aggregate) (760). Still other studies suggest that the expression of the bcl-2 oncogene product may be preferentially observed in neoplastic as opposed to reactive marrow B-cell lymphoid aggregates (761). As previously noted in this chapter, however, whenever immunoreactivity for bcl-2 is relied upon in distinguishing re-

active from neoplastic B-cell proliferations, the findings should be evaluated in conjunction with immunostains highlighting the reactive, bcl-2 positive T cells interspersed in the same areas. Lastly, however promising these results might be, one has to acknowledge that some histologically "borderline" cases of lymphoid lesions remain unsolved even after paraffin immunohistochemistry. This can be an issue, particularly in patients with previous history of low-grade B cell lymphoma undergoing a bone marrow examination for staging purposes or to ascertain the existence and extent of residual disease after cytoreductive treatment. In our opinion, these diagnostic problems are best approached when the combined use of traditional histology and flow cytometry immunophenotyping (and, if necessary, gene rearrangement studies) is planned ahead of time.

Because of their peculiar morphological appearance, RPLL may closely resemble the focal lesions of PTCL and HD. Despite their biological diversity, these three entities share some features, such as a polymorphous cellular infiltrate often rich in epithelioid histiocytes and the immunohistochemical finding of a predominance of T lymphocytes. However, in PTCL there usually is a spectrum of atypical lymphoid cells of different size and shape, nuclear pleomorphism may be pronounced and mitoses are often seen. On the other side, one of the distinguishing features of HD is the sharp hiatus between the abundant polycellular reactive component and the large, frankly atypical Reed–Sternberg cells or mononuclear variants. In contrast, RPLLs as a rule lack the pleomorphism, nuclear atypia, and mitotic activity of PTCLs or the diagnostic cells of HD. Immunohistochemical stains may also help in demonstrating the T-cell nature of the atypical lymphoid infiltrate of PTCL or in recognizing the immunophenotypic profile typical of HD. This notwithstanding, in an occasional case the differential diagnosis may be difficult. Therefore, thorough knowledge of the clinical history, review of the original diagnostic specimens, and correlation of the morphologic features with the results of additional (e.g., immunophenotypic) findings are always necessary. Aside from cases in which the overall morphologic features are unequivocally diagnostic of malignancy, the possibility that focal "polymorphous" marrow lymphoid infiltrates may be secondary to reactive processes should always be considered, particularly in patients affected by immunologic disorders.

Although most bone marrow GCs are readily recognized as reactive, they may be difficult to distinguish from some unusual instances of involvement by *follicular lymphomas (FLs)* and *mantle cell lymphomas (MCLs)*. *FLs* of predominantly small cleaved and mixed (small cleaved and large cell) types involve the bone marrow in about 50–60% of cases (747). The most frequent pattern is focal paratrabecular with a predominance of small cleaved cells, regardless of the lymph node histology. At times, however, FLs in the bone marrow become manifest as nodular foci composed of a mixed population of large cleaved and noncleaved cells, often surrounded by small cleaved cells spreading into the surrounding marrow spaces. These nodular infiltrates may occur in the setting of extensive involvement or, rarely, as isolated lesions (Fig. 45E, F). In the latter instance, their distinction from reactive GCs can be difficult, and requires a careful evaluation of the cytologic features observed in multiple sections as well as the review of the original lymph node biopsy. The finding of immunohistochemical reactivity for *bcl-2* in the follicular center cells supports a diagnosis of malignancy. If the bone marrow biopsy is the first diagnostic procedure and the overall findings are "atypical" but not unequivocally diagnostic, clinical evidence of lymphadenopathy or of a tissue mass should be sought and, if possible, a biopsy obtained. Otherwise, a repeat (possibly bilateral) bone marrow biopsy is advisable, and a sample of marrow aspirate should be submitted for flow cytometry or gene rearrangement studies. Marrow involvement by *MCL* is also common, being present in approximately 65% of cases at the time of diagnosis (762). In most instances, the features are those of a small cell lymphoproliferation with a focal, interstitial, or diffuse growth pattern, and are characterized by a degree of cytologic atypia "intermediate" between small lymphocytic and small cleaved cell lymphomas. Occasionally, the neoplastic infiltrate exhibits small and atrophic GCs

surrounded by thick cuffs of small lymphocytes (Fig. 45G). The diagnosis of lymphoma is based on the abnormal morphology of the lesions as well as on the comparison with the features of the initial diagnostic material. Flow cytometry and immunogenotypic analysis are important adjuncts to morphology.

### Evolution, Treatment, and Prognosis

Marrow RLLs require no treatment other than that appropriate for the disorder with which they may be associated. However, their presence has been associated with subsequent progression to overtly neoplastic lymphoproliferations in approximately one third of cases (763).

### Reactive Plasmacytosis

In normal conditions, plasma cells account for approximately 2% of the marrow elements, and in adult individuals an upper normal limit of 2–3% is generally accepted (767,768). In infants and children, they are even less conspicuous. In the marrow biopsy sections, normal plasma cells occur singly or in small aggregates in the interstitial spaces or clustered around capillaries. More than half of them contain cytoplasmic immunoglobulins of the IgG type, about a third produce IgA, and the remainder express IgM (769). Stains for immunoglobulin light chains show that both kappa- and lambda-positive plasma cells are present in a ratio of approximately 2:1 ("polyclonal" pattern).

In reactive plasmacytosis (RP), polyclonal marrow plasma cells are increased due to systemic antigenic stimulation. RP is not uncommon, and in one study it was detected in 28.6% of bone marrow specimens (767).

### Clinical Features

The conditions associated with RP are numerous, and include hematologic and nonhematologic neoplasia, nonneoplastic hematologic diseases, drug reactions, and infectious diseases and inflammatory processes, as well as heterogeneous disorders such as cirrhosis, cardiovascular disease, renal failure, and diabetes mellitus (767). An increase in reactive plasma cells is also frequently seen in postchemotherapy marrow specimens and in HIV-positive individuals.

### Morphologic Findings

**Peripheral blood.** No specific pattern of changes is recognized. If abnormalities are present, they reflect the associated disease process. Circulating activated lymphocytes, immunoblasts, and/or plasmacytoid cells may be seen when the response to an antigenic stimulus is intense.

**Bone marrow.** In RP plasma cells do not usually exceed 20% of all nucleated marrow elements, although occasionally higher values may be encountered. The plasma cells retain their interstitial and/or pericapillary location, and may form small aggregates (Fig. 46A). Mature plasma cells predominate, even though rare bi- or even trinucleated forms can be noted. Eosinophilic, PAS-positive cytoplasmic or intranuclear immunoglobulin inclusions (Russell or Dutcher bodies, respectively), or plasma cells with multiple cytoplasmic globules (Mott cells) can be present (Fig. 46B). Although these features are more commonly observed in clonal plasma cell processes, their occurrence as occasional findings does not necessarily imply malignancy. However, substantial atypia, immaturity, or nucleocytoplasmic dyssynchrony are not observed. Additional findings in RP include the presence of lymphoid follicles and lipid granulomas, noted in 25% and 12% of RP cases, respectively (767). A peculiar feature of RP is the "plasmocytic satellitosis," a morphologic unit composed of a central histiocyte surrounded by three or more plasma cells. This finding, which is best appreciated in the marrow aspirate smears, may be noted in up to 10% of bone marrows without RP and in about 45% of those with RP, and is only occasionally present in true, clonal plasma cell proliferations (770). Lastly, in RP immunostains show a polyclonal pattern of cytoplasmic immunoglobulin light chain expression.

### Differential Diagnosis

*Plasma cell dyscrasias (PCDs)* comprise a group of hematopoietic disorders characterized by the proliferation of a clone of immunoglobulin-producing plasma cells. The bone marrow is most often the primary site of involvement. The PCDs to be considered in the differential diagnosis with RP are *multiple myeloma (MM)* and its *smoldering* variant *(SMM)* as well as the *monoclonal gammopathies of unknown significance (MGUS)*. In addition, plasma cell differentiation is by definition present in *small lymphocytic lymphoma, lymphoplasmacytoid (SLL-LP)*; this entity is also included in

the differential diagnosis of marrow plasma cell proliferations. The essential features of these clonal plasma cell processes are briefly outlined before discussing their differential diagnosis with RP.

Patients with *MM* are usually adult or elderly individuals with anemia, bone pain, renal failure, or recurrent infections. The criteria for the diagnosis include an increase in abnormal marrow plasma cells along with evidence of a serum and/or urinary paraprotein or radiologically detectable multiple bony lesions. In general, a minimum of 10% bone marrow plasma cells and 3 g/dl of monoclonal serum paraprotein or more than 1 g/day of kappa or lambda immunoglobulin light chain proteinuria are required (771). The paraprotein is an IgG in approximately 50–60% of cases and an IgA in 20–25%; about 15% of MMs produce only light chains; nonsecretory myelomas are very rare. In approximately 20% of patients the abnormal paraprotein is found in the urine only. Additional laboratory findings include an elevated ESR, hypercalcemia, and abnormal renal function indices. The extent of bone marrow replacement is variable, but usually plasma cells account for 20% or more of the myelogram. The pattern of infiltration may be focal, interstitial, or diffuse. Plasma cells may range from well differentiated to highly atypical (Fig. 47A, B). Intranuclear or intracytoplasmic immunoglobulin inclusions are common. Evidence of bone damage can be seen, either due to direct destruction or consequent to the plasma cell production of "osteoclast-activating factors" such as TNFβ or IL-1 (772–774). The estimation of the tumor burden as judged from the biopsy sections may be useful for staging purposes (775). The unusual variant of *SMM* accounts for about 2% of all cases of MM (776). Patients usually have 10% or more bone marrow plasma cells with a monoclonal spike of at least 3 g/dl and/or small amounts of light chain proteinuria, but have a stable, prolonged clinical course without anemia, renal failure, or bone lesions. In this respect, their disease resembles *MGUS*. This too is a disease of the elderly and is indeed the most common

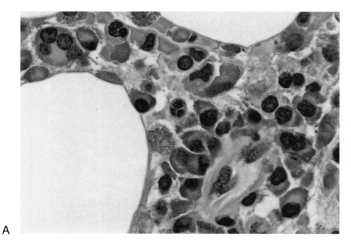
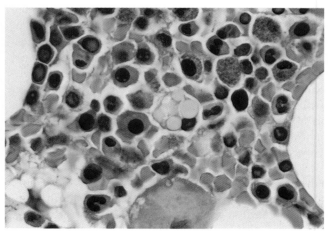

A                                                                                                                                                      B

**FIG. 46.** Reactive plasmacytosis in the marrow biopsy. **A:** A pericapillary plasma cell aggregate with a trinucleated form *(upper left field)*. **B:** A Mott cell *(center)*.

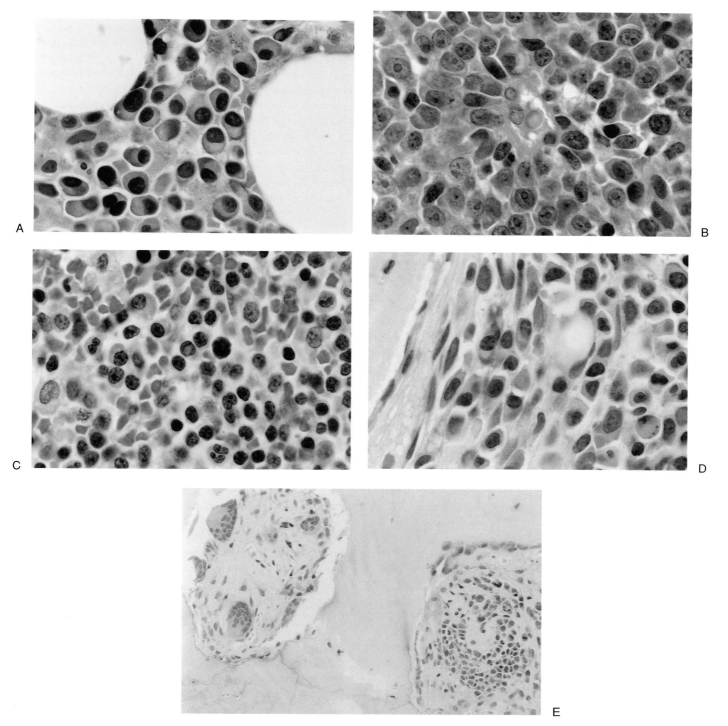

**FIG. 47.** Plasma cell dyscrasias in the marrow biopsy. **A:** A well-differentiated multiple myeloma. **B:** A case of myeloma with marked plasma cell atypia. **C:** Small lymphocytic lymphoma, plasmacytoid. A Dutcher body is present in the center. **D:** Plasmacytosis in a patient with monoclonal gammopathy of un- known significance and Paget's disease of the bone. Note paratrabecular fibrosis. **E:** Same case as D. Bone thickening, osteoblastic activation, and osteoclastic bone reabsorption are present; cement lines are seen in the lower left field.

form of PCD (777). Its main features are a stable serum paraprotein of <3 g/dl with no or negligible amounts of urinary paraprotein and no anemia, bone lesions, hypercalcemia, or renal failure. Plasma cells most often do not exceed 5% of the marrow elements, generally appear morphologically mature, and exhibit a perivascular or interstitial location, with the possible formation of small aggregates. Despite the indolent clinical behavior of their disease, approximately 25% of patients with MGUS eventually progress to overt MM, amyloidosis, Waldenstrom's macroglobulinemia, or other lymphoproliferative disorders (777). Lastly, *SLL-LP* is a morphologically and immunophenotypically distinct small B-lymphocyte disorder in which plasmacytoid differentiation is a defining feature (778). Patients are mostly adult or elderly individuals with lymphadenopathy and/or splenomegaly (about 50% of the cases) or peripheral blood cytopenias due to bone marrow disease. A "leukemic" blood picture due to circulating small lymphocytes and plasmacytoid forms is seen in about 30% of cases. In addition, a monoclonal paraprotein (most often of the IgM type) is frequently detected. SLL-LP is indeed the most frequent morphologic substrate of the clinicopathologic entity known as Waldenstrom's macroglobulinemia (WM), whose signs and symptoms are due to peripheral blood hyperviscosity consequent on the physicochemical properties of the secreted paraprotein. Bone marrow involvement is present in about 70% of cases of SLL-LP, and may be focal (paratrabecular or random), interstitial, or diffuse. The neoplastic population typically consists of an admixture of small B lymphocytes, plasmacytoid cells (cells with abundant, plasma cell–like cytoplasm but lymphocyte-like nuclei), and mature-looking plasma cells (Fig. 47C). Both the lymphoid and the plasma cell components may display some atypia, and intranuclear and/or cytoplasmic inclusions are frequently observed. An increase in mast cells is also often seen. The coexistence of an atypical small B-lymphocyte infiltrate bearing clonally restricted surface immunoglobulins with a population of plasmacytoid elements and plasma cells expressing the same cytoplasmic immunoglobulins is the hallmark of this disease.

The distinction between RP and the various types of PCD requires the evaluation of multiple parameters, and cannot be based on morphology or plasma cell counts alone because in some cases of RP plasma cells are considerably increased and may exhibit cytologic features (e.g., multinuclearity, intranuclear or cytoplasmic inclusions) more commonly associated with clonal processes. On morphologic grounds, however, the recognition of some abnormal growth patterns such as large and/or paratrabecular plasma cell foci or a pronounced interstitial plasma cell infiltrate certainly indicates the need for further investigation, particularly when distinct cytologic atypia is present. The combination of bony lesions and marrow plasmacytosis is also abnormal, but it has to be considered that the association between the two can be purely coincidental and due to the possible coexistence of primary diseases of the skeletal system such as Paget's disease of the bone (Fig. 47D, E). In addition to a careful consideration of the clinical setting, laboratory studies aimed at the detection and characterization of monoclonal paraproteins in serum or urine samples are essential in the diagnosis and classification of the PCD and in its differentiation from RP. In reactive conditions associated with RP and polyclonal hypergammaglobulinemia, a serum protein electrophoresis shows a broad-based peak in the densitometer tracing or a broad band on the cellulose membrane, usually limited to the $\gamma$ region. In contrast, a monoclonal paraprotein is identified as a narrow peak in the $\gamma$, $\beta$, or $\alpha_2$ regions of the densitometer tracing or as a dense, discrete band on the cellulose membrane. Both immunoelectrophoresis and immunofixation (particularly the latter) are more sensitive than conventional electrophoresis in the detection of monoclonal components (779).

Immunohistochemistry is another extremely useful tool in the differential diagnosis of bone marrow plasma cell processes. Evaluating the pattern of cytoplasmic immunoglobulin light chain expression frequently allows one to formulate a judgment concerning plasma cell clonality. As mentioned, the polyclonal staining pattern typical of RP consists of the presence of $\kappa$- and $\lambda$-positive plasma cells in a ratio of about 2:1. Even considering some normal interindividual variability, $\kappa/\lambda$ ratios of >4:1 or <1:2 are generally regarded as abnormal, and justify further investigation. Indeed, in many cases of PCD immunohistochemistry shows that the proliferating plasma cells predominantly express either one of the two possible immunoglobulin light chains. Several studies have established the importance of a quantitative evaluation of the light chain ratio by means of bone marrow immunohistology as a tool to distinguish the various forms of PCD from one another and from RP. In one report, for instance, cases of RP were characterized by a $\kappa/\lambda$ ratio of 1.5 ± 0.7, in contrast with light chain ratios >11.2 or <0.1 in cases of MM producing abnormal immunoglobulins of $\kappa$ or $\lambda$ type, respectively (780). In contrast, in MGUS the quantitative light chain ratios, when abnormal, are less markedly altered than in MM, and the values observed in these two types of PCD tend not to overlap (780,781). In addition, it has to be mentioned that in about one third of patients with MGUS immunohistochemical studies will result in a polyclonal staining pattern despite the existence of a serum or urinary monoclonal paraprotein. This finding can be explained assuming that in these patients the emergent clone of abnormal plasma cells is too small to be visualized, and the diagnosis is impossible without the support of adequate laboratory data. Discordance between the immunohistochemical and the serum/urine immunoelectrophoretic findings can, in fact, be expected when the percentage of bone marrow plasma cells is <5% (782). On the other side, bone marrow immunohistology is essential in those rare cases of nonsecretory clonal plasma cell proliferations, in which a serum or urinary paraprotein is undetectable, as well as in the evaluation of residual disease in patients with MM in whom the serum or urine paraprotein is no longer present after treatment (782).

Lastly, RP associated with reactive lymphoid aggregates

may simulate *SLL-LP*. The differential diagnosis is based on the abnormal morphology of the lymphoplasmacellular infiltrate observed in the latter as well as on the different clinical setting and immunophenotypic and electrophoretic studies.

### Evolution, Treatment, and Prognosis

Reactive marrow plasmacytosis is related to an underlying stimulus, the nature of which determines the therapeutic approach.

### Angioimmunoblastic Lymphadenopathy

Angioimmunoblastic lymphadenopathy (AIL) has already been described earlier in this chapter; only the peripheral blood and bone marrow findings are discussed here.

### Morphologic Findings

**Peripheral blood.** No specific pattern of changes exists. Anemia, lymphocytopenia, neutrophilia, and eosinophilia are more frequent. Circulating immunoblasts and plasma cells may be observed.

**Bone marrow.** Bone marrow involvement is seen in about 60–70% of cases (764–766). The pattern may be diffuse or focal. Focal lesions may be paratrabecular or randomly scattered in the marrow spaces. AIL lesions consist of loosely structured polymorphous lymphoid infiltrates often associated with prominent vascularity, reticulin fibrosis, and the presence of interstitial eosinophilic material. The cytology of the lymphoid infiltrates is identical to that seen in the lymph node lesions (Fig. 48A, B). Epithelioid histiocytes may be numerous, imparting a "granulomatoid" appearance to the infiltrates. In some cases, a fibroblastic reaction re-

placing large areas of hematopoietic tissue occurs. The uninvolved marrow is usually hypercellular.

### Differential Diagnosis

The histology of AIL lesions in the bone marrow is nonspecific. The presence of a spectrum of lymphoid cells of different size and shape and the absence of typical, diagnostic Reed–Sternberg cells help to distinguish AIL from Hodgkin's disease, but review of the lymph node histopathology is essential. Distinction of reactive AIL from AIL-like peripheral T-cell lymphomas is usually impossible based on morphology alone, particularly if clusters of immunoblasts with clear cytoplasm are not present. Review of the initial diagnostic specimen is necessary; gene rearrangement and cytogenetic studies are often needed as well. Lastly, the polymorphous histology of the AIL lesions bears strong similarities to the previously described reactive lymphohistiocytic lesions typically associated with immunologic disorders. This is not surprising if one considers that abnormalities of the immune system are believed to play an important role in the pathogenesis of AIL. The distinction between the two relies on the clinical setting and lymph node histopathology rather than on the bone marrow examination.

### Systemic Polyclonal Immunoblastic Proliferations

This atypical lymphoproliferative disorder has already been discussed elsewhere in this chapter. The following description is limited to the most common peripheral blood and bone marrow findings.

### Morphologic Findings

**Peripheral blood.** Systemic polyclonal immunoblastic proliferations (SPIP) are associated with a distinct peripheral

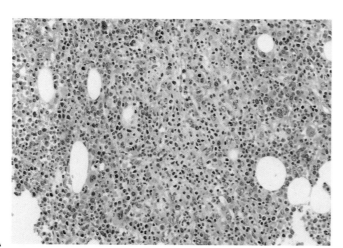
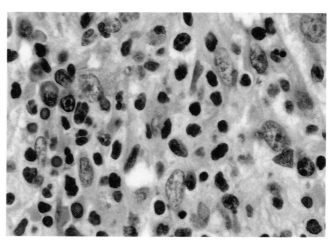

**FIG. 48.** Angioimmunoblastic lymphadenopathy in the marrow biopsy. **A:** A relatively hypocellular focus of involvement within a hypercellular bone marrow. **B:** At a higher power, the cellularity is polymorphous; some lymphoid cells have clear cytoplasm. Nuclear atypia in this case is mild.

blood picture. The absolute leukocyte count is generally elevated, often markedly so. A defining feature of this disorder is the presence of numerous circulating "immunocytes," i.e., immunoblasts, plasma cells, and intermediate forms. Neutrophilia with a left shift and toxic changes in the mature neutrophils are common; anemia and thrombocytopenia are frequently seen as well. Abnormal laboratory data include polyclonal hypergammaglobulinemia, elevated ESR, and positive Coombs' test.

**Bone marrow.** The marrow is usually hypercellular. The most prominent feature is a diffuse hyperplasia of immunoblasts and plasma cells, the latter including both mature and immature forms. Distinct cytologic atypia, however, is not observed. An increase in small lymphocytes, either scattered in the interstitial spaces or arranged in focal aggregates, may be seen as well. Immunophenotypic studies (including paraffin immunostains for cytoplasmic immunoglobulin light chains) show that the immunocytic infiltrate is *polyclonal.*

### Differential Diagnosis

In some respects, the peripheral blood and bone marrow changes of SPIP resemble those observed in *de novo plasma cell leukemia (PCL).* This rare entity is essentially a variant of plasma cell myeloma characterized by a prominent leukemic picture. The criteria for the diagnosis include an absolute peripheral blood plasma cell count exceeding $2000/\mu l$ or a plasma cell percentage of 20% or more of the differential count (783,784). In comparison with patients affected by multiple myeloma, those with *de novo* PCL tend to be younger, and more often have lymphadenopathy or organomegaly. Bone lesions are frequent, and a monoclonal paraprotein is present. PCL is an aggressive disorder, with an average survival of <1 year. Despite its unusual peripheral blood and bone marrow findings, SPIP is distinguished from PCL by virtue of the lack of a monoclonal paraprotein, absence of frank cytologic atypia, immunophenotypic demonstration of polyclonality, and an altogether different clinical setting.

### Immature Bone Marrow B-Cell Precursors: The "Hematogones"

The term "hematogones" (HGs) designates a population of immature, nonneoplastic B-cell lymphoid precursors with unique characteristics. These immature B cells are numerous in the bone marrow of normal infants and children affected by a number of disorders (785,786). Refined flow cytometry studies have shed light on the nature of the HG. During the various stages of normal B-cell differentiation, sequential antigen acquisitions and losses occur (787). The surface antigens CD19 and CD10 (CALLA) and intranuclear terminal deoxynucleotidyltransferase (Tdt) are acquired early, CD10

and Tdt being subsequently lost. Surface CD20, CD22, and polyclonal surface immunoglobulins (sIg) appear at later stages. Recent studies suggest that HGs are immunophenotypically heterogeneous, and that a number of HG subsets are likely to exist, corresponding to different B-cell maturational stages (788,789). Most HGs are characterized by the coexpression of surface CD19 and CD10; Tdt is detected in only a fraction of them, presumably the most immature ones. The expression of other B-cell-associated markers such as CD20, CD22, and polyclonal surface immunoglobulins is also limited to minor HG subpopulations, and is believed to indicate more advanced maturational stages.

### Clinical Features

In pediatric patients, disease states associated with an increase in HGs include iron deficiency anemia, congenital or immune-mediated cytopenias, and solid tumors such as retinoblastomas or neuroblastomas (785). In addition, HGs are frequently increased following cytotoxic chemotherapy or bone marrow transplantation. Recent observations have documented that HGs may also be increased in the bone marrow of adult patients with previously documented B-cell lymphomas, autoimmune diseases, HIV infection, or cytopenias of unknown cause (788,789).

### Morphologic Findings

*HGs generally do not recirculate in the blood.* In the *marrow* aspirate, they appear as small to medium-sized cells with round or notched nuclei, uniformly condensed chromatin, and inapparent nucleoli (Fig. 49A, B). The cytoplasm is very scant, deeply basophilic, and agranular. In the marrow core or clot sections HGs have the morphology of small lymphocytes that are scattered in the interstitial spaces or arranged in small clusters.

### Differential Diagnosis

Particularly in pediatric patients, HGs may represent a considerable proportion (even 50% or more) of the marrow nucleated cells (785). Since their cytologic features may be confused with those of lymphoblasts, a diagnosis of *de novo acute lymphoblastic leukemia (ALL)* may be entertained, especially in young patients presenting with peripheral blood cytopenias of uncertain origin. In addition, distinction of HGs from *residual lymphoblasts following chemotherapy for ALL* may be challenging. A careful correlation with the clinical setting and numerous other differential diagnostic criteria may be useful. Morphologically, HGs differ from lymphoblasts by virtue of their uniformly condensed nuclear chromatin with no or inconspicuous nucleoli. HGs have normal DNA content, show no evidence of clonal immunoglobulin gene rearrangement on molecular analysis, and are karyotypically normal (785). Both conventional cytogenetics and interphase cytogenetic analysis (also known as "fluorescence *in situ* hybridization," or *FISH*) may be useful in distinguishing HGs from residual neoplastic cells when chromosome abnormalities have been detected in the original diagnostic specimen. FISH, in particular, allows the direct correlation of the morphologic and cytogenetic findings on a cell-to-cell basis, and is sometimes even more sensitive than conventional chromosome studies in detecting minimal residual disease (790,791). Immunophenotypically, HGs may resemble the most common precursor B-cell ALL variant because of their characteristic profile (typically CD19/CD10 double-positive, surface immunoglobulin usually negative), but expression of intranuclear Tdt (present in the majority of the cells of most cases of ALL) is limited to only a proportion of them. This may be of use in those precursor B-cell ALL cases characterized by a CD19/CD10/Tdt phenotype but lacking detectable numeric or structural chromosome abnormalities.

*Evolution, Treatment, and Prognosis*

These are related to the conditions associated with an increase in marrow HGs. Admittedly, the biological function of these immature B-cell progenitors is still unknown. Their presence in increased numbers in association with immune-mediated cytopenias or bone marrow regeneration might reflect a possible stimulatory action of HGs on the other hematopoietic cells in response to cell destruction. However, the exact relationship between increased HGs and abnormal immune states or coexistent neoplastic lymphoproliferations is at the moment far from being understood. Further studies are needed to clarify the functional role of this unusual population of lymphoid precursors.

## HISTIOCYTIC HYPERPLASIAS SIMULATING NEOPLASMS

### Bone Marrow Granulomas

In the bone marrow as in any other tissue, granulomas appear as circumscribed, avascular aggregates of modified, "epithelioid" histiocytes usually surrounded by a cuff of small lymphocytes. Multinucleated giant cells of either the Langerhans or foreign body type are also characteristic of granulomas, but are not always present. Granuloma formation can be regarded as a distinctive pattern of chronic inflammation, and is thought to be a T-cell-dependent phenomenon. *In vitro* studies have indeed shown that cytokines such as IFNγ or IL-4 produced by activated T lymphocytes stimulate the transformation of bloodborne monocytes to multinucleated giant cells (792,793).

Bone marrow granulomas are a somewhat infrequent finding, being identifiable in 0.5–2% of all bone marrow specimens (794,795).

*Clinical Features*

Granulomas in the bone marrow may be associated with a broad spectrum of conditions. These include infectious processes of diverse origin, immunologic disorders such as sarcoid malignancies (particularly Hodgkin's disease and non-Hodgkin's lymphomas, and irrespective of bone marrow involvement), administration of drugs, and reaction to foreign substances (796). Quite often, however, they represent an unexpected finding for which no specific etiology can be established. In one series (794), the most common complaints associated with bone marrow granulomas were fever, fatigue, chills or sweats, loss of weight and anorexia, and in

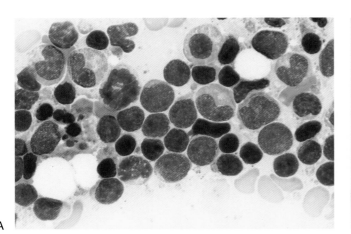

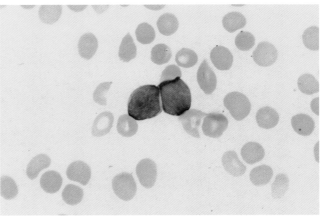

A      B

**FIG. 49.** Hematogones and malignant lymphoblasts. **A:** Numerous small to medium-sized lymphoid cells (hematogones) in the marrow smear of a young man following bone marrow transplant for Hodgkin's disease. Flow cytometry showed increased numbers of B cells coexpressing CD19 and CD10 antigens but lacking surface immunoglobulins. **B:** Small blasts in the peripheral blood smear of a child with precursor B-cell acute lymphoblastic leukemia.

the majority of the cases the symptoms had been present for several weeks before the bone marrow examination.

## Morphologic Findings

**Peripheral blood.** The peripheral blood changes are nonspecific and reflect an underlying disease. Anemia and lymphocytopenia are common (794). When the granulomatous response is extensive, pancytopenia with a leukoerythroblastic picture can be observed.

**Bone marrow.** In the core sections, granulomas might be single or multiple and of various size (Fig. 50A, B). Lesions randomly scattered in the marrow spaces are more common than paratrabecular ones. Occasionally, they are confluent and replace large areas of hematopoietic tissue. Granulomas are primarily composed of epithelioid histiocytes with bland nuclei and abundant eosinophilic cytoplasm with poorly defined borders. They are intermixed with small lymphocytes, occasional giant cells, and, at times, some eosinophils. Caseating necrosis is rare, and is more frequently associated with tuberculosis or histoplasmosis (794). Special stains to detect microorganisms are essential. In most cases the marrow aspirate smears appear unremarkable because of the reticulin fibrosis associated with the granulomatous foci. Occasionally, clusters of histiocytes can be observed; appropriate procedures can demonstrate the presence of infectious agents.

## Differential Diagnosis

In general, bone marrow granulomas are easily identified as part of a nonneoplastic process. However, occasional cases in which granulomas are very large, or confluent, or exhibit a more heterogeneous cellularity need to be distinguished from the lesions of *Hodgkin's disease* (HD) or non-Hodgkin's lymphomas. This is particularly true of *peripheral T-cell lymphomas (PTCLs)*. In both of these disorders, the neoplastic marrow infiltrates tend to be polymorphous, and epithelioid histiocytes are often abundant. However, nonneoplastic granulomas lack the Reed–Sternberg cells or mononuclear variants of HD, and the spectrum of atypical lymphoid cells seen in PTCL is not present. Comparison of the bone marrow histopathology with that of the previous biopsies is always necessary, and additional studies (e.g., special stains for microorganisms or paraffin immunostains) can be of further help. In other instances, small granulomas can be associated with foci of malignant lymphomas, but the neoplastic component is readily appreciated.

## Evolution, Treatment, and Prognosis

These are related to the underlying disease process. The significance of the granulomas found in the bone marrow of patients with HD or non-Hodgkin's lymphomas in the absence of infectious complications is debatable. In some older studies, marrow granulomas in patients with HD were thought to possibly represent either a consequence of altered delayed hypersensitivity (797) or evidence of a host response to the neoplasm with a favorable prognostic significance (798). In patients with non-Hodgkin's lymphomas, marrow granulomas associated with neoplastic infiltrates may represent a direct immunologic response to the tumor (799).

## Hemophagocytic Syndromes

The essential features of the hemophagocytic syndromes (HPSs) have already been outlined elsewhere in this chapter. Only the peripheral blood and bone marrow changes are discussed here.

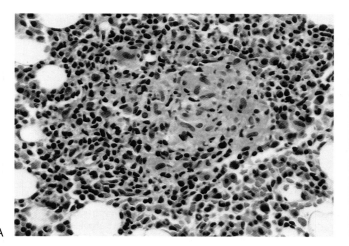 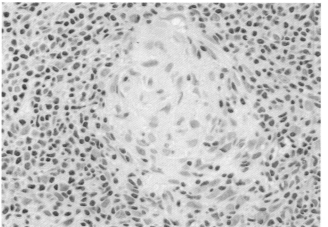

A                                                                                                                                         B

**FIG. 50.** Granulomas in the marrow biopsy. **A:** A nonnecrotizing granuloma in a patient with sarcoid. **B:** A similar lesion in a patient with marrow involvement by follicular lymphoma.

48. Poppema S, Kaleta J, Hugh J, Visser L. Neoplastic changes involving follicles: morphological, immunophenotypic and genetic diversity of lymphoproliferations derived from germinal center and mantle zone. *Immunol Rev* 1992;126:163–178.

49. Osborne BM, Butler JJ. Clinical implications of progressive transformation of germinal centers. *Am J Surg Pathol* 1984;8:725–733.

50. Ferry JA, Zukerberg LR, Harris NL. Florid progressive transformation of germinal centers. A syndrome affecting young men, without early progression to nodular lymphocyte predominance Hodgkin's disease. *Am J Surg Pathol* 1992;16:252–258.

51. Burns BF, Wood GS, Dorfman RF. The varied histopathology of lymphadenopathy in the homosexual male. *Am J Surg Pathol* 1985; 9:287–297.

52. Stanley MW, Frizzera G. Diagnostic specificity of histologic features in lymph node biopsy specimens from patients at risk for the acquired immunodeficiency syndrome. *Hum Pathol* 1986;17:1231–1239.

53. O'Murchadha MT, Wolf BC, Neiman RS. The histologic features of hyperplastic lymphadenopathy in AIDS-related complex are nonspecific. *Am J Surg Pathol* 1987;11:94–99.

54. Burns BF, Colby TV, Dorfman RF. Differential diagnostic features of nodular L&H Hodgkin's disease, including progressive transformation of germinal centers. *Am J Surg Pathol* 1984;8:253–261.

55. Lukes RJ, Butler JJ. The pathology and nomenclature of Hodgkin's disease. *Cancer Res* 1966;26:1063–1081.

56. Timens W, Visser L, Poppema S. Nodular lymphocyte predominance type of Hodgkin's disease is a germinal center lymphoma. *Lab Invest* 1986;54:457–461.

57. Stein H, Hansmann ML, Lennert K, Brandtzaeg P, Gatter KC, Mason D. Reed–Sternberg and Hodgkin cells in lymphocyte predominant Hodgkin's disease of nodular subtype contain J chain. *Am J Clin Pathol* 1986;86:292–297.

58. Sundeen JT, Cossman J, Jaffe ES. Lymphocyte predominant Hodgkin's disease nodular subtype with coexistent "large cell lymphoma." Histological progression or composite malignancy? *Am J Surg Pathol* 1988;12:599–606.

59. Hansmann ML, Wacker HH, Radzun HJ. Paragranuloma is a variant of Hodgkin's disease with predominance of B-cells. *Virchows Arch A Path Anat* 1986;409:171–181.

60. Schmid C, Sargent C, Isaacson PG. L and H cells of nodular lymphocyte predominant Hodgkin's disease show immunoglobulin light-chain restriction. *Am J Pathol* 1991;139:1281–1289.

61. Hansmann ML, Goedde-Salz E, Hui PK, Mueller-Hermelink HK, Lennert K. Cytogenetic findings in nodular paragranuloma (Hodgkin's disease with lymphocytic predominance; nodular) and in progressively transformed germinal centers. *Cancer Genet Cytogenet* 1986;21:319–325.

62. Griesser H, Feller AC, Mak TW, Lennert K. Clonal rearrangements of T-cell receptor and immunoglobulin genes and immunophenotypic antigen expression in different subclasses of Hodgkin's disease. *Int J Cancer* 1987;40:157–160.

63. Linden MD, Fishleder AJ, Katzin WE, Tubbs RR. Absence of B-cell or T-cell clonal expansion in nodular lymphocyte predominant Hodgkin's disease. *Hum Pathol* 1988;19:591–594.

64. Said JW, Sassoon AF, Shintaku IP, Kurtin PJ, Pinkus GS. Absence of bcl-2 major breakpoint region and Jh gene rearrangement in lymphocyte predominant Hodgkin's disease. Results of Southern blot analysis and polymerase chain reaction. *Am J Pathol* 1991;138:261–264.

65. Castleman B, Iverson L, Menendez VP. Localized mediastinal lymph node hyperplasia resembling thymoma. *Cancer* 1956;9:822–830.

66. Keller AR, Hochholzer L, Castleman B. Hyaline-vascular and plasma-cell types of giant lymph node hyperplasia of the mediastinum and other locations. *Cancer* 1972;29:670–683.

67. Frizzera G, Banks PM, Massarelli G, Rosai J. A systemic lymphoproliferative disorder with morphologic features of Castleman's disease. Pathological findings in 15 patients. *Am J Surg Pathol* 1983; 7:211–231.

68. Frizzera G, Peterson BA, Bayrd ED, Goldman A. A systemic lymphoproliferative disorder with morphologic features of Castleman's disease: clinical findings and clinicopathologic correlations in 15 patients. *J Clin Oncol* 1985;3:1202–1216.

69. Weisenburger DD, Nathwani BN, Winberg CD, Rappaport H. Multicentric angiofollicular lymph node hyperplasia: a clinicopathologic study of 16 cases. *Hum Pathol* 1985;16:162–172.

70. Frizzera G. Castleman's disease and related disorders. *Semin Diagn Pathol* 1988;5:346–364.

71. Danon AD, Krishnan J, Frizzera G. Morpho-immunophenotypic diversity of Castleman's disease, hyaline-vascular type: with emphasis on a stroma-rich variant and a new pathogenetic hypothesis. *Virchows Arch A Path Anat* 1993;423:369–382.

72. Nguyen DT, Diamond LW, Hansmann ML, et al. Castleman's disease. Differences in follicular dendritic network in the hyaline vascular and plasma cell variants. *Histopathology* 1994;24:437–443.

73. Abell MR. Lymphnodal hamartoma versus thymic choristoma of pulmonary hilum. *Arch Pathol* 1957;64:584–588.

74. Ruco LP, Gearing AJH, Pigott R, et al. Expression of ICAM-1, VCAM-1 and ELAM-1 in angiofollicular lymph node hyperplasia (Castleman's disease): evidence for dysplasia of follicular dendritic reticulum cells. *Histopathology* 1991;19:523–528.

75. Harris NL, Bhan AK. "Plasmacytoid T cells" in Castleman's disease: immunohistologic phenotype. *Am J Surg Pathol* 1987;11:109–113.

76. Hunt SJ, Anderson WD. Giant lymph node hyperplasia of the hyaline vascular type with plasmacytoid T-cells and presentation in infancy. *Am J Clin Pathol* 1989;91:344–347.

77. Brado B, Moeller P. The plasmacytoid T cell or plasmacytoid monocyte—a sessile lymphoid cell with unique immunophenotype and unknown function, still awaiting lineage affiliation. In: Grundmann E, Vollmer R, eds. *Reaction patterns of the lymph node. Part 1. Cell types and functions.* Berlin: Springer Verlag, 1990;179–192.

78. Facchetti F, de Wolf-Peeters C, Mason DY, Pulford K, van den Oord JJ, Desmet VJ. Plasmacytoid T cells. Immunohistochemical evidence for their monocyte/macrophage origin. *Am J Pathol* 1988;133:15–21.

79. Facchetti F, de Wolf-Peeters C, van den Oord JJ, de Vos R, Desmet VJ. Plasmacytoid T cells: a cell population normally present in the reactive lymph node. An immunohistochemical and electronmicroscopic study. *Hum Pathol* 1988;19:1085–1092.

80. Madero S, Onate JM, Garzon A. Giant lymph node hyperplasia in an angiolipomatous mediastinal mass. *Arch Pathol Lab Med* 1986;110: 853–855.

81. Ordi J, Grau JM, Junque A, Nomdedeu B, Palacin A, Cardesa A. Secondary (AA) amyloidosis associated with Castleman's disease. Report of two cases and review of the literature. *Am J Clin Pathol* 1993;100: 394–397.

82. Duijvestijn AM, Horst E, Pals ST, et al. High endothelial differentiation in human lymphoid and inflammatory tissues defined by monoclonal antibody HECA-452. *Am J Pathol* 1988;130:147–155.

83. Streeter PR, Rouse BTN, Butcher EC. Immunohistologic and functional characteristics of a vascular addressin involved in lymphocyte homing into peripheral lymph nodes. *J Cell Biol* 1988;107: 1853–1862.

84. Mueller-Hermelink HK, von Gaudecker B, Drenckhahn D, Jaworsky K, Feldmann C. Fibroblastic and dendritic reticulum cells of lymphoid tissue. Ultrastructural, histochemical, and $^3$H-thymidine labeling studies. *J Cancer Res Clin Oncol* 1981;101:149–164.

85. Pinkus GS, Warhol MJ, O'Connor EM, Etheridge CL, Fujiwara K. Immunohistochemical localization of smooth muscle myosin in human spleen, lymph node, and other lymphoid tissues. Unique staining pattern in splenic white pulp and sinuses, lymphoid follicles, and certain vasculature, with ultra-structural correlations. *Am J Pathol* 1986; 123:440–453.

86. Toccanier-Pelte M-F, Skalli O, Kapanci Y, Gabbiani G. Characterization of stromal cells with myoid features in lymph nodes and spleen in normal and pathologic conditions. *Am J Pathol* 1987;129:109–118.

87. Flendrig JA. Benign giant lymphoma: clinicopathologic correlation study. In: Clark RL, Cumley RW, eds. *The year book of cancer.* Chicago: Year Book Medical, 1970;296–299.

88. Hall PA, Donaghy M, Cotter FE, Stansfeld AG, Levison DA. An immunohistological and genotypic study of the plasma cell form of Castleman's disease. *Histopathology* 1989;14:333–346.

89. Isaacson PG. Commentary: Castleman's disease. *Histopathology* 1989;14:429–432.

90. Gherardi RK, Belec L, Fromont G, et al. Elevated levels of interleukin-1β (IL-1β) and IL-6 in serum and increased production of IL-1β mRNA in lymph nodes of patients with polyneuropathy, organomegaly, endocrinopathy, M protein, and skin changes (POEMS) syndrome. *Blood* 1994;83:2587–2593.

91. Leger-Ravet MB, Peuchmaur M, Devergne O, et al. Interleukin-6 gene expression in Castleman's disease. *Blood* 1991;78:2923–2930.

92. Yoshizaki K, Matsuda T, Nishimoto N, et al. Pathogenetic significance of interleukin-6 (IL-6/BSF-2) in Castleman's disease. *Blood* 1989;74:1360–1367.

93. Lattes R, Pachter MR. Benign lymphoid masses of probable hamartomatous nature. Analysis of 12 cases. *Cancer* 1962;15:197–214.

94. Symmers WSC. The lymphoreticular system. In: Symmers WSC, ed. *Systemic pathology.* Edinburgh: Churchill Livingstone, 1978; 504–924.

95. Weisenburger DD, Lipscomb Grierson H, Purtilo D. Immunologic studies of multicentric (M) and unicentric (U) angiofollicular lymphoid hyperplasia (ALH). *Lab Invest* 1986;54:68A.

96. Harris NL, Bhan AK. Immunohistology of Castleman's disease: a monoclonal antibody study. *Lab Invest* 1985;52:28A.

97. Nagai M, Irino S, Uda H, Ohtsu T, Tobinai K, Shimoyama M. Molecular genetic and immunohistochemical analyses of a case of multicentric Castleman's disease. *Jap J Clin Oncol* 1988;18:149–157.

98. Gerald W, Kostianovsky M, Rosai J. Development of vascular neoplasia in Castleman's disease. Report of seven cases. *Am J Surg Pathol* 1990;14:603–614.

99. Chan JKC, Tsang WYW, Ng CS. Follicular dendritic cell tumor and vascular neoplasm complicating hyaline-vascular Castleman's disease. *Am J Surg Pathol* 1994;18:517–525.

100. Weisenburger DD, Chan CW. Lymphomas of the follicles: mantle cell and follicle center cell lymphomas. *Am J Clin Pathol* 1993;99: 409–420.

101. Manconi R, Poletti A, Volpe R, Sulfaro S, Carbone A. Dendritic reticulum cell pattern as a microenvironmental indicator for a distinct origin of lymphoma of follicular mantle cells. *Br J Haematol* 1988;68: 213–218.

102. Monda L, Warnke R, Rosai J. A primary lymph node malignancy with features suggestive of dendritic reticulum cell differentiation. A report of 4 cases. *Am J Pathol* 1986;122:562–572.

103. Weiss LM, Berry GJ, Dorfman RF, et al. Spindle cell neoplasm of lymph nodes of probably reticulum cell lineage. True reticulum cell sarcoma? *Am J Surg Pathol* 1990;14:405–414.

104. Perez-Ordonez B, Erlandson RA, Rosai J. Follicular dendritic cell tumor. Report of 13 additional cases of a distinctive entity. *Am J Surg Pathol* 1996;20:944–955.

105. Xerri L, Guigou V, Lepidi H, Horschowski N, Lejeune C, Hassoun J. Lymphadenopathic tumor exhibiting intermingled features of Kaposi's sarcoma, malignant lymphoma, and angiofollicular hyperplasia. *Arch Pathol Lab Med* 1991;115:1162–1166.

106. Lin O, Frizzera G. Angiomyoid and follicular dendritic cell proliferative lesions in Castleman's disease of hyaline-vascular type: a study of ten cases. Submitted.

107. Van Wyk JJ, Hoffmann CR. Periarteritis nodosa: a case of fatal exfoliative dermatitis resulting from "Dilantin Sodium" sensitization. *Arch Intern Med* 1948;81:605–611.

108. Buijs L, Wijermans PW, van Groningen K, Gerrits WBJ, Kluin P, Haak HL. Hyaline-vascular type Castleman's disease with concomitant malignant B-cell lymphoma. *Acta Haematol* 1992;87:160–162.

109. McAloon EJ. Hodgkin's disease in a patient with Castleman's disease. *N Engl J Med* 1985;313:758.

110. Anonymous. Case records of the Massachusetts General Hospital. Case 39–1990. *N Engl J Med* 1990;323:895–908.

111. Drut R, Larregina A. Angiofollicular lymph node transformation in Hodgkin's lymphoma. *Pediatr Pathol* 1991;11:903–908.

112. Pettit C, Ferry JA, Harris NL. Simultaneous occurence of Hodgkin's disease and angiofollicular hyperplasia (Castleman's disease): report of 3 cases. *Mod Pathol* 1991;4:81A.

113. Zarate-Osorno A, Medeiros LJ, Danon AD, Neiman RS. Hodgkin's disease with coexistent Castleman-like histologic features. A report of three cases. *Arch Pathol Lab Med* 1994;118:270–274.

114. Maheswaran PR, Ramsay AD, Norton AJ, Roche WR. Hodgkin's disease presenting with the histological features of Castleman's disease. *Histopathology* 1991;18:249–253.

115. Harris NL. Hypervascular follicular hyperplasia and Kaposi's sarcoma in patients at risk for AIDS. *N Engl J Med* 1984;310:462–463.

116. Lowenthal DA, Filippa DA, Richardson ME, Bertoni M, Straus DJ. Generalized lymphadenopathy with morphologic features of Castleman's disease in an HIV-positive man. *Cancer* 1987;60:2454–2458.

117. Kimura T, Yoshimura S, Ishikawa E. On the unusual granulation combined with hyperplastic changes of lymphatic tissue (in Japanese). *Trans Soc Pathol Jpn* 1948;37:179–180.

118. Ishikawa E, Tanaka H, Kakimoto S, et al. A pathological study on eosinophilic lymphofolliculoid granuloma (Kimura's disease). *Acta Pathol Jpn* 1981;31:767–781.

119. Kung ITM, Gibson JB, Bannatyne PM. Kimura's disease: a clinicopathological study of 21 cases and its distinction from angiolymphoid hyperplasia with eosinophilia. *Pathology* 1984;16:39–44.

120. Hui PK, Chan JKC, Ng CS, Kung ITM, Gwi E. Lymphadenopathy of Kimura's disease. *Am J Surg Pathol* 1989;13:177–186.

121. Chan JKC, Hui PK, Ng CS, Yuen NWF, Kung ITM, Gwi E. Epithelioid haemangioma (angiolymphoid hyperplasia with eosinophilia) and Kimura's disease in Chinese. *Histopathology* 1989;15:557–574.

122. Googe PB, Harris NL, Mihm MCJ. Kimura's disease and angiolymphoid hyperplasia with eosinophilia: two distinct histopathological entities. *J Cutan Pathol* 1987;14:263–271.

123. Rosai J, Gold J, Landy R. The histiocytoid hemangiomas. A unifying concept embracing several previously described entities of skin, soft tissue, large vessels, bone and heart. *Hum Pathol* 1979;10:707–730.

124. Weiss SW, Ishak KG, Dail DH, Sweet DE, Enzinger FM. Epithelioid hemangioendothelioma and related lesions. *Semin Diagn Pathol* 1986;3:259–287.

125. Shimamoto C, Takao Y, Hirata I, Ohshiba S. Kimura's disease (angiolymphoid hyperplasia with eosinophilia) associated with ulcerative colitis. *Gastroenterologia Jpn* 1993;28:298–303.

126. Akosa AB, Ali MH, Khoo CTK, Evans DM. Angiolymphoid hyperplasia with eosinophilia associated with tetanus toxoid vaccination. *Histopathology* 1990;16:589–593.

127. Hallam LA, MacKinlay GA, Wright AMA. Angiolymphoid hyperplasia with eosinophilia: possible aetiological role of immunisation. *J Clin Pathol* 1989;42:944–949.

128. Terada N, Konno A, Shirotori K, et al. Mechanism of eosinophil infiltration in the patient with subcutaneous angioblastic lymphoid hyperplasia with eosinophilia (Kimura's disease). Mechanism of eosinophil chemotaxis mediated by candida antigen and IL-5. *Int Arch Allergy Immunol* 1994;104 Suppl 1:18–20.

129. Fetsch JF, Weiss SW. Observations concerning the pathogenesis of epithelioid hemangioma (angiolymphoid hyperplasia). *Mod Pathol* 1991;4:449–455.

130. Suster S. Nodal angiolymphoid hyperplasia with eosinophilia. *Am J Clin Pathol* 1987;88:236–239.

131. Wright DH, Padley NR, Judd MA. Angiolymphoid hyperplasia with eosinophilia simulating lymphadenopathy. *Histopathology* 1981; 5:127–140.

132. Razquin S, Mayayo E, Citores MA, Alvira R. Angiolymphoid hyperplasia with eosinophilia of the tongue: report of a case and review of the literature. *Hum Pathol* 1991;22:837–839.

133. Kuo T-T, Shih L-Y, Chan H-L. Kimura's disease. Involvement of regional lymph nodes and distinction from angiolymphoid hyperplasia with eosinophilia. *Am J Surg Pathol* 1988;12:843–854.

134. Urabe A, Tsuneyoshi M, Enjoji M. Epithelioid hemangioma versus Kimura's disease. A comparative clinicopathologic study. *Am J Surg Pathol* 1987;11:758–766.

135. Allen PW, Ramakrishna B, MacCormac LB. The histiocytoid hemangiomas and other controversies. *Pathol Annu* 1992;27, Pt 2:51–87.

136. Chun SI, Ji HG. Kimura's disease and angiolymphoid hyperplasia with eosinophilia: clinical and histopathologic differences. *J Am Acad Dermatol* 1992;27:954–958.

137. Motoi M, Wahid S, Horie Y, Akagi T. Kimura's disease: clinical, histological and immunohistochemical studies. *Acta Medica Okayama* 1992;46:449–455.

138. Inoue C, Ichikawa A, Hotta T, Saito H. Constitutive gene expression of interleukin-5 in Kimura's disease. *Br J Haematol* 1990;76: 554–559.

139. Enokihara H, Koike T, Arimura H, et al. IL-5 mRNA expression in blood lymphocytes from patients with Kimura's disease and parasite infection. *Am J Hematol* 1994;47:69–73.

140. Yamada A, Mitsuhashi K, Miyakawa Y, et al. Membranous glomerulonephritis associated with eosinophilic lymphofolliculosis of the skin (Kimura's disease): report of a case and review of the literature. *Clin Nephrol* 1982;18:211–215.

141. Matsuda O, Makiguchi K, Ishibashi K, et al. Long-term effects of steroid treatment on nephrotic syndrome associated with Kimura's disease and a review of the literature. *Clin Nephrol* 1992;37:119–123.

142. Akosa AB, Sherif A, Maidment CG. Kimura's disease and membranous nephropathy. *Nephron* 1991;58:472–474.

143. Tabata H, Ishikawa O, Ohnishi K, Ishikawa H. Kimura's disease with marked proliferation of HLA-DR-CD4-T cells in the skin, lymph node and peripheral blood. *Dermatology* 1992;184:145–148.

144. Sundaresan M, Rhodes T, Akosa AB. Immunoglobulin heavy chain patterns in reactive lymphadenopathy. *J Clin Pathol* 1991;44: 753–755.

145. Saita N, Ueno M, Yoshida M, Kimura T, Ando M, Hirashima M. Chemotactic heterogeneity of eosinophils in Kimura's disease. *Int Arch Allergy Immunol* 1994;104 (Suppl 1):21–23.

146. Stringfellow HF, Howat AJ. Postimmunization (vaccination) injection-site reactions. *Am J Surg Pathol* 1994;18:1179–1180.

147. Tsang WYW, Chan JKC, Dorfman RF, Rosai J. Vasoproliferative lesions of the lymph node. *Pathol Annu* 1994;29, Pt 1:63–133.

148. Chan JKC, Frizzera G, Fletcher CDM, Rosai J. Primary vascular tumors of lymph nodes other than Kaposi's sarcoma. Analysis of 39 cases and delineation of two new entities. *Am J Surg Pathol* 1992;16: 335–350.

149. Person JR. Angiolymphoid hyperplasia with eosinophilia may respond to pentoxifylline. *J Am Acad Dermatol* 1994;31:117–118.

150. Straus SE, Fleisher GR. Infectious mononucleosis: epidemiology and pathogenesis. In: Schlossberg D, ed. *Infectious mononucleosis.* 2nd ed. New York: Springer-Verlag, 1989;8–28.

151. Miller G. Epstein–Barr virus: biology, pathogenesis, and medical aspects. In: Fields B, Knipe D, eds. *Virology.* 2nd ed. New York: Raven Press, 1990;1921–1958.

152. Straus SE, Cohen JI, Tosato G, Meier J. Epstein–Barr virus infections: biology, pathogenesis, and management. *Ann Intern Med* 1993;118: 45–58.

153. Purtilo DT. Immunopathology of infectious mononucleosis and other complications of Epstein–Barr virus infections. *Pathol Annu* 1980;15, Part 1:253–299.

154. Strickler JG, Fedeli F, Horwitz CA, Copenhaver CM, Frizzera G. Infectious mononucleosis in lymphoid tissue. Histopathology, in situ hybridization, and differential diagnosis. *Arch Pathol Lab Med* 1993; 117:269–278.

155. Nahmias JA. Disseminated herpes simplex infection. *N Engl J Med* 1970;282:684–695.

156. Tamaru J-I, Mikata A, Horie H, et al. Herpes simplex lymphadenitis. Report of two cases with review of the literature. *Am J Surg Pathol* 1990;14:571–577.

157. Taxy JB, Tillawi I, Goldman PM. Herpes simplex lymphadenitis. An unusual presentation with necrosis and viral particles. *Arch Pathol Lab Med* 1985;109:1043–1044.

158. Miliauskas JR, Leong AS-Y. Localized herpes simplex lymphadenitis: report of three cases and review of the literature. *Histopathology* 1991;19:355–360.

159. Audouin J, Le Tourneau A, Aubert J-P, Diebold J. Herpes simplex virus lymphadenitis mimicking tumoral relapse in a patient with Hodgkin's disease in remission. *Virchows Arch A Path Anat* 1985; 408:313–321.

160. Howat AJ, Campbell AR, Stewart DJ. Generalized lymphadenopathy due to herpes simplex virus type I. *Histopathology* 1991;19:563–564.

161. Lapsley M, Kettle P, Sloan JM. Herpes simplex lymphadenitis: a case report and review of the published work. *J Clin Pathol* 1984;37: 1119–1122.

162. Abraham A, Manko M. Disseminated herpes virus hominis 2 infection following drug overdose. *Arch Intern Med* 1977;137:1198–1200.

163. Hillard P, Seeds J, Cefalo R. Disseminated herpes simplex in pregnancy: two cases and a review. *Obstet Gynecol Surv* 1982;37: 449–453.

164. Ramsey P, Fife K, Hackman R, Meyers J, Corey B. Herpes simplex virus pneumonia. Clinical, virologic and pathologic features in 20 patients. *Ann Intern Med* 1982;97:813–820.

165. Sutton A, Smithwick E, Seligman S, Kim D. Fatal disseminated herpes virus hominis type 2 infection in an adult with associated thymic dysplasia. *Am J Med* 1974;56:545–553.

166. Epstein JI, Ambinder RF, Kuhajda FP, Pearlman SH, Reuter VE, Mann RB. Localized herpes simplex lymphadenitis. *Am J Clin Pathol* 1986;86:444–448.

167. Gaffey MJ, Ben-Ezra JM, Weiss LM. Herpes simplex lymphadenitis. *Am J Clin Pathol* 1991;95:709–714.

168. Alford CAJ, Britt WJ. Cytomegalovirus. In: Fields BN, ed. *Virology.* New York: Raven Press, 1985;629–660.

169. Patterson SD, Larson EB, Corey L. Atypical generalized zoster with lymphadenitis mimicking lymphoma. *N Engl J Med* 1980;302: 848–851.

170. Fries LF, Sveum RJ. Adverse responses to immunization. In: Samter M, Talmage DW, Frank MM, et al, eds. *Immunological diseases.* 4th ed. Boston: Little, Brown, 1988;945–961.

171. Dorfman RF, Herweg JC. Live, attentuated measles virus vaccine. Inguinal lymphadenopathy complicating administration. *JAMA* 1966; 198:320–321.

172. Nakazono N. Studies on rubella vaccination in adult females. II. Hormonal influence on clinical reactions. *Hokkaido Igaku Zasshi* 1984; 59:192–201.

173. Gold JA, Sibbald RG, Phillips MJ, Edwards V. Angioimmunoblastic lymphadenopathy following typhoid AB vaccination and terminating in disseminated infection. *Arch Pathol Lab Med* 1985;109: 1085–1088.

174. Hartsock RJ. Postvaccinial lymphadenitis. Hyperplasia of lymphoid tissue that simulates malignant lymphomas. *Cancer* 1968;21: 632–649.

175. McKenna KE, Burrows D. Leucopenia, thrombocytopenia and lymphadenopathy associated with sulphasalazine. *Clin Exp Dermatol* 1994;19:419–420.

176. Kaufman D, Pichler W, Beer JH. Severe episode of high fever with rash, lymphadenopathy, neutropenia, and eosinophilia after minocycline therapy for acne. *Arch Intern Med* 1994;154:1983–1984.

177. Wolf R, Tamir A, Werbin N, Brenner S. Methyldopa hypersensitivity syndrome. *Ann Allergy* 1993;71:166–168.

178. D'Incan M, Souteyrand P, Bignon YJ, Fonck Y, Roger H. Hydantoin-induced cutaneous pseudolymphoma with clinical, pathologic, and immunologic aspects of Sezary syndrome. *Arch Dermatol* 1992;128: 1371–1374.

179. Saltzstein SL, Ackerman LV. Lymphadenopathy induced by anticonvulsant drugs and mimicking clinically and pathologically malignant lymphomas. *Cancer* 1959;12:164–182.

180. de Ponti F, Lecchini S, Cosentino M, Castelletti CM, Malesci A, Frigo GM. Immunological adverse effects of anticonvulsants. What is their clinical relevance? *Drug Safety* 1993;8:235–250.

181. Frizzera G. The clinico-pathological expression of Epstein–Barr virus infection in lymphoid tissues. *Virchows Arch B Cell Pathol* 1987;53: 1–12.

182. Salvador AH, JR HEG, Kyle RA. Lymphadenopathy due to infectious mononucleosis: its confusion with malignant lymphoma. *Cancer* 1971;27:1029–1040.

183. Tindle BH, Parker JW, Lukes RJ. "Reed–Sternberg cells" in infectious mononucleosis? *Am J Clin Pathol* 1972;58:607–617.

184. Gowing NFC. Infectious mononucleosis: histopathologic aspects. *Pathol Annu* 1975;10:1–20.

185. Childs CC, Parham DM, Berard CW. Infectious mononucleosis. The spectrum of morphologic changes simulating lymphoma in lymph nodes and tonsils. *Am J Surg Pathol* 1987;11:122–132.

186. Weisenburger DD, Purtilo DT. Failure in immunological control of the virus infection: fatal infectious mononucleosis. In: Epstein MA, Achong BG, eds. *The Epstein–Barr virus: recent advances.* New York: John Wiley and Sons, 1986;127–161.

187. Seemayer TA, Grierson H, Pirruccello SJ, et al. X-linked lymphoproliferative disease. *Am J Dis Child* 1993;147:1242–1245.

188. Sohier R, Lenoir GM, Lamelin J-P. Les formes mortelles de l'infection primaire a virus Epstein–Barr avec ou sans mononucleose infectieuse. *Annales de Medicine Interne* 1981;132:48–57.

189. Tazawa Y, Nishinomiya F, Noguchi H, et al. A case of fatal infectious mononucleosis presenting with fulminant hepatic failure associated with an extensive CD9-positive lymphocyte infiltration in the liver. *Hum Pathol* 1993;24:1135–1139.

190. Iijima T, Sumazaki R, Mori N, et al. A pathological and immunohistological case report of fatal infectious mononucleosis, Epstein–Barr virus infection, demonstrated by in situ and Southern blot hybridization. *Virchows Arch A Path Anat* 1992;421:73–78.

191. Rushin JM, Riordan GP, Heaton RB, Sharpe RW, Cotelingam JD, Jaffe ES. Cytomegalovirus-infected cells express Leu-M1 antigen. A potential source of diagnostic error. *Am J Pathol* 1990;136:989–995.

192. Younes M, Podesta A, Helie M, Buckley P. Infection of T but not B lymphocytes by cytomegalovirus in lymph node. An immunophenotypic study. *Am J Surg Pathol* 1991;15:75–80.

193. Abramowitz A, Livni N, Morag A, Ravid Z. An immunoperoxidase study of cytomegalovirus mononucleosis. *Arch Pathol Lab Med* 1982; 106:115–118.

194. Ioachim HL. *Lymph node biopsy.* Philadelphia: JB Lippincott, 1982.

195. Lucia HL, Griffith BP, Hsiung GD. Lymphadenopathy during cytomegalovirus-induced mononucleosis in guinea pigs. *Arch Pathol Lab Med* 1985;109:1019–1023.

196. Tajima M, Kudow S. Morphology of Warthin-Finkeldey giant cells in monkeys with experimentally induced measles. *Acta Pathol Jpn* 1976; 26:367–380.

197. Gaulier A, Sabatier P, Prevot S, Fournier JG. Do measles early giant cells result from fusion of non-infected cells? An immunohistochemical and in situ hybridization study in a case of morbillous appendicitis. *Virchows Arch A Path Anat* 1991;419:245–249.

198. Kamel OW, LeBrun DP, Berry GJ, Dorfman RF, Warnke RA. Warthin-Finkeldey polykaryocytes demonstrate a T-cell immunophenotype. *Am J Clin Pathol* 1992;97:179–183.

199. Gay RG, Fielder KL, Grogan TM. Quinidine-induced reactive lymphadenopathy. *Am J Med* 1987;82:143–145.

200. Zidar BL, Mendelow H, Winkelstein A, Shattuck RK. Diphenylhydantoin-induced serum sickness with fibrin-platelet thrombi in lymph node microvasculature. *Am J Med* 1975;58:704–707.

201. Frizzera G, Moran EM, Rappaport H. Angio-immunoblastic lymphadenopathy. Diagnosis and clinical course. *Am J Med* 1975;59: 803–818.

202. Lukes RJ, Tindle BH. Immunoblastic lymphadenopathy: a hyperimmune entity resembling Hodgkin's disease. *N Engl J Med* 1975;292: 1–8.

203. Diebold J, James J-M, Dao C, et al. Hyperplasie lymphoide immunoblastique pseudo-tumorale par hypersensibilite medicamenteuse. *Archives d'Anatomie et Cytologie Pathologiques* 1976;24: 189–194.

204. Steinberg AD, Seldin MF, Jaffe ES, et al. NIH conference. Angioimmunoblastic lymphadenopathy with dysproteinemia. *Ann Intern Med* 1988;108:575–584.

205. Katzin WE, Julius CJ, Tubbs RR, McHenry MC. Lymphoproliferative disorders associated with carbamazepine. *Arch Pathol Lab Med* 1990; 114:1244–1248.

206. Cullen MH, Stansfeld AG, Oliver RTD, Lister TA, Malpas JS. Angioimmunoblastic lymphadenopathy: report of ten cases and review of the literature. *Q J Med* 1979;48:151–177.

207. Sinnige HAM, Boender CA, Kuypers EW, Ruitenberg HM. Carbamazepine-induced pseudolymphoma and immune dysregulation. *J Intern Med* 1990;227:355–358.

208. Tosato G, Blaese RM. Epstein–Barr virus infection and immunoregulation in man. *Adv Immunol* 1985;37:99–149.

209. Shin SS, Berry GJ, Weiss LM. Infectious mononucleosis. Diagnosis by in situ hybridization in two cases with atypical features. *Am J Surg Pathol* 1991;15:625–631.

210. Niedobitek G, Hamilton-Dutoit SJ, Herbst H, et al. Identification of Epstein–Barr virus infected cells in tonsils of acute infectious mononucleosis by in situ hybridisation. *Hum Pathol* 1989;20:796–799.

211. Weiss LM, Movahed LA. In situ demonstration of Epstein–Barr viral genomes in viral-associated B cell lymphoproliferations. *Am J Pathol* 1989;134:651–659.

212. Fellbaum C, Hansmann ML, Parwaresch MR, Lennert K. Monoclonal antibodies Ki-B3 and Leu-M1 discriminate giant cells of infectious mononucleosis and of Hodgkin's disease. *Hum Pathol* 1988;19: 1168–1173.

213. Uehara T, Miyawaki T, Ohta K, et al. Apoptotic cell death of primed CD45RO-T lymphocytes in Epstein–Barr virus-induced infectious mononucleosis. *Blood* 1992;80:452–458.

214. De Waele M, Thielemans C, Van Camp BKG. Characterization of immunoregulatory T cells in EBV-induced infectious mononucleosis by monoclonal antibodies. *N Engl J Med* 1981;304:460–462.

215. Reynolds DJ, Banks PM, Gulley ML. New characterization of infectious mononucleosis and a phenotype comparison with Hodgkin's disease. *Am J Pathol* 1995;146:379–388.

216. Isaacson PG, Schmid C, Pan L, Wotherspoon AC, Wright DH. Epstein–Barr virus latent membrane protein expression by Hodgkin and Reed–Sternberg-like cells in acute infectious mononucleosis. *J Pathol* 1992;167:267–271.

217. Ambinder RF, Mann RB. Detection and characterization of Epstein–Barr virus in clinical specimens. *Am J Pathol* 1994;145: 239–252.

218. Prange E, Trautmann JC, Kreipe H, Radzun HJ, Parwaresch MR. Detection of Epstein–Barr virus in lymphoid tissues of patients with infectious mononucleosis by in situ hybridization. *J Pathol* 1992;166: 113–119.

219. Niedobitek G, Agathanggelou A, Finerty S, et al. Latent Epstein–Barr virus infection in cottontop tamarins. A possible model for Epstein–Barr virus infection in humans. *Am J Pathol* 1994;145:969–978.

220. Pallesen G, Hamilton-Dutoit SJ, Zhou X. The association of Epstein–Barr virus (EBV) with T cell lymphoproliferations and Hodgkin's disease: two new developments in the EBV field. *Adv Cancer Res* 1993;62:179–239.

221. Falk K, Ernberg I, Sakthivel R, et al. Expression of Epstein–Barr virus-encoded proteins and B-cell markers in fatal infectious mononucleosis. *Int J Cancer* 1990;46:976–984.

222. Anagnostopoulos I, Hummel M, Kreschel C, Stein H. Morphology, immunophenotype, and distribution of latently and/or productively Epstein–Barr virus-infected cells in acute infectious mononucleosis: implications for the interindividual infection route of Epstein–Barr virus. *Blood* 1995;85:744–750.

223. Braun RW, Teute HK, Kirchner H, Munk K. Replication of herpes simplex virus in human T lymphocytes; characterization of the viral target cell. *J Immunol* 1984;132:914–919.

224. Chehab FF, Xiao X, Kan YW, Yen TSB. Detection of cytomegalovirus infection in paraffin embedded tissue specimens with the polymerase chain reaction. *Mod Pathol* 1989;2:75–78.

225. Myerson D, Hackman RC, Nelson JA, Ward DC, McDougall JK. Widespread presence of histologically occult cytomegalovirus. *Hum Pathol* 1984;15:430–439.

226. Shuttleworth D, Graham-Brown RAC, Williams AJ, Campbell AC, Sewell H. Pseudo-lymphoma associated with carbamazepine. *Clin Exp Dermatol* 1984;9:421–423.

227. Gennis MA, Vemuri R, Burns EA, Hills JV, Miller MA, Spielberg SP. Familial occurrence of hypersensitivity to phenytoin. *Am J Med* 1991; 91:631–634.

228. Abbondanzo SL, Sato N, Straus SE, Jaffe ES. Acute infectious mononucleosis. CD30 (Ki-1) antigen expression and histologic correlations. *Am J Clin Pathol* 1990;93:698–702.

229. Grierson H, Purtilo DT. Epstein–Barr virus infections in males with the X-linked lymphoproliferative syndrome. *Ann Intern Med* 1987; 106:538–545.

230. Li FP, Willard DR, Goodman R, Vawter G. Malignant lymphoma after diphenylhantoin (Dilantin) therapy. *Cancer* 1975;36:1359–1362.

231. Starzl TE, Nalesnik MA, Porter KA, et al. Reversibility of lymphomas and lymphoproliferative lesions developing under cyclosporin-steroid therapy. *Lancet* 1984;1:583–587.

232. Shapiro RS, McClain K, Frizzera G, et al. Epstein–Barr virus-associated B-cell lymphoproliferative disorders following bone marrow transplantation. *Blood* 1988;71:1234–1243.

233. Young LS, Finerty S, Brooks L, Scullion F, Rickinson AB, Morgan AJ. Epstein–Barr virus gene expression in malignant lymphomas induced by experimental virus infection of cottontop tamarins. *J Virol* 1989;63:1967–1974.

234. Fischer A, Blanche S, Le Bidois J, et al. Anti-B-cell monoclonal antibodies in the treatment of severe B-cell lymphoproliferative syndrome following bone marrow and organ transplantation. *N Engl J Med* 1991;324:1451–1456.

235. Schwarzmeier JD, Reinisch WW, Kurkciyan IE, et al. Interferon-alpha induces complete remission in angioimmunoblastic lymphadenopathy (AILD): late development of aplastic anaemia with cytokine abnormalities. *Br J Haematol* 1991;79:336–337.

236. Nezelof C, Virelizier JL. Long lasting lymphadenopathy in childhood as an expression of a severe hyperimmune B lymphocyte disorder. *Hematol Oncol* 1983;1:227–242.

237. Koo CH, Nathwani BN, Winberg CD, Hill LR, Rappaport H. Atypical lymphoplasmacytic and immunoblastic proliferation in lymph nodes of patients with autoimmune disease (autoimmune-disease-associated lymphadenopathy). *Medicine* 1984;63:274–290.

238. Knecht H, Schwarze EW, Lennert K. Histological, immunohistological and autopsy findings in lymphogranulomatosis X (including angioimmunoblastic lymphadenopathy). *Virchows Arch A Path Anat* 1985;406:105–124.

239. Frizzera G, Moran EM, Rappaport H. Angio-immunoblastic lymphadenopathy with dysproteinaemia. *Lancet* 1974;1:1070–1073.

240. Suchi T. Atypical lymph node hyperplasia with fatal outcome. A report on the histopathological, immunological and clinical investigations of the cases. *Rec Adv RES Res* 1974;14:13–34.

241. Radaszkiewicz T, Lennert K. Lymphogranulomatosis X. Klinisches bild, therapie und prognose. *Dtsch Med Wochenschr* 1975;100: 1157–1163.

242. Shimoyama M, Minato K, Saito H, et al. Immunoblastic lymphadenopathy (IBL)-like T-cell lymphoma. *Jap J Clin Oncol* 1979;9 (Suppl):347–356.

243. Knecht H. Angioimmunoblastic lymphadenopathy: ten years' experience and state of current knowledge. *Semin Hematol* 1989;26:208–215.

244. Freter CE, Cossman J. Angioimmunoblastic lymphadenopathy with dysproteinemia. *Semin Oncol* 1993;20:627–635.

245. Dellagi K, Brouet J-C, Seligmann M. Antivimentin autoantibodies in angioimmunoblastic lymphadenopathy. *N Engl J Med* 1984;310:215–218.

246. Pizzolo G, Stein H, Josimovic-Alasevic O, et al. Increased serum levels of IL-2 receptor, CD30 and CD8 molecules and gamma-interferon in angioimmunoblastic lymphadenopathy: possible pathogenetic role of immunoactivation mechanisms. *Br J Haematol* 1990;75:485–488.

247. Ohshima K, Kikuchi M, Hashimoto M, et al. Genetic changes in atypical hyperplasia and lymphoma with angioimmunoblastic lymphadenopathy and dysproteinaemia in the same patients. *Virchows Arch A Path Anat* 1994;425:25–32.

248. Feller AC, Griesser H, Schilling CV, et al. Clonal gene rearrangement patterns correlate with immunophenotype and clinical parameters in patients with angioimmunoblastic lymphadenopathy. *Am J Pathol* 1988;133:549–556.

249. Nathwani BN, Rappaport H, Moran EM, Pangalis GA, Kim H. Malignant lymphoma arising in angio-immunoblastic lymphadenopathy. *Cancer* 1978;41:578–606.

250. Lukes RJ. The pathology of the white pulp of the spleen. In: Lennert K, Harms D, eds. *The spleen*. Berlin: Springer-Verlag, 1970;130–138.

251. Namikawa R, Suchi T, Ueda R, et al. Phenotyping of proliferating lymphocytes in angioimmunoblastic lymphadenopathy and related lesions by the double immunoenzymatic staining technique. *Am J Pathol* 1987;127:279–287.

252. Weiss LM, Strickler JO, Dorfman RF, Horning SJ, Warnke RA, Sklar J. Clonal T-cell populations in angioimmunoblastic lymphadenopathy and angioimmunoblastic lymphadenopathy-like lymphoma. *Am J Pathol* 1986;122:392–397.

253. Ohno T, Kita K, Miwa H, Shirakawa S. Immunophenotypical and molecular genetical examination of angioimmunoblastic lymphadenopathy. *Nippon Ketsueki Gakkai Zasshi* 1987;50:1657–1667.

254. Jaffe ES. Morphologic features. In: Steinberg, AD, moderator. Angioimmunoblastic lymphadenopathy with dysproteinemia. *Ann Intern Med* 1988;108:577–579.

255. Knecht H, Odermatt BF, Maurer R, Ruettner JR. Diagnosis and prognostic value of monoclonal antibodies in immunophenotyping of angioimmunoblastic lymphadenopathy/lymphogranulomatosis X. *Br J Haematol* 1987;67:19–24.

256. Nakamura S, Suchi T. A clinicopathologic study of node-based, low grade, peripheral T-cell lymphoma. Angioimmunoblastic lymphoma, T-zone lymphoma, and lymphoepithelioid lymphoma. *Cancer* 1991;67:2565–2578.

257. Ohsaka A, Saito K, Sakai T, et al. Clinicopathologic and therapeutic aspects of angioimmunoblastic lymphadenopathy-related lesions. *Cancer* 1992;69:1259–1267.

258. Leung CY, Ho FCS, Srivastava G, Loke SL, Liu YT, Chan ACL. Usefulness of follicular dendritic cell pattern in classification of peripheral T-cell lymphomas. *Histopathology* 1993;23:433–437.

259. Kon S, Sato T, Onodera K, et al. Detection of Epstein–Barr virus DNA and EBV-determined nuclear antigen in angioimmunoblastic lymphadenopathy with dysproteinemia type T cell lymphoma. *Pathol Res Pract* 1993;189:1137–1144.

260. Lorenzen J, Li G, Zhao-Hohn M, Wintzer C, Fischer R, Hansmann ML. Angioimmunoblastic lymphadenopathy type of T-cell lymphoma and angioimmunoblastic lymphadenopathy: a clinicopathological and molecular biological study of 13 Chinese patients using polymerase chain reaction and paraffin-embedded tissues. *Virchows Arch* 1994;424:593–600.

261. Lipford EH, Smith HR, Pittaluga S, Jaffe ES, Steinberg AD, Cossman J. Clonality of angioimmunoblastic lymphadenopathy and implications for its evolution to malignant lymphoma. *J Clin Invest* 1987;79:637–642.

262. Goedde-Salz E, Feller AC, Lennert K. Chromosomal abnormalities in lymphogranulomatosis X/angioimmunoblastic lymphadenopathy (AILD). *Leuk Res* 1987;11:181–190.

263. Cosimi MF, Casagranda I, Ghiazza G, Rossi G, Galvani P. Rearrangements on chromosomes 7 and 14 with breakpoints at 7q35 and 14q11 in angioimmunoblastic lymphadenopathy and IBL-like T-cell lymphoma. *Pathologica* 1990;82:391–397.

264. Kaneko Y, Maseki N, Sakurai M, et al. Characteristic karyotypic pattern in T-cell lymphoproliferative disorders with reactive "angioimmunoblastic lymphadenopathy with dysproteinemia-type" features. *Blood* 1988;72:413–421.

265. Schlegelberger B, Himmler A, Goedde E, Grote W, Feller AC, Lennert K. Cytogenetic findings in peripheral T-cell lymphomas as a basis for distinguishing low-grade and high-grade lymphomas. *Blood* 1994;83:505–511.

266. Schlegelberger B, Zhang Y, Weber-Matthiesen K, Grote W. Detection of aberrant clones in nearly all cases of angioimmunoblastic lymphadenopathy with dysproteinemia-type T-cell lymphoma by combined interphase and metaphase cytogenetics. *Blood* 1994;84:2640–2648.

267. Schlegelberger B, Feller A, Goedde E, Grote W, Lennert K. Stepwise development of chromosomal abnormalities in angioimmunoblastic lymphadenopathy. *Cancer Genet Cytogenet* 1990;50:15–29.

268. O'Connor NTJ, Crick JA, Wainscoat JS, et al. Evidence for monoclonal T lymphocyte proliferation in angioimmunoblastic lymphadenopathy. *J Clin Pathol* 1986;39:1229–1232.

269. Abruzzo LV, Schmidt K, Weiss LM, et al. B-cell lymphoma after angioimmunoblastic lymphadenopathy: a case with oligoclonal gene rearrangements associated with Epstein–Barr virus. *Blood* 1993;82:241–246.

270. Khan G, Norton AJ, Slavin G. Epstein–Barr virus in angioimmunoblastic T-cell lymphomas. *Histopathology* 1993;22:145–149.

271. Anagnostopoulos I, Hummel M, Finn T, et al. Heterogeneous Epstein–Barr virus infection patterns in peripheral T-cell lymphoma of angioimmunoblastic lymphadenopathy type. *Blood* 1992;80:1804–1812.

272. Weiss LM, Jaffe ES, Liu XF, Chen YY, Shibata D, Medeiros LJ. Detection and localization of Epstein–Barr viral genomes in angioimmunoblastic lymphadenopathy and angioimmunoblastic lymphadenopathy-like lymphoma. *Blood* 1992;79:1789–1795.

273. Hamilton-Dutoit SJ, Pallesen G. A survey of Epstein–Barr virus gene expression in sporadic non-Hodgkin's lymphomas. Detection of Epstein–Barr virus in a subset of peripheral T cell lymphomas. *Am J Pathol* 1992;140:1315–1325.

274. de Bruin PC, Jiwa M, Oudejans JJ, et al. Presence of Epstein–Barr virus in extranodal T-cell lymphomas: differences in relation to site. *Blood* 1994;83:1612–1618.

275. Borisch B, Caioni M, Hurwitz N, et al. Epstein–Barr virus subtype distribution in angioimmunoblastic lymphadenopathy. *Int J Cancer* 1993;55:748–752.

276. Yu AM, Song RL, Yu Z, et al. Detection of human cytomegalovirus antigen and DNA in lymph nodes and peripheral blood mononuclear cells of patients with angioimmunoblastic lymphadenopathy with dysproteinemia. *Arch Pathol Lab Med* 1992;116:490–494.

277. Newcom SR, Kadin ME. Prednisone in treatment of allergen-associated angio-immunoblastic lymphadenopathy. *Lancet* 1979;1:462–464.

278. Coupland RW, Pontifex AH, Salinas FA. Angioimmunoblastic lymphadenopathy with dysproteinemia. Circulating immune complexes and the review of 18 cases. *Cancer* 1985;55:1902–1906.

279. Archimbaud E, Coiffier B, Bryon PA, Vasselon C, Brizard CP, Viala JJ. Prognostic factors in angioimmunoblastic lymphadenopathy. *Cancer* 1987;59:208–212.

280. Hsu SM, JR WJA, Fink L, et al. Pathogenic significance of interleukin-6 in angioimmunoblastic lymphadenopathy-type T-cell lymphoma. *Hum Pathol* 1993;24:126–131.

281. Knecht H, Lennert K. Vorgeschichte und klinisches bild der lymphogranulomatosis X (einschliesslich (angio) immunoblastischer lymphadenopathie). *Schweiz Med Wochenschr* 1981;111:1108–1121.

282. Frizzera G, Kaneko Y, Sakurai M. Angioimmunoblastic lymphadenopathy and related disorders: a retrospective look in search of definitions. *Leukemia* 1989;3:1–5.

283. Siegert W, Agthe A, Griesser H, et al. Treatment of angioimmunoblastic lymphadenopathy (AILD)-type T-cell lymphoma using prednisone with or without the COPBLAM/IMVP-16 regimen. A multicenter study. Kiel Lymphoma Study Group. *Ann Intern Med* 1992;117:364–370.

284. Siegert W, Neri C, Meuthen I, et al. Recombinant human interferon-α in the treatment of angioimmunoblastic lymphadenopathy: results in 12 patients. *Leukemia* 1991;5:892–895.

285. Murayama T, Imoto S, Takahashi T, Ito M, Matozaki S, Nakagawa T. Successful treatment of angioimmunoblastic lymphadenopathy with dysproteinemia with cyclosporin A. *Cancer* 1992;69:2567–2570.

286. Pangalis GA, Moran EM, Nathwani BN, Zelman RJ, Kim H, Rappaport H. Angioimmunoblastic lymphadenopathy. Long-term follow-up study. *Cancer* 1983;52:318–321.

287. Donhuijsen K, Nabavi D, Leder LD. Angioimmunoblastische lLymphadenopathie (AILD): Histologie und uberlebenszeit. *Verhandlungen der Deutschen Gesellschaft fur Pathologie* 1992;76:117–121.

288. Diebold J, Tulliez M, Bernadou A, et al. Angiofollicular and plasmacytic polyadenopathy: a pseudotumorous syndrome with dysimmunity. *J Clin Pathol* 1980;33:1068–1976.

289. Mori S, Mohri N, Uchida T, Shimamine T. Idiopathic plasmacytic lymphadenopathy with polyclonal hyperimmunoglobulinemia. A syndrome related to giant lymph node hyperplasia of plasma cell type. *J Jpn Soc RES* 1981;20 (Suppl):85–94.

290. Mori N, Tsunoda R, Kojima K. Multicentric lymphadenopathy histologically simulating Castleman's disease. *J Jpn Soc RES* 1981; 20(suppl):55–66.

291. Kojima M, Sakuma H, Mori N. Histopathological features of plasma cell dyscrasia with polyneuropathy and endocrine disturbances, with special reference to germinal center lesions. *Jap J Clin Oncol* 1983; 13:557–576.

292. Ben-Chetrit F, Flusser D, Okon E, Ackerman Z, Rubinow A. Multicentric Castleman's disease associated with rheumatoid arthritis: a possible role of hepatitis B antigen. *Ann Rheum Dis* 1989;48:326–330.

293. Lachant NA, Sun NC, Leong LA, Oseas RS, Prince HE. Multicentric angiofollicular lymph node hyperplasia (Castleman's disease) followed by Kaposi's sarcoma in two homosexual males with the acquired immunodeficiency syndrome (AIDS). *Am J Clin Pathol* 1985; 83:27–33.

294. Rywlin AM, Rechner L, Hoffman EP. Lymphoma-like presentation of Kaposi's sarcoma. Three cases without characteristic skin lesions. *Arch Dermatol* 1966;93:554–561.

295. Lubin J, Rywlin AM. Lymphoma-like lymph node changes in Kaposi's sarcoma. Two additional cases. *Arch Pathol* 1971;92:338–341.

296. Peterson BA, Frizzera G. Multicentric Castleman's disease. *Semin Oncol* 1993;20:636–647.

297. Massey GV, Kornstein MJ, Wahl D, Huang XL, McCrady CW, Carchman RA. Angiofollicular lymph node hyperplasia (Castleman's disease) in an adolescent female. Clinical and immunologic findings. *Cancer* 1991;68:1365–1372.

298. Carrington PA, Anderson H, Harris M, Walsh SE, Houghton JB, Morgenstern GR. Autoimmune cytopenias in Castleman's disease. *Am J Clin Pathol* 1990;94:101–104.

299. Salisbury JR. Castleman's disease in childhood and adolescence: report of a case and review of literature. *Pediatr Pathol* 1990;10: 609–615.

300. O'Reilly PEJ, Joshi VV, Holbrook CT, Weisenburger DD. Multicentric Castleman's disease in a child with prominent thymic involvement: a case report and brief review of the literature. *Mod Pathol* 1993;6:776–780.

301. Chan JK, Fletcher CDM, Hicklin GA, Rosai J. Glomeruloid hemangioma. A distinctive cutaneous lesion of multicentric Castleman's disease associated with POEMS syndrome. *Am J Surg Pathol* 1990;14: 1036–1046.

302. Kitamura K, Tamura N, Hatano H, Toyama K, Mikata A, Watanabe S. A case of plasmacytosis with multiple peculiar eruptions. *J Dermatol* 1980;7:341–349.

303. Watanabe S, Ohara K, Kukita A, Mori S. Systemic plasmacytosis. A syndrome of peculiar multiple skin eruptions, generalized lymphadenopathy, and polyclonal hypergammaglobulinemia. *Arch Dermatol* 1986;122:1314–1320.

304. Marsh JH, Colbourn DS, Donovan V, Staszewski H. Systemic Castleman's disease in association with Evan's syndrome and vitiligo. *Med Pediatr Oncol* 1990;18:169–172.

305. Gaba AR, Stein RS, Sweet DL, Variakojis D. Multicentric giant lymph node hyperplasia. *Am J Clin Pathol* 1978;69:86–90.

306. Feigert JM, Sweet DL, Coleman M, et al. Multicentric angiofollicular lymph node hyperplasia with peripheral neuropathy, pseudotumor cerebri, IgA dysproteinemia, and thrombocytosis in women. A distinct syndrome. *Ann Intern Med* 1990;113:362–367.

307. Gianaris PG, Leestma JE, Cerullo LJ, Butler A. Castleman's disease manifesting in the central nervous system: case report with immunological studies. *Neurosurgery* 1989;24:608–613.

308. Lacombe M, Poirer J, J-P C. Intracranial lesion resembling giant lymph node hyperplasia. *Am J Clin Pathol* 1983;80:721–723.

309. Stanley MW, Frizzera G, Dehner LP. Castleman's disease, plasma cell type. Diagnosis of central nervous system involvement by cerebrospinal fluid cytology. *Acta Cytol* 1986;30:481–486.

310. Hineman VL, Phyliky RL, Banks PM. Angiofollicular lymph node hyperplasia and peripheral neuropathy. Association with monoclonal gammopathy. *Mayo Clin Proc* 1982;57:379–382.

311. Okuda K, Himeno Y, Toyama T, Ohta M, Kitagawa M, Sugai S. Gamma heavy chain disease and giant lymph node hyperplasia in a patient with impaired T cell function. *Jap J Med* 1982;21:109–114.

312. Kessler E, Beer R. Multicentric giant lymph node hyperplasia clinically simulating angioimmunoblastic lymphadenopathy. Associated Kaposi's sarcoma in two of three cases. *Isr J Med Sci* 1983;19: 230–234.

313. Chen KTK. Multicentric Castleman's disease and Kaposi's sarcoma. *Am J Surg Pathol* 1984;8:287–293.

314. Chan KW, Lo WK, Cheng IK. Nephrotic syndrome associated with angiofollicular lymph node hyperplasia, and subsequent amyloidosis [letter]. *Pathology* 1992;24:229–230.

315. Karcher DS, Pearson CE, Butler WM, Hurwitz MA, Cassell PF. Giant lymph node hyperplasia involving the thymus with associated nephrotic syndrome and myelofibrosis. *Am J Clin Pathol* 1982;77: 100–104.

316. Weisenburger DD. Membranous nephropathy. Its association with multicentric angiofollicular lymph node hyperplasia. *Arch Pathol Lab Med* 1979;103:591–594.

317. Tsukamoto Y, Hanada N, Nomura Y, et al. Rapidly progressive renal failure associated with angiofollicular lymph node hyperplasia. *Am J Nephrol* 1991;11:430–436.

318. Takatsuki K, Sanada I. Plasma cell dyscrasia with polyneuropathy and endocrine disorder: clinical laboratory features of 109 reported cases. *Jap J Clin Oncol* 1983;13:543–556.

319. Nakanishi T, Sobue I, Toyokura Y, et al. The Crow-Fukase syndrome: a study of 102 cases in Japan. *Neurology (Cleveland)* 1984;34: 712–720.

320. Bardwick PA, Zvaifler NJ, Gill GN, Newman D, Greenway GD, Resnick DL. Plasma cell dyscrasia with polyneuropathy, organomegaly, endocrinopathy, M protein, and skin changes: the POEMS syndrome. Report on two cases and a review of the literature. *Medicine (Baltimore)* 1980;59:311–322.

321. Farhangi M, Merlini G. The clinical implications of monoclonal immunoglobulins. *Semin Oncol* 1986;13:366–379.

322. Anonymous. Case records of the Massachusetts General Hospital. Case 10-1987. *N Engl J Med* 1987;316:606–618.

323. Bitter MA, Komaiko W, Franklin WA. Giant lymph node hyperplasia with osteoblastic bone lesions and the POEMS (Takatsuki's) syndrome. *Cancer* 1985;56:188–194.

324. Munoz G, Geijo P, Moldenhauer F, Perez-Moro E, Razquin J, Piris MA. Plasmacellular Castleman's disease and POEMS syndrome. *Histopathology* 1990;17:172–174.

325. Rolon PG, Audouin J, Diebold J, A RP, Gonzalez A. Multicentric angiofollicular lymph node hyperplasia associated with a solitary osteolytic costal IgG lambda myeloma. POEMS syndrome in a South American (Paraguayan) patient. *Pathol Res Pract* 1989;185:468–475.

326. Myers BM, Miralles GD, Taylor CA, Gastineau DA, Pisani RJ, Talley NJ. POEMS syndrome with idiopathic flushing mimicking carcinoid syndrome. *Am J Med* 1991;90:646–648.

327. Gherardi R, Baudrimont M, Kujas M, et al. Pathological findings in three non-Japanese patients with the POEMS syndrome. *Virchows Arch A Path Anat* 1988;413:357–365.

328. Radaszkiewicz T, Hansmann M-L, Lennert K. Monoclonality and polyclonality of plasma cells in Castleman's disease of the plasma cell variant. *Histopathology* 1989;14:11–24.

329. Miller RT, Mukai K, Banks PM, Frizzera G. Systemic lymphoproliferative disorder with morphologic features of Castleman's disease. Immunoperoxidase study of cytoplasmic immunoglobulins. *Arch Pathol Lab Med* 1984;108:626–630.

330. Tanda F, Massarelli G, Costanzi G. Multicentric giant lymph node hyperplasia: an immunohistochemical study. *Hum Pathol* 1983;14: 1053–1058.

331. Ohyashiki JH, Ohyashiki K, Kawakubo K, et al. Molecular genetic, cytogenetic, and immunophenotypic analyses in Castleman's disease of the plasma cell type. *Am J Clin Pathol* 1994;101:290–295.

332. York JC, Taylor CR, Lukes RJ. Monoclonality in giant lymph node hyperplasia. *Lab Invest* 1981;44:77A.

721. Zsebo KM, Yuschenkoff VN, Schiffer S et al. Vascular endothelial cells and granulopoiesis: Interleukin-1 stimulates release of G-CSF and GM-CSF. *Blood* 1988;71:99–103.

722. Freund M, Kleine HD. The role of GM-CSF in infection. *Infection* 1992;20 (Suppl 2):84–92.

723. Kitamura M, Kodama F, Odagiri S, Nagahara N, Inoue T, Kanisawa M. Granulocytosis associated with malignant neoplasms: a clinical pathologic study and demonstration of colony-stimulating activity in tumor extracts. *Hum Pathol* 1989;20:878–885.

724. Nishihara H, Tanaka Y, Kigasawa H, Sasaki Y, Fujimoto J. Ki-1 lymphoma producing G-CSF. *Br J Haematol* 1992;80:556–557.

725. Bagby GJ. Leukocytosis and leukemoid reactions. In: Wyngaarden JB, Smith LH, eds. *Cecil textbook of medicine.* 18th ed. Philadelphia: WB Saunders, 1988;967–970.

726. McCall CE, Katayama I, Cotran RS, Finland M. Lysosomal and ultrastructural changes in human "toxic" neutrophil during bacterial infections. *J Exp Med* 1969;129:267–293.

727. Thiele J, Holgado S, Choritz H, Georgii A. Density distribution and size of megakaryocytes in inflammatory reactions of the bone marrow (myelitis) and chronic myeloproliferative disorders. *Scand J Haematol* 1983;31:329–341.

728. Nowell PC, Hungerford DA. A minute chromosome in human chronic granulocytic leukemia. *Science* 1960;132:1497–1498.

729. Rowley JD. A new consistent chromosomal abnormality in chronic myelogenous leukemia identified by quinacrine fluorescence and Giemsa staining. *Nature* 1973;243:290–293.

730. Rowley JD. Chromosome abnormalities in human leukemia. *Annu Rev Genet* 1980;14:17–39.

731. Hooberman AL, Westbrook CA. Molecular methods to detect the Philadelphia chromosome. *Clin Lab Med* 1990;10:839–855.

732. Shepherd PCA, Ganesan TS, Galton DAG. Haematological classification of the chronic myeloid leukemias. *Bailliere's Clin Haematol* 1987;4:887–906.

733. Kamada N, Uchino H. Chronologic sequence in appearance of clinical and laboratory findings characteristic of chronic myelocytic leukemia. *Blood* 1978;51:843–850.

734. You W, Weisbrot IM. Chronic neutrophilic leukemia. Report of two cases and review of the literature. *Am J Clin Pathol* 1979;72:233–242.

735. Lugassi G, Fahri R. Chronic neutrophilic leukemia associated with polycythemia vera. *Am J Hematol* 1989;31:300–301.

736. Foa P, Iurlo A, Saglio G, Guerrasio A, Capsoni F, Maiolo AT. Chronic neutrophilic leukemia associated with polycythemia vera: pathogenetic implications and therapeutic approach. *Br J Haematol* 1991;78:286–288.

737. Lieschke GJ, Burgess AW. Drug therapy: granulocyte colony-stimulating factor and granulocyte-*monocyte* colony-stimulating factor (first of two parts). *N Engl J Med* 1992;327:28–33.

738. Schmitz LL, McClure JS, Litz CE et al. Morphologic and quantitative changes in blood and bone marrow cells following growth factor therapy. *Am J Clin Pathol* 1994;101:67–75.

739. Schmitz LL, Litz CE, Brunning RD. The morphologic and quantitative alterations in hematopoietic cells associated with growth factor therapy: a review of the literature. *Hematol Pathol* 1994;8:55–73.

740. Harris AC, Todd WM, Hacney MH, Ben-Ezra J. Bone marrow changes associated with recombinant granulocyte-macrophage and granulocyte colony-stimulating factors. Discrimination of granulocytic regeneration. *Arch Pathol Lab Med* 1994;118:624–629.

741. Takamatsu H, Nakao S, Ohtake S et al. Granulocyte colony-stimulating factor-dependent leukemic cell proliferations in vivo in acute promyelocytic leukemia. *Blood* 1993;81:3485–3486.

742. Lowenberg B, Touw IP. Hematopoietic growth factors and their receptors in acute leukemia. *Blood* 1993;81:281–292.

743. Tohyama K, Ueda T, Yoshida Y, Nakamura T. Altered response of purified blast cells from the myelodysplastic syndromes to colony-stimulating factors in vitro: comparison with normal blast cells. *Exp Hematol* 1994;222:539–545.

744. Kojima S, Tsuchida M, Matsuyama T. Myelodysplasia and leukemia after treatment of aplastic anemia with G-CSF. *N Engl J Med* 1992;326:1294–1295.

745. Brunning RD, McKenna RW. Lesions simulating lymphoma and miscellaneous tumor-like lesions in the bone marrow. In: Brunning RD, McKenna RW, eds. *Atlas of tumor pathology. Third Series. Fascicle 9. Tumors of the bone marrow.* Washington, DC: Armed Forces Institute of Pathology, 1994;409–419.

746. Li CJ, Yam LT. Cytochemical, histochemical and immunohistochem-

ical analysis of the bone marrow. In: Knowles DM, ed. *Neoplastic hematopathology.* Baltimore: Williams and Wilkins, 1992;1097–1134.

747. Foucar K, McKenna RW, Frizzera G, Brunning RD. Bone marrow and blood involvement by lymphoma in relationship to the Lukes–Collins classification. *Cancer* 1982;49:888–897.

748. Hu E, Thompson J, Horning S et al. Detection of B-cell lymphoma in peripheral blood by DNA hybridisation. *Lancet* 1985;2:1092–1094.

749. Nakano M, Kawanishi Y, Kuge S et al. Clinical and prognostic significance of monoclonal small cells in the peripheral blood and bone marrow of various B-cell lymphomas. *Blood* 1992;12:3253–3260.

750. Fahri DC. Germinal centers in the bone marrow. *Hematol Pathol* 1989;3:133–136.

751. McKenna RW. The bone marrow manifestations of Hodgkin's disease, the non-Hodgkin's lymphomas and lymphoma-like disorders. In: Knowles DM, ed. *Neoplastic hematopathology.* Baltimore: Williams and Wilkins, 1992;1137–1180.

752. Rappaport H, Berard CW, Butler JJ et al. Report on the committee on histopathological criteria contributing to staging of Hodgkin's disease. *Cancer Res* 1971;31:1864–1865.

753. Varjakojis D, Anastasi J. Unresolved issues concerning Hodgkin's disease and its relationship to non-Hodgkin's lymphoma. *Am J Clin Pathol* 1993;99:436–444.

754. The non-Hodgkin's lymphoma pathologic classification project: National Cancer Institute-sponsored study of classifications of non-Hodgkin's lymphomas. Summary and description of a Working Formulation for clinical usage. *Cancer* 1982;49:2112–2135.

755. Weiss LM, Crabtree GS, Rouse RV, Warnke RA. Morphologic and immunologic characterization of 50 peripheral T-cell lymphomas. *Am J Pathol* 1985;118:316–324.

756. Cabecadas JM, Isaacson PG. Phenotyping of T-cell lymphomas in paraffin sections-which antibodies? *Histopathology* 1991;19:419–424.

757. Hanson CA, Brunning RD, Gajl KJ, Frizzera G, McKenna RW. Bone marrow manifestations of peripheral T-cell lymphoma. A study of 30 cases. *Am J Clin Pathol* 1986;86:449–460.

758. Gaulard P, Kanavaros P, Farcet JP et al. Bone marrow histologic and immunohistochemical findings in peripheral T-cell lymphoma: a study of 38 cases. *Hum Pathol* 1991;22:331–338.

759. Horny HP, Wehrmann M, Griesser H, Tiemann M, Bultmann B, Kaiserling E. Investigation of bone marrow lymphocyte subsets in normal, reactive and neoplastic states using paraffin-embedded biopsy specimens. *Am J Clin Pathol* 1993;99:142–149.

760. Bluth RF, Casey T, McCurley T. Differentiation of reactive from neoplastic small cell lymphoid aggregates in paraffin-embedded marrow particle preparations using L26 (CD20) and UCHL-1 (CD45R0) monoclonal antibodies. *Am J Clin Pathol* 1993;99:150–156.

761. Ben-Ezra J, King BE, Harris AC, Todd WM, Kornstein MJ. Staining for bcl-2 protein helps to distinguish benign from malignant lymphoid aggregates in bone marrow biopsies. *Mod Pathol* 1994;7:560–564.

762. Weisenburger DD, Duggan MJ, Perry DA, Sanger WG, Armitage JO. Non-Hodgkin's lymphomas of mantle cell origin. *Pathol Annu* 1991;26 (Pt. 1):139–158.

763. Faulkner-Jones B, Howie AJ, Boughton BJ, Franklin IM. Lymphoid aggregates in bone marrow: study of eventual outcome. *J Clin Pathol* 1988;41:768–775.

764. Pangalis GA, Moran EM, Rappaport H. Blood and bone marrow findings in angioimmunoblastic lymphadenopathy. *Blood* 1978;51:71–83.

765. Schnaidt U, Vykoupil KF, Thiele J, Georgii A. Angioimmunoblastic lymphadenopathy. Histopathology of bone marrow involvement. *Virchows Arch A Path Anat* 1980;389:369–380.

766. Ghani AM, Krause JR. Bone marrow biopsy findings in angioimmunoblastic lymphadenopathy. *Br J Haematol* 1985;61:203–213.

767. Hyun BH, Kwa D, Gabaldon H, Ashton JK. Reactive plasmacytic lesions of the bone marrow. *Am J Clin Pathol* 1976;65:921–928.

768. Kjeldsberg C. Normal blood and bone marrow values in man. In: Lee GR, Bithell TC, Foerster J, Athens JW, Lukens JN, eds. *Wintrobe's clinical hematology.* 9th ed. Philadelphia: Lea and Febiger, 1993;2298–2309.

769. Crocker J, Curran RC. Quantitative study of the immunoglobulin-containing cells in trephine samples of bone marrow. *J Clin Pathol* 1981;34:1080–1082.

770. Pillay TS, Sayers G, Bird AR, Jacobs P. Plasmacyte-reticulum cell satellitism in multiple myeloma associated with amyloidosis. *J Clin Pathol* 1992;45:623–624.

771. Kyle RA. Diagnostic criteria for multiple myeloma. *Hematol Oncol Clin North Am* 1992;251:1849–1854.
772. Garrett LR, Durie BGM, Nedwin GE et al. Production of the bone resorbing cytokine lymphotoxin by cultured human myeloma cells. *N Engl J Med* 1987;317:526–532.
773. Kawano M, Yamamoto I, Iwato K et al. Interleukin-1 beta rather than lymphotoxin as the major bone resorbing activity in human multiple myeloma. *Blood* 1989;73:1646–1649.
774. Cozzolino F, Torcia M, Aldinucci D, et al. Production of interleukin-1 by bone marrow myeloma cells: its role in the pathogenesis of lytic bone lesions. *Blood* 1989;74:380–387.
775. Bartl R, Frisch B, Fateh-Moghadam A, Kettner G, Jaeger K, Sommerfeld W. Histological classification and staging of multiple myeloma. A retrospective and prospective study of 674 cases. *Am J Clin Pathol* 1987;87:342–355.
776. Kyle RA, Greipp PR. Smoldering multiple myeloma. *N Engl J Med* 1980;302:1347–1349.
777. Kyle RA. "Benign" monoclonal gammopathy—After 20 to 35 years of follow-up. *Mayo Clin Proc* 1993;68:26–36.
778. Pangalis GA, Boussiotis VA, Kittas C. Malignant disorders of small lymphocytes. *Am J Clin Pathol* 1993;99:402–408.
779. Kyle RA. The monoclonal gammopathies. *Clin Chem* 1994;40:2154–2161.
780. Eckert F, Schmid L, Kradolfer D, Schmid U. Bone marrow plasmacytosis—an immunohistological study. *Blut* 1986;53:11–19.
781. Peterson LC, Brown BA, Crosson JT, Mladenovic J. Application of the immunoperoxidase technic to bone marrow trephine biopsies in the classifications of monoclonal gammopathies. *Am J Clin Pathol* 1986;85:688–693.
782. Wolf B, Brady K, O'Murchadcha MT, Neiman R. An evaluation of immunoglobulin light chain in bone marrow biopsies in benign and malignant plasma cell proliferations. *Am J Clin Pathol* 1990;94:742–746.
783. Kosmo MA, Gale RP. Plasma cell leukemia. *Semin Hematol* 1987;24:202–208.
784. Noel P, Kyle RA. Plasma cell leukemia: an evaluation of response to therapy. *Am J Med* 1987;83:1062–1068.
785. Longacre TA, Foucar K, Crago S et al. Hematogones: a multiparametric analysis of bone marrow precursor cells. *Blood* 1989;73:543–552.
786. Caldwell CW, Poje E, Helikson MA. B-cell precursors in normal pediatric bone marrow. *Am J Clin Pathol* 1991;95:816–823.
787. Loken MR, Shah VO, Dattilio KL, Civin CI. Flow cytometric analysis of human bone marrow, II: Normal B lymphocyte development. *Blood* 1987;70:1316–1324.
788. Vanderstenhoven AM, Williams JE, Borowitz MJ. Marrow B-cell precursors are increased in lymphomas and systemic diseases associated with B-cell dysfunction. *Am J Clin Pathol* 1993;100:60–66.
789. Davis RE, Longacre TA, Cornbleet PJ. Hematogones in the bone marrow of adults. Immunophenotypic features, clinical settings and differential diagnosis. *Am J Clin Pathol* 1994;102:202–211.
790. Anastasi J, Thanghavelu M, Vardiman JW et al. Interphase cytogenetic analysis detects minimal residual disease in a case of acute lymphoblastic leukemia and resolves the question of origin of relapse after allogeneic bone marrow transplantation. *Blood* 1991;77:1087–1091.
791. Anastasi J, Vardiman JW, Rudinsky R et al. Direct correlation of cytogenetic findings with cell morphology using in situ hybridization: an analysis of suspicious cells in bone marrow specimens of two patients completing therapy for acute lymphoblastic leukemia. *Blood* 1991;77:2456–2462.
792. Weinberg JB, Hobbs MM, Misukonis MA. Recombinant human gamma-interferon induces human monocyte polykaryon formation. *Proc Natl Acad Sci USA* 1984;81:4554–4557.
793. McInnes A, Rennick DM. Interleukin-4 induces cultured monocytes/macrophages to form giant multinucleated cells. *J Exp Med* 1988;167:598–611.
794. Bodem CR, Hamory BH, Taylor HM, Kleopfer L. Granulomatous bone marrow disease. A review of the literature and clinico-pathological analysis of 58 cases. *Medicine* 1983;62:372–383.
795. Bhargava V, Fahri DC. Bone marrow granulomas: clinicopathological findings in 72 cases and review of the literature. *Hematol Pathol* 1988;2:43–50.
796. Bain BJ, Clark DM, Lampert IA. Bone marrow granulomas. In: Bain BJ, Clark DM, Lampert IA, eds. *Bone marrow pathology.* Oxford: Blackwell Scientific, 1992;46–52.

797. Kadin ME, Donaldson SS, Dorfman RF. Isolated granulomas in Hodgkin's disease. *N Engl J Med* 1970;283:859–861.
798. Sacks EL, Donaldson SS, Gordon J, Dorfman RF. Epithelioid granulomas associated with Hodgkin's disease: clinical correlation in 55 previously untreated patients. *Cancer* 1978;41:562–567.
799. Yu NC, Rywlin AM. Granulomatous lesions of the bone marrow in non-Hodgkin's lymphoma. *Hum Pathol* 1982;13:905–910.
800. Warnke RA, Kim H, Dorfman RF. Malignant histiocytosis (histiocytic medullary reticulosis): I. Clinico-pathological study of 29 cases. *Cancer* 1975;35:215–230.
801. Wilson MS, Weiss LM, Gatter KC, Mason DY, Dorfman RF, Warnke RA. Malignant histiocytosis. A reassessment of cases previously reported in 1975 based on paraffin section immunophenotyping studies. *Cancer* 1990;66:530–536.
802. Fraga M, Brousset P, Schlaifer D et al. Bone marrow involvement in anaplastic large cell lymphoma. Immunohistochemical detection of minimal residual disease and its prognostic significance. *Am J Clin Pathol* 1995;103:82–89.
803. Wong KF, Chan JKC, Ng CS, Chu YC, Lam PWY, Yuen HL. Anaplastic large cell Ki-1 lymphoma involving bone marrow: marrow findings and association with reactive hemophagocytosis. *Am J Hematol* 1991;37:112–119.

## ADDENDUM REFERENCES

### *Atypical Lymphoid Hyperplasias and Lymphoproliferative Diseases*

Beltrami CA. The atypical lymphoproliferative disorders: tissue expression. *Clin Exp Rheumatol* 1996;14(Suppl 14):S15–S19.
Luppi M, Torelli G. The new lymphotropic herpesviruses (HHV-6, HHV-7, HHV-8) and hepatitis C virus (HCV) in human lymphoproliferative diseases: an overview. *Haematologica* 1996;81:265–281.
Rojo J, Ferrer-Argote VE, Klueppelberg U, Kureger GR, Eidt E, Ablashi DV, Luka J, Tesch H. Semiquantitative in situ hybridization and immunohistology for antigen expression of human herpesvirus-6 in various lymphoproliferative diseases. *In Vivo* 1994;8:517–526.
Segal GH, Perkins SL, Kjeldsberg CR. Benign lymphadenopathies in children and adolescents. *Semin Diagn Pathol* 1995;12:288–302.

### *Angioimmunoblastic Lymphadenopathies*

Jaffe ES. Angioimmunoblastic T-cell lymphoma: new insights, but the clinical challenge remains. *Ann Oncol* 1995;6:631–632.
Luppi M, Barozzi P, Maiorana A, Artusi T, Trovato R, Marasca R, Savarino M, Ceccerini-Nelli L, Torelli G. Human herpesvirus-8 DNA sequences in human immunodeficiency virus-negative angioimmunoblastic lymphadenopathy and benign lymphadenopathy with giant germinal center hyperplasia and increased vascularity. *Blood* 1996;87:3903–3909.
Schlegelberger B, Zwingers T, Hohenadel K, Henne-Bruns D, Schmitz N, Haferlach T, Tirier C, Bartels H, Sonnen R, Kuse R, et al. Significance of cytogenetic findings for the clinical outcome in patients with T-cell lymphoma of angioimmunoblastic lymphadenopathy. *J Clin Oncol* 1996;14:593–599.
Siegert W, Nerl C, Agthe A, Engelhard M, Brittinger G, Tiemann M, Lennert K, Huhn D. Angioimmunoblastic lymphadenopathy (AILD)-type T-cell lymphoma: prognostic impact of clinical observations and laboratory findings at presentation. *Ann Oncol* 1995;6:659–664.

### *Systemic Immunoblastic Proliferations*

Okuyama R, Ichinohasama R, Tagami H. Carbamazepine induced erythroderma with systemic lymphadenopathy. *J Dermatol* 1996;23:489–494.

### *Castleman's Disease*

Gossios K, Nikolaides C, Bai M, Fountzilas G. Widespread Castleman disease: CT findings. *Eur Radiol* 1996;6:95–98.
MacDonald SR, Lurain JR, Hoff F, Variakojis D, Fishman DA. Castleman disease presenting as a pelvic mass. *Obstet Gynecol* 1996;87:875–877.
Menke DM, Tiemann M, Camoriano JK, Chang SF, Madan A, Chow M, Habermann TM, Parwaresch R. Diagnosis of Castleman's disease by identification of an immunophenotypically aberrant population of man-

tle zone B lymphocytes in paraffin-embedded lymph node biopsies. *Am J Clin Pathol* 1996;105:268–276.

Soulier J, Grollet L, Oksenhendler E, Cacoub P, Cazals-Hatem D, Babinet P, d'Agay MF, Clauvel JP, Raphael M, Degos L, et al. Kaposi's sarcoma-associated herpesvirus-like DNA sequences in multicentric Castleman's disease. *Blood* 1995;86:1276–1280.

Soulier J, Grollet L, Oksenhendler E, Miclea JM, Cacoub P, Baruchel A, Brice P, Clauvel JP, d'Agay MF, Raphael M, et al. Molecular analysis of clonality in Castleman's disease. *Blood* 1995;86:1131–1138.

### Kimura's Disease

Takagi K, Harada T, Ishikawa E. Kimura's disease (eosinophilic lympho-folliculoid granuloma). *Jpn J Clin Med* 1993;51:785–788.

Taskin M, Gokaslan T, Kakani R, DaSilva M. Kimura disease. *Arch Otolaryngol Head Neck Surg* 1996;122:892–895.

### Kikuchi's Disease

Klinger M, Danter J, Siegert R, Moubayed P. Kikuchi lymphadenitis: a contribution to the differential diagnosis of cervical lymph node swelling of unknown origin. *HNO* 1995;43:253–256.

Sever CE, Leith CP, Appenzeller J, Foucar K. Kikuchi's histiocytic necrotizing lymphadenitis associated with ruptured silicone breast implant. *Arch Pathol Lab Med* 1996;120:380–385.

### Hemophagocytic Syndromes

Balduini CL, Belletti S. A single cell summarizing the pathogenesis of cytopenias in hemophagocytic syndrome. *Hematologica* 1996;81:190.

Braun MC, Cohn RA, Kletzel M. Nephrotic syndrome accompanying familial hemophagocytic syndrome. *J Pediatr Hematol Oncol* 1996;18:195–197.

Syruckova Z, Stary J, Sedlacek P, Smisek P, Vavrinec J, Komrska V, Roubalova K, Vandasova J, Sintakova B, Houskova J, Hassan M. Infection-associated hemophagocytic syndrome complicated by infectious lymphoproliferation: a case report. *Pediatr Hematol Oncol* 1996;13:143–150.

Tiab M, Mechinaud F, Hamidou M, Gaillard F, Raffi F, Harousseau JL. Hemophagocytic syndromes: a series of 23 cases. *Ann Med Interne* 1996;147:138–144.

### Mycobacterial Spindle Cell Pseudotumors

Wolf DA, Wu CD, Medeiros LJ. Mycobacterial pseudotumors of lymph node: a report of two cases diagnosed at the time of intraoperative consultation using touch imprint preparations. *Arch Pathol Lab Med* 1995;119:811–814.

### Inflammatory Pseudotumors of Lymph Node

Arber DA, Kamel OW, van de Rijn M, Davis RE, Medeiros LJ, Jaffe ES, Weiss LM. Frequent presence of the Epstein-Barr virus in inflammatory pseudotumor. *Hum Pathol* 1995;26:1093–1098.

Dogusoy G, Erdogan N, Gulhan Y, Gulmen M, Tuzuner N, Ulku B. Inflammatory pseudotumor of pelvic lymph nodes. *Arch Anat Cytol Pathol* 1996;44:122–124.

### Vascular Transformation of Lymph Nodes

Cook PD, Czerniak B, Chan JKC, Mackay B, Ordonez NG, Ayala AG, Rosai J. Nodular spindle cell vascular transformation of lymph nodes. *Am J Surg Pathol* 1995;19:1010–1020.

### Inflammatory Pseudotumor of the Spleen

McHenry CR, Perzy-Gall HB, Mardini G, Chung-Park M. Inflammatory pseudotumor of the spleen: a rare entity that may mimic hematopoietic malignancy. *Am Surg* 1995;61:1067–1071.

### Splenic Peliosis

Lam KY, Chan AC, Chan TM. Peliosis of the spleen: possible association with chronic renal failure and erythropoietin therapy. *Postgrad Med J* 1995;71:493–496.

### Splenic Hamartoma

Kumar PV. Splenic hamartoma: a diagnostic problem on fine needle aspiration cytology. *Acta Cytol* 1995;39:391–395.

Wirbel RJ, Uhlig U, Futterer KM. Splenic hamartoma with hematologic disorders. *Am J Med Sci* 1996;311:243–246.

### Megaloblastic Anemia

Campbell BA. Megaloblastic anemia in pregnancy. *Clin Obstet Gynecol* 1995;38:455–462.

Davenport J. Macrocytic anemia. *Am Fam Phys* 1996;53:155–162.

Wollman MR, Penchansky L, Shekhter-Levin S. Transient 7q- in association with megaloblastic anemia due to dietary folate and vitamin B12 deficiency. *J Pediatr Hematol Oncol* 1996;18:162–165.

### Leukemoid Reactions

Calhoun DA, Kirk JF, Christensen RD. Incidence, significance, and kinetic mechanism responsible for leukemoid reactions in patients in the neonatal intensive care unit: a prospective evaluation. *J Pediatr* 1996;129:403–409.

Kan M, Tamura M, Kojima K, Naruo S, Kanayama H, Kagawa S. A case of renal cell carcinoma producing granulocyte-macrophage colony-stimulating factor. *J Urol* 1996;155:2022–2023.

Kinawa N. Positional cloning of the putative gene responsible for transient abnormal myelopoiesis and that for multiple cartilaginous exostoses. *Jpn J Clin Pathol* 1996;44:13–18.

### Lymphoid Hyperplasia of the Bone Marrow

Thiele J. Differential "lymphoid cell infiltrate" diagnosis in bone marrow. *Pathologe* 1995;16:106–119.

### Pseudoneoplastic Plasmacytosis of the Bone Marrow

Kawano MM, Mihara K, Tsujimoto T, Huang N, Kuramoto A. A new phenotypic classification of bone marrow plasmacytosis. *Int J Hematol* 1995;61:179–188.

Koduri PR, Naides SJ. Transient blood plasmacytosis in parvovirus B19 infection: a report of two cases. *Ann Hematol* 1996;72:49–51.

Molina T, Brouland JP, Bigorgne C, LeTourneau A, Delmer A, Audouin J, Diebold J. Pseudomyelomatous plasmacytosis of the bone marrow in multicentric Castleman's disease. *Ann Pathol* 1996;16:133–136.

### Bone Marrow Granulomas

Eid A, Carion W, Nystrom JS. Differential diagnosis of bone marrow granuloma. *West J Med* 1996;164:510–515.

sis, blastomycosis, sporotrichosis, syphilis (Fig. 12), and actinomycosis, as well as rare examples of other transmissible diseases (51–59).

### Potential Mechanisms for Cutaneous PEH

Freeman (37) has reviewed the potential pathogenetic evolution of PEH in general. Based on studies of associated conditions in varying sequential phases of their development, he concluded that the epidermal hyperplasia had a potentially binary origin. It could be a reflection of the continued growth of entrapped surface epithelium in resurfacing ulcers or scars, or, alternatively, a manifestation of appendageal metaplasia and acanthosis. In all likelihood, these mechanisms both play roles in individual cases.

### Pathologic Findings in PEH

The basic morphologic hallmark of PEH is that of irregular acanthosis of the epidermis, centered on the rete ridges, the acrosyringia, or the pilosebaceous units. The proliferating keratinocytes form broad "tongues" of downward-growing epithelium, which often have extremely irregular interfaces with the subjacent dermal stroma (34,36). However, it is notable that there is no localized eosinophilia, fibromyxoid change, desmoplasia, or lymphatic or perineural permeation in this zone, as expected in well-differentiated carcinomas. The constituent cells in PEH demonstrate one of two cytomorphotypes: either they are fully keratinized polygonal cells with abundant eosinophilic cytoplasm and well-seen intercellular "bridges" (34,36,37) (Figs. 13–15), or they resemble basaloid cells of the normal epidermis with compact hyperchromatic nuclei and scanty amphophilic cytoplasm (61) (Fig. 16). Nucleoli and mitoses are variably seen in both

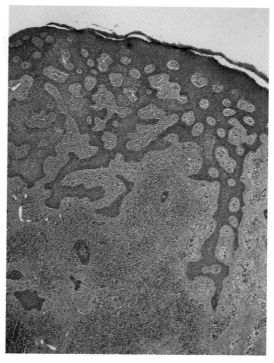

**FIG. 16.** Pseudoepitheliomatous hyperplasia. A darker image is imparted to this pseudoepitheliomatous expansion due to a proliferation of basaloid cells of the epidermis.

PEH and carcinomas; thus, they cannot be reliably used in differential diagnosis between these conditions. Fully keratinized PEH that is associated with several chronic infections—as well as halogenodermas of various types—often shows keratolytic microabscesses composed of polymorphonuclear leukocytes in the proliferative squamous epithelium, as well as neutrophilic collections in the subjacent corium (Figs. 17 and 18) that might contain identifiable infectious organisms (Figs. 19 and 20) or foreign bodies (38,

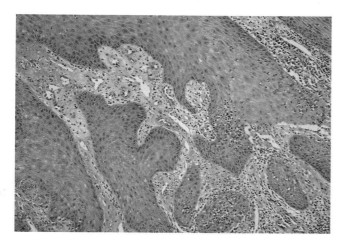

**FIG. 15.** The morphologic differential diagnosis for this case of pseudoepitheliomatous hyperplasia includes a well-differentiated squamous cell carcinoma. Particularly disconcerting are the nests of squamous cells within the inflamed fibrous stroma. However, the epithelium–stroma interface in pseudoepitheliomatous hyperplasia might be quite irregular, and tangential sectioning might result in apparently isolated islands of hyperplastic squamous cells.

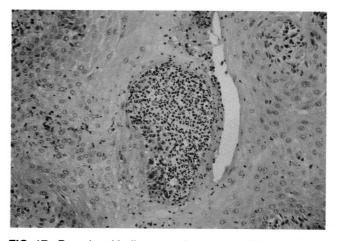

**FIG. 17.** Pseudoepitheliomatous hyperplasia. Keratolytic microabscess in the proliferative squamous epithelium of pseudoepitheliomatous hyperplasia secondary to infection.

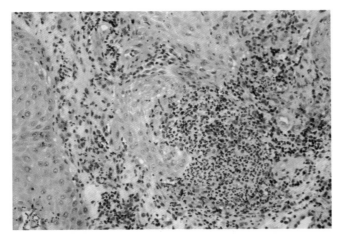

FIG. 18. Pseudoepitheliomatous hyperplasia. The collections of polymorphonuclear leukocytes in pseudoepitheliomatous hyperplasia secondary to infection may also be found in the adjacent dermis.

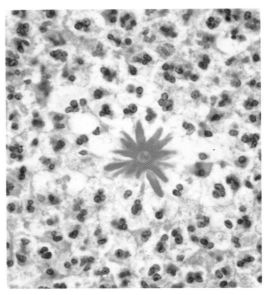

FIG. 20. Pseudoepitheliomatous hyperplasia. "*Sporothrix asteroid*" in a microabscess in pseudoepitheliomatous hyperplasia. This type of yeast form (blastospore), with its distinctive starburst likeness, may be found in most suppurative foci in *Sporothrix* infection of the skin, if serial sections are prepared (60).

42,51–60). These findings are unexpected in true neoplasms of the integument. In a similar vein, basaloid PEH can be separated diagnostically from BCC by attention to the nature of its supporting matrix. The former of these proliferations is associated with mature collagenous stroma in the subjacent dermis, with or without concurrent inflammation, whereas BCC exhibits more loosely arranged fibromyxoid supporting tissue (58). Exophytic papillomatous growth of the epidermis is also evident in many cases of PEH, and the subtype known as "prurigo nodularis" might also feature associated dermal neural hyperplasia (52,63).

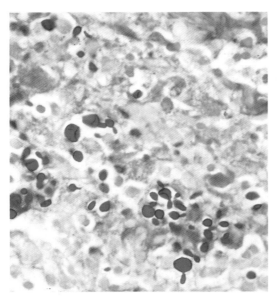

FIG. 19. Pseudoepitheliomatous hyperplasia. Yeast forms of *Sporothrix shenckii* identified by periodic acid–Schiff (PAS) stain, in a case of pseudoepitheliomatous hyperplasia with microabscess formation. Multiple serial sections may need to be stained with PAS to demonstrate the fungal elements (60).

A particularly challenging differential diagnosis involving the fully keratinized and "verruciform" (papillomatous) form of PEH concerns its distinction from verrucous squamous carcinoma. The latter condition is still confused with nonneoplastic conditions by many physicians, owing in part to the persistence of such antiquated terms as "giant condyloma of Buschke and Loewenstein" (64) or "pseudoepitheliomatous keratotic micaceous balanitis" (65) to describe this unusual form of squamous carcinoma. Verrucous carcinoma is characterized by its invasive and irregular interface with the dermis, featuring broad and often interanastomosing columns of fully mature keratinocytes. There is little or no associated inflammation in this tumor, and striking overlying papillomatosis and hyperkeratosis are apparent. Data on the *macroscopic* characteristics of verrucous carcinoma are also critical because the pathologist's diagnostic consideration of a wart is not shared by knowledgeable clinicians in such cases (66).

Some authors in the past have attempted to address histologically difficult diagnostic cases in this sphere by employing the term "atypical pseudoepitheliomatous hyperplasia" (67). Use of the latter designation undoubtedly emanated from the inability of some observers to decide whether or not a particular proliferation was benign or malignant. However, this practice and the rubric in question should be deplored. As indicated by Johnston et al. (68), most if not all examples of "atypical" PEH act in an aggressive fashion, and doubtlessly represent well-differentiated carcinomas.

It is worth reiterating the admonition that the possibility of an underlying neoplasm should be considered in all examples of PEH that are only superficially sampled. Pathologic reports in such cases may include a disclaimer stating that the specified association may exist but cannot be adequately assessed, making the desirability of a deeper biopsy self-evident.

Occasional studies on PEH have also focused on submicroscopic attributes of the condition that might be employed in the differential diagnosis. Holden and colleagues (69) suggested, for example, that immunostains for $\beta_2$-microglobulin ($\beta_2$M) could be employed to distinguish PEH (which is $\beta_2$M$^+$) from verrucous carcinoma ($\beta_2$M$^-$). However, we would urge the exercise of caution in relying exclusively on such paradigms. This reservation stems in part from the results of other evaluations that have shown a great deal of biological similarity between the lesions under discussion. Lee et al. (70) demonstrated p53 antioncogene expression in PEH, "keratoacanthoma," and well-differentiated squamous cell carcinomas alike, reflecting a shared biochemical nuclear abnormality at a subcellular level. Also, basing a malignant diagnosis on a negative immunostain is unwise due to the possibility of technical staining problems of poor antigen preservation. Thus, it stands to reason that these proliferations will continue to be difficult to separate from one another, regardless of the modality of study that is chosen.

## PSEUDONEOPLASTIC MESENCHYMAL LESIONS

The dermis and subcutis are formed by mesenchymal tissues of several diverse types. Hence, one should not be surprised that a multiplicity of mesodermal proliferations may be encountered in this anatomic compartment. These include lesions of an inflammatory nature, as well as myofibroblastic, vascular, myogenous, and neural "pseudotumors."

### Pseudosarcomatous Polyps

A recent report (71) has detailed three cases of acquired polypoid lesions of the skin. The lesions clinically mimicked fibroepithelial polyps or nevus lipomatosis. All patients were >50 years old. All cases demonstrated marked degrees of cytologic atypia. One case, with a core of fatty tissue admixed with nodules of pleomorphic spindle cells, was felt to represent a lesion with similarities to smooth muscle hamartomas. The other two cases had cores of hyalinized vessels, with bizarre spindle cells. In this regard, they resembled pleomorphic soft tissue tumors, such as pleomorphic lipoma or fibroma, or the vaginal pseudosarcomatous polyp. The behavior of all three lesions has been uniformly benign; for that reason, it is felt that the cellular atypia is likely degenerative in nature.

## "Inflammatory Pseudotumors" of the Skin

As discussed in several other chapters in this text, the pathologic entity known as "inflammatory pseudotumor" (IPT) or "inflammatory myofibroblastic tumor" has been described in a diversity of organ sites. The skin is no exception to this statement, but there has been only one formal report on cutaneous IPT in the English literature to date. Hurt and Santa Cruz (72) described four examples of that lesion in adult patients, all of whom presented with nontender dermal and subcuticular masses of variable duration. The clinical impressions of these proliferations included adnexal tumors, dermatofibromas, and inflammatory conditions.

In likeness to the pathologic features of IPT in extracutaneous locations (73), the basic histologic structure of these lesions in the skin is that of a dermal fibroblastic-myofibroblastic proliferation with variable numbers of superimposed inflammatory cells. These cells primarily include lymphocytes, plasma cells, macrophages, and neutrophils. The spindle cells in IPT are cytologically bland, although mitotic figures may certainly be observed in them; these elements may assume a focally storiform growth pattern. Foam cells and deposits of hemosiderin are absent, and the overlying epidermis is unremarkable. The density of matrical collagen is variable, as is the number of stromal blood vessels. Another feature observed in several of the cases reported by Hurt and Santa Cruz (72) was the nodular aggregation of lymphocytes at the peripheral aspects of the lesions, with focal germinal center formation (Figs. 21–24). This observa-

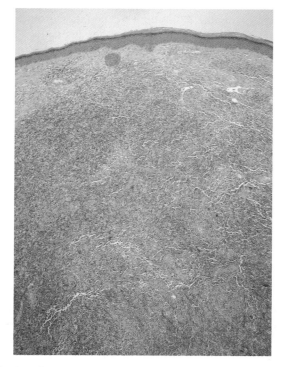

**FIG. 21.** Survey of cutaneous inflammatory pseudotumor showing a dermal fibroinflammatory mass, with sparing of the epidermis.

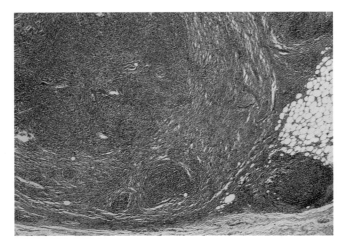

FIG. 22. Lymphoid aggregates at the periphery of a cutaneous inflammatory pseudotumor, with focal extension into subcutaneous adipose tissue.

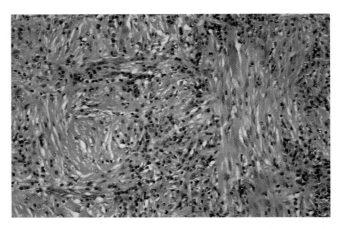

FIG. 24. Inflammatory pseudotumor of the skin with a vague storiform pattern of spindle cell arrangement. Chronic inflammatory cells, predominantly lymphocytes, permeate the mass. Dermatofibroma is in the differential diagnosis, but note the lack of foam cells, multinucleated histiocytes, hemosiderin, and keloidal collagen.

tion contributed to a diagnostic misinterpretation of "intra-dermal lymph node" in one instance.

The differential diagnosis of cutaneous IPT is relatively broad. It includes "pseudolymphoma" of the skin and other dermal lymphoreticular hyperplasias; inflamed dermatofibroma; angiolymphoid hyperplasia with eosinophilia; Kimura's disease; and late-stage arthropod bite reactions (74–80). Some of these disorders are discussed further; however, as a synoptical approach to separating this generic group of lesions from IPT, it is prudent to focus on the fundamentally spindle cell nature of the latter proliferation, which is not shared by any of the other alternatives except dermatofibroma. In comparison, that neoplasm commonly contains foam cells, multinucleated histiocytes, and tissue iron deposits, and it is surrounded by keloidal-type dermal collagen bundles with fragmented, rounded profiles (81,82). Those attributes are not part of the morphologic spectrum of

cutaneous inflammatory pseudotumors as they are currently understood.

### Proliferative Noninfectious Granulomatous Lesions

Selected noninfectious granulomatous lesions of the skin and superficial soft tissue are capable of such exuberant histiocytic proliferation that they may be mistaken for neoplasms. In particular, isolated rheumatoid nodules or necrobiotic granulomas ("deep granuloma annulare") have a great potential to simulate the histopathologic features of epithelioid sarcoma (EPS) (83–87). All of these disorders favor the distal extremities; although patients in the first three decades of life are preferentially affected by EPS, this demographic attribute cannot be used in individual cases to distinguish

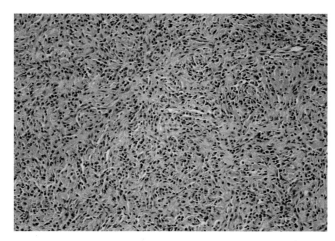

FIG. 23. Inflammatory pseudotumor of the skin with haphazard arrangement of fibroblasts/myofibroblasts, with an intimately admixed inflammatory cell population.

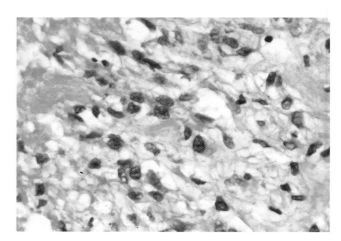

FIG. 25. Isolated necrobiotic granuloma with cytologic features of constituent cells similar to those of epithelioid sarcoma.

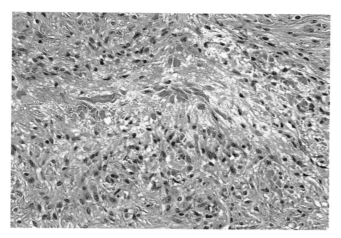

**FIG. 26.** Isolated necrobiotic granuloma exhibiting collagenolysis with surrounding peripheral palisade of lesional histiocytic cells.

that tumor from necrobiotic granulomas (87). Both of these conditions usually manifest as painless or only slightly tender nodules of variable duration, and are therefore relatively nondescript clinically.

Histologically, EPS and isolated necrobiotic granulomas (INGs) may likewise be quite similar. In fact, the title of the seminal paper on EPS by Enzinger (88) emphasized that fact. These lesions each show a circumscribed aggregation of polygonal cells that may demonstrate only slightly elevated nucleocytoplasmic ratios, vesicular chromatin, small nucleoli, variable mitotic activity, and a moderate amount of amphophilic cytoplasm (Fig. 25). A central lesional area of collagenolysis is potentially common to both, and palisading of the peripherally disposed cells may be evident in either ING or EPS (88,89) (Figs. 26 and 27). The most effective means of separating the two proliferations diagnostically is that of immunohistologic study. The tumor cells of EPS are reproducibly reactive for keratin, with or without epithelial mem-

brane antigen (EMA), whereas the histiocytic elements of ING instead express CD45 and CD68 (90) (Fig. 28).

Additional clinical information is also valuable in the assessment of the specified problem. If positive serologic results are obtained for rheumatoid factor or other indicators of systemic autoimmunity, one may strongly favor rheumatoid nodule as the probable diagnosis in this context. Conversely, magnetic resonance imaging of the extremity may disclose "skip" lesions along fascial planes or tendons in cases of EPS, whereas these findings are not expected in diseases featuring INGs.

## Pseudoneoplastic Vascular Proliferations of the Skin

Because of the impact of the acquired immunodeficiency syndrome (AIDS) epidemic on dermatopathology, there has been intense interest in Kaposi's sarcoma (KS) and other proliferative endothelial lesions of the skin in recent years. This focus has resulted in the characterization of several pseudoneoplastic pathologic mimics of KS, as detailed below.

### Reactions to Monsel's Solution

Monsel's solution (MS) is a styptic preparation used by dermatologists after shave biopsies of the skin or other minor surgical procedures in order to control bleeding. Its principal ingredient is ferric sulfate. In selected individuals, an idiosyncratic dermal reaction to MS may be seen that manifests as a nodule at the operative site (91). Biopsies of these lesions show proliferations with a superficial morphologic resemblance to KS. They feature the growth of spindle cells that are arranged in loose fascicles or in a haphazard fashion, admixed with capillary-sized blood vessels (91,92) (Figs. 29 and 30). In florid form, this condition can be extremely worrisome to the dermatopathologist in terms of the differential

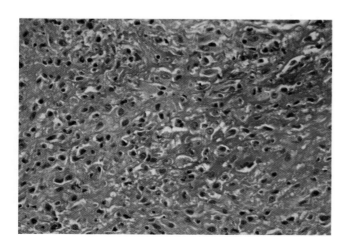

**FIG. 27.** Isolated necrobiotic granuloma with characteristic regional necrosis.

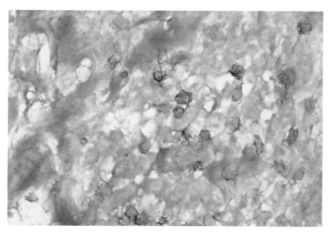

**FIG. 28.** Isolated necrobiotic granuloma: CD45-positive histiocytes by immunohistochemical analysis.

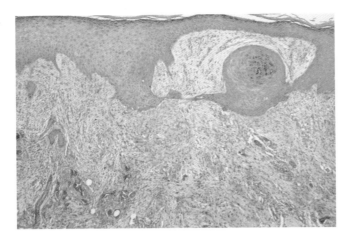

**FIG. 29.** Reaction to Monsel's solution might mimic a spindle cell neoplasm such as Kaposi's sarcoma.

diagnosis of a true endothelial neoplasm. However, the lack of the hyaline globular bodies that are commonly seen in the tumor cells of KS—as well as the stromal deposition of large "chunks" of iron salt—distinguish reactions to MS from the latter sarcoma (93,94). Obviously, it is most helpful to obtain the historical information that a dermatologic procedure has been done in the recent past, with application of the solution in question. Unfortunately, however, these facts are often withheld by submitting physicians.

### Acroangiodermatitis

The condition that is variously known as "acroangiodermatitis of Mali," "dermatitis hemostatica," "Bluefarb–Stewart syndrome," or a form of "pseudo-Kaposi's sarcoma" is in actuality a proliferative dermal mesenchymal reaction seen in the setting of long-standing stasis dermatitis (95–99). Thus, as one might predict, this disorder is most common in

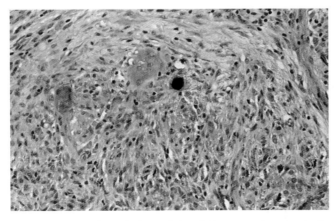

**FIG. 30.** Monsel's solution might elicit a prominent spindle cell proliferation, with histiocytes and sometimes multinucleated giant cells being apparent, as evident here. Iron, often in large aggregates, might be identified as an encrustation of collagen fibers and within histiocytes.

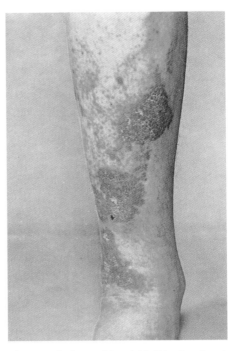

**FIG. 31.** Acroangiodermatitis of Mali in its classical clinical presentation as red and violaceous, scaly plaques extending to the lateral aspects of the lower part of the leg. There is a background of brawny pigmentation, which is typical of stasis dermatitis. These lesions occur as a consequence of increased venous pressure.

the lower extremities of older individuals, where it assumes the form of red–blue macules and plaques that are commonly confluent (Fig. 31). The latter clinical description is, perplexingly, one that could easily be applied to "classical" (Mediterranean) KS as well (100).

Microscopically, both acroangiodermatitis (AAD) and KS may contain zones of proliferating spindle cells and extravasated stromal erythrocytes, admixed with small blood vessels of venular size (Figs. 32 and 33). Nevertheless, AAD

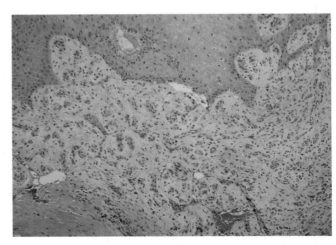

**FIG. 32.** Acroangiodermatitis. A dermal spindle cell proliferation and neovascularity are prominent.

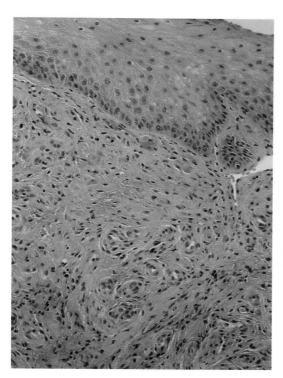

**FIG. 33.** Acroangiodermatitis. The vessels in acroangiodermatitis have regular and rounded profiles, and lack the "dissecting" quality of the neoplastic vessels of Kaposi's sarcoma.

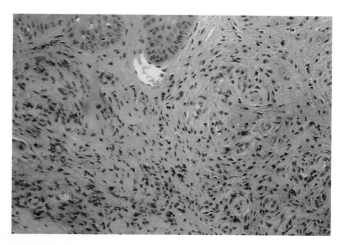

**FIG. 34.** Acroangiodermatitis with abundant dermal hemosiderin pigment deposition.

does not exhibit the disorganized proliferation of sinusoidal vascular spaces seen in KS, nor does it show the formation of new blood vessels around preexisting ones (the so-called promontory sign of KS) or the intralesional hyaline globules, peritumoral lymphatic dilatation, or aggregates of plasma cells that are commonly observed in KS (92–94,98,99). Conversely, biopsies of AAD contain much more hemosiderin pigment than those of KS, and the former of these two lesions has a more fibromyxoid background stroma (99) (Figs. 34 and 35).

Histologic findings that are similar to those of AAD are observed in biopsies taken from children or young adult patients who have "acral capillary angiomatosis" (ACA), regarded as another type of "pseudo-KS" (101,102). It is represented by the progressive growth of painful red–violet nodular lesions on the skin of the feet. One may also see associated regional hyperhidrosis and hypertrichosis. The condition is thought to be to due to minute arteriovenous shunts or other microscopic vascular malformations (102).

### Pigmented Purpura (Majocchi–Schamberg Disease; Progressive Pigmentary Dermatosis; Purpura Annularis Telangiectoides)

The "pigmented purpuras" (PPs) comprise a group of vasculopathies that present themselves as "cayenne pepper"–colored macules and patches, usually on the extremities

(103–105). They may affect patients of both genders and over a wide range of ages, and are therefore indistinguishable from the recognized variants of KS at a macroscopic level. Histopathologically, however, PPs show only a limited degree of capillary proliferation, with abundant stromal hemosiderin and erythrocyte extravasation (104). This microscopic profile is much like that of early AAD; it could conceivably be confused with the appearance of "patch stage" KS, but the promontory sign, perilesional lymphangiectasia, and plasmacytosis of the latter condition (93,94, 100) are again lacking in PPs.

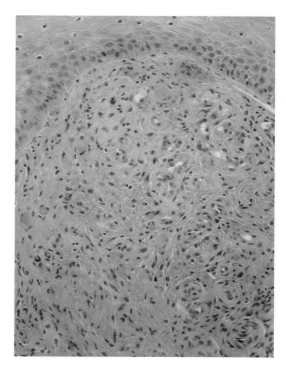

**FIG. 35.** Acroangiodermatitis showing a fibromyxoid stroma that is more extensive than that usually seen in Kaposi's sarcoma.

*Proliferative Scars*

In similarity to patients who develop the aforementioned reactions to Monsel's solution, others may manifest a peculiarly proliferative cutaneous scarring process that could potentially be confused with KS. Quite obviously, knowledge that the skin site in question has been traumatized recently would provide the necessary means to avoid this problem. Short of that, one can also rely on reproducible points of microscopic dissimilarity between scars and vascular sarcomas. The fibroblastic proliferation in cutaneous scars is cytologically bland; moreover, it is arranged in a parallel fashion under the skin surface, transected by tubular blood vessels that tend to be aligned vertically (93,94) (Figs. 36 and 37). Extravasated red blood cells, stromal hemosiderin, and plasmacytic inflammation may or may not be present. On the other hand, the ancillary histologic features of KS cited above are consistently lacking.

### Intravascular Papillary Endothelial Hyperplasia (Masson's Lesion)

In 1923, Masson described a peculiar secondary proliferative change in the lumina of hemorrhoids, which mimicked the histopathologic appearance of angiosarcoma (106). This phenomenon is now known to occur within dilated vascular channels in a variety of lesions of the skin, subcutis, or deep soft tissues (107–112). It is felt to be a consequence of thrombosis and endoluminal reendothelialization; the pro-

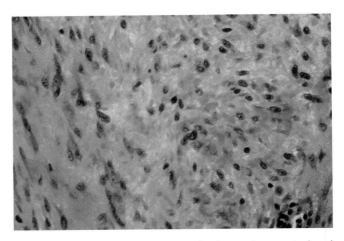

**FIG. 37.** Proliferative scars may harbor extravasated red blood cells but the nuclei of the fibroblasts lack pleomorphism.

cess may follow trauma to a blood vessel, or it may occur apparently spontaneously. Although Masson originally called the proliferation in question "intravascular vegetant hemangioendothelioma" (106) the currently preferred designation is "intravascular papillary endothelial hyperplasia" (IPEH) or, more simply, "Masson's lesion." Clinically, the presenting symptoms and signs of IPEH are principally related to changes in the vascular structures within which the lesion is contained. These may include preexisting vascular neoplasms, such as cavernous hemangiomas, or ectatic veins, which, as stated above, have undergone superimposed

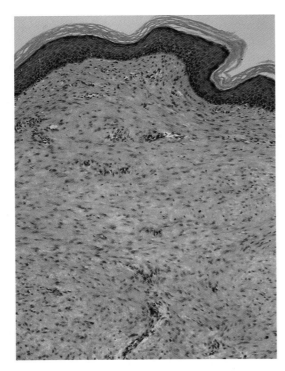

**FIG. 36.** Proliferative scar. The reactive fibroblastic cells are horizontally oriented under the epidermis.

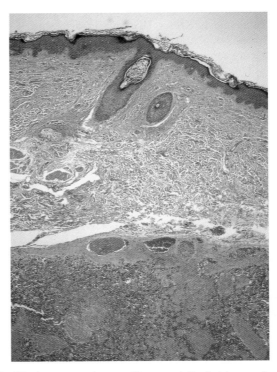

**FIG. 38.** Intravascular papillary endothelial hyperplasia in the lower dermis, representing a recanalized thrombus.

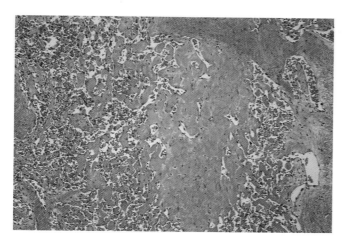

**FIG. 39.** Intravascular papillary endothelial hyperplasia with clusters of papillary processes.

thrombosis. Patients of all ages are potentially affected, and cutaneous IPEH shows a topographic predilection for the head, neck, and extremities (109,111).

Microscopically, this condition is typified by the formation of racemose channels inside a preformed blood vessel, reflecting the recanalization of a fibrin thrombus (Fig. 38). The neovascular endoluminal spaces are lined with plump but cytologically bland endothelial cells that can form small papillary structures (Figs. 39 and 40), and "normal" mitotic figures may be observed therein. However, there is never any extravascular extension of the cellular proliferation in IPEH, nor is there nuclear atypia, as would be expected in true angiosarcoma.

### "Reactive Angioendotheliomatosis"

In 1959, Pfleger and Tappeiner (113) described a young woman who had developed disseminated cutaneous patches and plaques with a purpura-like clinical appearance (Fig. 41). Biopsy of these lesions disclosed a peculiar vasocentric proliferation of bluntly spindled and oval cells, associated with intravascular microthrombi. The authors coined a new name for this disorder—"angioendotheliomatosis proliferans systemisata"—and they proposed that it represented a unique form of endothelial proliferation that was only questionably neoplastic (114).

Subsequently, other examples of this syndrome were tentatively recorded in the dermatology literature, but with a notable difference. Most of those patients manifested a progressive disease that proved fatal, despite the fact that biopsies from their cutaneous lesions were thought to show similar features to those of the seminal case (115–117). Accordingly, a dogma was crystallized that held that there were two forms of "angioendotheliomatosis"—reactive and malignant—and that histologic findings were unreliable in distinguishing between them.

The latter maxim is only a half-truth. If one chooses to continue using the term "angioendotheliomatosis," it is accurate to state that there are two forms of that condition. However, these are quite different from one another microscopically, and it is furthermore currently recognized that they are composed of cells of entirely different lineages of differentiation. "Malignant angioendotheliomatosis" features the presence of loose dermal and subcuticular intravascular collections of blatantly atypical cells with high nuclear-to-cytoplasmic ratios, prominent nucleoli, and vesicular chromatin, and these elements are strongly reactive for CD45 (the leukocyte common antigen) (118–120). Hence, that disorder is more properly called "intravascular lymphomatosis" (IVL), and is undeniably a variant of non-Hodgkin's lymphoma. On the other hand, "reactive angioendotheliomatosis" (RAE) (121–124) features the proliferation of only modestly atypical and enlarged endothelial cells in blood vessels of the dermis (Figs. 42–44). These are regularly accompanied by perivascular pericytic proliferations as

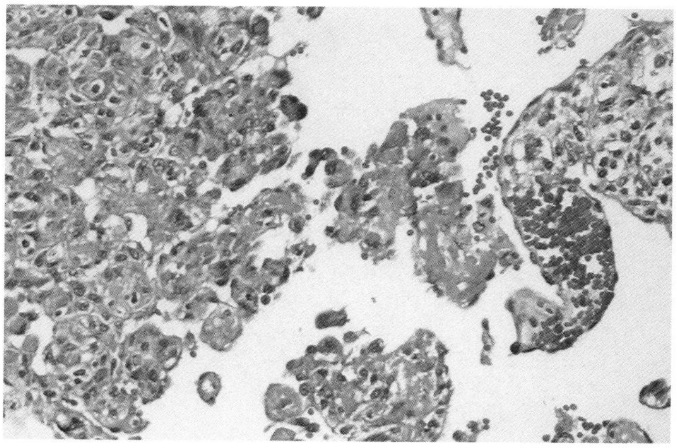

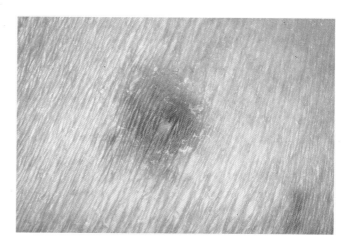

**FIG. 41.** Reactive angioendotheliomatosis. The clinical appearance is that of a red, poorly marginated papule with peripheral scaling.

**FIG. 40.** Intravascular papillary endothelial hyperplasia. The papillary arrangements are lined with enlarged, but not pleomorphic, endothelial cells. This reactive neovascularization has also been termed "Masson's pseudoangiosarcoma."

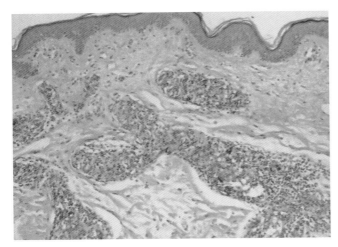

FIG. 42. Reactive angioendotheliomatosis. There are expanded blood vessels in the dermis.

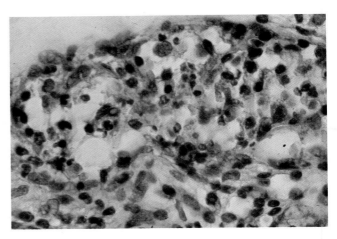

FIG. 44. Reactive angioendotheliomatosis. Modest cytologic atypia and nuclear enlargement of the reactive, proliferating endothelial cells.

well, yielding a "glomeruloid" appearance to the affected vessels (120), whereas that attribute is not part of the spectrum of IVL. Both conditions may show the presence of intravascular microthrombi in dermal blood vessels. However, these are thought to possibly represent an *inciting etiologic factor* in RAE (125) (possibly associated with cryoglobulinemia or vasculitis), whereas thrombosis is probably a secondary event in IVL (120). In concordance with these premises, it would be expected that RAE should usually be a self-limited or, at least, chronic process, whereas IVL should have the behavior of a full-blown malignancy. These predictions have, in fact, been validated.

Although we believe that the dissimilar degree of cellular atypia in IVL and RAE allows for their diagnostic separation, as does the presence of pericytic proliferations in the latter disease, some observers prefer to confirm the divergent lineages of the intravascular cells in these two conditions with adjunctive studies. As stated above, the proliferating

cells of IVL are seen to be CD45+ by immunohistochemistry (118,119), whereas those of RAE are not. Conversely, immunostains for blood group isoantigens, factor VIII–related antigen, and CD31 confirm the endothelial identity of the constituent cells in RAE (120) (Fig. 45).

### Angiokeratoma

Angiokeratomas are commonly confused with true hemangiomas of the skin, both clinically and pathologically. However, as summarized by Cooper (126), these lesions are thought to represent reactive (possibly posttraumatic) telan-

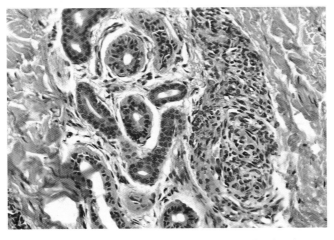

FIG. 43. Reactive angioendotheliomatosis. Whorls of reactive endothelial cells may suggest a vaguely "glomeruloid" structure.

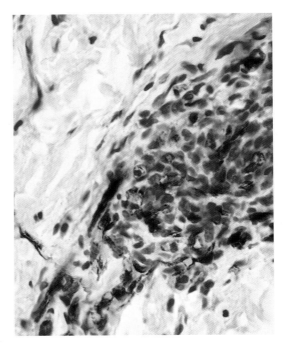

FIG. 45. Reactive angioendotheliomatosis. Immunoreactivity for blood group isoantigens is characteristic.

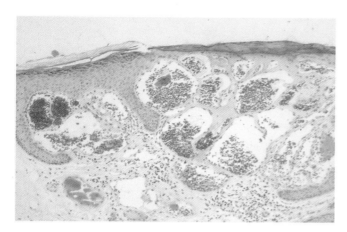

**FIG. 46.** Angiokeratoma. Ectatic vascular channels in the superficial dermis are the hallmark of this disorder.

giectasias rather than neoplasms. There are two forms of these papular reddish lesions—peripheral and central—with the latter affecting the truncal (particularly genital) skin and being potentially associated with Fabry's disease (127,128).

Histologically, angiokeratomas feature the presence of greatly dilated vascular spaces in the upper dermis, filled with erythrocytes (Fig. 46). The overlying epidermis appears to enclose such "blood lakes" completely, but it is separated from them by a narrow zone of collagenous matrix (Fig. 47). Endothelial cells in angiokeratomas are flattened and inconspicuous, and papillary proliferation is never observed. In a minority of cases, dilated blood vessels are also present in the subjacent dermis.

### Bacillary Angiomatosis

"Bacillary angiomatosis" (BA) is a generic term that is used to describe pseudoneoplastic endothelial proliferations, which are generally caused by infections with various rickettsial and bacterial microorganisms. The most well-known

of these are selected *Rochalimaea* species (*henselae, quintana*) and *Bartonella bacilliformis*, although some *Afipia* species (e.g., *A. felis*) also have been implicated (127–138). The clinical disorders that may be associated with such agents are represented by immunosuppression-related bacillary angiomatosis and bacillary peliosis, verruga peruana of Carrion's disease (bartonellosis), and cat-scratch disease (135,137). All of these conditions might feature the presence of lesions that could be confused with those of KS pathologically (Fig. 48). The common thread accounting for this peculiarity is the propensity for all of the specified organisms to infect endothelial cells and to stimulate their subsequent growth and proliferation (139).

On histologic grounds, the attributes of BA lesions that might foster confusion with KS include a potential for densely cellular growth with mitotic figures and nuclear atypia (132,133,136,138). However, as outlined by Adal et al. (128), there are more microscopic differences than similarities between these two groups of lesions. Cutaneous BA [including both immunosuppression-related forms and verruga peruana (137,138)] is usually sharply demarcated from the surrounding dermis; it shows a lobulated architectural pattern on low-power microscopy (Fig. 49); constituent endothelial cells are plump [accounting for the alternative designation of "epithelioid angiomatosis" (133)] (Fig. 50), and may contain visible clumps of purplish granular material, which represents microorganisms (which are verifiable with silver impregnation stains such as the Steiner method) (Fig. 51); there are no hyaline globular inclusions; and intralesional neutrophilia (Fig. 52) is common even in the absence of surface ulceration. None of these features is expected in the usual case of KS, regardless of tumoral subtype (93,100).

### Other Pseudoneoplastic Reactions to Infection

In addition to vasogenic proliferations, other pseudoneoplastic mesenchymal lesions of the skin may be associated with infectious diseases. The two that are most well charac-

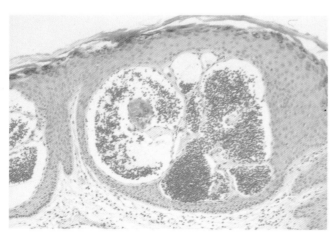

**FIG. 47.** Angiokeratoma. The epidermis may partially or completely encircle the dilated vessels.

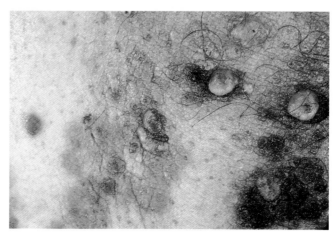

**FIG. 48.** Bacillary angiomatosis. Tan to black nodules and plaques are evident.

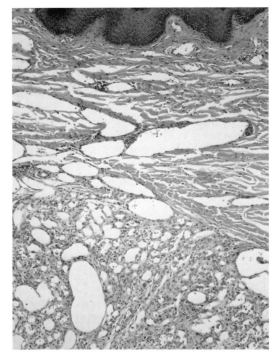

**FIG. 49.** Bacillary angiomatosis. In contrast to Kaposi's sarcoma, bacillary angiomatosis exhibits a well-circumscribed or lobular growth pattern, more akin to that of pyogenic granuloma.

terized are "histoid" leprosy and nonlepromatous mycobacterial spindle cell pseudotumors.

### "Histoid" Leprosy

In 1963, Wade (140) reported a peculiar variant of lepromatous leprosy in which nodular dermal or subcutaneous lesions were represented histologically by circumscribed proliferations of spindle cells and polygonal cells, arranged in

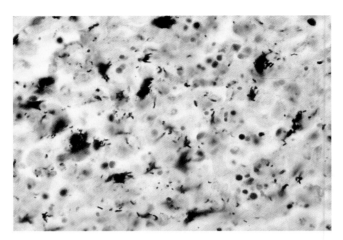

**FIG. 51.** Identification of bacteria in bacillary angiomatosis by the Warthin–Starry method.

fascicular or storiform arrays. Patients of both genders and over a wide range of ages were affected. The typically vacuolated "lepra" or "Virchow" cells of lepromatous disease were lacking, but acid-fast stains nonetheless demonstrated a large number of mycobacteria in the constituent cellular elements. Because this lesional subtype simulated the appearance of a "fibrohistiocytic" neoplasm, the term chosen to describe it was "histoid." We have recently documented another example of this proliferation that demonstrated an unusual degree of permeation of dermal nerves, blood vessels, and appendages by the spindle cells (Figs. 53–55), which showed a "histiocytic" phenotype immunohistologically (141). Hence, microscopic simulation of a neoplasm was striking. The patient in question was not immunocompromised, as is true of many individuals with histoid leprosy in published series on that disease (142).

The mechanisms underlying the peculiar proliferative cellular response to infection with *Mycobacterium leprae* are as yet uncharacterized in histoid leprosy (143–145). Although it is largely restricted to areas of the world that are endemic

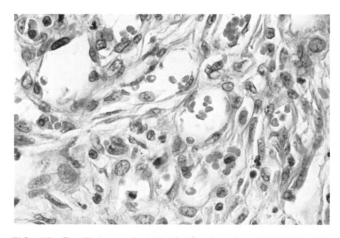

**FIG. 50.** Bacillary angiomatosis. Lesional endothelial cells have enlarged and rounded ("epithelioid") nuclei.

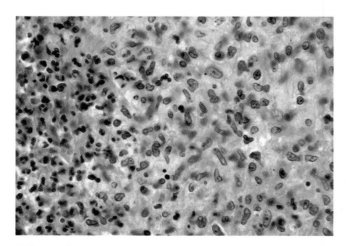

**FIG. 52.** Bacillary angiomatosis with a neutrophilic cell response to the infection.

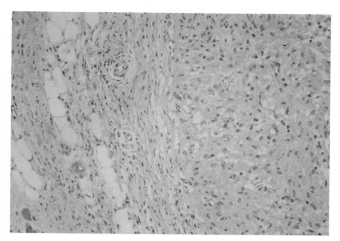

**FIG. 53.** Histoid leprosy. Pseudoneoplastic nodule formation is created by the lesional histiocytes.

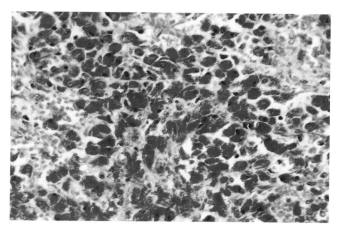

**FIG. 55.** Numerous acid-fast bacilli are present in the histiocytes of histoid leprosy.

for that organism, pathologists everywhere must be aware of this disease variant in light of current international travel patterns. Mistaken diagnoses of fibrohistiocytic neoplasia are tragic in cases of histoid leprosy because they deprive the patient of potentially curative therapy with sulfone-type antibiotics (144).

### Nonlepromatous Mycobacterial Pseudotumors of the Skin

Wood et al. (146) first described a case of "atypical" cutaneous mycobacteriosis (infection with *Mycobacterium avium-intracellulare*) that simulated the clinicopathologic profile of histoid leprosy in an immunocompromised individual who had received a cardiac transplant. Since that time, additional examples of this phenomenon have been documented in other patients with dysfunctional immunity, most notably in the context of AIDS (147). Infection-related pseudotumors may be encountered not only in the skin but

also in the lymph nodes and viscera (148–151).

Histologically, nonlepromatous mycobacterial pseudotumors (NLMP) are virtually identical to the profile presented above, in reference to histoid leprosy. Fascicles of plump spindle cells—often with hyperchromatic nuclei and nucleoli, and abundant foamy or granular cytoplasm—are admixed with polygonal cells resembling histiocytes, as well as a modest number of lymphocytes and neutrophils (146,149) (Figs. 56 and 57). Mitotic activity is often brisk, but atypical division figures are not observed. The proliferation may assume a permeative character in the dermis and subcutis, or, alternatively, it may be sharply demarcated by a fibrous pseudocapsule. Histochemical stains for acid-fast bacilli (in

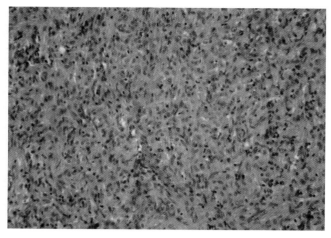

**FIG. 54.** Histoid leprosy simulating a fibrohistiocytic neoplasm.

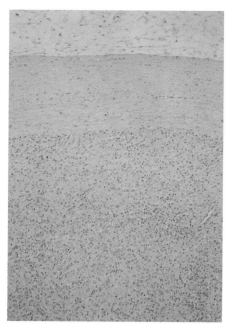

**FIG. 56.** Mycobacterial pseudotumor. Spindled and epithelioid cells may prompt a differential diagnostic consideration of dermatofibroma.

**FIG. 57.** Mycobacterial pseudotumor. Focal microabscesses constitute a diagnostic clue for consideration of the possibility of infection.

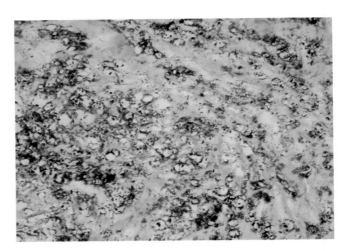

**FIG. 59.** Silver impregnation histochemical stains, such as the Steiner stain shown here, may also be utilized to highlight the microorganisms in mycobacterial pseudotumor.

particular, the Fite method) and silver impregnation techniques show that the fusiform cells of NLMP are teeming with masses of mycobacteria (Figs. 58 and 59). On touch-imprint preparations of the lesions that are stained with Romanowsky's methods, these microorganisms may appear as "negative images" in the cytoplasm.

The differential diagnosis of these proliferations includes fibrohistiocytic neoplasms such as dermatofibroma, "atypical fibrous histiocytoma," dermatofibrosarcoma protuberans, and xanthogranuloma. The peculiar granular nature of the cytoplasm in the cells of NLMP distinguishes it from these other tumors; obviously, the presence of microorganisms on special stains does so as well.

### Hamartomatous Mesenchymal Lesions of the Skin

Several forms of hamartomatous growth in the skin are capable of imitating other lesions. While acknowledging the fact that the entire concept of hamartomas (as developmen-

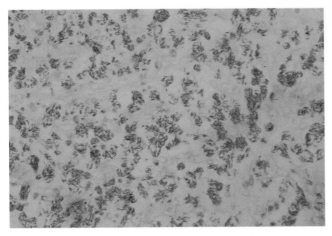

**FIG. 58.** Acid-fast bacilli in mycobacterial pseudotumor, non-lepromatous type, as demonstrated by Fite stain.

tal anomalies that are distinct from autonomously-replicating neoplasms) is still not universally accepted, we discuss five cutaneous proliferations in this general category.

#### *Fibrous Hamartoma of Infancy*

Fibrous hamartomas are confined to infancy and childhood, where they show a predilection for males. These lesions present as nodules in the dermis or subcutis that are relatively rapidly enlarging and that may attain a size of several centimeters (152–156). Preferred sites of origin are the upper trunk and proximal arms, but many other topographic locations for fibrous hamartoma, including the hands and feet, have been documented as well. Multiplicity is not a feature of this lesion, and simple excision constitutes adequate treatment.

At a microscopic level, fibrous hamartoma has permeative peripheral borders, and it is tripartite in constituency. Bands of cellular fibrous tissue—composed of bland but mitotically active myofibroblastic elements—are interspersed with myxoid zones containing nondescript stellate cells, as well as areas of fetal or mature adipose tissue (152,153) (Figs. 60 and 61). These are arranged haphazardly, and vary in proportion from case to case. Thus, a resemblance to lipomas, lipoblastomas, myofibromatoses, and even fibrosarcomas is possible in selected cases (6,152). Nevertheless, the distinction between these entities can be made by attention to the specific threefold composition of fibrous hamartoma, which is not shared by the diagnostic alternatives just cited.

#### *Smooth Muscle Hamartomas and "Becker's Nevi"*

Smooth muscle hamartomas (SMHs) of the skin may either be congenital or acquired in early life (158–162), and in all likelihood they also form part of the spectrum of

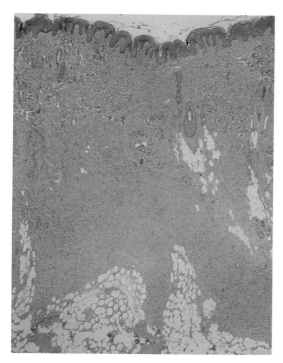

**FIG. 60.** Fibrous hamartoma of infancy. The three components include fibrocollagenous tissue, myxoid zones, and regions of adipose tissue.

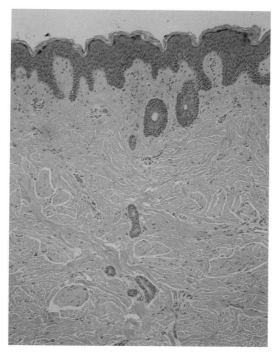

**FIG. 62.** Smooth muscle hamartoma. In contrast to cutaneous leiomyoma, which is often a well-delineated nodule of smooth muscle, smooth muscle hamartomas show a disorganized arrangement of smooth muscle bundles, with collagenous separation.

"Becker's nevi" (165–167). These lesions are solitary and arise most often on the trunk or the extremities, where they take the form of lightly pigmented patches or plaques measuring up to several centimeters in greatest dimension. Hypertrichosis in or around SMHs is a commonly associated finding. Slight rubbing may produce "pseudo-Darier's sign" in that temporary elevation ("pseudourtication") of the lesion occurs, but SMHs are not painful (158,163). Simple excision is curative, but usually no therapeutic intervention is needed unless the patient desires improved cosmesis.

Microscopic examination of SMHs shows abnormal bundles of smooth muscle in the reticular dermis and even in the hypodermis, configured in haphazardly arranged or widely separated fascicles (Figs. 62 and 63). These often have an attachment to adjacent *arrector pilorum* muscles and are immunoreactive for desmin and several actin isoforms (Fig. 64). In "pure" myogenous hamartomas, there are no associated abnormalities in the overlying epidermis. However, Slifman et al. (161) have shown that some examples of Becker's nevi—in which surface acanthosis, papillomatosis, hypertrichosis, and hyperpigmentation are expected—do indeed show deep myogenic proliferations that are indistinguishable from those of SMHs.

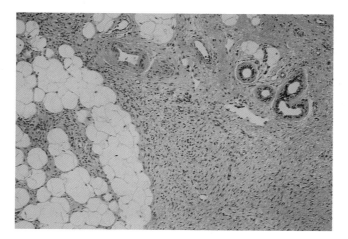

**FIG. 61.** Fibrous hamartoma of infancy. Elongated and stellate myofibroblastic cells populate the myxoid zones.

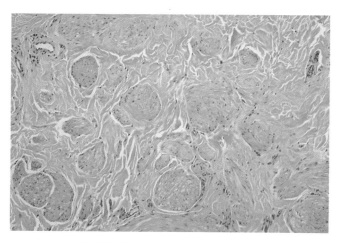

**FIG. 63.** Smooth muscle hamartoma.

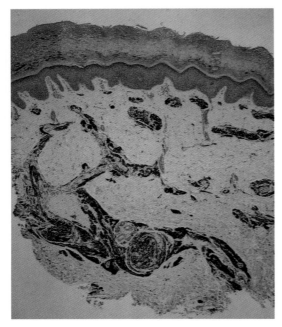

**FIG. 64.** Desmin immunoreactivity in a smooth muscle hamartoma.

First, differential diagnosis between SMHs and leiomyoma cutis or cutaneous leiomyosarcoma depends on a correlation between clinical data and histologic findings (168,169). True myogenous neoplasms of the skin are exceedingly rare in children, whereas SMHs are typically found in pediatric patients. Second, smooth muscle tumors usually have a relatively sharp microscopic interface with surrounding connective tissue, whereas SMHs show a "ragged" peripheral margin and features more disorganized fascicular growth. Mitotic activity, nuclear atypia, and spontaneous necrosis are not features of SMHs, but one or several of those findings are expected in cutaneous leiomyosarcomas. Lastly, true myogenous neoplasms are not associated with the specified abnormalities of the epidermis that are seen in examples of SMHs.

### Neurovascular Hamartomas of the Skin

Perez-Atayde et al. (170) recently described an unusual congenital dermal mesenchymal lesion in two children who had concomitant neoplasms of the kidney and soft tissue with the features of "malignant rhabdoid tumor." The cutaneous abnormalities were represented by reddish plaques on the trunk with irregular surfaces and borders, and "satellite" papules around them.

Microscopic examination of the lesions showed epidermal papillomatosis, increased capillary-sized blood vessels in the dermis, and an intervascular proliferation of bland spindle cells that tended to be arranged in fascicles. Immunostains for S-100 protein were positive in the latter cellular elements, suggesting that they were Schwannian in nature. Because of the presence of these cutaneous abnormalities at birth and the particular histologic profiles, Perez-Atayde and colleagues suggested that the abnormalities were malformative rather than neoplastic (170). These "neurovascular hamartomas" are thought to be markers of risk for the development of rhabdoid tumors. In that regard, it is of interest that the soft tissue neoplasm in case 2 of the cited paper appeared to arise directly from the base of the cutaneous lesion. Both of the affected infants died of their malignancies.

If one focuses on isolated components of its histologic image, the cutaneous neurovascular hamartoma could be confused with epidermal nevi, hemangiomas, or neurofibromas. However, when considered together in aggregate, the features of this unusual "marker" lesion of the skin appear to be diagnostically distinctive.

### "Pleomorphic" (Possibly Neuromuscular) Hamartoma of the Skin

Shitabata et al. (171) reported a nodular, flesh-colored lesion of the subcutis in an adult male. It had been present for some time, was slowly enlarging, and had attained a size of 5 cm, but produced no other complaints. There were likewise no other abnormal clinical findings.

Microscopic examination of the excised mass showed a sharply circumscribed subcutaneous spindle cell proliferation with abundantly collagenized stroma (Fig. 65). Narrow fascicles of plump spindle cells—some of which had "ser-

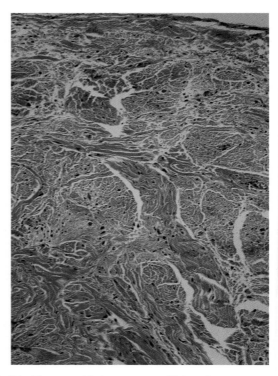

**FIG. 65.** Pleomorphic hamartoma. This subcutaneous mass was remarkable for a spindle cell proliferation with a densely collagenized stromal background.

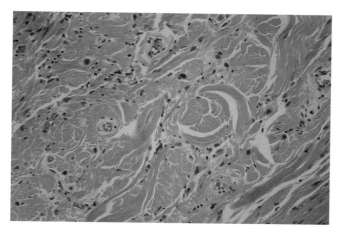

**FIG. 66.** Pleomorphic hamartoma.

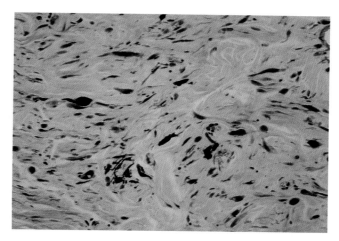

**FIG. 68.** S-100 protein was identified in the pleomorphic hamartoma by immunohistochemical means.

piginous" nuclear contours—were interposed between the collagen bundles, as were randomly scattered floret-type multinucleated giant cells and aggregates of mature adipocytes (Figs. 66 and 67). There was no nuclear atypia, mitotic activity, or necrosis. The overall appearance of the lesion incorporated features of "pleomorphic fibroma" (172), "pleomorphic lipoma" (173), and neurofibroma. Immunohistologic evaluation likewise showed a hybrid immunophenotype; the spindle cells of the mass were concurrently reactive for vimentin, S-100 protein, CD57, myelin basic protein, and desmin (Figs. 68 and 69). Based on these results, the authors concluded that the lesion was best considered a neuromuscular hamartoma, and posited that it perhaps represented a superficial counterpart of the so-called deep neuromuscular hamartoma or "benign triton tumor" (174).

### Rhabdomyomatous Mesenchymal Hamartomas

Rhabdomyomatous mesenchymal hamartomas are polypoid lesions that appear to be confined to the facial skin of infants. Only a few examples have been reported, as pedunculated, soft, flesh-colored excrescences measuring no more than a few centimeters in greatest dimension (175–177).

Histologically, rhabdomyomatous mesenchymal hamartoma demonstrates the haphazard disposition of variably sized fascicles or single fibers of mature striated muscle throughout, and otherwise unremarkable dermis and superficial subcutis. The muscular bands mold themselves to cutaneous adnexae and may be associated with nerve branches. A polypoid lesional configuration is reproducibly seen in these cases. The bases of the excrescences are narrower than their distal aspects, yielding a club-shaped image. Immunostains confirm the presence of striated muscle cells, with reactivity for desmin, muscle-specific actin, and myoglobin.

Diagnostic misinterpretation of this malformative lesion of the skin as a rhabdomyoma is obviated by attention to its diffuse, disorganized growth pattern, contrasting with the cohesive and discrete nature of true but benign striated muscle neoplasms (178,179). Rhabdomyosarcomas conversely show a primitive level of differentiation and are predomi-

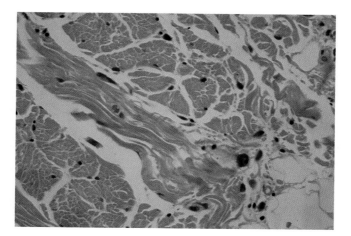

**FIG. 67.** Pleomorphic hamartoma with focal mature adipose tissue.

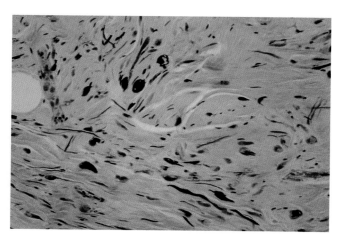

**FIG. 69.** The immunophenotype of subcutaneous pleomorphic hamartoma includes desmin reactivity.

nantly composed of small round or modestly pleomorphic cells (6).

### Idiosyncratic Proliferative Mesenchymal Reactions to Injury

Selected cutaneous lesions that are related to injury have already been considered above, including some vascular proliferations and pseudoepitheliomatous hyperplasia. Additional conditions that may be placed in this pathogenetic category are nodular fasciitis and "postoperative spindle cell nodule," as discussed below.

### Nodular (Proliferative; Pseudosarcomatous; Infiltrative) Fasciitis

Despite the fact that nodular fasciitis (NF) was first described as a clinicopathologic entity 40 years ago (180), it is still underrecognized by some pathologists. This disorder is thought to represent an idiosyncratic mesenchymal "overreaction" to an injury (which is many times slight and unnoticed by the patient), and it is therefore most often observed in skin areas that are likely to be traumatized. These principally include the surfaces of the upper extremities; however, NF has been described in virtually every topographic location (180–188). There is no gender predilection, but patients under the age of 50 years are preferentially affected. The lesions manifest as rapidly growing nodules—which are sometimes tender—that typically have been present for less than 1 month. They are located in the deep dermis and subcutis, commonly with attachment to subjacent fascial planes or aponeuroses, and range in size from 1 to 4 cm (181,182). Simple excision is curative, but if the diagnosis is established by nonexcisional biopsies [such as fine needle aspiration (189)], simple "benign neglect" shows that spontaneous resolution of the lesions often eventuates. As Enzinger and Weiss (190) have indicated, the recurrence of a mass thought to represent NF should prompt its diagnostic reassessment, with an alternative interpretation of a true neoplasm being likely.

The microscopic characteristics of NF are distinctive (181–183). They feature the loose apposition of haphazardly arranged, large, proliferating, fusiform, and stellate myofibroblasts producing the so-called tissue culture appearance. These cells have an open nuclear chromatin pattern and discernible nucleoli (Figs. 70 and 71). Because of the latter attributes, some cells in NF are said to be "ganglionoid," and others may resemble multinucleated osteoclast-like elements. Mitotic activity is abundant (Fig. 72), but pathologic division figures are never seen. Cytoplasm is abundant and amphophilic. The stroma of NF is characteristically myxedematous, with numerous capillary-sized blood vessels surrounded at least focally by extravasated erythrocytes (Fig. 73). At the center of the lesions, it is common to see zones of denser cellularity with a more fibrous matrix; indeed, the lat-

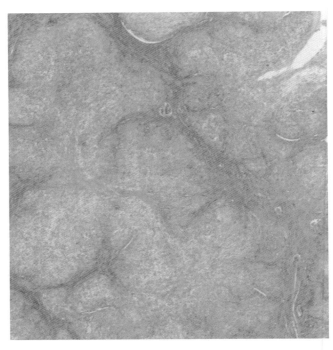

**FIG. 70.** Nodular fasciitis. Cases of this reparative process have been misdiagnosed as sarcomas.

ter may assume a keloidal character in some examples. The peripheral aspects of NF show an irregular, permeative interface with adjacent connective tissue. One variant of NF with particular pertinence to dermatopathology is a type in which a proliferation with the features just cited is seen in an exclusively intravascular location (184). Usually a large vein is affected.

The differential diagnosis of NF usually centers on a form of fibromatosis or a fibrohistiocytic neoplasm [e.g., myxoid malignant fibrous histiocytoma or dermatofibrosarcoma pro-

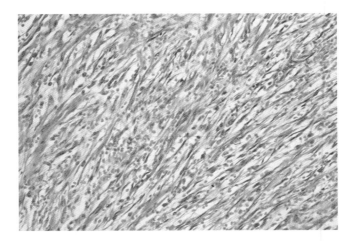

**FIG. 71.** Nodular fasciitis is characterized by a spindle cell proliferation with a myxoid stromal background. This image has been likened to a tissue culture-like appearance.

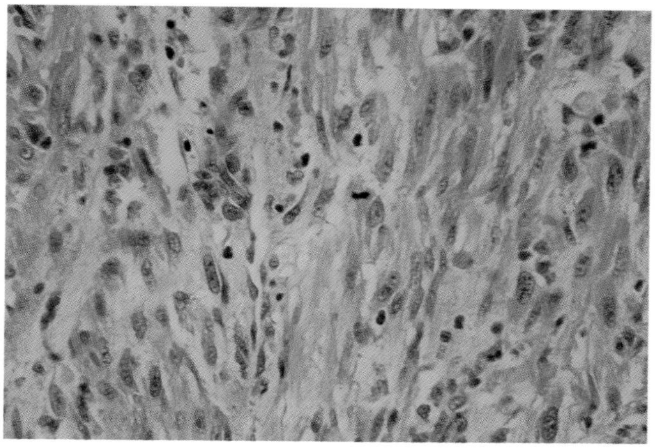

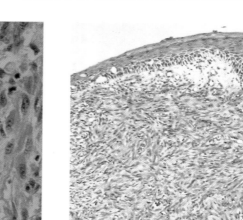

**FIG. 72.** Mitotic figures might be numerous in nodular fasciitis but atypical mitoses are not present.

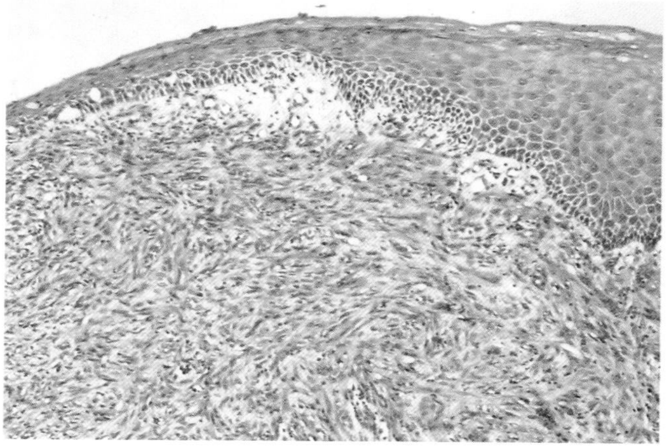

**FIG. 74.** Cutaneous postoperative spindle cell nodule with a hypercellular, dermal, spindle cell proliferation.

tuberans (191)]. Indeed, a distinction between these conditions might be nearly impossible in some cases if NF is sampled in the late stages of its evolution. Under other circumstances, the observation of spontaneous necrosis, pathologic mitoses, significant nuclear atypia, or areas of extremely dense cellularity should direct diagnostic opinion away from fasciitis.

### Postoperative Spindle Cell Nodules

Another reactive mesenchymal lesion that is probably closely related to NF on mechanistic grounds is known as "postoperative spindle cell nodule" (PSCN) (192). This condition was first described in the genitourinary tract, following such procedures as transurethral bladder biopsy or prostatic resection (192–194) (see chapter on urinary tract), but we have also seen two histologically identical cases in mucocutaneous locations. One case concerned an adult woman who had previously had a punch biopsy of the vulva done for

the diagnosis of extramammary Paget's disease (Figs. 74 and 75), and the other involved a young man who had an abdominal cutaneous nodule develop adjacent to a colostomy stoma (Figs. 76 and 77). In general, affected patients may be of either gender and any age. In analogy to our earlier discussion of reactions to Monsel's solution, the typical clinical presentation of PSCN is that of a rapidly enlarging nodule at the site of a prior surgical procedure. If this history is provided, the recognition of this entity is uncomplicated. However, it may prove to be a diagnostic trap for the pathologist if no accessory clinical information is received.

The microscopic appearance of PSCN shares many points of similarity with NF in that it features a zonal proliferation of large, mitotically active myofibroblastic cells set in a myxedematous stroma that contains extravascular red blood cells (194) (see Figs. 74–77). Nonetheless, cellularity tends to be more dense in PSCN than in NF; also, there is a more fascicular growth pattern and stromal blood vessels are less

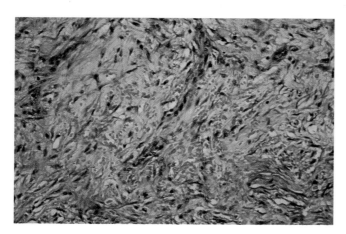

**FIG. 73.** Neovascularity and extravasated red blood cells might be conspicuous findings in nodular fasciitis.

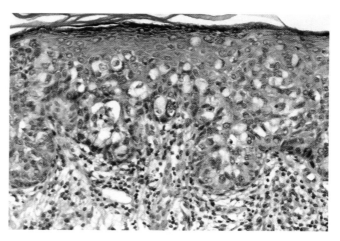

**FIG. 75.** A previous punch biopsy of the extramammary (vulvar) Paget's disease, shown here, resulted in the postoperative spindle cell nodule formation.

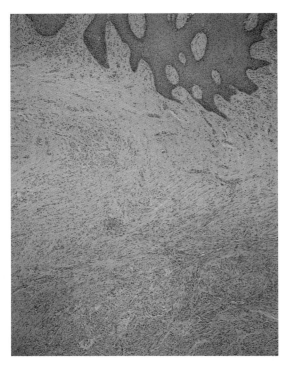

**FIG. 76.** Postoperative spindle cell nodule of the skin. A mass developed adjacent to a colostomy stroma.

conspicuous. Modest nuclear atypia may also be apparent. Unlike NF, the proliferating elements in PSCN have the unexplained and maddening ability to express keratin "aberrantly" (195), potentially causing immunohistologic confusion with a sarcomatoid carcinoma. Nevertheless, concurrent diffuse immunoreactivity for desmin and actin should cause one to reconsider the latter interpretation in favor of PSCN (194,195). Other differential diagnostic possibilities are as outlined above in connection with NF. However, it should be emphasized that the separation between a

true sarcoma and PSCN is often difficult and is therefore critically dependent on accurate and complete clinical information.

## PSEUDONEOPLASTIC NEUROCUTANEOUS RESTS AND ECTOPIAS

Rarely, tissue "rests" or ectopic elements from the developing nervous system may be entrapped in the skin and may proliferate over time. As such, they sometimes simulate the microscopic appearances of selected neoplastic entities.

### Rudimentary Meningocele (Primary Cutaneous Meningioma; Meningotheliomatous Hamartoma)

In 1974, Lopez et al. reviewed the clinicopathologic attributes of several apparently meningothelial cutaneous lesions, and adopted the term "acoelic meningeal hamartoma" to describe them (196). This rubric implies that the masses in question had no connection to the central nervous system or its coverings, and it also indicates that they were thought to be nonneoplastic. The latter issues were reviewed by Sibley and Cooper (197) in 1989, yielding the similar interpretation that a subset of cutaneous meningothelial lesions probably represented developmental malformations. These were called "rudimentary meningoceles" (RMs), signifying the premise that they were formed by nonneoplastic rests of the meninges that had become entrapped in the integument early

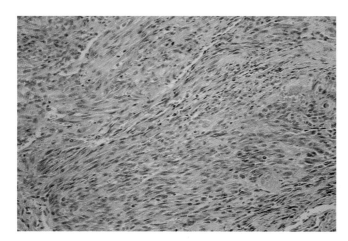

**FIG. 77.** The postoperative spindle cell nodule is more cellular than nodular fasciitis, with a more organized arrangement of the spindle cells, which may resemble fascicles.

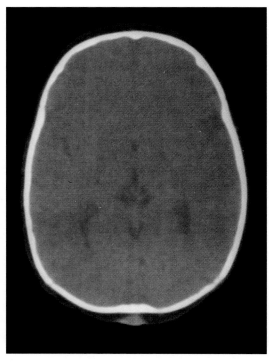

**FIG. 78.** Rudimentary meningocele. Computerized tomogram of skull showing soft tissue mass adjacent to skull (arrow).

in life. This same interpretation was espoused by Suster and Rosai (198), except that the alternative term "meningotheliomatous hamartoma" was chosen for the lesion under discussion.

Whichever of these designations is preferred to describe them, RMs show reproducible clinical features. Unlike true meningoceles, which are typically noted in the neonatal period and which show radiographic evidence of continuity with the cerebral investments, RMs manifest later in childhood; although there may be subjacent defects in cranial suture lines (Fig. 78), no underlying nervous system abnormalities are evident (197—200). These same features distinguish RMs from secondary cutaneous meningiomas. The latter are typically seen in the frontal or superior scalp in middle-aged or elderly patients, and the lesions derive from direct cutaneous extension by true neoplasms of the meninges (196,197).

RMs are characteristically seen in the posterior scalp as asymptomatic, nondescript, flesh-colored nodules that measure up to 3 cm. Simple excision of such masses is curative (200).

The microscopic appearance of RMs is potentially deceptive. It features the deep dermal and subcuticular proliferation of polygonal cells with oval nuclei, dispersed chromatin, and a moderate amount of amphophilic cytoplasm, arranged in a dyscohesive, "dissecting," permeative pattern in the supporting connective tissue (Figs. 79–81). Like meningothelial

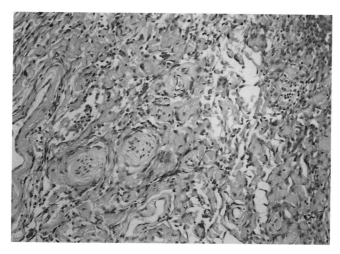

**FIG. 80.** Rudimentary meningocele. The cleft-like spaces associated with the meningothelial cell proliferation can, at this magnification, be easily misinterpreted as a malignant vascular neoplasm.

cells in general, the proliferating elements of RMs are immunoreactive for EMA (Fig. 82) and vimentin (197–199).

The intercellular spaces that are formed in RMs and the overall image that is produced are reminiscent of the features of angiosarcomas or, at least, atypical hemangiomas (198). Nevertheless, there are no erythrocytes in the first-named of these lesions, and serial sections may demonstrate the presence of small psammomatoid calcifications. The latter findings are not expected in vascular tumors, as is also true of EMA immunoreactivity. Another differential diagnostic consideration is the neoplasm known as "giant cell fibroblastoma" (201), which similarly features the presence of intratumoral angiectid channels. However, that lesion is found preferentially on the extremities of adolescents; it has a second constituent growth pattern composed of a more solid fibroblastic proliferation, and is EMA-negative as well (199).

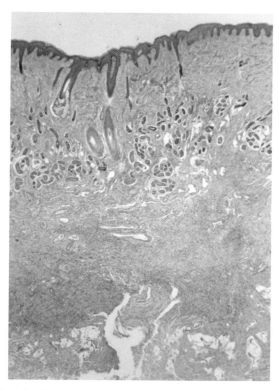

**FIG. 79.** Rudimentary meningocele type of cutaneous "meningioma." A meningotheliomatous proliferation is found in the deep dermis and subcutis.

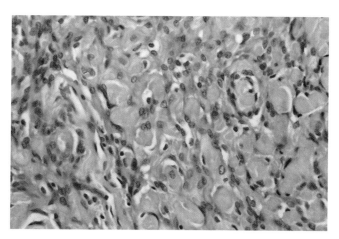

**FIG. 81.** Rudimentary meningocele. The polygonal meningothelial cells are cytologically bland and are disposed as strands and clusters in a collagenous stroma.

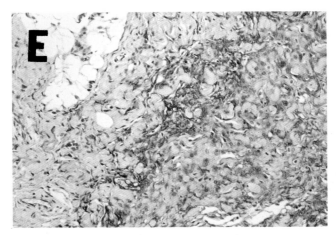

**FIG. 82.** The meningothelial cells of the rudimentary meningocele bind antibodies reactive against epithelial membrane antigen.

### Cutaneous Glial Heterotopia ("Nasal Glioma")

Another malformation that is pathogenetically similar to RMs is the cutaneous glial heterotopia (CGH), also known inaccurately as "nasal glioma" (202–207). This lesion is seen in children; in its pure form, it represents the growth of cerebral matter that has become completely detached from the subjacent brain during development. Other clinically similar masses are instead accompanied by patent subjacent meningeal tracts through the skull that are definable radio-

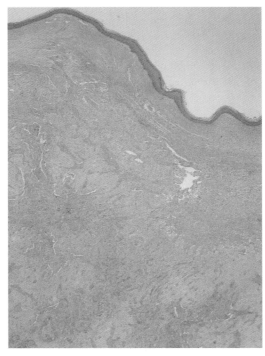

**FIG. 83.** Nasal glioma. This nodule of heterotopic glial tissue has replaced normal dermal structures.

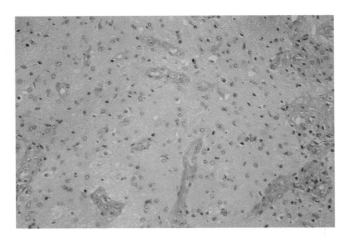

**FIG. 84.** Nasal glioma. Glial cells are enmeshed within a neurofibrillary background.

graphically; these should be regarded technically as encephaloceles rather than heterotopias (207). Because gross examination is incapable of distinguishing CGH from an encephalocele, and casual excision of the latter lesion carries a major risk of iatrogenic meningitis, all patients with these abnormalities should be given a thorough neuroradiologic evaluation (208).

Both CGH and encephaloceles characteristically present in the skin of the nasal bridge as single, asymptomatic, firm, pink/tan/violaceous nodules. Extension of the masses into the nasal cavity is also seen in a minority of cases. Aside from the caveat stated above, there are no associated neural defects in these patients (202–204,207).

The microscopic attributes of CGH are responsible for its having been assigned the erroneous designation "glioma." A proliferation of astrocytes—with or without a minor population of oligodendroglia or the formation of "Rosenthal fibers"—is observed histologically, with compartmentalization by delicate fibrovascular stroma (Figs. 83 and 84).

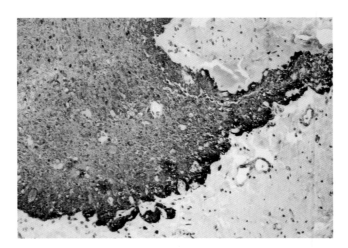

**FIG. 85.** Immunoreactive glial fibrillary acidic protein in the nasal glioma.

There is a fibrillary background neuropil, and scattered ganglion cells are apparent in a minority of cases. No "secondary" features of true gliomas, such as perivascular hypercellularity or submeningeal astrocytic proliferation, are evident in CGH. Mitoses and necrosis are also uniformly absent (203–207).

If a demonstration of the nonneoplastic nature of CGH is desired, the proliferating glial cells can be labeled for glial fibrillary acidic protein immunohistologically (Fig. 85), and the matrical neuropil is reactive for neurofilament protein. Ganglion cells are recognizable by stains for synaptophysin. These conjoint observations are incompatible with the diagnosis of a true glioma (206).

## PSEUDONEOPLASTIC LYMPHORETICULAR INFILTRATES OF THE SKIN

There are few other lesions in dermatopathology that are as anxiety-provoking as cutaneous lymphoreticular infiltrates. Indeed, the complexity of this topical area is so great that entire textbooks have been devoted specifically to it (209). In the following sections, we summarize the most salient points regarding the diagnostic separation of pseudoneoplastic (benign) and neoplastic (malignant) diseases in this broad category.

### Pseudoneoplastic Lymphoreticular Infiltrates: General Considerations

The general features of cutaneous "pseudolymphomas" have been artfully summarized by Rijlaarsdam and Willemze (210). As defined by those authors, these disorders are recognized by procurement of cutaneous biopsy findings that suggest a malignant lymphoid infiltrate in the absence of other evidence for such an interpretation. The most convincing clinical data that might be used in the latter context include an identification of a specific etiology for the cutaneous lesions in question or spontaneous resolution of the condition in the absence of any therapy. Unfortunately, the application of such precepts can best be done in a retrospective manner, making the task of the pathologist in this setting a difficult one indeed.

Broadly speaking, there are few if any clinical findings that can be used with certainty to distinguish many true lymphomas of the skin from their microscopic simulators. In specific reference to cutaneous T-cell lymphoma (CTCL), many other conditions are capable of mimicking its various macroscopic presentations, which potentially include multifocal erythematous patches, plaques, and nodules; diffuse erythroderma; verrucous lesions; pustules; bullae; alopecia; acanthosis nigricans–like lesions; hypopigmented foci; and pigmented purpura-like eruptions (210,211). With regard to other cutaneous lymphoreticular malignancies, it is likewise extremely challenging on clinical grounds to separate the lesions of "benign lymphocytic infiltrates" or other various

clinical "pseudolymphomas" from true lymphomas, regardless of their particular cellular lineages. Hence, the degree of reliance placed by dermatologists on the interpretation of skin biopsies in these contexts is great.

### Nonneoplastic Conditions Producing "Lichenoid" Infiltrates Capable of Simulating CTCL

The two major forms of CTCL—mycosis fungoides and Sezary's syndrome—are initially manifested by erythroderma or the development of multiple eczematoid scaly patches that are often pruritic (Fig. 86). As such, these conditions closely mirror the clinical findings seen in a panoply of chronic spongiotic dermatitides (211).

This same capacity for imitation pertains to the histologic findings that are observed in such disorders as well. Both early CTCL and various pseudo-CTCLs may exhibit a band-like (lichenoid) upper dermal infiltrate of lymphocytes with indeterminate degrees of nuclear atypia and irregularity, as well as limited permeation of the epidermis by the same cells with little or no associated spongiosis (Figs. 87–89) and "basket-weave" hyalinosis of the papillary dermal collagen (212). Parakeratosis and acanthosis may likewise be present indiscriminately, and eosinophils may be found in the cellular infiltrate. As such, this microscopic profile lacks the intraepidermal collections of obviously atypical lymphoid cells (so-called Pautrier's microabscesses) that typify CTCL in classical form (210,214), but conversely it does not allow for the elimination of lymphoma as a possible diagnosis. Clinicopathologic entities with the potential to simulate CTCL in this way include "actinic reticuloid" [an unusual form of photosensitivity dermatitis (213)]; lymphomatoid contact dermatitis; idiosyncratic drug eruptions after ingestion of allopurinol, beta-blocking cardiovascular medications, phenytoin, phenothiazines, and penicillin; and other idiopathic forms of "pseudo-CTCL" (210,214).

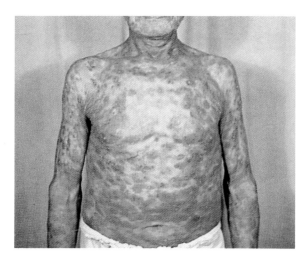

**FIG. 86.** Mycosis fungoides. Clinical presentation as diffuse orange–brown to violaceous papules and plaques that coalesce.

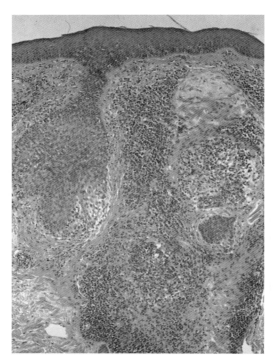

FIG. 87. Pseudomycosis fungoides. A dense dermal lymphocytic infiltrate is apparent. The patient had a history of a drug rash.

It would be tempting to expect the application of special pathologic studies to be capable of resolving the aforementioned uncertainties. Unfortunately, this is not so. The variants of CTCL and its biologically benign simulators might

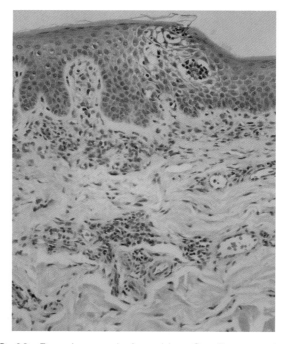

FIG. 88. Pseudomycosis fungoides. Small aggregates of lymphocytes in the epidermis may simulate Pautrier's microabscesses of mycosis fungoides.

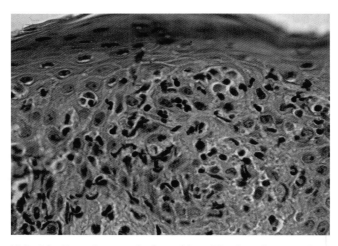

FIG. 89. Pseudomycosis fungoides. The lymphocytes in a drug reaction sometimes appear hyperchromatic, with slight cytologic atypia.

show identical T-cell immunophenotypes—whether they are physiologic or "aberrant" (215)—and even genotypic analyses have demonstrated an unexpected sharing of results (with potential rearrangements of T-cell receptor genes) among these diseases (216). Thus, the pathologist is left with the reality that he or she must reserve a definitive diagnosis of CTCL for those cases in which unequivocal pathologic and clinical data exist to support that interpretation. Otherwise, as suggested by Banks (217), more descriptive diagnoses such as "atypical psoriasiform dermatitis" or "atypical lymphoid infiltrate with epidermotropism" should be employed, with disclaimers in the body of the pathology report regarding the conditions that are capable of imitating CTCL.

### Nonneoplastic Conditions Producing Nodular or Diffuse Lymphoid Infiltrates Capable of Simulating B-Cell Lymphomas and Peripheral T-Cell Lymphomas

Traditionally, the term "pseudolymphoma" has had a more restrictive meaning in dermatopathology than that implied in the foregoing discussion. This designation has usually been employed in connection with nodular dermal lymphoid infiltrates rather than in connection with lichenoid lesions. Even so, "pseudolymphoma" of the skin has not been regarded as a single disease but rather as a polyglot of disorders with both B-cell and T-cell lineages. These include "Spiegler–Fendt sarcoid," "lymphocytoma cutis," "lymphadenosis benigna cutis" and other cutaneous lesions of Lyme disease, Kimura's disease, "benign lymphocytic infiltrate of Jessner–Kanof," lupus profunda, persistent arthropod bite reactions, and nodular lymphoid lesions that appear after administration of anticonvulsant medications, injections of gold, or tattooing (79,217–227).

In prototypical form, the latter disorders feature the presence of "tight" lymphoid cellular aggregates in the dermis, in the absence of epidermal involvement. The cell groups have their epicenters in the upper dermis, but with little or no

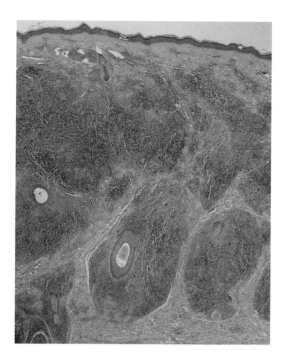

**FIG. 90.** Cutaneous lymphoid hyperplasia simulating lymphoma. This is the benign lymphocytic infiltrate of Jessner–Kanof with well-demarcated perivascular and periappendageal benign lymphocytic cell infiltrates, with absence of epidermal involvement.

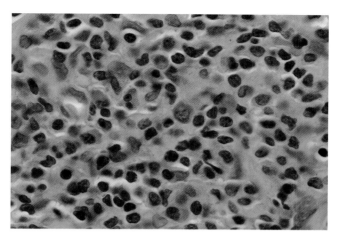

**FIG. 92.** Cutaneous lymphoid hyperplasia. The cellular composition of the infiltrate is mixed, with several types of mature hematolymphoid cells identified.

infiltration of the surface epithelium; they tend to surround blood vessels, nerves, and appendages discretely, and show a relatively sharp interface with the surrounding dermal collagen (Figs. 90 and 91). There is usually little or no involvement of the subcutaneous adipose tissue. Moreover, cytologic heterogeneity is common, with a mixture of small mature and larger activated lymphocytes, as well as scattered immunoblasts, eosinophils, neutrophils, and a few plasma cells (Fig. 92). Germinal centers may be evident as well, containing tingible body macrophages (Fig. 93). Occasion-

ally, either loose collections of histiocytes or sterile epithelioid granulomas are apparent in the infiltrate. In all of these scenarios, it is worthwhile obtaining a Steiner or Warthin–Starry stain to evaluate the possible presence of *Borrelia burgdorferii* (the causative agent of Lyme disease) (78).

Predictably, however, cases are not uncommon in which the aforementioned stylized histologic features are absent, or they are obfuscated by other findings that are suggestive of lymphoreticular malignancies. The latter include multifocal and confluent infiltration of the dermal interstitium by the lymphoid cells, slight nuclear atypia, and a lack of clear-cut organization into reactive follicles (212,217) (Figs. 94 and 95); shallow biopsies may not allow assessment of the depth of the lesions.

In this particular setting, special studies might provide valuable diagnostic information. If the lymphoid cell population is composed predominantly of B cells, the demonstration of monotypism for lambda or kappa light chain immunoglobulins—on frozen section immunostains—provides

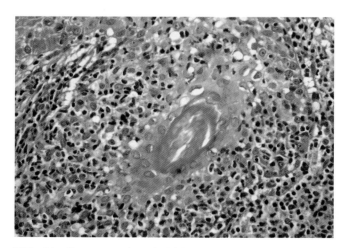

**FIG. 91.** Cutaneous lymphoid hyperplasia. The infiltrate in cutaneous lymphoid hyperplasia does not destroy the appendageal structures.

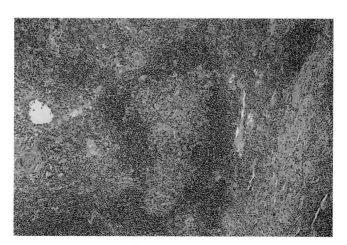

**FIG. 93.** Germinal centers are observed in a minority of cases of cutaneous lymphoid hyperplasia. This finding favors a diagnosis of a benign lymphoproliferative process.

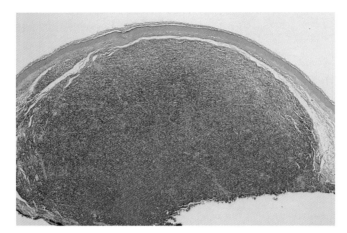

**FIG. 94.** Atypical lymphoid hyperplasia in the skin. A more sheet-like arrangement of a lymphoid infiltrate in the dermis.

strong evidence favoring a diagnosis of malignancy, as does rearrangement of immunoglobulin genes (228,229). We have likewise shown that the coexpression of CD20 and CD43, with or without aberrant CD45RA labeling, correlates with an interpretation of cutaneous B-cell lymphoma in paraffin section immunohistochemistry (230,231). The same diagnostic conclusion is also suggested by a predominance (>75%) of cells labeling as B lymphocytes in that context (232). Interestingly, immunostains for the *bcl-2* oncoprotein, which is highly expressed as a consequence of chromosomal translation in follicular small-cleaved cell lymphomas, are not of particular differential diagnostic assistance in cutaneous B-cell infiltrates that lack a nodular histologic configuration (232).

In fact, most "pseudolymphomas" are composed of either a majority of T cells or discrete zones of B and T cells. Nodular dermal T-cell infiltrates are less amenable to definitive biological characterization using immunohistology. Flow cytometric or frozen section immunostains that demonstrate

the loss of "pan-T-cell" antigens such as CD2, CD3, CD5, or CD7 are suggestive of immunophenotypic aberrancy in the proper histologic context. Nevertheless, this finding is best used as a potential indicator of malignancy in conjunction with genotypic data that demonstrate concurrent T-cell gene rearrangements in the same cell population (233,234).

### Plasma Cell Infiltrates of the Skin and Mucosae That Simulate Plasmacytoma

There are basically two clinical conditions in which dermal plasma cell infiltrates are so dense that serious histopathologic consideration is given to a diagnosis of cutaneous plasmacytoma. These are secondary syphilis (condylomalata) (51,52) and idiopathic plasma cell cheilitis/mucositis (235–238). Both of these disorders feature the presence of confluent sheets of mature plasma cells in the corium or in the subepithelial tissue of modified mucosal surfaces such as the lips, mouth, and genital skin (Figs. 96 and 97). Occasional binucleation of the plasmacytes may be apparent, but overt nuclear atypia is lacking. There is no clinical evidence of a paraproteinemia in examinations of the serum or urine, as expected in plasmocytic neoplasms. Also, immunostains for immunoglobulin light chains should show a mixed kappa/lambda population. In fact, plasma cells routinely maintain reactivity in paraffin sections, in a cytoplasmic pattern, as opposed to the membrane immunoglobulin reactiv-

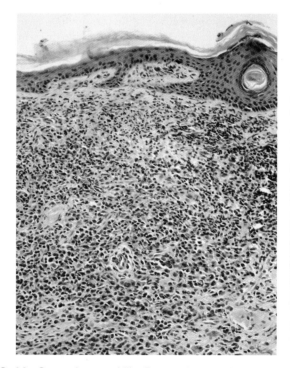

**FIG. 96.** Secondary syphilis. Dense dermal plasmocytic cell infiltrate, which, as is typical for condylomalata, is superficial and deep in its dermal distribution.

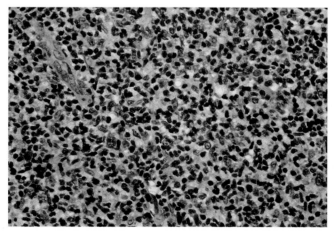

**FIG. 95.** Atypical cutaneous lymphoid hyperplasia. Cytologically, the lymphoid infiltrate is monomorphous.

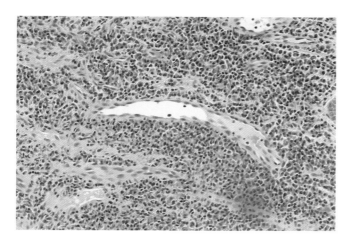

**FIG. 97.** Secondary syphilis. An extensive perivascular plasma cell proliferation is apparent.

ity of B cells, which are often lost in paraffin sections. Histochemical stains for *Treponema pallidum* are floridly positive in the lesions of secondary lues (51,52) (Fig. 98), and these should always be obtained in cases showing the specified histologic characteristics.

## Histiocytic (Macrophage/Monocyte) Infiltrates of the Skin Capable of Simulating Malignant Neoplasms

The very existence of cells known as "histiocytes" has been called into serious question by some observers in recent years (239). However, it is clear that certain proliferations of cells in the macrophage/monocyte series potentially affect the skin. Two of these in particular—"sinus histiocytosis with massive lymphadenopathy" (SHML; Rosai–Dorfman disease) and cutaneous malakoplakia—may be confused with lymphomas or other malignant neoplasms.

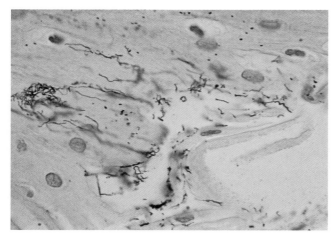

**FIG. 98.** *Treponema pallidum* organisms in secondary syphilis as visualized by the Warthin–Starry stain are thin, delicate, spiral structures.

## Sinus Histiocytosis with Massive Lymphadenopathy

As reviewed recently by Foucar et al. (240), sinus histiocytosis with massive lymphadenopathy (SHML) is not considered a clonal and autonomous process. Instead, it is felt to represent a localized or systemic lesion of dysfunctional immunity, and is therefore included in this book on pseudoneoplastic conditions. The typical patient profile in this disease is that of a young adult—more likely to be male than female—who develops marked lymphadenopathy, fever or other systemic complaints, elevations in erythrocyte sedimentation rate, and laboratory indicators of disturbed humoral or cellular immunity in up to 80% of cases.

These abnormalities might be accompanied by the formation of mass lesions in tissues other than the lymph nodes. The skin is the foremost of these, being affected in 7% of all patients with the disease. Furthermore, cutaneous involvement may be preferential and may occur in the absence of nodal infiltrates. The skin lesions in SHML are typically described as plaque-like or nodular and yellowish, resembling xanthomas; they are often multiple and do not exhibit a strong predilection for any given topographic site (240,241).

Histologic examination of biopsy specimens in cutaneous SHML demonstrates a peculiar low-power microscopic similarity of the lesions to intradermal lymph nodes. They are characterized by a peripheral, at times circumferential, fibrous pseudocapsule, inside of which there is a sinusoidal arrangement of spaces in which large, pale, polygonal histiocytes reside. These elements contain abundant "glassy" or granular eosinophilic cytoplasm (Figs. 99 and 100), and

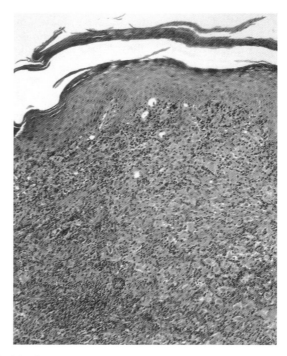

**FIG. 99.** Sinus histiocytosis with massive lymphadenopathy in the skin is characterized by a dense dermal infiltrate.

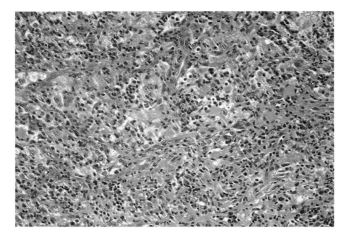

**FIG. 100.** Sinus histiocytosis with massive lymphadenopathy. Groups of large histiocytes are prominent.

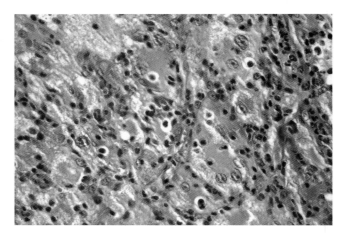

**FIG. 102.** Sinus histiocytosis with massive lymphadenopathy. Lymphocytes are often localized within the cytoplasm of the histiocytes.

show the distinctive morphologic feature known as "emperipolesis," wherein other intact inflammatory cells (usually mature lymphocytes) are identified within their cellular confines (Figs. 101 and 102). There is a heterogeneous population of other hematopoietic cells (e.g., neutrophils, eosinophils, lymphocytes, and banal histiocytes) in the background, often with fibrosis and formation of lymphoid follicles, but the constituent large histiocytes fail to show more than modest nuclear hyperchromasia or mitotic activity (240–243). Immunostains for both S-100 protein and CD68 are strongly positive in the large pale histiocytic cells. This conjoint phenotype is unusual and virtually pathognomonic in this context (240).

Differential diagnosis with lymphoma, melanoma, and carcinoma of the skin (any of which may be composed of large pale tumor cells) is usually attainable by attention to

the histologic nuances of SHML, although immunohistologic analyses might be desired to objectify this process. S-100 protein reactivity is shared only rarely by lymphomas; moreover, these usually express CD20, CD30, or CD45R0, whereas SHML does not (233,234,243). HMB45—a melanocyte marker—and the keratin proteins of carcinomas are both lacking in SHML (86,225).

### Cutaneous Malakoplakia

Malakoplakia—as described in the chapters on several other organ systems in this text—is a rare condition of the skin (244–249). It has been reported in both immunocompetent and immunodeficient patients of all ages as red–yellow papules or nodules. Affected mucocutaneous sites have included the periurethral area, the perineum, and the uvula, and the subcutis may also be involved. This disease is thought to reflect defective intracellular processing of encapsulated

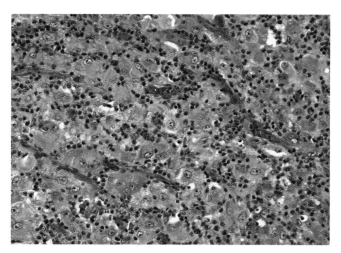

**FIG. 101.** The characteristic cell of sinus histiocytosis with massive lymphadenopathy is a large histiocyte with abundant amphophilic, glassy cytoplasm and vesicular nucleus. Numerous small mature lymphocytes are scattered among the histiocytes.

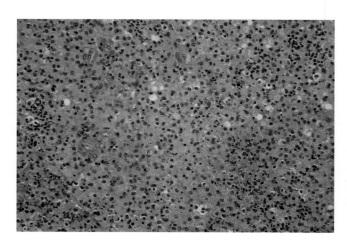

**FIG. 103.** Malakoplakia of the skin is a histiocyte cell–rich chronic inflammatory disorder.

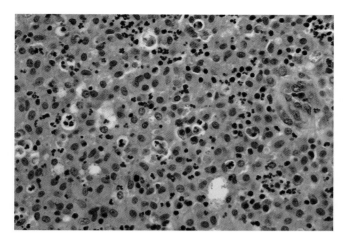

**FIG. 104.** Cutaneous malakoplakia. There are sheets of macrophages, with scattered plasma cells and neutrophils.

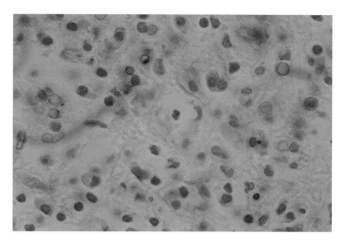

**FIG. 106.** Michaelis–Guttmann bodies in cutaneous malakoplakia are positive for iron by histochemical staining (Perl's stain).

bacteria by elements of the macrophage/monocyte series (246).

Either in cytologic preparations, e.g., obtained via fine needle aspiration (245), or excisional biopsy specimens, the proliferating cells of malakoplakia are large and polygonal with abundant eosinophilic or amphophilic cytoplasm (247, 249). They are arranged in the dermis in confluent sheets, often punctuated by infiltrates of neutrophils, mature lymphocytes, and other inflammatory cells (Figs. 103 and 104). Nuclei in the large cells may be enlarged and moderately hyperchromatic, and mitotic activity is not uncommon. The overlying epidermis may either be ulcerated or intact.

The differential diagnosis of this disorder is similar to that outlined above for SHML, and it also includes reticulohistiocytoma and xanthogranuloma of the skin. However, close inspection of routinely stained sections will demonstrate characteristic and diagnostically exclusive inclusions in the histiocytes of malakoplakia, called "Michaelis–Guttmann bodies." These are small, spherical, sometimes concentri-

cally laminated cytoplasmic organelles, representing complex lysosomal forms. They are labeled with the periodic acid–Schiff method after diastase digestion (Fig. 105), and they stain black with the von Kossa technique for calcium salt or blue with the Prussian blue method for iron (250,251) (Fig. 106).

## CONCLUSIONS

As outlined here, the spectrum of pseudoneoplastic conditions encountered in the skin is a broad one. In order to successfully address differential diagnosis in this context, it is desirable to employ a systematic approach to histologic analysis—along the lines suggested by the authors—as well as stylized procedures for tissue procurement and processing. Because special studies are often desired in the evaluation of the lesions discussed here, representative portions of biopsy specimens should be frozen or placed in special fixatives in the appropriate clinical settings.

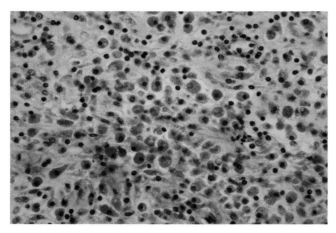

**FIG. 105.** Michaelis–Guttmann bodies in cutaneous malakoplakia as highlighted by the periodic acid–Schiff method, with diastase digestion.

## REFERENCES

1. Nuovo G. Diseases related to infection with human papillomaviruses. *Adv Pathol Lab Med* 1995;8:119–148.
2. Willman CL, Busque L, Griffith BB, et al. Langerhans' cell histiocytosis (histiocytosis-X): a clonal proliferative disease. *N Engl J Med* 1994;331:154–160.
3. Lever WF. Localized mycosis fungoides with prominent epidermotropism (Woringer–Kolopp disease). *Arch Dermatol* 1977;113:1254–1256.
4. McMillan EM, Wasik R, Martin D, et al. T-cell nature of exocytic and dermal lymphoid cells in atrophic parapsoriasis. *J Cutan Pathol* 1981;8:355–360, 385–391.
5. Kaudewitz P, Burg G. Lymphomatoid papulosis and Ki-1 (CD30)–positive cutaneous large cell lymphomas. *Semin Diagn Pathol* 1991;8:117–124.
6. Coffin CM, Dehner LP. Soft tissue neoplasms in childhood: a clinicopathologic overview. In: Finegold M, ed. *Pathology of neoplasia in children and adolescents*. Philadelphia: WB Saunders, 1986;223–255.
7. Reed RJ, Ichinose H, Clark WH, et al. Common and uncommon

melanocytic nevi and borderline melanomas. *Semin Oncol* 1975; 2:119–147.

8. Kuehnl-Petzoldt C, Volk B. Histology of congenital nevi during the first year of life: a study by conventional and electron microscopy. *Am J Dermatopathol* 1984;6(Suppl):81–88.

9. Weiss SW, Enzinger FM. Spindle-cell hemangioendothelioma. *Am J Surg Pathol* 1986;10:521–530.

10. Fletcher CDM, Beham A, Schmid C. Spindle cell hemangioendothelioma: a clinicopathological and immunohistochemical study indicative of a non-neoplastic lesion. *Histopathology* 1991;18:291–301.

11. Rogers M, McCrossin I, Commens C. Epidermal nevi and the epidermal nevus syndrome. *J Am Acad Dermatol* 1989;20:476–481.

12. Submoke S, Piamphongsant P. Clinicohistopathologic study of epidermal nevi. *Aust J Dermatol* 1983;24:130–136.

13. Su WPD. Histopathological varieties of epidermal nevus: a study of 160 cases. *Am J Dermatopathol* 1982;4:161–171.

14. Arnold HL, Odom RB, James WD, eds. *Andrews' diseases of the skin.* 8th ed. Philadelphia: WB Saunders, 1990;745–807.

15. Hurwitz S. Epidermal nevi and tumors of epidermal origin. *Pediatr Clin North Am* 1983;30:483–494.

16. Kennedy C. Inflammatory linear verrucous epidermal nevus (eczematous linear naevus). *Clin Exp Dermatol* 1980;5:471–473.

17. Zeligman I, Pomeranz J. Variation of congenital ichthyosiform erythroderma: report of cases of ichthyosis hystrix and nevus unius lateris. *Arch Dermatol* 1965;91:120–125.

18. Goldstein N. Ephidrosis (local hyperhidrosis): nevus sudoriferus. *Arch Dermatol* 1967;96:67–71.

19. Kin JH, Hur H, Lee CW, Kim YT. Apocrine nevus. *J Am Acad Dermatol* 1988;18:579–581.

20. Wick MR, Swanson PE. *Cutaneous adnexal tumors: a guide to pathologic diagnosis.* Chicago: ASCP Press, 1991;1–77, 113–167.

21. Wolf R, Krakowski A, Dorfman B, Baratz M. Eccrine angiomatous hamartoma. *Arch Dermatol* 1959;125:1489–1490.

22. Challa VR, Jona J. Eccrine angiomatous hamartoma: a rare skin lesion with diverse histological features. *Dermatologica* 1977;155:206–209.

23. Mehregan AH. Proliferation of sweat ducts in certain diseases of the skin. *Am J Dermatopathol* 1981;3:27–31.

24. Lerner TH, Barr RJ, Dolezal JF, Stagnone JJ. Syringomatous hyperplasia and eccrine squamous syringometaplasia association with benoxaprofen therapy. *Arch Dermatol* 1987;123:1202–1204.

25. Bhawan J, Malhotra R. Syringosquamous metaplasia: a distinctive eruption in patients receiving chemotherapy. *Am J Dermatopathol* 1990;12:1–6.

26. Leshin B, White WL. Folliculocentric basaloid proliferation; the bulge (der Wulst) revisited. *Arch Dermatol* 1990;126:900–906.

27. Mehregan AH. Hair follicle tumors of the skin. *J Cutan Pathol* 1985; 12:189–195.

28. Mehregan AH, Baker S. Basaloid follicular hamartoma: report of three cases with localized and systematized unilateral lesions. *J Cutan Pathol* 1985;12:55–65.

29. Ridley CM, Smith N. Generalized hair follicle hamartoma associated with alopecia and myasthenia gravis: report of a second case. *Clin Exp Dermatol* 1981;6:283–289.

30. Imai S, Nitto H. Trichogenic trichoblastoma. *Hautarzt* 1982;33: 609–611.

31. Gilks CB, Clement PB, Wood WS. Trichoblastic fibroma: a clinicopathologic study of three cases. *Am J Dermatopathol* 1989;11: 397–402.

32. McGibbon DH. Malignant epidermal tumors. *J Cutan Pathol* 1985; 12:224–238.

33. Wade TR, Ackerman AB. The many faces of basal cell carcinoma. *J Dermatol Surg Oncol* 1978;4:23–28.

34. Winer LH. Pseudoepitheliomatous hyperplasia. *Arch Dermatol Syphilol* 1940;42:856–867.

35. Ju DMC. Pseudoepitheliomatous hyperplasia of the skin. *Dermatol Int* 1967;6:82–92.

36. Sommerville J. Pseudoepitheliomatous hyperplasia. *Acta Dermatol Venereol* 1953;33:236–251.

37. Freeman RG. On the pathogenesis of pseudoepitheliomatous hyperplasia. *J Cutan Pathol* 1974;1:231–237.

38. Su WPD, Duncan SC, Perry HO. Blastomycosis-like pyoderma. *Arch Dermatol* 1979;115:170–173.

39. Wagner RF Jr, Grande DJ. Pseudoepitheliomatous hyperplasia versus squamous cell carcinoma. *J Dermatol Surg Oncol* 1986;12:632–635.

40. Elton RF. Complications of cutaneous cryosurgery. *J Am Acad Dermatol* 1983;8:513–519.

41. Weber PJ, Johnson BL, Dzubow LM. Pseudoepitheliomatous hyperplasia following Mohs micrographic surgery. *J Dermatol Surg Oncol* 1989;15:557–560.

42. Teller H. Bromoderma und jododerma tuberosum. *Dermatol Wochenschr* 1961;143:273–282.

43. Hoover EL, Williams W, Koger L, et al. Pseudoepitheliomatous hyperplasia and pyoderma gangrenosum after a brown recluse spider bite. *South Med J* 1990;83:243–246.

44. Schoenfeld RJ. Epidermal proliferations overlying histiocytomas. *Arch Dermatol* 1964;90:266–270.

45. Lack EE, Worsham GF, Callihan MD, et al. Granular cell tumor: a clinicopathologic study of 110 patients. *J Surg Oncol* 1980;13: 301–316.

46. Taylor HB, Helwig EB. Dermatofibrosarcoma protuberans. *Cancer* 1961;15:717–725.

47. Scott G, Chen KTK, Rosai J. Pseudoepitheliomatous hyperplasia in Spitz nevi. *Arch Pathol Lab Med* 1989;113:61–63.

48. Sagebiel RW, Chinn EK, Egbert BM. Pigmented spindle cell nevus: clinical and histologic review of 90 cases. *Am J Surg Pathol* 1984; 8:645–653.

49. Weedon D, Little JH. Spindle and epithelioid cell nevi in children and adults. *Cancer* 1977;40:217–225.

50. Krasne DL, Warnke RA, Weiss LM. Malignant lymphoma presenting as pseudoepitheliomatous hyperplasia. *Am J Surg Pathol* 1988;12: 835–842.

51. Abell E, Marks R, Wilson-Jones E. Secondary syphilis: a clinicopathological review. *Br J Dermatol* 1975;93:53–61.

52. Jeerapaet P, Ackerman AB. Histologic patterns of secondary syphilis. *Arch Dermatol* 1973;107:373–377.

53. Wong KD, Lee KP, Chiu SF. Tuberculosis of the skin in Hong Kong. *Br J Dermatol* 1968;80:424–429.

54. Cott RE, Carter DM, Sall T. Cutaneous disease caused by atypical mycobacteria. *Arch Dermatol* 1967;95:259–268.

55. Santa Cruz DJ, Strayer DS. The histologic spectrum of the cutaneous mycobacterioses. *Hum Pathol* 1982;13:485–495.

56. Fisher ER, Dimling C. Rhinoscleroma. *Arch Pathol* 1964;78: 501–512.

57. Witorsch P, Utz JP. North American blastomycosis: a study of 40 patients. *Medicine* 1968;47:169–200.

58. Brown JR. Human actinomycosis: a study of 181 subjects. *Hum Pathol* 1973;4:319–330.

59. Carr RD, Storken MA, Wilson JW, et al. Extensive verrucous sporotrichosis of long duration. *Arch Dermatol* 1964;89:124–130.

60. Ballpitt P, Weedon D. Sporotrichosis: a review of 39 cases. *Pathology* 1978;10:249–256.

61. Goette DK, Helwig EB. Basal cell carcinomas and basal cell carcinoma–like changes overlying dermatofibromas. *Arch Dermatol* 1975; 111:589–592.

62. Miyauchi H, Urchara M. Follicular occurrence of prurigo nodularis. *J Cutan Pathol* 1988;15:208–211.

63. Doyle JA, Connolly SM, Hunziker N, et al. Prurigo nodularis: a reappraisal of the clinical and histologic features. *J Cutan Pathol* 1979; 6:392–403.

64. Balazs M. Buschke–Loewenstein tumor: a histologic and ultrastructural study of six cases. *Virchows Arch A Path Anat* 1986;410:83–92.

65. Bargman H. Pseudoepitheliomatous keratotic and micaceous balanitis. *Cutis* 1985;35:77–79.

66. Kao GF, Graham JH, Helwig EB. Carcinoma cuniculatum (verrucous carcinoma of the skin). *Cancer* 1982;49:2395–2403.

67. Johnson LL, Kempson RL. Epidermoid carcinoma in chronic osteomyelitis. *J Bone Joint Surg (Am)* 1965;47A:133–143.

68. Johnston WH, Miller TA, Frileck SP. Atypical pseudoepitheliomatous hyperplasia and squamous cell carcinoma in chronic cutaneous sinuses and fistulas. *Plast Reconstr Surg* 1980;66:395–400.

69. Holden CA, Horton JJ, McKee PH, MacDonald DM. The discriminatory diagnostic ability of beta-2-microglobulin labeling in viral warts, pseudoepitheliomatous hyperplasia, and verrucous carcinoma of the skin. *Clin Exp Dermatol* 1985;10:217–221.

70. Lee YS, Teh M. p53 expression in pseudoepitheliomatous hyperplasia, keratoacanthoma, and squamous cell carcinoma of the skin. *Cancer* 1994;73:2317–2323.

71. Williams B, Barr R, Barrett T, et al. Cutaneous pseudosarcomatous

polyps. Abstract presented at the American Society of Dermatology Conference, February 1995.

72. Hurt MA, Santa Cruz DJ. Cutaneous inflammatory pseudotumor. *Am J Surg Pathol* 1988;14:764–773.

73. Pettinato G, Manivel JC, DeRosa N, Dehner LP. Inflammatory myofibroblastic tumor (plasma cell granuloma): clinicopathologic study of 20 cases with immunohistochemical and ultrastructural observations. *Am J Clin Pathol* 1990;94:538–546.

74. Lange-Wantzin G, Hou-Jensen K, Nielsen M, et al. Cutaneous lymphocytomas. *Acta Dermatol Venereol* 1982;62:119–124.

75. Wirt DP, Grogen TM, Jolley CS, et al. The immunoarchitecture of cutaneous pseudolymphoma. *Hum Pathol* 1985;16:492–510.

76. Clark WH, Mihm MC Jr, Reed RJ, et al. The lymphocytic infiltrates of the skin. *Hum Pathol* 1974;5:25–43.

77. Weber K, Schierz G, Wilske B, et al. Das lymphozytom—eine borreliose? *Z Hautkr* 1985;60:1585–1598.

78. Duray PH. The surgical pathology of human Lyme disease. *Am J Surg Pathol* 1987;11(Suppl):47–60.

79. Googe PB, Harris NL, Mihm MC Jr. Kimura's disease and angiolymphoid hyperplasia with eosinophilia: two distinct histopathological entities. *J Cutan Pathol* 1987;14:263–271.

80. Barker SM, Winkelmann RK. Inflammatory lymphadenoid reactions with dermatofibroma/histiocytoma. *J Cutan Pathol* 1986;13:222–226.

81. Niemi KM. The benign fibrohistiocytic tumors of the skin. *Acta Dermatol Venereol* 1970;50(Suppl):1–66.

82. Gonzalez S, Duarte I. Benign fibrous histiocytoma of the skin: a morphologic study of 290 cases. *Pathol Res Pract* 1982;174:379–391.

83. Beatty EC. Rheumatic-like nodules occurring in non-rheumatic children. *Arch Pathol* 1959;68:154–159.

84. Lowney ED, Simons HM. "Rheumatoid" nodules of the skin. *Arch Dermatol* 1963;88:853–858.

85. Patterson JW. Rheumatoid nodule and subcutaneous granuloma annulare: a comparative histologic study. *Am J Dermatopathol* 1988;10:1–8.

86. Salomon RJ, Gardepe SF, Woodley DT. Deep granuloma annulare in adults. *Int J Dermatol* 1986;25:109–112.

87. Shmookler BM, Gunther SF. Superficial epithelioid sarcoma: a clinical and histologic simulant of benign cutaneous disease. *J Am Acad Dermatol* 1986;14:893–898.

88. Enzinger FM. Epithelioid sarcoma: a sarcoma simulating a granuloma or a carcinoma. *Cancer* 1970;26:1029–1041.

89. Heenan PJ, Quirk CJ, Papadimitriou JM. Epithelioid sarcoma: a diagnostic problem. *Am J Dermatopathol* 1986;8:95–104.

90. Wick MR, Kaye VN. The role of diagnostic immunohistochemistry in dermatology. *Semin Dermatol* 1986;5:346–358.

91. Amazon K, Robinson MD, Rywlin AM. Ferrugination caused by Monsel's solution. *Am J Dermatopathol* 1980;2:197–205.

92. Wick MR, Manivel JC. Vascular neoplasms of the skin: a current perspective. *Adv Dermatol* 1989;4:185–254.

93. Chor PJ, Santa Cruz DJ. Kaposi's sarcoma: a clinicopathologic review and differential diagnosis. *J Cutan Pathol* 1992;19:6–20.

94. Blumenfeld W, Egbert BM, Sagebiel RW. Differential diagnosis of Kaposi's sarcoma. *Arch Pathol Lab Med* 1985;109:123–127.

95. Mali JWH, Kuiper JP, Hamers AA. Acroangiodermatitis of the foot. *Arch Dermatol* 1965;92:515–518.

96. Earhart RN, Aeling JA, Nuss DD, et al. Pseudo-Kaposi's sarcoma. *Arch Dermatol* 1974;110:907–910.

97. DeVillez RL, Roberts LC. Acroangiodermatitis of Mali. *South Med J* 1984;77:255–258.

98. Yi JU, Lee CW. Acroangiodermatitis: a clinical variant of stasis dermatitis. *Int J Dermatol* 1990;29:515–516.

99. Rao B, Unis M, Poulos E. Acroangiodermatitis: a study of ten cases. *Int J Dermatol* 1994;33:179–183.

100. Wick MR. Kaposi's sarcoma unrelated to the acquired immunodeficiency syndrome. *Curr Opin Oncol* 1991;3:377–383.

101. Rusin LJ, Harrell ER. Arteriovenous fistula: cutaneous manifestations. *Arch Dermatol* 1976;112:1135–1138.

102. Marshall ME, Hatfield ST, Hatfield DR. Arteriovenous malformation simulating Kaposi's sarcoma (pseudo-Kaposi's sarcoma). *Arch Dermatol* 1985;121:99–101.

103. Schamberg JF. A peculiar progressive pigmentary disease of the skin. *Br J Dermatol* 1901;13:1–5.

104. Randall SJ, Kierland RR, Montgomery H. Pigmented purpuric eruptions. *Arch Dermatol* 1951;64:177–191.

105. Newton RC, Raimer SS. Pigmented purpuric eruptions. *Dermatol Clin* 1985;3:165–169.

106. Masson P. Hemangioendotheliome vegetant intravasculaire. *Bull Soc Anat* 1923;93:517–523.

107. Barr RJ, Graham JH, Sherwin LA. Intravascular papillary endothelial hyperplasia. *Arch Dermatol* 1978;114:723–726.

108. Clearkin KP, Enzinger FM. Intravascular papillary endothelial hyperplasia. *Arch Pathol Lab Med* 1976;100:441–444.

109. Kreutner A Jr, Smith RM, Trefny FA. Intravascular papillary endothelial hyperplasia. *Cancer* 1978;42:2304–2310.

110. Kuo TT, Gomez LG. Papillary endothelial proliferation in cystic lymphangioma. *Arch Pathol Lab Med* 1979;103:306–308.

111. Kuo TT, Sayers P, Rosai J. Masson's "vegetant intravascular hemangioendothelioma": a lesion often mistaken for angiosarcoma. *Cancer* 1976;38:1227–1236.

112. Paslin DA. Localized primary cutaneous intravascular papillary endothelial hyperplasia. *J Am Acad Dermatol* 1981;4:316–318.

113. Pfleger L, Tappeiner J. Zur Kenntnis der systemisierten endotheliomatose der cutanen blutgefasse (reticulo-endotheliose?). *Hautarzt* 1959;10:359–363.

114. Tappeiner J, Pfleger L. Angioendotheliomatosis proliferans systemisata. *Hautarzt* 1963;14:67–70.

115. Braverman IM, Lerner AB. Diffuse malignant proliferation of vascular endothelium. *Arch Dermatol* 1961;84:22–30.

116. Ruiter M, Mandema E. New cutaneous syndrome in subacute bacterial endocarditis. *Arch Intern Med* 1964;113:283–290.

117. Kauh VC, McFarland JP, Carnabuci GG, et al. Malignant proliferating angioendotheliomatosis. *Arch Dermatol* 1980;116:803–806.

118. Bhawan J, Wolff SM, Ucci AA, et al. Malignant lymphoma and malignant angioendotheliomatosis: one disease. *Cancer* 1985;55:570–576.

119. Wrotnowski U, Mills SE, Cooper PH. Malignant angioendotheliomatosis: an angiotropic lymphoma. *Am J Clin Pathol* 1985;83:244–248.

120. Wick MR, Mills SE. Intravascular lymphomatosis: clinicopathologic features and differential diagnosis. *Semin Diagn Pathol* 1991;8:91–101.

121. Martin S, Pitcher D, Tschen J, et al. Reactive angioendotheliomatosis. *J Am Acad Dermatol* 1980;2:117–123.

122. Eisert J. Skin manifestations of subacute bacterial endocarditis. *Cutis* 1980;25:394–400.

123. Pasyk K, Depowski M. Proliferating systematized angioendotheliomatosis in a 5 month old infant. *Arch Dermatol* 1978;114:1513–1515.

124. Amantea A, Gaudio E, Donati P, et al. Benign reactive proliferating angioendotheliomatosis. *G Ital Dermatol Venereol* 1988;123:245–248.

125. LeBoit PE, Solomon AR, Santa Cruz DJ, Wick MR. Angiomatosis with luminal cryoprotein deposition. *J Am Acad Dermatol* 1992;27:969–973.

126. Cooper PH. Vascular tumors. In: Farmer ER, Hood AF, eds. *Pathology of the skin.* Norwalk, CT: Appleton and Lange, 1990;804–846.

127. Imperial R, Helwig EB. Angiokeratoma: a clinicopathological study. *Arch Dermatol* 1967;95:166–175.

128. Imperial R, Helwig EB. Angiokeratoma of the scrotum (Fordyce type). *J Urol* 1967;98:379–387.

129. Adal KA, Cockerell CJ, Petri WA Jr. Cat scratch disease, bacillary angiomatosis, and other infections due to *Rochalimaea. N Engl J Med* 1994;330:1509–1515.

130. Tappero JW, Mohle-Boetani J, Koehler JE, et al. The epidemiology of bacillary angiomatosis and bacillary peliosis. *JAMA* 1993;269:770–775.

131. Haught WH, Steinbach J, Zander DS, Wingo CS. Case report: bacillary angiomatosis with massive visceral lymphadenopathy. *Am J Med Sci* 1993;306:236–240.

132. Cockerell CJ, Tierno PM, Friedman-Kien AE, Kim KS. Clinical, histologic, microbiologic, and biochemical characterization of the causative agent of bacillary (epithelioid) angiomatosis: a rickettsial illness with features of bartonellosis. *J Invest Dermatol* 1991;97:812–817.

133. Cockerell CJ, Whitlow MA, Webster GF, Friedman-Kien AE. Epithelioid angiomatosis: a distinct vascular disorder in patients with the acquired immunodeficiency syndrome or AIDS-related complex. *Lancet* 1987;2:654–656.

134. Mulvany NJ, Billson VR. Bacillary angiomatosis of the spleen. *Pathology* 1993;25:398–401.

135. Koehler JE, Tappero JW. Bacillary angiomatosis and bacillary peliosis in patients infected with human immunodeficiency virus. *Clin Infect Dis* 1993;17:612–624.

136. Cotell SL, Noskin GA. Bacillary angiomatosis: clinical and histologic features, diagnosis, and treatment. *Arch Intern Med* 1994;143: 524–528.

137. Arias-Stella J, Lieberman PH, Erlandson RA, Arias-Stella J Jr. Histology, immunohistochemistry, and ultrastructure of the verruga in Carrion's disease. *Am J Surg Pathol* 1986;10:595–610.

138. Arias-Stella J, Lieberman PH, Garcia-Caceros U, et al. Verruga peruana mimicking malignant neoplasms. *Am J Dermatopathol* 1987; 9:279–291.

139. Garcia FU, Wojta J, Broadley KN, et al. *Bartonella bacilliformis* stimulates endothelial cells in vitro and is angiogenic in vivo. *Am J Pathol* 1990;136:1125–1135.

140. Wade HW. The histoid variety of lepromatous leprosy. *Int J Leprosy* 1963;31:129–142.

141. Triscott JA, Nappi O, Ferrara G, Wick MR. Pseudoneoplastic leprosy: leprosy revisited. *Am J Dermatopathol* 1995;117:297–302.

142. Sehgal VN, Srivastava G, Saha K. Immunological status of histoid leprosy. *Lepr Rev* 1985;56:27–33.

143. Mansfield RE. Histoid leprosy. *Arch Pathol* 1969;87:580–585.

144. Sehgal VN, Srivastava G. Histoid leprosy: a prospective diagnostic study in 38 patients. *Dermatologica* 1988;177:212–217.

145. Janniger CK, Rajendra K, Schwartz RA, et al. Histoid lepromas of lepromatous leprosy. *Int J Dermatol* 1990;29:494–496.

146. Wood C, Nickoloff BJ, Todes-Taylor NR. Pseudotumor resulting from atypical mycobacterial infection: a "histoid" variety of *Mycobacterium avium-intracellulare* complex infection. *Am J Clin Pathol* 1985;83:524–527.

147. LeBoit PE. Dermatopathologic findings in patients infected with human immunodeficiency virus. *Dermatol Clin* 1992;10:59–71.

148. Brandwein M, Choi HSH, Strauchen J, Stoler M. Spindle cell reaction to nontuberculous mycobacteriosis in AIDS mimicking a spindle cell neoplasm. *Virchows Arch A Path Anat* 1990;416:281–286.

149. Umlas J, Federman M, Crawford C, et al. Spindle cell pseudotumor due to *Mycobacterium avium-intracellulare* in patients with acquired immunodeficiency syndrome (AIDS). *Am J Surg Pathol* 1991;15: 1181–1187.

150. Suster S, Moran CA, Blanco M. Mycobacterial spindle-cell pseudotumor of the spleen. *Am J Clin Pathol* 1994;101:539–542.

151. Sekosan M, Cleto M, Senseng C, et al. Spindle cell pseudotumors in the lungs due to *Mycobacterium tuberculosis* in a transplant patient. *Am J Surg Pathol* 1994;18:1065–1068.

152. Paller AS, Gonzalez-Crussi F, Sherman JO. Fibrous hamartoma of infancy. *Arch Dermatol* 1989;125:88–91.

153. Enzinger FM. Fibrous hamartoma of infancy. *Cancer* 1965;18: 241–248.

154. Mitchell ML, Di Sant' Agnese PA, Gerber JE. Fibrous hamartoma of infancy. *Hum Pathol* 1982;13:586–588.

155. Maung R, Lindsay R, Trevener C, et al. Fibrous hamartoma of infancy. *Hum Pathol* 1987;18:652–653.

156. Mehregan AH. Superficial fibrous tumors in childhood. *J Cutan Pathol* 1981;8:321–334.

157. Harris CJ, Das S, Vogt PJ. Fibrous hamartoma of infancy in the scrotum. *J Urol* 1982;127:781–782.

158. Johnson MD, Jacobs AH. Congenital smooth muscle hamartoma. *Arch Dermatol* 1989;125:820–822.

159. Tsambaos D, Orfanos CE. Cutaneous smooth muscle hamartoma. *J Cutan Pathol* 1982;9:33–42.

160. Bronson DM, Fretzin DF, Farrell LN. Congenital pilar and smooth muscle nevus. *J Am Acad Dermatol* 1983;8:111–114.

161. Slifman NR, Harrist TJ, Rhodes AR. Congenital arrector pili hamartoma. *Arch Dermatol* 1985;121:1034–1037.

162. Goldman MP, Kaplan RP, Heng MCY. Congenital smooth muscle hamartoma. *Int J Dermatol* 1987;26:448–452.

163. Darling TN, Kamino H, Murray JC. Acquired cutaneous smooth muscle hamartoma. *J Am Acad Dermatol* 1993;28:844–845.

164. Wong RC, Solomon AR. Acquired dermal smooth muscle hamartoma. *Cutis* 1985;35:369–370.

165. Chapel TA, Tavafoghi V, Mehregan AH, et al. Becker's melanosis: an organoid hamartoma. *Cutis* 1981;27:405–415.

166. Karo KR, Gange RW. Smooth muscle hamartoma: possible congenital Becker's nevus. *Arch Dermatol* 1981;117:678–679.

167. Urbanek RW, Johnson WC. Smooth muscle hamartoma associated with Becker's nevus. *Arch Dermatol* 1978;114:104–106.

168. Fisher WG, Helwig EB. Leiomyomas of the skin. *Arch Dermatol* 1963;88:78–88.

169. Swanson PE, Stanley MW, Scheithauer BW, Wick MR. Primary cutaneous leiomyosarcoma. *J Cutan Pathol* 1988;15:129–141.

170. Perez-Atayde AR, Newbury R, Fletcher JA, et al. Congenital "neurovascular hamartoma" of the skin: a possible marker of malignant rhabdoid tumor. *Am J Surg Pathol* 1994;18:1030–1038.

171. Shitabata PK, Ritter JH, Fitzgibbon JF, et al. Pleomorphic hamartoma of the subcutis: a lesion with possible myogenous and neural lineages. *J Cutan Pathol* 1995;22:269–275.

172. Kamino H, Lee JYY, Berke A. Pleomorphic fibroma of the skin: a benign neoplasm with cytologic atypia. *Am J Surg Pathol* 1989;13: 107–113.

173. Shmookler BM, Enzinger FM. Pleomorphic lipoma: a benign tumor simulating liposarcoma. *Cancer* 1981;47:126–135.

174. Markel SF, Enzinger FM. Neuromuscular hamartoma: a benign "triton" tumor composed of mature neural and striated muscle elements. *Cancer* 1982;49:140–144.

175. Ashfaq R, Timmons CF. Rhabdomyomatous mesenchymal hamartoma of skin. *Pediatr Pathol* 1992;12:731–735.

176. Sahn EE, Garen PD, Pai GS, et al. Multiple rhabdomyomatous mesenchymal hamartomas of skin. *Am J Dermatopathol* 1990;12: 485–491.

177. Mills AE. Rhabdomyomatous mesenchymal hamartoma of skin. *Am J Dermatopathol* 1989;11:58–63.

178. Dehner LP, Enzinger FM, Font RL. Fetal rhabdomyoma: an analysis of nine cases. *Cancer* 1972;30:160–166.

179. Kapadia SB, Meis JM, Frisman DM, et al. Adult rhabdomyoma of the head and neck: a clinicopathologic and immunophenotypic study. *Hum Pathol* 1993;24:608–617.

180. Konwaler BE, Keasbey L, Kaplan L. Subcutaneous pseudosarcomatous fibromatosis (fasciitis). *Am J Clin Pathol* 1955;25:241–252.

181. Allen PW. Nodular fasciitis. *Pathology* 1972;4:9–26.

182. Shimizu S, Hashimoto H, Enjoji M. Nodular fasciitis: an analysis of 250 patients. *Pathology* 1984;16:161–166.

183. Montgomery EA, Meis JM. Nodular fasciitis: its morphologic spectrum and immunohistochemical profile. *Am J Surg Pathol* 1991;15: 942–948.

184. Price SK, Kahn LB, Saxe N. Dermal and intravascular fasciitis: unusual variants of nodular fasciitis. *Am J Dermatopathol* 1993;15: 539–543.

185. Goodlad JR, Fletcher CDM. Intradermal variant of nodular fasciitis. *Histopathology* 1990;17:569–571.

186. Lai FMM, Lam WY. Nodular fasciitis of the dermis. *J Cutan Pathol* 1993;20:66–69.

187. Zuber TJ, Finley JL. Nodular fasciitis. *South Med J* 1994;87:842–844.

188. Batsakis JG, El-Naggar AK. Pseudosarcomatous proliferative lesions of soft tissues. *Ann Otol Rhinol Laryngol* 1994;103:578–582.

189. Stanley MW, Skoog L, Tani EM, Horwitz CA. Nodular fasciitis: spontaneous resolution following diagnosis by fine needle aspiration. *Diagn Cytopathol* 1993;9:322–324.

190. Enzinger FM, Weiss SW. *Soft tissue tumors.* 3rd ed. St. Louis: CV Mosby, 1994;167–176.

191. Oshiro Y, Fukuda T, Tsuneyoshi M. Fibrosarcoma versus fibromatoses and cellular nodular fasciitis. *Am J Surg Pathol* 1994;18: 712–719.

192. Proppe KH, Scully RE, Rosai J. Postoperative spindle cell nodules of genitourinary tract resembling sarcomas: a report of eight cases. *Am J Surg Pathol* 1984;8:101–108.

193. Huang WL, Ro JY, Grignon DJ, et al. Postoperative spindle cell nodule of the prostate and bladder. *J Urol* 1990;143:824–826.

194. Jones EC, Young RH. Non-neoplastic and neoplastic spindle cell proliferations and mixed tumors of the urinary bladder. *J Urol Pathol* 1994;2:105–134.

195. Wick MR, Brown BA, Young RH, Mills SE. Spindle cell proliferations of the urinary tract: an immunohistochemical study. *Am J Surg Pathol* 1988;12:379–389.

196. Lopez DA, Silvers DN, Helwig EB. Cutaneous meningioma: a clinicopathologic study. *Cancer* 1974;34:728–744.

197. Sibley DA, Cooper PH. Rudimentary meningocele: a variant of "primary cutaneous meningioma." *J Cutan Pathol* 1989;16:72–80.

198. Suster S, Rosai J. Hamartoma of the scalp with ectopic meningothelial elements. *Am J Surg Pathol* 1990;14:1–11.
199. Marrogi AJ, Swanson PE, Kyriakos M, Wick MR. Rudimentary meningocele of the skin. *J Cutan Pathol* 1991;18:178–188.
200. Stone MS, Walker PS, Kennard CD. Rudimentary meningocele presenting with a scalp hair tuft: report of two cases. *Arch Dermatol* 1994;130:775–777.
201. Dymock RB, Allen PW, Stirling JW, et al. Giant cell fibroblastoma: a distinctive recurrent tumor of childhood. *Am J Surg Pathol* 1987;11:263–271.
202. Brunsting HA. Nasal glioma. *Cutis* 1981;27:43–46.
203. Gebhart W, Hohlbrugger H, Lassmann H, Ramadan W. Nasal glioma. *Int J Dermatol* 1982;21:212–215.
204. Fletcher CDM, Carpenter G, McKee PH. Nasal glioma: a rarity. *Am J Dermatopathol* 1986;8:341–346.
205. Mirra SS, Pearl GS, Hoffman JC, Campbell WG Jr. Nasal glioma with prominent neuronal component. *Arch Pathol Lab Med* 1981;105:540–541.
206. Patterson K, Kapur S, Chandra RS. "Nasal glioma" and related brain heterotopias. *Pediatr Pathol* 1986;5:353–362.
207. Younis M, Coode PE. Nasal glioma and encephalocele: two separate entities. *J Neurosurg* 1986;64:516–519.
208. Barkovich AJ, Vandermarck P, Edwards MSB, Cogen PH. Congenital nasal masses: CT and magnetic resonance imaging features in 16 cases. *Am J Neuroradiol* 1991;12:105–116.
209. Murphy GF, Mihm MC Jr, eds. *Lymphoproliferative disorders of the skin.* Boston: Butterworth, 1986.
210. Rijlaarsdam JU, Eillemze R. Cutaneous pseudo-T-cell lymphomas. *Semin Diagn Pathol* 1991;8:102–108.
211. LeBoit PE. Variants of mycosis fungoides and related cutaneous T-cell lymphomas. *Semin Diagn Pathol* 1991;8:73–81.
212. LeBoit PE. Cutaneous lymphomas and their histopathologic imitators. *Semin Dermatol* 1986;5:322–333.
213. Toonstra J. Actinic reticuloid. *Semin Diagn Pathol* 1991;8:109–116.
214. Wolf R, Kahane E, Sandbank M. Mycosis fungoides-like lesions associated with phenytoin therapy. *Arch Dermatol* 1985;121:1181–1182.
215. Rijlaarsdam JU, Boorsma DM, De Haan P, et al. The significance of Leu-8 negative T-cells in lymphoid skin infiltrates. *Br J Dermatol* 1990;123:587–593.
216. Bignon YJ, Souteyrand P. Genotyping of cutaneous T-cell lymphomas and pseudolymphomas. *Curr Prob Dermatol* 1990;19:114–123.
217. Banks PM. Lymphoid neoplasms. In: Wick MR, ed. *Pathology of unusual malignant cutaneous tumors.* New York: Marcel Dekker, 1985;299–356.
218. Evans HL, Winkelmann RK, Banks PM. Differential diagnosis of malignant and benign cutaneous lymphoid infiltrates. *Cancer* 1979;44:699–717.
219. Burke JS. Malignant lymphomas of the skin: their differentiation from lymphoid and nonlymphoid cutaneous infiltrates that simulate lymphoma. *Semin Diagn Pathol* 1985;2:169–182.
220. Caro WA, Helwig EB. Cutaneous lymphoid hyperplasia. *Cancer* 1969;24:487–502.
221. Medeiros LJ, Picker LJ, Abel EA, et al. Cutaneous lymphoid hyperplasia: immunologic characteristics and assessment of criteria recently proposed as diagnostic of malignant lymphoma. *J Am Acad Dermatol* 1989;21:929–942.
222. McDonald DM. Histopathological differentiation of benign and malignant cutaneous lymphocytic infiltrates. *Br J Dermatol* 1982;107:715–718.
223. Van Hale HM, Winkelmann RK. Nodular lymphoid disease of the head and neck: lymphocytoma cutis, benign lymphocytic infiltrate of Jessner, and their distinction from malignant lymphoma. *J Am Acad Dermatol* 1985;12:455–461.
224. Ashworth J, Turbitt M, Mackie R. A comparison of the dermal infiltrates in discoid lupus erythematosus and Jessner's lymphoid infiltrate of the skin using the monoclonal antibody Leu 8. *J Cutan Pathol* 1987;14:198–201.
225. Iwatsuki K, Tagami H, Moriguchi T, Yamada M. Lymphadenoid structure induced by gold hypersensitivity. *Arch Dermatol* 1982;118:608–611.
226. Silverman AK, Fairley J, Wong RC. Cutaneous and immunologic reactions to phenytoin. *J Am Acad Dermatol* 1988;18:721–741.
227. Blumenthal G, Okun MR, Ponitch JA. Pseudolymphomatous reaction to tattoos. *J Am Acad Dermatol* 1982;6:485–488.

228. Hammer E, Sangueza O, Suwanjindar P, et al. Immunophenotypic and genotypic analysis in cutaneous lymphoid hyperplasias. *J Am Acad Dermatol* 1993;28:426–433.
229. Weinberg JM, Rook AH, Lessin SR. Molecular diagnosis of lymphocytic infiltrates of the skin. *Arch Dermatol* 1993;129:1491–1500.
230. Wick MR, Swanson PE, Ritter JH, Fitzgibbon JF. Immunohistology of cutaneous neoplasia: a practical perspective. *J Cutan Pathol* 1993;20:481–497.
231. Ritter JH, Adesokan PN, Fitzgibbon JF, Wick MR. Paraffin section immunohistochemistry as an adjunct to morphologic analysis in the diagnosis of cutaneous lymphoid infiltrates. *J Cutan Pathol* 1994;21:481–493.
232. Triscott JA, Ritter JH, Swanson PE, Wick MR. Immunoreactivity for bcl-2 protein in cutaneous lymphomas and lymphoid hyperplasias. *J Cutan Pathol* 1995;22:2–10.
233. Wood GS, Weiss LM, Warnke RA, Sklar J. The immunopathology of cutaneous lymphomas: immunophenotypic and immunogenotypic characteristics. *Semin Diagn Pathol* 1986;5:334–345.
234. Ralfkiaer E. Immunohistological markers for the diagnosis of cutaneous lymphomas. *Semin Diagn Pathol* 1991;8:62–72.
235. White JW Jr, Olsen KD, Banks PM. Plasma cell orificial mucositis. *Arch Dermatol* 1986;122:1321–1324.
236. Luger A. Cheilitis plasmacellularis. *Hautarzt* 1966;17:244–248.
237. Batsakis JG. Plasma cell tumors of the head and neck. *Ann Otol Rhinol Laryngol* 1983;92:311–313.
238. Ferreiro JA, Egorshin EV, Olsen KD, et al. Mucous membrane plasmacytosis of the upper aerodigestive tract: a clinicopathologic study. *Am J Surg Pathol* 1994;18:1048–1053.
239. Headington JT. The histiocyte: in memoriam. *Arch Dermatol* 1986;122:532–533.
240. Foucar E, Rosai J, Dorfman R. Sinus histiocytosis with massive lymphadenopathy (Rosai–Dorfman disease): review of the entity. *Semin Diagn Pathol* 1990;7:19–73.
241. Thawerani H, Sanchez RL, Rosai J, et al. The cutaneous manifestations of sinus histiocytosis with massive lymphadenopathy. *Arch Dermatol* 1978;114:191–197.
242. Suster S, Cartagena N, Cabello-Inchausti B, Robinson MJ. Histiocytic lymphophagocytic panniculitis: an unusual extranodal presentation of sinus histiocytosis with massive lymphadenopathy (Rosai–Dorfman disease). *Arch Dermatol* 1988;124:1246–1251.
243. Chu P, LeBoit PE. Histologic features of cutaneous sinus histiocytosis with massive lymphadenopathy (Rosai–Dorfman disease): study of cases both with and without systemic involvement. *J Cutan Pathol* 1992;19:201–206.
244. Palou J, Torres H, Baradad M, et al. Cutaneous malakoplakia. *Dermatologica* 1988;176:288–292.
245. Chan ACL, Lorentz TG, Ma L, et al. Fine needle aspiration of cutaneous malakoplakia. *Diagn Cytopathol* 1993;9:576–580.
246. Nieland ML, Silverman AR, Borochovitz D, Saferstein AL. Cutaneous malakoplakia. *Am J Dermatopathol* 1981;3:287–301.
247. Moore WM III, Stokes TL, Cabanas VY. Malakoplakia of the skin. *Am J Clin Pathol* 1973;60:218–221.
248. Singh M, Kaur S, Vajpayee BK, Banerjee AK. Cutaneous malakoplakia with dermatomyositis. *Int J Dermatol* 1987;26:190–191.
249. Palazzo JP, Ellison DJ, Garcia IE, et al. Cutaneous malakoplakia simulating relapsing malignant lymphoma. *J Cutan Pathol* 1990;17:171–175.
250. Price HM, Hanrahan JB, Florida RG. Morphogenesis of calcium laden cytoplasmic bodies in malakoplakia of the skin. *Hum Pathol* 1973;4:381–394.
251. Sencer O, Sencer H, Uluoglu O, et al. Malakoplakia of the skin: ultrastructural and quantitative x-ray microanalysis of Michaelis–Gutmann bodies. *Arch Pathol Lab Med* 1979;103:446–450.

## ADDENDUM REFERENCES

### *Epidermal Nevi*

Cohen MM Jr. Perspectives on craniofacial asymmetry. VI. The hamartoses. *Int J Oral Maxillofac Surg* 1995;24:195–200.
Gurecki PJ, Holden KR, Sahn EE, Dyer DS, Cure JK. Developmental neural abnormalities and seizures in epidermal nevus syndrome. *Devel Med Child Neurol* 1996;38:716–723.

Hamanaka S, Otsuka F. Multiple malignant eccrine poroma and a linear epidermal nevus. *J Dermatol* 1996;23:469–471.

Happle R. Epidermal nevus syndromes. *Semin Dermatol* 1995;14:111–121.

Happle R, Mittag H, Kuster W. The CHILD nevus: a distinct skin disorder. *Dermatology* 1995;19:210–216.

Oram Y, Arisoy AE, Hazneci E, Gurer I, Muezzinoglu B, Arisoy ES. Bilateral inflammatory linear verrucous epidermal nevus associated with psoriasis. *Cutis* 1996;57:275–278.

Paller AS, Syder AJ, Chan YM, Yu QC, Hutton E, Tadini G, Fuchs E. Genetic and clinical mosaicism in a type of epidermal nevus. *N Engl J Med* 1994;331:140.

### Appendageal Nevi & Hamartomas

Alessi E, Azzolini A. Localized hair follicle hamartoma. *J Cutan Pathol* 1993;20:364–367.

Brownstein MH. Basaloid follicular hamartoma: solitary and multiple types. *J Am Acad Dermatol* 1992;27:237–240.

Choi EH, Ahn SK, Lee SH, Bang D. Hair follicle nevus. *Int J Dermatol* 1992;31:578–581.

De Viragh PA. Hair follicle nevus: an entity of its own? *Dermatology* 1993;187:213–214.

Goldhahn RT Jr. Basaloid follicular hamartoma. *J Am Acad Dermatol* 1994;31:131–132.

Hermann JJ, Eramo LR. Congenital apocrine hamartoma: an unusual clinical variant of organoid nevus with apocrine differentiation. *Pediatr Dermatol* 1995;12:248–251.

Kato N, Ueno H, Nakamura J. Localized basaloid follicular hamartoma. *J Dermatol* 1992;19:614–617.

Komura A, Tani M. Hair follicle nevus. *Dermatology* 1992;185:154–155.

Mori O, Hachisuka H, Sasai Y. Apocrine nevus. *Int J Dermatol* 1993;32:448–449.

Neill JS, Park HK. Apocrine nevus: light microscopic, immunohistochemical, and ultrastructural studies of a case. *J Cutan Pathol* 1993;20:79–83.

Nelson BR, Johnson TM, Waldinger T, Gillard M, Lowe L. Basaloid follicular hamartoma: a histologic diagnosis with diverse clinical presentations. *Arch Dermatol* 1993;129:915–917.

Nishikawa Y, Tokusashi Y, Saito Y, Ogawa K, Miyokawa N, Katagiri M. A case of apocrine adenocarcinoma associated with hamartomatous apocrine gland hyperplasia of both axillae. *Am J Surg Pathol* 1994;18:832–836.

### Pseudoepitheliomatous Epidermal Hyperplasia

Calhoun KH, Wagner RF Jr, Kumar D, Hokanson JA. Pseudoepitheliomatous hyperplasia mistaken for cancer after delayed reconstruction. *South Med J* 1995;88:454–457.

Gattuso P, Candel AG, Castelli MJ, Kowal-Vern A, Gamelli RL, Hermann C. Pseudoepitheliomatous hyperplasia in chronic cutaneous wounds: a flow cytometric study. *J Cutan Pathol* 1994;21:312–315.

### Sarcoma-like Proliferations of the Dermis

Samaratunga H, Searle J, O'Loughlin B. Nodular fasciitis and related pseudosarcomatous lesions of soft tissue. *Austr NZ J Surg* 1996;66:22–25.

### "Der Wulst" (Follicular "Bulge")

Akiyama M, Dale BA, Sun TT, Holbrook KA. Characterization of hair follicle bulge in human fetal skin: the human fetal bulge is a pool of undifferentiated keratinocytes. *J Invest Dermatol* 1995;287:279–284.

DeViragh PA, Meuli M. Human scalp hair follicle development from birth to adulthood: statistical study with special regard to putative stem cells in the bulge and proliferating cells in the matrix. *Arch Dermatol Res* 1995;287:279–284.

### Pseudoneoplastic Necrobiotic Granulomas and Differential Diagnoses

Golden BD, Wong DC, Diconstanzo D, Solomon G. Rheumatoid papules in a patient with acquired immune deficiency syndrome and symmetric polyarthritis. *J Rheumatol* 1996;23:760–762.

Halling AC, Wollan PC, Pritchard DJ, Vlasak R, Nascimento AG. Epithelioid sarcoma: a clinicopathologic review of 55 cases. *Mayo Clin Proc* 1996;71:636–642.

Hollowood K, Fletcher CDM. Soft tissue sarcomas that mimic benign lesions. *Semin Diagn Pathol* 1995;12:87–97.

Von Hochstetter AR, Cserhati MD. Epithelioid sarcoma presenting as chronic synovitis and mistaken for osteosarcoma. *Skel Radiol* 1995;24:636–638.

### Acroangiodermatitis (Pseudo-Kaposi's Sarcoma)

Kanitakis J, Narvaez D, Claudy A. Expression of the CD34 antigen distinguishes Kaposi's sarcoma from pseudo-Kaposi's sarcoma (acroangiodermatitis). *Br J Dermatol* 1996;134:44–46.

### Pigmented Purpura (Majocchi-Schamberg Disease)

Ghersetich I, Lotti T, Bacci S, Comacchi C, Campanile G, Romagnoli P. Cell infiltrate in progressive pigmented purpura (Schamberg's disease): immunophenotype, adhesion receptors, and intercellular relationships. *Int J Dermatol* 1995;34:846–850.

### Intravascular Papillary Endothelial Hyperplasia (Masson's Lesion)

Cisco RW, McCormac RM. Intravascular papillary endothelial hyperplasia of the foot. *J Foot Ankle Surg* 1994;33:610–616.

Del Rio E, Aguilar A, Sanchez-Yus E. Intravascular papillary endothelial hyperplasia: a reorganizing thrombus. *Int J Dermatol* 1992;31:713–714.

Levere SM, Barsky SH, Meals RA. Intravascular papillary endothelial hyperplasia: a neoplastic "actor" representing an exaggerated attempt at recanalization mediated by basic fibroblast growth factor. *J Hand Surg (A)* 1994;19:559–564.

Renshaw AA, Rosai J. Benign atypical vascular lesions of the lip: a study of 12 cases. *Am J Surg Pathol* 1993;17:557–565.

Stewart M, Smoller BR. Multiple lesions of intravascular papillary endothelial hyperplasia (Masson's lesion). *Arch Pathol Lab Med* 1994;118:315–316.

### Reactive Angioendotheliomatosis

Judge MR, McGibbon DH, Thompson RP. Angioendotheliomatosis associated with Castleman's lymphoma and POEMS syndrome. *Clin Exp Dermatol* 1993;18:360–362.

Krell JM, Sanchez RL, Solomon AR. Diffuse dermal angiomatosis: a variant of reactive cutaneous angioendotheliomatosis. *J Cutan Pathol* 1994;21:363–370.

### Pseudoneoplastic (Histoid) Leprosy

Kontochristopoulos GJ, Aroni K, Panteleos DN, Tosca AD. Immunohistochemistry in histoid leprosy. *Int J Dermatol* 1995;34:777–781.

### Mycobacterial Pseudotumors of the Skin

Perrin C, Michiels JF, Bernard E, Hofman P, Rosenthal E, Loubiere R. Cutaneous spindle cell pseudotumors due to *Mycobacterium gordonae* and *Leishmania infantum*: an immunophenotypic study. *Am J Dermatopathol* 1993;15:553–558.

### Fibrous Hamartoma of Infancy

Effem SE, Ekpo MD. Clinicopathological features of untreated fibrous hamartoma of infancy. *J Clin Pathol* 1993;46:522–524.

Michal M, Mukensnabl P, Chlumska A, Kodet R. Fibrous hamartoma of infancy: a study of eight cases with immunohistochemical and electron microscopical findings. *Pathol Res Pract* 1992;188:1049–1053.

Popek EJ, Montgomery EA, Fourcroy JL. Fibrous hamartoma of infancy in the genital region: findings in 15 cases. *J Urol* 1994;152:990–993.

Sotelo-Avila C, Bale PM. Subdermal fibrous hamartoma of infancy: pathology of 40 cases and differential diagnosis. *Pediatr Pathol* 1994;14:39–52.

Stock JA, Niku SD, Packer MG, Krous H, Kaplan GW. Fibrous hamartoma of infancy: a report of two cases in the genital region. *Urology* 1995;45:130–131.

Zogno C, Berti E, Coci A, Schiaffino E. Fibrous hamartoma in childhood. *Pathologica* 1994;86:319–323.

### Smooth Muscle Hamartoma and Becker's Nevus

De La Espirella J, Grossin M, Marinho E, Belaich S. Smooth muscle hamartoma: anatomoclinical characteristics and nosological limits. *Ann Dermatol Venereol* 1993;120:879–883.

Gagne EJ, Su WPD. Congenital smooth muscle hamartoma of the skin. *Pediatr Dermatol* 1993;10:142–145.

Hsiao GH, Chen JS. Acquired genital smooth muscle hamartoma: a case report. *Am J Dermatopathol* 1995;17:67–70.

Prigent F. Smooth muscle hamartoma and congenital hypertrichosis. *Ann Dermatol Venereol* 1992;119:489.

Zarate-Moysen A, Feregrino-Hernandez HE, Delgado-Fernandez A, Vega-Memije E. Becker's melanosis: a case report. *Bol Med Hosp Infant Mex* 1992;49:762–765.

### *Neurofollicular and Neurocristic Hamartomas of the Skin*

Crowson AN, Magro CH, Clark WH Jr. Pilar neurocristic hamartoma. *J Am Acad Dermatol* 1996;34:715.

Pearson JP, Weiss SW, Headington JT. Cutaneous malignant melanotic neurocristic tumors arising in neurocristic hamartomas: a melanocytic tumor morphologically and biologically distinct from common melanoma. *Am J Surg Pathol* 1996;20:665–677.

Sangueza OP, Requena L. Neurofollicular hamartoma: a new histogenetic interpretation. *Am J Dermatopathol* 1994;16:150–154.

### *Rhabdomyomatous Mesenchymal Hamartoma of the Skin*

Farris PE, Manning S, Vuitch F. Rhabdomyomatous mesenchymal hamartoma. *Am J Dermatopathol* 1994;16:73–75.

### *Nodular Fasciitis*

Samaratunga H, Searle J, O'Loughlin B. Nodular fasciitis and related pseudosarcomatous lesions of soft tissues. *Austr NZ J Surg* 1996;66:22–25.

### *Rudimentary Meningoceles and Glial Heterotopias of the Skin*

Miyamoto T, Mihara M, Hagari Y, Shimao S. Primary cutaneous meningioma on the scalp: report of two siblings. *J Dermatol* 1995;22:611–619.

Stone MS, Walker PS, Kennard CD. Rudimentary meningocele presenting with a scalp hair tuft: report of two cases. *Arch Dermatol* 1994;130:775–777.

Tashiro Y, Sueishi K, Nakao K. Nasal glioma: an immunohistochemical and ultrastructural study. *Pathol Int* 1995;45:393–398.

Thomson HG, Al-Qattan MM, Becker LE. Nasal glioma: is dermis involvement significant? *Ann Plast Surg* 1995;34:168–172.

### *Benign Lymphoid and Plasmacytic Infiltrates of the Skin*

Don PC, Rubinstein R, Christie S. Malignant syphilis (lues maligna) and concurrent infection with HIV. *Int J Dermatol* 1995;34:403–407.

Fan K, Kelly R, Kendrick V. Nonclonal lymphocytic proliferation in cutaneous lymphoid hyperplasia: a flow-cytometric and morphological analysis. *Dermatology* 1992;185:113–119.

Martin DH, Mroczkowski TF. Dermatologic manifestations of sexually transmitted diseases other than HIV. *Infect Dis Clin N Am* 1994;8:533–582.

Norgard MV, Riley BS, Richardson JA, Radolf JD. Dermal inflammation elicited by synthetic analogs of *Treponema pallidum* and *Borrelia burgdorferi* lipoproteins. *Infect Immun* 1995;63:1507–1515.

Pandhi RK, Singh N, Ramam M. Secondary syphilis: a clinicopathologic study. *Int J Dermatol* 1995;34:240–243.

### *Rosai-Dorfman Disease of the Skin*

Foss HD, Herbst H, Araujo L, Hummel M, Berg E, Schmitt-Graff A, Stein H. Monokine expression in Langerhans' cell histiocytosis and sinus histiocytosis with massive lymphadenopathy (Rosai-Dorfman disease). *J Pathol* 1996;179:60–65.

Perez A, Rodriguez M, Febrer I, Aliaga A. Sinus histiocytosis confined to the skin: case report and review of the literature. *Am J Dermatopathol* 1995;17:384–388.

Perrin C, Michiels JF, Lacour JP, Chagnon A, Fuzibet JG. Sinus histiocytosis (Rosai-Dorfman disease) clinically limited to the skin: an immunohistochemical and ultrastructural study. *J Cutan Pathol* 1993;20:368–374.

*Pathology of Pseudoneoplastic Lesions,*
edited by M. R. Wick, P. A. Humphrey, and J. H. Ritter.
Lippincott-Raven Publishers, Philadelphia © 1997.

# CHAPTER 15

# Pseudoneoplastic Lesions of the Heart

Mark R. Wick, Jon H. Ritter, Jeffrey E. Saffitz, and Henry D. Tazelaar

Secondary tumors—usually representing metastatic melanomas, mammary carcinomas, and lung cancers—are by far the most often encountered tumors of the heart (1–4). Truly primary neoplasms of this organ and its investments are uncommon. Most of them are benign, and the majority are myxomas (5–9); these are seen with sufficient frequency that surgical pathologists are familiar with their morphologic characteristics (10). Malignant lesions arising in the endocardium, myocardium, or pericardium are exceedingly rare; however, fibrosarcomas, rhabdomyosarcomas, angiosarcomas, neurogenic sarcomas, malignant fibrous histiocytomas, liposarcomas, leiomyosarcomas, extraosseous osteosarcomas, synovial sarcomas, non-Hodgkin's lymphomas, and malignant mesotheliomas have been observed in such sites (1,7–9).

Aside from the above-cited proliferations, there remain a number of tumefactive intracardiac disorders that are capable of simulating neoplasms at both clinical and pathologic levels. Hamartomas, other developmental anomalies, inflammatory conditions, and selected hyperplasias and hypertrophies of endogenous tissue elements are included in this group. This chapter considers the pathologic characteristics of such lesions.

## HAMARTOMAS AND CHORISTOMAS OF THE HEART

At least three tumefactive lesions of the heart were originally described with the assumption that they represented truly neoplastic proliferations; however, with the passage of time and the accrual of clinicopathologic details on these disorders, it now appears virtually certain that they are hamartomatous growths. The conditions in question include rhabdomyomatous hamartoma (so-called cardiac rhabdomyoma), fibroelastomatous hamartoma (papillary fibroelastoma), and endodermal choristoma of the atrioventricular septum (mesothelioma of the atrioventricular node).

### Rhabdomyomatous Hamartomas

So-called rhabdomyomas of the heart are well known in the context of the tuberous sclerosis complex (TSC; Bourneville's disease), a multiorgan phakomatosis that also potentially affects the kidneys, lungs, central nervous system, and skin (1). Cardiac lesions occur in up to 50% of patients with TSC. The lesions may be single or multiple, and are characteristically nodular, measuring from 1 mm to several cm in maximal dimension. These may project into one of the four cardiac chambers or be totally intramural. Such rhabdomyomatous hamartomas (RHs) are presumably present from birth, inasmuch as they have been seen in TSC patients who die during infancy (11–13).

M.R. Wick, J.H. Ritter, and J.E. Saffitz: Department of Pathology, Washington University School of Medicine, St. Louis, Missouri 63110.
H.D. Tazelaar: Division of Anatomic Pathology, Mayo Medical School, Rochester, Minnesota 55905.

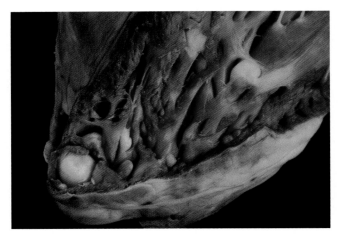

**FIG. 1.** Rhabdomyomatous hamartomas. Multiple white nodules are present in the right ventricle of a 2-year-old boy with tuberous sclerosis.

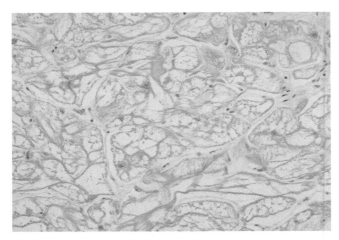

**FIG. 3.** Rhabdomyomatous hamartoma with large oval-to-polygonal cells containing vacuolated cytoplasm.

As summarized by McAllister and Fenoglio (1), RHs also may develop sporadically. Most of these patients are asymptomatic, and the lesions are discovered incidentally during cardiac angiography or echocardiography done for other reasons; but a minority present with symptoms and signs of congestive heart failure that are presumably attributable to the effects of the hamartoma(s) on myocardial contractility. Most non-TSC-related RHs affect individuals who are 25 years old or younger. Therapeutic intervention is necessary only if the lesions interfere with cardiac function; there have been no documented reports of malignant transformation in RHs.

Macroscopically, RHs are tan or tan–pink, homogeneous, and solid nodules (Fig. 1) that may exhibit a fascicular substructure on close inspection. They have a variably distinct interface with the surrounding myocardium, and virtually never show internal necrosis or hemorrhage.

Histologic examination shows broadly lobulated aggregates of large polygonal myogenic cells that focally show mature cardiac-type cytoplasmic cross-striations. Nuclei are

generally centrally located, with evenly distributed chromatin and small chromocenters (Figs. 2 and 3). Nuclear atypia and mitotic activity are virtually never encountered in RHs. A characteristic feature of "adult" or cardiac RHs is the presence of so-called "spider" cells (1,11–13). These are rhabdomyocytes in which artifactual retraction of the cytoplasm has occurred in a centripetal manner, leaving several radially disposed strands that are attached to the plasmalemma. These resemble the legs of a spider (Fig. 4).

Interestingly, two other patterns of "rhabdomyoma" that are seen in other topographic locations—namely, the "fetal" and "juvenile" types (14–16)—have not been reported in the heart. It may be that these lesions are truly neoplastic, thus accounting for the cited lack of anatomic overlap with cardiac RHs. Alternatively, one might posit that selected extracardiac "rhabdomyomas" are hamartomas that are indigenous only to skeletal-type striated muscle.

Selected examples of RHs with numerous "spider cells" might be confused with metastatic clear cell carcinomas or melanomas. In comparison with the latter neoplasms, however, the immunophenotype of RHs is distinctive. It features

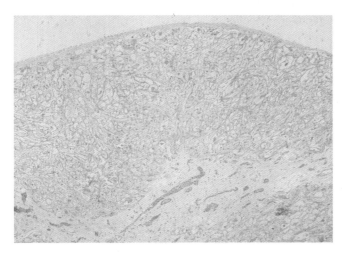

**FIG. 2.** Rhabdomyomatous hamartoma, seen at low power. Note the lobulated architecture of this subendocardial lesion.

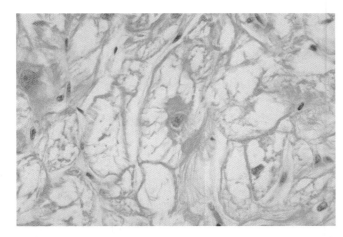

**FIG. 4.** Rhabdomyomatous hamartoma, showing a prominent "spider" cell with retraction of the cytoplasm.

without interspersed fetal fat or myocytes. They are typically located on the epicardial surface but have been rarely seen within the ventricular myocardium as well.

## BRONCHOGENIC CYSTS

Very uncommonly, tissue from the developing lung buds may be aberrantly entrapped in the fetal heart during embryogenesis. Later in life, these ectopic implants then become evident through the formation of an intracardiac bronchogenic cyst (IBC). In the experience of the Armed Forces Institute of Pathology (AFIP), all but one patient with IBC were adults between the ages of 35 and 75; however, the remaining individual was a 6-month-old baby who had tricuspid dysfunction because of displacement of the valve by an IBC of the superior interventricular septum (1).

McAllister and Fenoglio (1) found that bronchogenic cysts of the heart were most commonly <2 cm in maximum diameter, and that they were usually intramural myocardial lesions. The ventricular walls, interatrial septum, and interventricular myocardium were equally affected as sites of origin for this malformation. In similarity to bronchogenic cysts of the mediastinum and lungs, the contents of IBCs are mucoid and highly viscous.

Microscopic evaluation shows that bronchogenic cysts of the heart have a reproducibly structured architecture. The lining is typically composed of pseudostratified columnar respiratory epithelium with scattered goblet cells; if the cyst is inflamed, focal squamous metaplasia may also be present. Immediately peripheral to the epithelial core of the lesion, there is usually a mantle of hyaline cartilage—recapitulating formation of the bronchial plates; laminae of smooth muscle may also be seen (46). There are never any ectodermal, neuroectodermal, or nonrespiratory mesodermal elements in IBCs. The latter findings are unlike those seen in the principal differential diagnostic alternative, intracardiac teratoma (47).

## MESOTHELIAL-MONOCYTIC INTRACARDIAC EXCRESCENCES

Veinot et al. (48) recently described four examples of a lesion previously reported as resembling histiocytoid (epithelioid) hemangiomas occurring in the cardiovascular system, particularly the heart (49–51). The most recent evidence suggests that these lesions are best regarded as a type of artifactually produced pseudotumor. Twenty examples of cardiac mesothelial-monocytic intracardiac excrescences (MICE) have been reported, occurring in patients from 5 to 76 years of age. All have been incidental findings; some have been found to be free-floating by the surgeon in cardiac chambers or on cardiac valves, in right ventricular endomyocardial biopsy specimens, in the pericardial sac, in the specimen jars submitted to pathology, or in the ascending aorta. The lesions range in size from microscopic (true of those found in

endomyocardial biopsy specimens) up to 3 cm in diameter. All have been solitary. Grossly, they are dark red to brown, and frequently are associated with an obvious thrombus (Fig. 15).

Histologically, these excrescences are composed of two cell types, set in a background of fibrin. The first type features cytologically bland histiocytes, often present in sheets, in which representatives of the second cell type—which is more cuboidal in shape—are enmeshed. These elements form cords and pseudoglandular spaces, and they show central oval nuclei, dispersed or slightly vesicular chromatin, small nucleoli, and a moderate amount of amphophilic cytoplasm (Fig. 16).

Immunohistochemical analysis of MICE shows that one population of constituent cells is keratin-negative but expresses CD68—supporting its histiocytic/monocytic nature—whereas the more cuboidal and pseudoglandular component demonstrates the converse of this immunophenotype (48) (Fig. 17). Ultrastructural studies (Fig. 18) and additional immunohistologic assessments (for CEA and TAG-72) suggest mesothelial participation in the lesions.

The initial hypothesis regarding the origin of MICE stated that they might represent a form of mesothelial hyperplasia. This was thought to possibly represent a reaction to previous cardiac catheterization (75% of the patients in one series had such a history).

An additional premise has been put forward by Courtice and co-workers (51), as a result of examination of material found in extracorporeal bypass pumps and adherent to mediastinal and pericardial drains. Based on their study (in which cardiac MICE were observed in the filters of 82% of bypass pumps investigated and 13% of mediastinal and pericardial drains), Courtice and colleagues (51) suggested that the lesions were produced during cardiac surgery by compaction of friable mesothelial strips, other tissue, debris, and fibers on the cardiotomy suction tip. The agglomerated mass could then be transported around and from the operative site, and

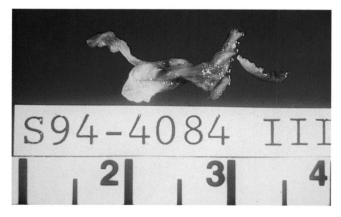

**FIG. 15.** Mesothelial/monocytic incidental cardiac excrescence (MICE). This heterogeneous mass is composed of an agglomeration of fibrin, erythrocytes, mesothelial cells, and monocytes.

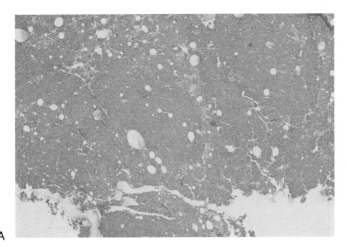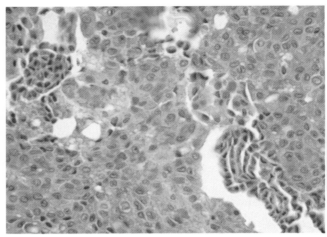

A                                                                                                    B

**FIG. 16.** MICE. Two cell types predominate in this lesion, represented by epithelioid histiocytes (**A**) and strips of cuboidal mesothelial cells (**B**).

thus be found free-floating by either the surgeon or the pathologist. This is certainly an intriguing hypothesis and may well explain the majority of examples of this lesion. It does not, however, account for cases found in right ventricular endomyocardial biopsy specimens; thus, rare examples of this lesion may result from perforation of the right ventricle and subsequent displacement of mesothelial cells into the cardiac chamber. Along with fibrin, previously circulating macrophages, and rare inflammatory cells, MICE probably form by cellular coalescence to yield a pseudoneoplasm, as emphasized by Courtice et al. (51). The lack of histologic attachment to underlying tissues and the absence of supporting stroma highlight the fact that the fibrin meshwork of MICE is not only a prominent feature of these lesions but is also likely an essential element in their formation and adherence to other tissues. The absence of stroma also makes it unlikely that these lesions actually have any capacity to grow other than by increasing the number of cells that adhere to the fibrinous matrix.

The importance of MICE lies in the potential for their mis-

diagnosis as metastatic adenocarcinoma, particularly in those examples that exhibit a prominent pseudoglandular component that is composed of cuboidal mesothelial cells. This mistake can be avoided by an awareness of their clinical presentation (they are usually incidental and unexpected) as well as by their biphasic cytologic features and characteristic immunophenotype. All of the latter points show consistent differences from the typical features of metastatic adenocarcinomas (52).

## INFLAMMATORY PSEUDOTUMOR (MYOFIBROBLASTIC TUMOR) OF THE HEART

Exceedingly rare accounts of intracardiac inflammatory pseudotumors (IIPT) have been reported. Grossly, these lesions have measured up to 3 cm in greatest dimension, and are typically smooth-surfaced, sessile lesions. They have been attached to the atrial or ventricular walls by a broad base, with projection into the lumina of the cardiac cham-

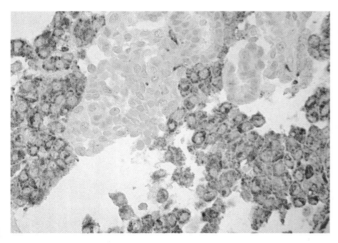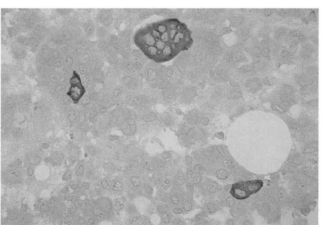

A                                                                                                    B

**FIG. 17.** MICE. The monocytes in this lesion express CD68 (**A**), whereas the cuboidal mesothelial cells are positive for keratin (**B**).

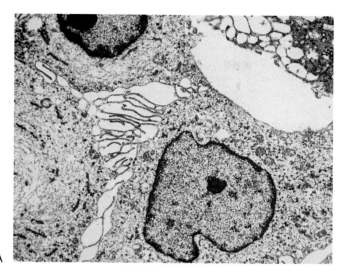
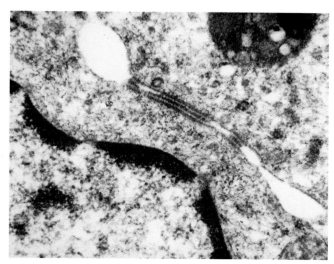

**FIG. 18.** MICE. Electron microscopy shows that the mesothelial cells in this lesion (**A**) possess long microvilli, cytoplasmic intermediate filaments, abundant rough endoplasmic reticulum, and desmosome-like intercellular junctions (**B**).

bers. The interface between an intracardiac IPT and the surrounding myocardium is usually indistinct. Children, adolescents, and young adults have typically been affected. In one case, a 17-year-old boy with an IIPT also developed leukocytoclastic (hypersensitivity) vasculitis, polyarteritis, and inferior vena caval thrombosis (53).

The histologic profile of cardiac inflammatory pseudotumor is no different than that of the same lesion in other topographic sites (Figs. 19 and 20). Therefore, it is not recounted at this point. The differential diagnosis focuses on true sarcomas of the heart (1), as well as lymphoreticular proliferations in examples of IIPT showing an abundance of lymphocytes and plasma cells. Distinguishing points between these lesions are similar to those outlined in reference to pseudotumors of the lungs (see Chapter 4).

## ATYPICAL ("PSEUDOLYMPHOMATOUS") LYMPHOID INFILTRATES OF THE MYOCARDIUM

There are several conditions wherein lymphoid infiltrates may be seen in the myocardium that simulate the histologic appearance of cardiac lymphoma. In endomyocardial biopsies, these often present challenging diagnostic problems.

### Severe Viral Myocarditis

Viral myocarditis [due to Coxsackie viruses, human immunodeficiency virus (HIV), or Epstein–Barr virus (EBV)] often becomes manifest with rapidly declining cardiac out-

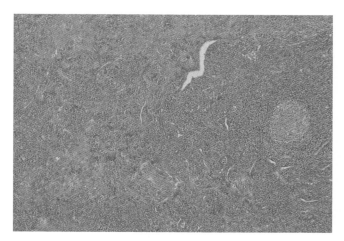

**FIG. 19.** Plasma cell granuloma (inflammatory pseudotumor) involving the myocardium. A germinal center is apparent, with an admixture of chronic inflammatory cells, including plasma cells and lymphocytes.

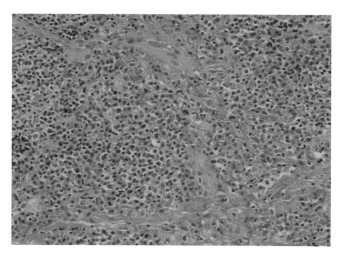

**FIG. 20.** Plasma cell granuloma (inflammatory pseudotumor) of the heart. Note the rich vascularity of the stroma and the heterogeneous cell population in this lesion.

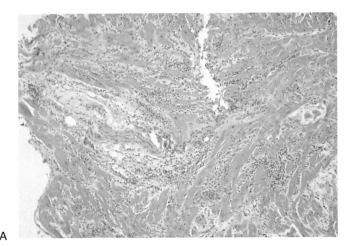

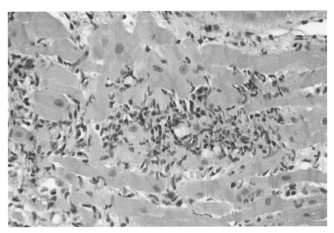

FIG. 21. T-cell malignant lymphoma involving the myocardium **(A)**. Myocyte damage is often associated with malignant hematopoietic infiltrates of the heart **(B)**.

put, progressive cardiomegaly, and corresponding symptoms and signs of congestive heart failure (54–56). Fever and other constitutional symptoms may or may not be evident, and patients of all ages are potentially affected.

Endomyocardial biopsy is often undertaken in such cases to obtain a histologic diagnosis, sometimes to justify immunosuppressive therapy (54–57). Although most of the problems with the histologic diagnosis of myocarditis revolve around its overdiagnosis (58), cases of diffuse severe myocarditis may resemble cardiac involvement by a lymphoproliferative process (59). This is particularly true when the lymphoid cells form partially confluent infiltrates of cytologically atypical, mitotic, "activated" lymphocytes. By definition, muscle cell damage or necrosis are present in myocarditis, but similar patterns of myocyte damage can be associated with hematopoietic malignancies as well (60,61) (Fig. 21).

A history of previous lymphoma or leukemia may be helpful in arriving at the correct diagnosis, but when the heart is the primary site of involvement, adjuvant studies may be necessary for definitive interpretation. The atypical but benign lymphoid infiltrates of typical viral myocarditis are composed of T cells (60), and the majority of cardiac lymphomas are B-cell in nature. B lymphocytes that are apparent in cases of myocarditis will be polytypic for light chain immunoglobulins by immunohistology or on molecular pathologic evaluation (e.g., using the polymerase chain reaction) for immunoglobulin light and heavy chain genes. In cases of suspected leukemic involvement, immunostains for myeloid determinants or the chloroacetate esterase stain may also be helpful (59).

Recipients of organ allografts and patients with the acquired immunodeficiency syndrome (AIDS) also can develop B-cell lymphoproliferative lesions of the myocardium that are "driven" by EBV (62,63). It can be particularly vexing to separate polyclonal examples of such disorders from monoclonal (overtly lymphomatous) proliferations, and molecular studies designed to assess the presence of episomal viral DNA might be valuable in such instances (64).

In a similar vein, in severe allograft rejection, which may feature atypical lymphocytes, a conjoint lack of immunoreactivity for CD20, CD43, and EBV latent membrane protein has been observed (64). In contrast, histologically similar

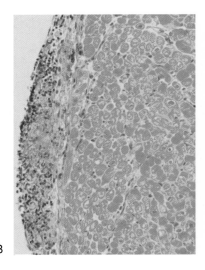
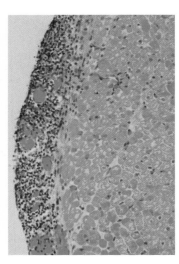

FIG. 22. Endocardial lymphocytic infiltrates ("Quilty" lesions). The infiltrates are often confined to the endocardium (**A,** trichrome stain) and usually have a rich capillary network **(B)**. They occasionally spill over into the underlying myocardium

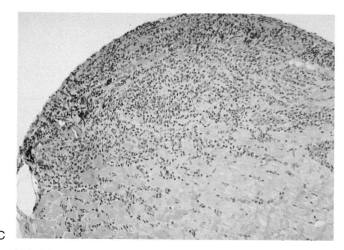

C

**FIG. 22.** *Continued* (**C**), where they might be associated with myocyte damage, and at least focally resemble lymphomas involving the heart.

posttransplant lymphoproliferative diseases do express these markers reproducibly (65). T-cell-mediated AIDS-related myocarditis can likewise be identified by positive immunostains for HIV p17 or p24 proteins in the infiltrating lymphocytes and cardiac interstitial cells (65).

### Florid "Quilty" Lesions in Cardiac Allografts

Approximately 10% of patients who have undergone cardiac transplantation develop a peculiar and brisk lymphocytic infiltrate in the endocardial surface of the allograft. This phenomenon has been named ELI (endocardial lymphocytic infiltrate) or the Quilty lesion, after the first patient who exhibited such a tissue response; it may be florid enough that the possibility of a posttransplantation lymphoproliferative disorder may enter the differential diagnosis (57,60). This may be particularly problematic in the form of the Quilty lesion, in which involvement of the underlying myocardium occurs (Fig. 22). These infiltrates are typically small (1–2 mm) nodular aggregates of lymphocytes (occa-

sionally with small numbers of plasma cells), punctuated by thin-walled dilated blood vessels. However, myocardial extension of the lymphoid cells may occur, and may be associated with myocyte damage. There is little mitotic activity or apoptosis, and immunoblasts are distinctly uncommon (57). These attributes differ from those of most cases of posttransplant lymphoproliferative disease, as well as *de novo* cardiac lymphoma. Immunohistology may prove useful in this differential diagnosis in that it shows a preponderance of T lymphocytes with small numbers of B cells in Quilty lesions (60) (Fig. 23). As stated above, such observations generally militate against a diagnosis of neoplastic lymphoproliferations in the posttransplant setting.

### PERICARDIAL MESOTHELIAL HYPERPLASIA

In likeness to reactions in the pleura, nonspecific or infectious pericarditis may incite florid mesothelial hyperplasia in association with a pericardial effusion (1). Focal lesions are typically inapparent on gross inspection of the external cardiac surface, but occasional examples of nodular hyperplasia have indeed been documented (66,67). Other cases might in fact simulate the macroscopic appearance of mesothelioma because the inflammatory response in the pericardium creates a dense fibrofibrinous rind involving both its visceral and parietal layers.

At a microscopic level, the distinction between reactive pericardial mesothelial hyperplasia and mesothelioma may also be a challenging one (Fig. 24). Reactive (but benign) mesothelial cells are capable of a striking degree of nuclear atypia (1,67), with prominent nucleoli and nuclear pleomorphism. Additionally, the presence of mesothelial cells nested deep within a thickened pericardium may also simulate invasion.

In cytologic preparations (without the benefit of architectural landmarks) one must rely on strict cytologic criteria for the separation of benign and malignant mesothelial proliferations (68,69). Numerous mitotic figures (especially if some are atypical) and any appreciable spindle cell growth favor the diagnosis of mesothelioma. Because one is dealing with

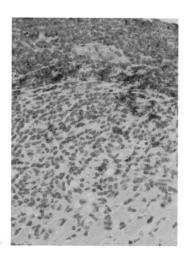
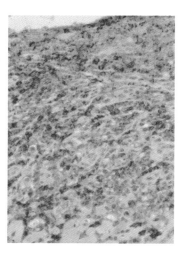

A, B

**FIG. 23.** Endocardial lymphocytic infiltrate. Small islands of B cells (**A**, CD20 stain) are interspersed among large numbers of T lymphocytes (**B**, CD45R0 stain).

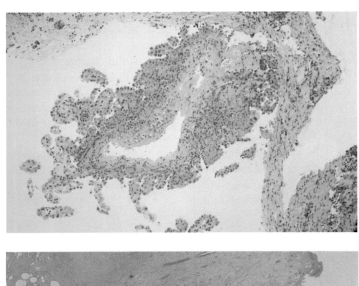

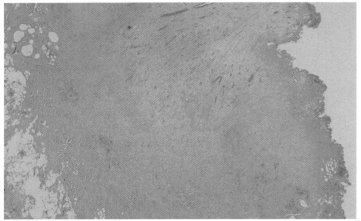

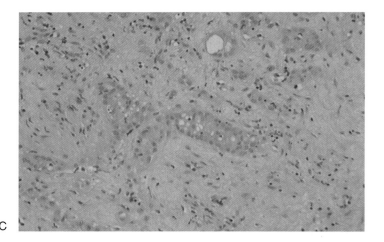

**FIG. 24.** Reactive mesothelial hyperplasia. The process may be papillary (**A**) or alternatively show deeply situated reactive mesothelium. The thickened pericardium shown (**B**) contains the deep tubular collections of mesothelial cells depicted (**C**).

mesothelial cells in both of these pathologic processes, histochemical and immunohistochemical stains have little or no value. However, some authors have suggested that adenocarcinoma and mesothelioma cells express EMA strongly, whereas reactive mesothelial cells are negative or only weakly positive for that marker (70). Mutant p53 protein has also recently been used to make this distinction, with p53 immunopositivity putatively being present in malignant

mesotheliomas and absent in reactive processes (71). Apparent invasion of adjacent tissue is occasionally seen in benign mesothelial proliferations, especially in the pericardium (72). The appearance of invasion must be interpreted with caution, particularly in small biopsies. Particularly with pericardial processes, the clinical history is often helpful. Patients may have idiopathic recurrent benign pericardial effusions for many years (68,72). Positive immunostains for

CEA, TAG-72, and the CD15 antigen would argue for the presence of yet another diagnostic alternative, namely that of metastatic adenocarcinoma in the pericardium (52).

## SUMMARY

Pseudoneoplastic lesions of the heart are limited in number, but they are important because of vast differences in the therapeutic approaches that attend their differential diagnostic alternatives. As is true of other entities discussed in this book, adjunctive pathologic studies may in some cases play a useful role in the recognition of cardiac pseudotumors. Nonetheless, the foundation of this process should still rest on thoroughness and skill in histologic evaluation.

## REFERENCES

1. Hanfling SM. Metastatic cancer to the heart. *Circulation* 1960;22:474-483.
2. Thurber DL, Edwards JE, Achor RW. Secondary malignant tumors of the pericardium. *Circulation* 1962;26:228–241.
3. Burnett RC, Shimkin MB. Secondary neoplasms of the heart. *Arch Intern Med* 1954;93:205–218.
4. McAllister HA Jr, Fenoglio JJ Jr. Tumors of the cardiovascular system. In: *Atlas of tumor pathology.* Series 2. Fascicle 15. Washington, DC: Armed Forces Institute of Pathology, 1978.
5. Fine G. Primary tumors of the pericardium and heart. *Cardiovasc Clin* 1973;5:207–238.
6. Prichard RW. Tumors of the heart: review of the subject and report of one hundred and fifty cases. *Arch Pathol* 1951;51:98–128.
7. Tazelaar HD, Locke TJ, McGregor CG. Pathology of surgically excised primary cardiac tumors. *Mayo Clin Proc* 1992;67:957–965.
8. Wiatrowska BA, Walley VM, Masters RG, et al. Surgery for cardiac tumors: the University of Ottawa Heart Institute experience. *Can J Cardiol* 1993;9:65–72.
9. Lund JT, Ehman RL, Julsrud PR, et al. Cardiac masses: assessment by MR imaging. *AJR* 1989;152:469–473.
10. Burke AP, Virmani R. Cardiac myxoma: a clinicopathologic study. *Am J Clin Pathol* 1993;100:671–680.
11. Fenoglio JJ Jr, McAllister HA Jr, Ferrans VJ. Cardiac rhabdomyoma: a clinicopathologic and electron microscopic study. *Am J Cardiol* 1976;38:241–251.
12. Taber RE, Lam CR. Diagnosis and surgical treatment of intracardiac myxoma and rhabdomyoma. *J Thorac Cardiovasc Surg* 1960;40:337–354.
13. Silverman JF, Kay S, McCue CM, Lower RR, et al. Rhabdomyomas of the heart: ultrastructural study of three cases. *Lab Invest* 1976;35:596–606.
14. Dehner LP, Enzinger FM, Font RL. Fetal rhabdomyoma: an analysis of nine cases. *Cancer* 1972;30:160–166.
15. Kapadia SB, Meis JM, Frisman DM, et al. Fetal rhabdomyoma of the head and neck: a clinicopathologic and immunophenotypic study of 24 cases. *Hum Pathol* 1993;24:754–765.
16. Crotty PL, Nakhleh RE, Dehner LP. Juvenile rhabdomyoma: an intermediate form of skeletal muscle tumor in children. *Arch Pathol Lab Med* 1993;117:43–47.
17. Lehtonen E, Asikainen U, Badley RA. Rhabdomyoma: ultrastructural features and distribution of desmin, muscle type of intermediate filament protein. *Acta Pathol Microbiol Immunol Scand* 1982;90:125–129.
18. Fishbein MC, Ferrans VJ, Roberts WC. Endocardial papillary fibroelastomas: histologic, histochemical, and electron microscopic findings. *Arch Pathol* 1975;39:335–341.
19. Pomerance A. Papillary tumors of the heart valves. *J Pathol* 1961;81:135–140.
20. Takahashi A, Kitaura K, Murayama Y, et al. A case of papillary fibroelastoma of the heart found 13 years after open mitral commisurotomy. *J Jpn Assoc Thorac Surg* 1993;41:2121–2125.
21. Wolfe JT III, Finck SJ, Safford RE, Persellin ST. Tricuspid valve papillary fibroelastoma: echocardiographic characterization. *Ann Thorac Surg* 1991;51:116–118.
22. Corbi P, Jebara V, Fabiani JN, et al. Benign tumors of the heart (excluding myxoma): experience with 9 surgically treated cases. *Ann Cardiol Angiol* 1990;39:433–436.
23. Gorton ME, Soltanzadeh H. Mitral valve fibroelastoma. *Ann Thorac Surg* 1989;47:605–607.
24. Seib HJ, Wildenauer M, Luther M, et al. Papillary fibroelastoma of the aortic valve: sudden death caused by an uncommon tumor of the heart. *Zeitschr Kardiol* 1984;73:409–413.
25. Almagro UA, Perry LS, Choi H, Pintar K. Papillary fibroelastoma of the heart: report of six cases. *Arch Pathol Lab Med* 1982;106:318–321.
26. Rubin MA, Snell J, Tazelaar HD, Lack EE, Austenfeld MD, Azumi N. Cardiac papillary fibroelastoma: an immunohistochemical investigation and unusual clinical manifestations. *Mod Pathol* 1995;8:402–407.
27. Raeburn C. Papillary fibroelastic hamartoma of the heart valves. *J Pathol* 1953;65:371–375.
28. Fine G, Morales AR. Mesothelioma of the atrioventricular node. *Arch Pathol* 1971;92:402–408.
29. Fenoglio JJ Jr, Jacobs DW, McAllister HA Jr. Ultrastructure of the mesothelioma of the atrioventricular node. *Cancer* 1977;40:721–727.
30. Manion WC, Nelson WP, Hall RJ, Brierty RE. Benign tumor of the heart causing complete heart block. *Am Heart J* 1972;83:535–542.
31. Burke AP, Anderson PG, Virmani R, et al. Tumor of the atrioventricular nodal region: a clinical and immunohistochemical study. *Arch Pathol Lab Med* 1990;114:1057–1062.
32. Franciosi RA, Singh A. Oncocytic cardiomyopathy syndrome. *Hum Pathol* 1988;19:1361–1362.
33. Keller BB, Mehta AV, Shamszadeh M, Marino TA, et al. Oncocytic cardiomyopathy of infancy with Wolff–Parkinson–White syndrome and ectopic foci causing tachydysrhythmias in children. *Am Heart J* 1987;114:782–792.
34. Silver MM, Burns JE, Sethi RK, Rowe RD. Oncocytic cardiomyopathy in an infant with oncocytosis in exocrine and endocrine glands. *Hum Pathol* 1980;11:598–605.
35. Kearney DL, Titus JL, Hawkins EP, et al. Pathologic features of myocardial hamartomas causing childhood tachyarrhythmias. *Circulation* 1987;75:705–710.
36. Ghargozloo F, Porter CJ, Tazelaar HD, Danielson GK. Multiple myocardial hamartomas causing ventricular tachycardia in young children: combined surgical modification and medical treatment. *Mayo Clin Proc* 1994;69:262–267.
37. Gelb AB, Van Meter SH, Billingham ME, Berry GJ, Rouse RV. Infantile histiocytoid cardiomyopathy—myocardial or conduction system hamartoma: what is the cell type involved? *Hum Pathol* 1993;24:1226–1231.
38. Ziegler VL, Gillette PC, Crawford FA, Wiles HB, Fyfe DA. New approaches to treatment of incessant ventricular tachycardia in the very young. *J Am Coll Cardiol* 1990;16:681–685.
39. Zimmerman A, Diem P, Cottier H. Congenital "histiocytoid" cardiomyopathy: evidence suggesting a developmental disorder of the Purkinje cell system of the heart. *Virchows Arch A Path Anat* 1982;396:187–195.
40. Basu S, Folliguet T, Anselmo M, et al. Lipomatous hypertrophy of the interatrial septum. *Cardiovasc Surg* 1994;2:229–231.
41. Shirani J, Roberts WC. Clinical, electrocardiographic, and morphologic features of massive fatty deposits ("lipomatous hypertrophy") in the atrial septum. *J Am Coll Cardiol* 1993;22:226–238.
42. Smith CE, Teague SM, Ameredes T, et al. Atrial septal lipomatous hypertrophy and ischemic heart disease: an unusual presentation. *J Clin Anesth* 1993;5:73–75.
43. Koehler U, Bittinger A. Lipomatous hypertrophy of the atrial septum: cardiac-induced syncope in hamartoma of the right heart atrium. *Deutsche Med Wochenschr* 1991;116:1393–1396.
44. Okel BB. The Wolff–Parkinson–White syndrome: report of a case with fatal arrhythmia and autopsy findings of myocarditis, interatrial lipomatous hypertrophy, and prominent right moderator band. *Am Heart J* 1968;75:673–678.
45. Roberts WC, Roberts JD. The floating heart or the heart too fat to sink: analysis of 55 necropsy patients. *Am J Cardiol* 1983;52:1286–1289.
46. Wick MR. Mediastinal cysts and intrathoracic thyroid tumors. *Semin Diagn Pathol* 1990;7:285–294.
47. Solomon RD. Malignant teratoma of the heart: report of a case with necropsy. *Arch Pathol* 1951;52:561–568.

48. Veinot JP, Tazelaar HD, Edwards WD, Colby TV. Mesothelial/mono-cytic incidental cardiac excrescences: cardiac MICE. *Mod Pathol* 1994; 7:9–16.
49. Luthringer DJ, Virmani R, Weiss SW, Rosai J. A distinctive cardiovas-cular lesion resembling histiocytoid (epithelioid) hemangioma. *Am J Surg Pathol* 1990;14:993–1000.
50. Rosai J, Gold S, Landy R. The histiocytoid hemangioma: a unifying concept embracing several previously described entities of skin, soft tissue, large vessels, bone, and heart. *Hum Pathol* 1979;10:707–730.
51. Courtice RW, Stinson WA, Walley VM. Tissue fragments recovered at cardiac surgery masquerading as tumoral proliferations: evidence sug-gesting iatrogenic or artefactual origin and common occurrence. *Am J Surg Pathol* 1994;18:167–174.
52. Wick MR. Immunohistochemistry in the diagnosis of solid malignant tumors. In: Jennette JC, ed. *Immunohistology in diagnostic pathology.* Boca Raton: CRC Press, 1989;161–191.
53. Stark P, Sandbank JC, Rudnicki C, Zahavi I. Inflammatory pseudotu-mor of the heart with vasculitis and venous thrombosis. *Chest* 1992; 102:1884–1885.
54. Edwards WD, Holmes DR Jr, Reeder GS. Diagnosis of active lympho-cytic myocarditis by endomyocardial biopsy. *Mayo Clin Proc* 1982;57: 419–428.
55. Aretz HT, Billingham ME, Edwards WD, et al. Myocarditis: a histopathologic definition and classification. *Am J Cardiovasc Pathol* 1987;1:3–10.
56. Aretz HT. Myocarditis: the Dallas classification. In: Virmani R, Atkin-son JB, Fenoglio JJ Jr, eds. *Cardiovascular pathology.* Philadelphia: WB Saunders, 1991; 246–256.
57. Fenoglio JJ Jr, Marboe CC. Endomyocardial biopsy. In: Sternberg SS, ed. *Diagnostic surgical pathology.* New York: Raven Press, 1989; 877–895.
58. Tazelaar HD. Surgical pathology of the heart: endomyocardial biopsy, valvular heart disease, and cardiac tumors. In: Schoen FJ, Gimbrone MA Jr, eds. *Cardiovascular pathology: clinicopathologic correlations and pathogenetic mechanisms.* Baltimore: Williams and Wilkins, 1995; 81–107.
59. Flipse TR, Tazelaar HD, Holmes DR Jr. Diagnosis of malignant cardiac disease by endomyocardial biopsy. *Mayo Clin Proc* 1990;65: 1415–1422.
60. Billingham ME. Cardiac transplant pathology. In: Hammond EH, ed. *Solid organ transplantation.* Philadelphia: WB Saunders, 1994;69–91.
61. Abu-Farsakh H, Cagle PT, Buffone GJ, et al. Heart allograft involve-ment with Epstein–Barr virus–associated posttransplant lymphoprolif-erative disorder. *Arch Pathol Lab Med* 1992;116:93–95.
62. Eisen HJ, Hicks D, Kant JA, et al. Diagnosis of posttransplantation lympholiferative disorder by endomyocardial biopsy in a cardiac allo-graft recipient. *J Heart Lung Transplant* 1994;13:241–245.
63. Cleary ML, Nalesnik MA, Shearer WT, et al. Clonal analysis of trans-plant-associated lymphoproliferations based on the structure of the ge-nomic termini of the Epstein–Barr virus. *Blood* 1988;72:349–352.
64. Ritter JH, Wick MR. Posttransplant lymphoproliferative disorders: im-munohistochemical differential diagnosis with severe allograft rejec-tion. *Int J Surg Pathol* 1994;2:105–116.
65. Ward JM, O'Leary TJ, Baskin GB, et al. Immunohistochemical local-ization of human and simian immunodeficiency viral antigens in fixed tissue sections. *Am J Pathol* 1987;127:199–205.
66. Sandhyamani S, Kartha CC, Pattankar VL, et al. Reactive mesothelial nodule of the pericardium. *Ind Heart J* 1984;36:169–172.
67. Rosai J, Dehner LP. Nodular mesothelial hyperplasia in hernia sacs: a benign reactive condition simulating a neoplastic process. *Cancer* 1975;35:165–175.
68. Wiener HG, Kristensen IB, Haubek A, et al. The diagnostic value of pericardial cytology: an analysis of 95 cases. *Acta Cytol* 1991;35: 149–153.
69. Leong ASY, Stevens MW, Mukherjee TM. Malignant mesothelioma: cytologic diagnosis with histologic, immunohistochemical, and ultra-structural correlation. *Semin Diagn Pathol* 1992;141–150.
70. Singh HK, Silverman JF, Berns L, Haddad ME, Park HK. Significance of epithelial membrane antigen in the workup of problematic serous ef-fusions. *Diagn Cytopathol* 1995;13:3–7.
71. Cagle PT, Brown RW, Lebovitz RM. p53 immunostaining in the dif-ferentiation of reactive processes from malignancy in pleural biopsy specimens. *Hum Pathol* 1994;25:443–448.
72. Fazekas T, Ungi I, Tiszlavicz L. Primary malignant mesothelioma of the pericardium. *Am Heart J* 1992;124:227–231.

## ADDENDUM REFERENCES

### *Rhabdomyomatous Hamartoma of the Heart*

Cowley CG, Tani LY, Judd VE, Shaddy RE. Sinus node dysfunction in tuberous sclerosis. *Pediatr Cardiol* 1996;17:51–52.
Demkow M, Sorensen K, Whitehead BF, Rees PG, Sullivan ID, Elliott MJ, de Leval MR. Heart transplantation in an infant with rhabdomyoma. *Pe-diatr Cardiol* 1995;16:204–206.
Green AJ, Smith M, Yates JR. Loss of heterozygosity on chromosome 16p13.3 in hamartomas from tuberous sclerosis patients. *Nature Genet* 1994;6:193–196.
Henske EP, Scheithauer BW, Short MP, Wollmann R, Nahmias J, Hornigold N, van Siegtenhorst M, Welsh CT, Kwiatkowski DJ. Allelic loss is frequent in tuberous sclerosis kidney lesions but rare in brain le-sions. *Am J Hum Genet* 1996;59:400–406.
Jozwiak S, Kawalec W, Diuzewska J, Daszkowska J, Mirkowicz-Malek M, Michalowicz R. Cardiac tumors in tuberous sclerosis: their incidence and course. *Eur J Pediatr* 1994;153:155–157.
Takach TJ, Reul GJ, Ott DA, Cooley DA. Primary cardiac tumors in infants and children: immediate and long-term operative results. *Ann Thorac Surg* 1996;62:559–564.

### *Fibroelastomatous Hamartoma of the Heart*

Shahian DM, Labib SB, Chang G. Cardiac papillary fibroelastoma. *Ann Thorac Surg* 1995;59:538–541.

### *Endodermal Choristoma ("Mesothelioma") of the Interatrial Septum*

Balasundaram S, Halees SA, Duran C. Mesothelioma of the atrioventricu-lar node: first successful followup after excision. *Eur Heart J* 1992;13: 718–719.
Bharati S, Bauernfeind R, Josephson M. Intermittent preexcitation and mesothelioma of the atrioventricular node: a hitherto undescribed entity. *J Cardiovasc Electrophysiol* 1995;6:823–831.
Matturri L, Nappo A, Varesi C, Rossi L. Cardiac block caused by metasta-sis of lung adenocarcinoma to the bundle of His. *Minerva Med* 1993;84: 141–144.
Monzon-Munoz FJ, Aguilera-Tapia B, Martinez-Penuela-Virseda JM, Oliva-Aldamiz H. Polycystic endodermal heterotopia of the atrioventric-ular node. *Med Clin* 1995;104:257–261.

### *Oncocytic Myocardial Metaplasia (Oncocytoma; Histiocytoid Cardiomyopathy)*

BirdLM, Krous HF, Eichenfield LF, Swalwell CI, Jones MC. Female infant with oncocytic cardiomyopathy and microphthalmia with linear skin de-fects (MLS): a clue to the pathogenesis of oncocytic cardiomyopathy? *Am J Med Genet* 1994;53:141–148.
Heifetz SA, Faught PR, Bauman M. Histiocytoid (oncocytic) cardiomyopa-thy. *Arch Pediatr Adolesc Med* 1995;149:464–465.
Koponen MA, Siegel RJ. Histiocytoid cardiomyopathy and sudden death. *Hum Pathol* 1996;27:420–423.
Otani M, Hoshida H, Saji T, Matsuo N, Kawamura S. Histiocytoid car-diomyopathy with hypotonia in an infant. *Pathol Int* 1995;45:774–780.
Ruszkiewicz AR, Vernon-Roberts E. Sudden death in an infant due to his-tiocytoid cardiomyopathy: a light microscopic, ultrastructural, and im-munohistochemical study. *Am J Forens Med Pathol* 1995;16:74–80.

### *Lipomatous Cardiac Hypertrophy*

Burke AP, Litovsky S, Virmani R. Lipomatous hypertrophy of the atrial septum presenting as a right atrial mass. *Am J Surg Pathol* 1996;20: 678–685.
Lam KY, Dickens P, Chan AC. Tumors of the heart: a 20 year experience with a review of 12,485 consecutive autopsies. *Arch Pathol Lab Med* 1993;117:1027–1031.

### *Bronchogenic Cysts of the Heart and Pericardium*

Hayashi AH, McLean DR, Peliowski A, Tierney AJ, Finer NN. A rare in-trapericardial mass in a neonate. *J Pediatr Surg* 1992;27:1361–1363.

### *Pseudoneoplastic Myocarditis*

Kuhl U, Noutsias M, Schultneiss HP. Immunohistochemistry in dilated car-diomyopathy. *Eur Heart J* 1995;16 (Suppl):100–106.

Schowengerdt KO, Ni J, Denfield SW, Gajarski RJ, Radovancevic B, Frazier HO, Demmier GJ, Kearney D, Bricker JT, Towbin JA. Diagnosis, surveillance, and epidemiologic evaluation of viral infections in pediatric cardiac transplant recipients with the use of the polymerase chain reaction. *J Heart Lung Transplant* 1996;15:111–123.

## Pseudoneoplastic Transplant-Related Lymphocytic Cardiac Infiltrates

Joshi A, Masek MA, Brown BW Jr, Weiss LM, Billingham ME. "Quilty" revisited: a 10-year perspective. *Hum Pathol* 1995;26:547–557.

Lozano MD, Pardo-Mindan FJ. Significance of endocardial infiltrates (Quilty effect) in the transplanted heart. *J Heart Lung Transplant* 1994; 13:733–734.

Luthringer DJ, Yamashita JT, Czer LS, Trento A, Fishbein MC. Nature and significance of epicardial lymphoid infiltrates in cardiac allografts. *J Heart Lung Transplant* 1995;14:537–543.

Sanchez-Vegazo I, Sanz E, Anaya A. Pathology of the heart transplant. *Rev Espan Cardiol* 1995;48(Suppl):65–70.

# Subject Index

*(Page references in **boldface** refer to illustrations.)*

## A

Abdomen
  cystic mesothelioma, 7
  inflammatory myofibroblastic tumors,
    134–136
  *See also specific anatomic structure*
Acroangiodermatitis, 9, **556**, 556–557,
  **557**
Acromegaly, 27, 347
Acrospiromas, 547
Actinomycosis
  female genital tract, 310, **311**
  pseudoepitheliomatous hyperplasia in,
    551
Adamantinoma, 425–426, **426**
Addison's disease, 361, 362
Adenocarcinoma, endometrial
  vs. adenomyosis-related change, 281
  vs. mucinous metaplasia, 278
Adenocarcinoma, heart
  vs. endodermal choristoma, 590–591
  vs. mesothelial-monocytic intracardiac
    excrescences, 594
Adenocarcinoma, pituitary gland, 344–345
Adenocarcinoma, prostate gland
  differential diagnosis, 223
  vs. adenosis, 223–225
  vs. atrophy, 223
  vs. sclerosing adenosis, 225
  vs. xanthoma, 230
Adenocarcinoma, uterine cervix
  intestinal metaplasia in, 276
  vs. changes secondary to extravasation
    of mucin, 275
  vs. clear cell change of pregnancy, 283
  vs. deep cysts, 268
  vs. mesonephric hyperplasia, 270,
    273–274
  vs. microglandular hyperplasia, 270
  vs. reactive atypia, 276
  vs. tubal/tuboendometrioid metaplasia,
    275–276
  vs. tunnel clusters, 268
Adenocarcinoma, vaginal, 295
Adenochondroma, pulmonary, 98
Adenofibrolipochondromyxoma,
  pulmonary, 98
Adenoma, adrenal, 362

Adenoma, basal cell, 233
Adenoma, bile duct, 173–174
Adenoma, breast, 325–326
Adenoma, hepatocellular
  clinical findings, 169
  differential diagnosis, 170
  pathologic features, 169–170, **170**
Adenoma, nephrogenic
  band-like tubule growth, **213**
  classic pattern, **211**
  complex branching of tubules, **213**
  cystic pattern, **211**
  differential diagnosis, 214–215
  diffuse pattern, **212**
  with edematous polyps, **214**
  of female urethra, **237**, 237–238, **238**
  gross pathology, 211
  histopathology, 211, 214
  hobnail cells in, **214**
  lesional cell arrangements, **213**
  of male urethra, 237, **237**
  papillary pattern, **214**
  polypoid pattern, **212**
  prominent basement membranes, **213**
  prostatic involvement, 225–227, **227**
  signet ring cell appearance in, 214,
    **215**
  solid tubular pattern, **212**
  thin cord pattern, **212**
  thin papillae, **212**
Adenoma, parathyroid
  parathyroid cysts and, 348
  vs. hyperplasia, 349–350
Adenoma, pituitary
  hemorrhage, 345
  vs. hyperplasia, 347
Adenoma, salivary gland, 85
Adenoma, thyroid, 355
Adenomatoid hyperplasia, salivary gland,
  **78**, 78–79
Adenomyoma, 13
Adenomyosis, 280–281, **281**, **282**
Adenosis, breast
  apocrine, 336–337, **337**
  diagnostic conceptualization, 333
  microglandular, 335–336, **336**
  sclerosing, **333**, 333–335, **334**, **335**
  tubular, 337

Adenosis, prostatic, 223–225, **224**, **225**,
  **226**
Adenosis, vaginal, 11
  diethylstilbestrol-related, 287–288, **288**
Adenovirus, 480
Adrenal tissue
  carcinoma, 360, 362
  congenital hyperplasia, 251–252,
    361–362
  cysts, **360**, 360–361
  cytomegaly, 360
  ectopias, 360
  functional pseudotumors, 13
  hamartoma, 360
  heterotopias, 53, 359–360
  hyperplasia, 361–362
  inflammatory myofibroblastic
    pseudotumor, 363
  lymphocytic infiltrates, 361
  myelolipoma, 361
Adrenogenital syndrome. *See* Adrenal
  tissue, congenital
  hyperplasia
*Afipia felis*, 490, 561
Agammaglobulinemia in pulmonary
  lymphoid hyperplasia, 110
AIDS/HIV
  atypical follicular hyperplasia in, 450,
    452
  bacillary angiomatosis in, 490, 491
  bacillary peliosis hepatis in, 174
  cryptococcomas infection and, 48
  ineffective hematopoiesis in, 503
  infection-related mesenchymal
    proliferations, 408–409
  lymphoid interstitial pneumonia and, 110
  megaloblastic state, 503
  mycobacterial spindle cell pseudotumor
    in, 483
  persistent generalized lymphadenopathy
    in, 82
  progressive multifocal
    leukoencephalopathy in, 41
  syphilis infection and, 46, 140
  systemic polyclonal immunoblastic
    proliferation and, 479
  tuberculous infection and, 46–47
  viral myocarditis in, 595, 596, 597